NEUROPSYCHOLOGY OF MEMORY
THIRD EDITION

D1319094

NEUROPSYCHOLOGY OF MEMORY

THIRD EDITION

Edited by

Larry R. Squire
Daniel L. Schacter

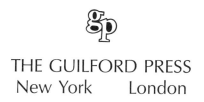

THE GUILFORD PRESS
New York   London

Library of Congress Cataloging-in-Publication Data

Neuropsychology of memory / edited by Larry R. Squire, Daniel L.
   Schacter.—3rd ed.
      p. ; cm.
   Includes bibliographical references and index.
   ISBN 1-57230-731-5 (hard)
      1. Memory. 2. Neuropsychology. 3. Amnesia. I. Squire, Larry R.
   II. Schacter, Daniel L.
      [DNLM: 1. Memory—physiology. 2. Memory disorders.
   3. Neuropsychology. WM 173.7 N494 2002]
   QP406 .N535   2002
   612.8'2—dc21   2001051230

To the memory of Nelson Butters, colleague and friend

ABOUT THE EDITORS

Larry R. Squire, PhD, is Research Career Scientist at the Veterans Affairs San Diego Healthcare System and Professor of Psychiatry, Neurosciences, and Psychology at the University of California, San Diego. He is a member of the National Academy of Sciences and the Institute of Medicine. Dr. Squire was past president of the Society for Neuroscience. His book, *Memory: From Mind to Molecules* (with Eric Kandel), was published in 1999.

Daniel L. Schacter, PhD, is Professor and Chair of Psychology at Harvard University. He is a member of the American Academy of Arts and Sciences and a recipient of the John Simon Guggenheim Memorial Fellowship. Dr. Schacter's books include *Searching for Memory: The Brain, the Mind, and the Past* (1996), *The Seven Sins of Memory: How the Mind Forgets and Remembers* (2001), and *Forgotten Ideas, Neglected Pioneers: Richard Semon and the Story of Memory* (2001).

CONTRIBUTORS

John P. Aggleton, PhD, School of Psychology, Cardiff University, Cardiff, Wales, United Kingdom

Marilyn S. Albert, PhD, Departments of Psychiatry and Neurology, Massachusetts General Hospital, Harvard Medical School, Charlestown, Massachusetts

Maria C. Alvarado, PhD, Department of Neurobiology and Anatomy, University of Texas Health Science Center, Houston, Texas

Jocelyne Bachevalier, PhD, Department of Neurobiology and Anatomy, University of Texas Health Science Center, Houston, Texas

Alan Baddeley, PhD, Centre for the Study of Learning and Memory, Bristol University, Bristol, United Kingdom

Mark G. Baxter, PhD, Department of Psychology, Harvard University, Cambridge, Massachusetts

Peter J. Brasted, PhD, Laboratory of Systems Neuroscience, National Institute of Mental Health, Bethesda, Maryland

Nicola J. Broadbent, PhD, Department of Psychiatry, University of California, San Diego, La Jolla, California

Malcolm W. Brown, PhD, Department of Anatomy, University of Bristol, Bristol, United Kingdom

Randy L. Buckner, PhD, Department of Psychology, Washington University in St. Louis, and Departments of Radiology and Anatomy and Neurobiology, Washington University School of Medicine and Howard Hughes Medical Center, St. Louis, Missouri

Elizabeth A. Buffalo, PhD, Laboratory of Neuropsychology, National Institute of Mental Health, National Institutes of Health, Bethesda, Maryland

Maria C. Carrillo, PhD, Department of Neurological Sciences, Cognitive Neuroscience Section, Rush–Presbyterian–St. Luke's Medical Center, Chicago, Illinois

Robert E. Clark, Department of Psychiatry, University of California, San Diego, La Jolla, California

Nicola S. Clayton, PhD, Department of Experimental Psychology, University of Cambridge, Cambridge, United Kingdom

Robert Desimone, PhD, Laboratory of Neuropsychology, National Institute of Mental Health, National Institutes of Health, Bethesda, Maryland

Mark D'Esposito, MD, Henry H. Wheeler, Jr., Brain Imaging Center and Helen Wills Neuroscience Institute, and Department of Psychology, University of California, Berkeley, Berkeley, California

John F. Disterhoft, PhD, Department of Physiology, Northwestern University Medical School, Chicago, Illinois

R. J. Dolan, MD, Wellcome Department of Cognitive Neurology, Institute of Neurology, University College London, London, United Kingdom

Julien Doyon, PhD, Department of Psychology, University of Montreal, Montreal, Quebec, Canada, and Laboratory of Brain and Cognition, National Institute of Mental Health, National Institutes of Health, Bethesda, Maryland

Howard Eichenbaum, PhD, Department of Psychology, Boston University, Boston, Massachusetts

Catherine B. Fortier, MA, Memory Disorders Research Center, Boston University School of Medicine, Boston, Massachusetts

John D. E. Gabrieli, PhD, Department of Psychology, Stanford University, Stanford, California

Michela Gallagher, PhD, Department of Psychology, Johns Hopkins University, Baltimore, Maryland

Paul E. Gilbert, BS, Department of Psychology, University of Utah, Salt Lake City, Utah

Elizabeth L. Glisky, PhD, Department of Psychology, University of Arizona, Tucson, Arizona

Paul E. Gold, PhD, Department of Psychology, University of Illinois at Urbana–Champaign, Champaign, Illinois

Daniel P. Griffiths, PhD, Department of Experimental Psychology, University of Cambridge, Cambridge, United Kingdom

Lynn Hasher, PhD, Rotman Research Institute, Baycrest Centre for Geriatric Care, Toronto, Ontario, Canada, and Department of Psychology, Trent University, Peterborough, Ontario, Canada

Jane E. Herron, BSc, Institute of Cognitive Neuroscience, London, United Kingdom

Stig A. Hollup, PhD, Neuroscience Unit, Norwegian University of Science and Technology, Trondheim, Norway

Alfred W. Kaszniak, PhD, Departments of Neurology and Psychology, University of Arizona, Tucson, Arizona

Margaret M. Keane, PhD, Department of Psychology, Wellesley College, Boston, Massachusetts

Raymond P. Kesner, PhD, Department of Psychology, University of Utah, Salt Lake City, Utah

Michael P. Kilgard, PhD, Department of Cognition and Neuroscience, School of Human Development, University of Texas at Dallas, Richardson, Texas

Barbara J. Knowlton, PhD, Department of Psychology, University of California, Los Angeles, Los Angeles, California

M-Grace Knuttinen, MD, PhD, Department of Cell and Molecular Biology, Northwestern University Medical School, Chicago, Illinois

Michael D. Kopelman, PhD, Department of Psychiatry and Psychology, King's College, and St. Thomas's Hospital, London, United Kingdom

Edward Korzus, PhD, Department of Neurosciences, University of California, San Diego, La Jolla, California

Wilma Koutstaal, PhD, Department of Psychology, University of Reading, Reading, United Kingdom

Inah Lee, PhD, Department of Psychology, University of Utah, Salt Lake City, Utah

Alex Martin, PhD, Laboratory of Brain and Cognition, National Institute of Mental Health, National Institutes of Health, Bethesda, Maryland

Andrew R. Mayes, DPhil, Department of Psychology, University of Liverpool, Liverpool, United Kingdom

Mark Mayford, PhD, The Scripps Research Institute, Department of Neurosciences, University of California, San Diego, La Jolla, California

Kathleen B. McDermott, PhD, Department of Psychology, Washington University in St. Louis, and Department of Radiology, Washington University School of Medicine, St. Louis, Missouri

James L. McGaugh, PhD, Center for the Neurobiology of Learning and Memory and Department of Neurobiology and Behavior, University of California at Irvine, Irvine, California

Regina McGlinchey-Berroth, PhD, Memory Disorders Research Center, Boston University School of Medicine, Boston, Massachusetts

Yasushi Miyashita, PhD, Department of Physiology, University of Tokyo School of Medicine, Tokyo, Japan

Alexa M. Morcom, PhD, Institute of Cognitive Neuroscience, London, United Kingdom

Edvard I. Moser, PhD, Neuroscience Unit, Norwegian University of Science and Technology, Trondheim, Norway

May-Britt Moser, PhD, Neuroscience Unit, Norwegian University of Science and Technology, Trondheim, Norway

Mark B. Moss, PhD, Department of Anatomy and Neurobiology, Boston University School of Medicine, Boston, Massachusetts

Stephanie L. Murg, AB, Department of Psychology, Harvard University, Cambridge, Massachusetts

Elisabeth A. Murray, PhD, Laboratory of Neuropsychology, National Institute of Mental Health, Bethesda, Maryland

Sarah Nemanic, MS, Department of Neurobiology and Anatomy, University of Texas Health Science Center, Houston, Texas

Lis Nielsen, MA, Department of Psychology, University of Arizona, Tucson, Arizona

Lars Nyberg, PhD, Department of Psychology, Umeå University, Umeå, Sweden

Ken A. Paller, PhD, Department of Psychology and Cognitive Neurology and Alzheimer Disease Center, Northwestern University, Evanston, Illinois

Bradley R. Postle, PhD, Department of Psychology, University of Wisconsin–Madison, Madison, Wisconsin

Alison Preston, BA, Department of Psychology, Stanford University, Stanford, California

Steven Z. Rapcsak, MD, Neurology Section, Veterans Affairs Medical Center, and Departments of Neurology and Psychology, University of Arizona, Tucson, Arizona

Michael D. Rugg, PhD, Institute of Cognitive Neuroscience, University College London, London, United Kingdom

Daniel L. Schacter, PhD, Department of Psychology, Harvard University, Cambridge, Massachusetts

Geoffrey Schoenbaum, MD, PhD, Department of Psychology, Johns Hopkins University, Baltimore, Maryland

Barry Setlow, PhD, Department of Psychology, Johns Hopkins University, Baltimore, Maryland

Arthur P. Shimamura, PhD, Department of Psychology, University of California, Berkeley, Berkeley, California

Larry R. Squire, PhD, Veterans Affairs Healthcare System, San Diego, and Departments of Psychiatry, Neurosciences, and Psychology, University of California, San Diego, La Jolla, California

Nicola Stanhope, PhD, Department of Psychology, Institute of Psychiatry, King's College, London, United Kingdom

B. A. Strange, PhD, Wellcome Department of Cognitive Neurology, Institute of Neurology, University College London, London, United Kingdom

Wendy A. Suzuki, PhD, Center for Neural Science, New York University, New York, New York

Emi Takahashi, BS, Department of Physiology, University of Tokyo School of Medicine, Tokyo, Japan

Miranda van Turennout, PhD, Laboratory of Brain and Cognition, National Institute of Mental Health, National Institutes of Health, Bethesda, Maryland, and Max Planck Institute for Psycholinguistics, Nijmegen, The Netherlands

Leslie G. Ungerleider, PhD, Laboratory of Brain and Cognition, National Institute of Mental Health, National Institutes of Health, Bethesda, Maryland

Mieke Verfaellie, PhD, Boston University School of Medicine and Memory Disorders Research Center, Boston Veterans Affairs Medical Center, Boston, Massachusetts

Anthony D. Wagner, PhD, Department of Brain and Cognitive Sciences, Massachusetts Institute of Technology, Cambridge, Massachusetts

Craig Weiss, PhD, Department of Cell and Molecular Biology, Northwestern University Medical School, Chicago, Illinois

Barbara A. Wilson, PhD, MRC Cognition and Brain Sciences Unit, Addenbrooke's Hospital, Cambridge, United Kingdom

Gordon Winocur, PhD, Department of Psychology, Trent University, and Rotman Research Institute, Baycrest Centre for Geriatric Care and Departments of Psychology and Psychiatry, University of Toronto, Toronto, Ontario, Canada

Steven P. Wise, PhD, Laboratory of Systems Neuroscience, National Institute of Mental Health, Bethesda, Maryland

Stuart Zola, PhD, Veterans Affairs Healthcare System, San Diego, and Departments of Psychiatry and Neuroscience, University of California, San Diego, La Jolla, California

PREFACE

Neuropsychology of Memory was published originally in 1984, with a second edition in 1992. The inspiration for these books came from the late Nelson Butters, who in the early 1980s invited Larry Squire to join him in this venture. The volumes have been popular, and have frequently been used as teaching texts. Nelson, we think, would have liked the idea of carrying this project forward, as he was quite proud of the first two editions. His friend and colleague Daniel Schacter has joined the venture, and the third edition was planned in the same spirit as the first two. Thus, we have again invited scientists to describe in brief chapters their current approaches to the study of memory and to summarize what they have learned. We have tried to include a broad spectrum of contemporary work on the neuropsychology of memory, as there have been enormous changes in the shape of the discipline since the appearance of the second edition. In this edition, for example, many chapters report findings using neuroimaging techniques (positron emission tomography [PET] and functional magnetic resonance imaging [fMRI]). In 1992, PET was just being applied to the study of memory for the first time, and fMRI was not yet available. Furthermore, in this edition one can find studies of memory with genetically modified mice, using techniques that first became available in the 1990s. We have organized the volume into three parts: "Studies of Normal and Abnormal Memory in Humans," "Studies of Memory in Nonhuman Primates," and "Studies of Memory in Rodents and Birds." Each part is prefaced by an introductory comment, and the chapters within each section have been ordered to provide additional structure. We hope that readers find the result both useful and interesting, and that comparisons to the first two editions will provide an indication of how the discipline has progressed.

LARRY R. SQUIRE
DANIEL L. SCHACTER

CONTENTS

PART I

STUDIES OF NORMAL AND ABNORMAL MEMORY IN HUMANS

The neuropsychology of human memory has evolved steadily during the past 50 years, and dramatically within the past decade. Beginning with the pioneering observations by William Beecher Scoville and Brenda Milner during the 1950s concerning patient H. M., who developed a severe and selective loss of recent memory after bilateral resection of the medial temporal lobes, the field focused intensively on patients with amnesia. Neuropsychological studies of such patients during the 1960s and 1970s attempted to locate the source of memory loss at the encoding, consolidation, or retrieval stages of memory.

In the 1980s and 1990s, the neuropsychology of memory focused increasingly on striking dissociations between impaired and preserved memory functions in amnesic patients. Stimulated by the early observation that H. M. could acquire motor skills in a relatively normal manner despite failing to recollect the experience of learning, numerous studies explored forms of memory that can be fully intact in patients with amnesia, including skill learning, priming, and conditioning. These observations, along with complementary studies of patients with memory disorders attributable to such conditions as Alzheimer's disease and Parkinson's disease, led to an explosion of research and to the important proposal that memory consists of multiple forms or systems.

During the early 1990s, new functional neuroimaging techniques, including a positron emission tomography (PET) and functional magnetic resonance imaging (fMRI), began to transform the study of memory. The second edition of *Neuropsychology of Memory*, published in 1992, did not contain a single chapter on functional neuroimaging of memory. Since that time, scores of imaging studies have been published, and increasing numbers appear in the journals each month. The chapters in this section reflect both the traditional concerns of the field as well as the new wave of neuroimaging research.

Chapters 1–11 focus primarily on neuropsychological studies of patients with memory disorders. Chapters 1 and 2 paint a broad picture of the role played by the medial temporal lobe in memory: Chapter 1 synthesizes work from humans and other animals, and Chapter 2 focuses on the relation between the medial temporal lobe and other brain regions in the representation of complex information. Chapter 3 contrasts impaired and preserved memory processes in patients with amnesia, focusing on the relationship between explicit or declarative memory (conscious recollection of previously acquired information), which is severely impaired by amnesia, and implicit or nondeclarative memory (nonconscious influences of experience on subsequent performance), which is usually preserved. Chapter 4 compares the effects of lesions to the temporal lobes, frontal lobes, and diencephalon on both anterograde amnesia and retrograde amnesia. The evidence reveals a number of similarities in the effects of the different lesions, but also points toward important differences. Chapters 5 and 6 draw on observations from patients with amnesia and neuroimaging studies in order to account for how various brain regions bind together and consolidate different types of information. Chapter 7 explores the theoretical implications of recently described cases of developmental amnesia, in which memory problems are attributable to medial temporal lobe damage incurred early in childhood. Studies of these patients have raised important questions concerning the relation between episodic memory (recollection of personal experiences) and semantic memory (knowledge of facts and concepts). Chapter 8 describes recent work on eyeblink conditioning in patients with amnesia and older adults, where important issues have arisen concerning the role of awareness in different forms of conditioning.

Chapters 9 and 10 report on a relatively new concern for neuropsychology: the experimental analysis of false or illusory memories. This topic has recently generated considerable interest among cognitive psychologists, and is attracting increasing attention from neuropsychologists. The two chapters describe findings and ideas concerning memory illusions that can be observed in patients with lesions to the medial temporal lobes (Chapter 9) and the frontal lobes (Chapter 10). Chapter 11 shifts the neuroanatomical focus to the basal ganglia and examines their involvement in such implicit/nondeclarative forms of memory as category learning and conditioning.

Chapters 12–19 are concerned with functional neuroimaging of memory. Chapters 12 and 13 explore the neural correlates of episodic memory retrieval, paying particular attention to the role of the frontal and parietal lobes. Chapter 12 focuses mainly on the electrophysiological technique of event-related potentials (ERPs), which allows fine-grained analyses of the time course of retrieval processes. Chapter 13 (and the others in this group) rely on findings from PET and fMRI, which provide greater spatial resolution than ERPs and therefore allow a more precise analysis of the functional neuroanatomy of retrieval processes. The next two chapters examine both encoding and retrieval processes. Chapter 14 discusses the contribution of specific regions within the frontal lobe to cognitive control processes that are important for both episodic encoding and semantic retrieval. Chapter 15 delineates similarities and differences in the brain regions that are involved in episodic encoding and retrieval. In Chapter 16, the focus returns to the medial temporal lobe. The authors provide a summary and theoretical analysis of neuroimaging studies that have documented a hippocampal response to novel stimuli.

Chapters 17–19 each examine a different type of memory. Chapter 17 summarizes fMRI studies of working memory in relation to evidence from studies of patients with brain damage. Chapter 18 discusses new insights from fMRI studies concerning increases and decreases in the activity of particular brain regions during motor skill learning. Chapter 19 focuses on the neural correlates of visual object priming, attempting to provide a theoretical account of priming-related increases and decreases observed in insular cortex and posterior cortical regions, respectively.

The final three chapters have a more pragmatic emphasis. Chapter 20 discusses neuropsychological test data and neuroimaging findings that can aid in the early identification of Alzheimer's disease. Chapter 21 considers different approaches to memory rehabilitation in brain-damaged patients, including environmental modification and techniques for promoting new learning. Chapter 22 considers evidence from circadian rhythms indicating that time of testing can influence memory performance in older humans and rats. By linking studies of human and nonhuman memory, the chapter also provides a helpful transition to the final two sections of the book, where attention shifts to memory in nonhuman primates, and then to memory in rodents and birds.

1

The Medial Temporal Lobe and Memory

NICOLA J. BROADBENT, ROBERT E. CLARK,
STUART ZOLA, and LARRY R. SQUIRE

In 1957, the profound effects of bilateral medial temporal lobe resection on memory were described in a patient who became known as H. M. (Scoville & Milner, 1957). This case established the important principle that the ability to acquire new memories is a distinct cerebral function, separable from intellect and personality. The case also demonstrated that the medial aspect of the temporal lobe is important for memory function. This seminal publication inaugurated a continuing tradition of neuropsychological research centered on amnesic patients with damage to medial temporal lobe structures, which has yielded an enormous amount of information about the organization of memory (cf. Mayes, 1988; Squire & Butters, 1992; Tulving & Craik, 2000). About 25 years after H. M. was described, the first successes were achieved in establishing an animal model of human amnesia in the monkey (Mishkin, 1978; Mishkin, Spiegler, Saunders, & Malamut, 1982; Squire & Zola-Morgan, 1983; Zola-Morgan, Squire, & Mishkin, 1982). Cumulative work with the animal model over a 10–year period succeeded in identifying the anatomical components of the medial temporal lobe memory system (Mishkin & Murray, 1994; Squire & Zola-Morgan, 1991; Zola-Morgan & Squire, 1993). The success of this effort in monkeys led to similar studies in the rodent aimed at understanding the contribution of the hippocampus and related structures to memory (Eichenbaum, 1997; Eichenbaum, Dudchenko, Wood, Shapiro, & Tanila, 1999; Jarrard, 1993; Steele & Morris, 1999). A key ingredient of this work with amnesic patients, monkeys, and rodents was the discovery that medial temporal lobe structures are essential for just one kind of memory (declarative memory), and that other kinds of (nondeclarative) memory depend on other brain systems (for reviews, see Squire, 1992; Schacter & Tulving, 1994).

This chapter reviews recent findings within this tradition. We first discuss the work with monkeys that led to identification of the anatomical components of the medial temporal lobe memory system. We then consider how the components of this system might contribute differently to memory. Next we consider this issue in more detail in humans, monkeys, and rodents, focusing on recognition memory, an elemental form of declarative memory. We then review work on the functions of the perirhinal cortex, which lies within the medial temporal lobe, and we compare and contrast the effects of perirhinal cortex lesions with the effects of lesions to the adjacent, unimodal visual area TE. Finally, we review recent work with human classical eyeblink conditioning, which has been useful in sharpening the distinction between declarative and nondeclarative memory.

AN ANIMAL MODEL OF HUMAN MEDIAL TEMPORAL LOBE AMNESIA

The development of an animal model of amnesia in the monkey relied especially on the trial-unique, delayed-nonmatching-to-sample (DNMS) task, a task of visual recognition memory. In this task, a sample object is presented, which the monkey displaces to receive a food reward. Following a variable delay interval, the sample object is presented together with a second unfamiliar object. To receive a food reward, the monkey must displace the novel object. Different objects are used on each trial.

Early work with the DNMS task revealed severe, delay-dependent memory impairment following large medial temporal lobe lesions that damaged the hippocampus, the amygdala, and the cortex underlying these structures (the H$^+$A$^+$ lesion) (Mishkin, 1978). The H$^+$A$^+$ lesion impaired memory more severely than when damage was restricted to the posterior medial temporal lobe (sparing the amygdala and perirhinal cortex), but including the hippocampus, the posterior entorhinal cortex, and most of the parahippocampal cortex (the H$^+$ lesion) (Mishkin, 1978; Zola-Morgan & Squire, 1985, 1986; Zola-Morgan, Squire, & Amaral, 1989a).

Subsequent studies revealed that the severity of memory impairment following H$^+$A$^+$ lesions could not be attributed to damage to the amygdala. Selective damage to the amygdala did not impair performance on the DNMS task and did not exacerbate the memory impairment associated with the H$^+$ lesion (Zola-Morgan, Squire, & Amaral 1989b). In contrast, extending the H$^+$ lesion forward to include the perirhinal cortex, but not the amygdala, did increase the severity of the memory impairment (the H^{++} lesion) (Zola-Morgan, Squire, Clower, & Rempel, 1993). Moreover, conjoint lesions of the perirhinal and parhippocampal cortices severely impaired memory (Zola-Morgan, Squire, Amaral, & Suzuki, 1989; Suzuki, Zola-Morgan, Squire, & Amaral, 1993). These findings, and others, led to the conclusion that the hippocampal formation (the CA fields of the hippocampus, the dentate gyrus, the subiculum, and the entorhinal cortex) and the adjacent perirhinal and parahippocampal cortices comprise the major components of the medial temporal lobe memory system (Squire & Zola-Morgan, 1991) (Figure 1.1). Large lesions of this system in the monkey produce a pattern of memory impairment that closely resembles what is observed when similar lesions occur in amnesic patients (e.g., patient H. M.—Corkin, 1984; Corkin, Amaral, Gonzalez, Johnson, & Hyman, 1997; Scoville & Milner, 1957; and patient E. P.—Stefanacci, Buffalo, Schmolck, & Squire, 2000). The impairment in monkeys is multimodal (Buffalo et al., 1999; Murray & Mishkin, 1984; Suzuki et al., 1993) and long-lasting (Zola-Morgan & Squire, 1985). In addition, monkeys with such lesions exhibit intact short-term memory (Overman, Ormsby, & Mishkin, 1990), intact skill-based memory, and intact habit-like memory (Malamut, Saunders, & Mishkin, 1984; Zola-Morgan & Squire, 1984).

Whether one assesses memory impairment only with the DNMS task, or with a battery of memory tasks, the impairment is more severe when more components of the medial temporal lobe are damaged. This conclusion was supported by an evaluation of behavioral data from 30 monkeys that completed testing in our laboratory during a 10-year period (Zola-Morgan, Squire, & Ramus, 1994). It is also supported by the observation that pa-

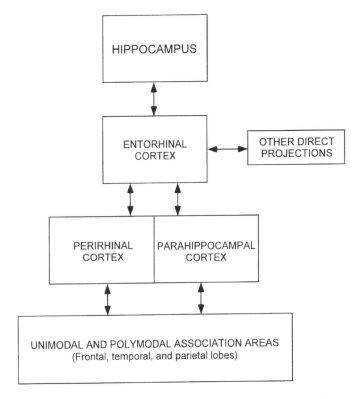

FIGURE 1.1. A schematic view of the medial temporal lobe memory system. The entorhinal cortex is the major source of cortical projections to the hippocampus. The perirhinal and parahippocampal cortices account for approximately 60% of the cortical input to the entorhinal cortex, and they in turn receive projections from unimodal and polymodal areas in the frontal, temporal, and parietal lobes. The entorhinal cortex also receives other direct inputs from the orbitofrontal cortex, cingulate cortex, insular cortex, and superior temporal gyrus. As indicated, all these projections are reciprocal. From Squire and Zola-Morgan (1991).

tients H. M. and E. P., who have large medial temporal lobe lesions, are much more severely amnesic than were patients R. B., G. D., L. M., and W. H., who had histologically confirmed lesions limited to the hippocampus or to the hippocampus and entorhinal cortex (Corkin et al., 1997; Rempel-Clower, Zola, Squire, & Amaral, 1996; Stefanacci et al., 2000; Zola-Morgan, Squire, & Amaral, 1986).

This set of facts has sometimes been taken to imply or require the view that the structures of the medial temporal lobe work together as a single functional unit (Murray & Bussey, 2001; Tulving & Markowitsch, 1998). However, early discussions of these findings emphasized that structures within the medial temporal lobe might make qualitatively different contributions to memory function, and that this possibility is consistent with the finding that larger lesions produce more impairment than smaller lesions (Zola-Morgan et al., 1994). Note that anatomical connections from different regions of the neocortex enter the medial temporal lobe at different points. Thus the higher visual areas TE and TEO project preferentially to the perirhinal cortex. Conversely, spatial information that comes to the medial temporal lobe from the parietal cortex arrives exclusively at the parahippocampal cortex. Consistent with these anatomical facts, damage to the parahippocampal cortex was found to impair spatial memory more than damage to the perirhinal cortex (Malkova &

Mishkin, 1997; Parkinson, Murray, & Mishkin, 1988), and damage to the perirhinal cortex impaired performance on the visual DNMS task, but damage to the parahippocampal cortex did not (Ramus, Zola-Morgan, & Squire, 1994).

The hippocampus lies at the end of the processing hierarchy of the medial temporal lobe, receiving input from both the perirhinal and parahippocampal cortices as well as the entorhinal cortex. If we reason again from anatomy, it seems plausible that the hippocampus extends and combines functions performed by the structures that project to it. There has also been interest in the possibility that some aspect of memory function might be associated specifically and uniquely with the hippocampus itself (e.g., episodic memory), or that some aspect of declarative memory might not depend on the hippocampus (e.g., recognition memory) (Aggleton & Brown, 1999; Brown & Aggleton, 2001; Vargha-Khadem et al., 1997). These ideas are currently active topics of experimental work.

RECOGNITION MEMORY AND THE HIPPOCAMPUS

One focus of investigation has concerned whether the hippocampus might be specialized for the recollective and associative aspects of episodic memory, and is not needed to make the judgments of familiarity involved in recognition memory. This issue has now been examined in humans, monkeys, and rodents with damage limited to the hippocampal region. Recognition memory is impaired following hippocampal damage. In humans, this point was established in amnesic patients with histologically confirmed damage to the CA1 region of the hippocampus (patients R. B. and G. D.), as well as in patients with histologically confirmed damage to all the CA fields of the hippocampus, plus limited cell loss in entorhinal cortex (patients L. M. and W. H.) (Reed & Squire, 1997). In another study, three patients with damage thought to be limited to the hippocampal region were impaired on both the recall and recognition portions of the Doors and People Test, a standardized test of memory (Manns & Squire, 1999).

In monkeys, five studies have assessed the effects of restricted hippocampal lesions made in adulthood on recognition memory performance, as measured by the DNMS task (Alvarez, Zola-Morgan, & Squire, 1995; Beason-Held, Rosene, Killiany, & Moss, 1999; Murray & Mishkin, 1998; Zola et al., 2000; Zola-Morgan, Squire, Rempel, Clower, & Amaral, 1992). Of these five studies, four found impaired performance following lesions to the hippocampus (Alvarez et al., 1995; Beason-Held et al., 1999; Zola et al., 2000; Zola-Morgan et al., 1992). Zola and colleagues (2000) brought together data from 18 monkeys with bilateral lesions of the hippocampus made either by an ischemic procedure, by radiofrequency, or by ibotenic acid. Significant recognition memory impairment was observed at all the delays that were tested from 15 seconds to 40 minutes (Figure 1.2). The one study that did not find impaired performance on the DNMS task involved conjoint amygdala–hippocampal lesions (Murray & Mishkin, 1998) and differed methodologically in at least two ways from the studies that found an impairment. First, monkeys were pretrained on the DNMS task prior to surgery. Extensive training on applying the DNMS rule across short delays (i.e., choosing the new object) might provide monkeys with a strategy that helps them to maintain memory of the sample object over extended delays (Zola-Morgan & Squire, 1986). Second, the monkeys were operated upon in two stages, once on each side, with surgery separated by at least 2 weeks. Two-stage surgery sometimes results in less impairment than one-stage surgery (Finger, 1978).

An additional difference between the study by Murray and Mishkin (1998) and the other studies is that the monkeys tested by Murray and Mishkin had relatively large hip-

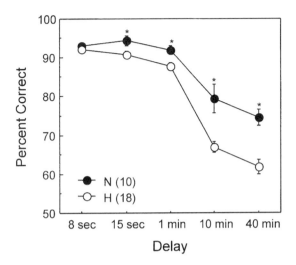

FIGURE 1.2. Performance on the delayed-nonmatching-to-sample (DNMS) task by 10 normal monkeys (N) and 18 monkeys with lesions limited to the hippocampal region (H). The monkeys of the H group consisted of four monkeys with ischemic lesions, nine monkeys with radiofrequency lesions, and five monkeys with ibotenic acid lesions. Asterisks indicate impaired performance of the lesion group relative to the N group. The ischemic monkeys were not tested at the 40-minute delay, so that the scores of 14 monkeys contributed to this data point. From Zola et al. (2000).

pocampal lesions. However, when the data from the available studies (Beason-Held et al., 1999; Murray & Mishkin, 1998; Zola et al., 2000) were analyzed together, lesion size was not a significant predictor of performance (Zola & Squire, 2001). In a multiple-regression analysis, most of the variance was explained by differences among the studies, and lesion size itself accounted for only a small amount of the variability in the data. Moreover, an analysis of covariance indicated that there were differences among the studies beyond lesion size that significantly affected performance. The relation between lesion size and performance has been addressed systematically in the water maze with rats, and the result was as one might expect. Increasing the size of the lesion increased the behavioral deficit up to a point, beyond which increasing the size of the lesion did not further increase the deficit (Moser, Moser, & Andersen, 1993; Moser, Moser, Forrest, Andersen, & Morris, 1995).

The DNMS task has also been adapted for use with rats (Mumby, Pinel, & Wood, 1990). Several studies have reported that bilateral damage to the hippocampus or to the fornix impairs DNMS performance (Clark, West, Zola, & Squire, 2001; Mumby, Pinel, Kornecook, Shen, & Redila, 1995; Mumby, Wood, & Pinel, 1992; Wiig & Bilkey, 1995). For example, rats with large ibotenic acid lesions of the hippocampus were impaired on the DNMS task at delays of 1 and 2 minutes, but not at delays of 30 seconds or less (Clark et al., 2001). Other studies of DNMS or similar tasks have failed to find an impairment following bilateral hippocampal or fornix lesions (Aggleton, Hunt, & Rawlins, 1986; Duva et al., 1997; Kesner, Bolland, & Dakis, 1993; Mumby et al., 1996; Rothblat & Kromer, 1991). A consideration of all the studies suggests that impaired performance on the DNMS task typically does occur following hippocampal damage if the delay is sufficiently long and if the hippocampal lesions are sufficiently large (see Clark et al., 2001). For example, in the study by Aggleton and colleagues (1986), animals were not tested at delays longer than 1 minute.

In summary, the data from humans, monkeys, and rats indicate that the hippocampus is essential for normal recognition performance. However, this conclusion is open to two kinds of qualifications. First, recent evidence suggests that patients who become amnesic early in life as a result of restricted hippocampal damage can perform well on some recognition tests (Baddeley, Vargha-Khadem, & Mishkin, 2001; Vargha-Khadem et al., 1997) For example, one such patient (Jon) performed in the normal range on the Doors and People Test (Baddeley et al., 2001)—the same test that was failed by patients with adult-onset amnesia and apparently similar lesions (Manns & Squire, 1999). Early-onset injury may permit some compensation during development, either as a result of functional reorganization or perhaps as a result of learned strategies (see also Baddeley, Chapter 7, this volume).

A second qualification turns on the view that recognition memory consists of two separate components, and that only one of these components depends on the integrity of the hippocampus (Brown & Aggleton, 2001). According to this view, the recollection of a stimulus as one that was encountered before (e.g., recollection of the learning episode) depends on the hippocampus, but the simple experience of familiarity does not require the hippocampus. This distinction is difficult to evaluate in experimental animals (but see below). In humans, however, the limited evidence available from amnesic patients with damage to the hippocampal formation suggests that both kinds of recognition (remembering and knowing) are affected (Knowlton & Squire, 1995; Squire & Zola, 1998). It has also been suggested that in patients with unilateral posterior cerebral artery occlusions, recollection may be more impaired than familiarity (Yonelinas, Kroll, Dobbins, Lazzara, & Knight, 1998). (For further discussion, see Schacter, Verfaellie, & Koutstaal, Chapter 9, this volume.)

Although much of the data concerning recognition memory and the hippocampus come from the DNMS task, other measures of recognition memory have also been used. The visual paired-comparison (VPC) task, which was originally designed for humans, measures how much time an individual spends looking at a new picture and a recently presented (now familiar) picture when the two pictures are presented together. Two identical pictures are first presented side by side (familiarization phase), and then after a variable delay, one of the old pictures is presented together with a new one (choice phase). Normal subjects prefer to look at the new picture, and this spontaneous preference shows that the familiar picture has been recognized and distinguished from the new picture. The task appears to depend on an individual's voluntary search of the environment, which is influenced by what is recognized as familiar or novel. In this sense, the task provides a measure of declarative memory (Manns, Stark, & Squire, 2000).

An early indication that the VPC task is sensitive to hippocampal damage came from work with amnesic patients (McKee & Squire, 1993). Amnesic patients performed normally on this task when the delay between the familiarization and choice phases was short (i.e., 0.5 second), but were impaired when the delay was extended to 2 minutes or 2 hours (Figure 1.3A). Impaired performance on the VPC task has also been reported for neonatal or adult monkeys with large medial temporal lobe lesions (Bachevalier, 1990; Bachevalier, Brickson, & Hagger, 1993) and for adult monkeys with neonatal lesions of the hippocampal formation and underlying cortex (Pascalis & Bachevalier, 1999). The VPC task has also been used to assess recognition memory in monkeys with selective damage to the hippocampus (Zola et al., 2000). Monkeys with radiofrequency lesions or fiber-sparing ibotenic acid lesions performed normally when the delay between the familiarization and the choice phases was only 1 second, but were impaired at longer delays of 10 seconds, 1 minute, or 10 minutes (Figure 1.3B).

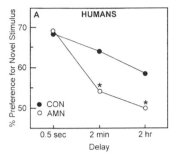 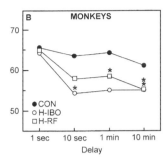 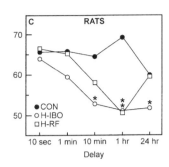

FIGURE 1.3. Performance of humans, monkeys, and rats on the visual paired-comparison (VPC) task, a task of recognition memory. Asterisks indicate impaired performance of the lesion group relative to the control (CON) group. Chance performance is 50%. (A) Performance of human amnesic patients (AMN) with damage to the hippocampal formation or the diencephalon and controls (CON). Data from 9–11 individuals contribute to each delay point. (B) Performance of 5 monkeys with radiofrequency (H-RF) lesions of the hippocampal region, 4 monkeys with ibotenic acid (H-IBO) lesions of the hippocampal region, and 5 control animals. (C) Performance of 8 rats with H-RF lesions, 8 rats with H-IBO lesions, and 16 controls. Data from McKee and Squire (1993), Zola et al. (2000), and Clark, Zola, and Squire (2000).

A rodent version of the VPC task has also been developed (Ennaceur & Delacour, 1988). Rats with radiofrequency or ibotenic acid lesions of the hippocampus performed normally when the delay was short (10 seconds), but performed poorly when the delay was longer than 1 minute (Clark, Zola, & Squire, 2000) (Figure 1.3C). Rats with ischemic damage to the CA1 region of the hippocampus also performed poorly on the VPC task (Wood & Phillips, 1991). Finally, impaired performance on the VPC task was reported in mice lacking the NMDAR-1 subunit in the CA1 region of the hippocampus (Rampon et al., 2000). These results indicate that disruption of hippocampal function impairs performance on the VPC task in humans, monkeys, and rodents (Figure 1.3). Because the VPC task depends on spontaneous reactions to novelty and familiarity, this task would seem to depend less on recollection of previous events and more on the simple detection of familiarity. If so, the finding that restricted hippocampal lesions impair performance on the VPC task would seem to favor the view that the hippocampus supports recognition performance generally, including the capacity for familiarity.

Functional imaging studies of human volunteers have also provided evidence for the importance of the hippocampal region in recognition memory (Gabrieli, Brewer, Desmond, & Glover, 1997; Schacter & Wagner, 1999; Stark & Squire, 2000a, 2000b). For example, Stark and Squire (2000b) asked volunteers to study 80 items and then, while in the scanner, to take recognition memory tests for the previously studied items. Either words or line drawings of nameable objects were used at both study and test. Robust hippocampal activation was recorded during the recognition memory tests when word stimuli were used at both study and test, and also when pictures of objects were used at both study and test. This finding shows that the hippocampal region is active during information retrieval in traditional tasks of recognition memory.

These findings are consistent with data from electrophysiological studies in animals. Single-cell recording studies have shown, for example, that cells in the hippocampus signal mnemonic information during recognition memory tasks (see Suzuki & Eichenbaum, 2000). For example, neurons recorded from the hippocampus during visual or olfactory recognition tasks can convey an abstracted match–nonmatch signal—that is, a signal that contains information about the outcome of the match–nonmatch comparison rather than information about the stimulus itself. Furthermore, the match–nonmatch signal can occur in conjunction with other task features, such as spatial position, odor, and other stimulus properties (Fried, MacDonald, & Wilson, 1997; Hampson, Heyser, & Deadwyler, 1993; Suzuki & Eichenbaum, 2000; Wiebe & Staubi, 1999; Wood, Dudchenko, & Eichenbaum, 1999). The hippocampus therefore appears to play a broad role in recognition memory.

It is perhaps not surprising that recognition memory is hippocampus-dependent. Recognition memory tasks require that an association be made between the item to be remembered and the learning event, or between the item to be remembered and the subject's interaction with it. It is this process of forming an association and maintaining it through time that is critical and that ties recognition memory to other forms of declarative memory.

THE PERIRHINAL CORTEX

Within the medial temporal lobe the perirhinal cortex has also been a focus of study (Murray & Richmond, 2001). The perirhinal cortex and area TE are immediately adjacent to each other in the temporal lobe and are reciprocally interconnected. These areas are thought to lie at the interface between visual perception and visual memory, but it has been unclear what their separate contributions might be. Recent studies of monkeys and humans suggest that the perirhinal cortex plays an important role in declarative memory, and that area TE is important for visual information processing (Buffalo, Ramus, Squire, & Zola, 2000; Buffalo, Reber, & Squire, 1998; Buffalo et al., 1999; Stark & Squire, 2000c). These conclusions are based in part on functional dissociations that have been demonstrated between the effects of damage to the perirhinal cortex and the effects of damage to visual area TE. For example, monkeys with damage limited to the perirhinal cortex exhibited a delay-dependent memory impairment on both visual and tactile versions of the DNMS task. In contrast, monkeys with damage limited to area TE were impaired on the visual DNMS task but not the tactile DNMS task (Buffalo et al., 1999).

A particularly important finding was that monkeys with perirhinal cortical lesions acquired an automated version of the visual DNMS task as quickly as normal animals when the delay between sample and choice was only 0.5 second (Buffalo et al., 2000). This finding shows that the ability to perceive the visual stimuli was not affected by perirhinal lesions. By contrast, monkeys with TE lesions were severely impaired at the 0.5-second delay, and three of the four animals could not learn the task within 3,000 trials. Thus monkeys with TE lesions failed even when the memory demands of the task were minimal. This result suggests that the monkeys with TE lesions had difficulty processing the visual stimuli. A similar finding was obtained with the VPC task. Monkeys with perirhinal lesions performed like monkeys with hippocampal lesions. Performance was intact when the delay between the familiarization and choice phases was only 1 second, but was impaired at longer delays (Figure 1.4). In contrast, monkeys with area TE lesions were impaired even at the shortest delay.

A dissociation between the effects of lesions to the perirhinal cortex and to area TE was also revealed by comparing the findings for simple object discrimination learning and concurrent discrimination learning. In the simple two-choice object discrimination task, the monkey is trained with one pair of objects at a time, and in just a few trials comes to learn which object of the pair is always rewarded. In the concurrent discrimination task, the monkey is presented with eight different pairs of objects within each testing session (five

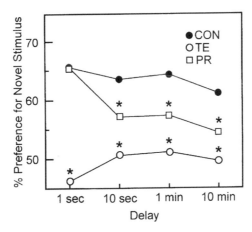

FIGURE 1.4. Performance on the VPC task by 13 control monkeys, 5 monkeys with lesions of the perirhinal cortex (PR), and 3 monkeys with lesions of area TE. Asterisks indicate impaired performance of the lesion group relative to the control (CON) group. Chance-level performance is 50%. Adapted from Buffalo et al. (1999).

presentations of each pair within a 40-trial session). One object in each pair is consistently rewarded, and the discriminations are learned gradually over a large number of trials.

Perirhinal cortex lesions impaired performance on the simple object discrimination task, but had no effect on concurrent discrimination learning. Lesions to area TE yielded the opposite pattern of performance: Performance was impaired on the concurrent discrimination task, but not on the simple object discrimination task (Figure 1.5). Why did perirhinal cortex lesions impair performance on the simple object discrimination task but spare learning of the concurrent discrimination task? For humans, the concurrent discrimination task is a task of declarative memory, dependent on the structure of the medial temporal lobe. The amnesic patient H. M. was severely impaired at concurrent discrimination learning (Hood, Postle, & Corkin, 1999). However, several investigators have suggested that for monkeys the concurrent discrimination task is a task of habit learning, not a test of declarative memory (Buffalo, Stefanacci, Squire, & Zola, 1998; Mishkin, Malamut, & Bachevalier, 1984; Phillips, Malmut, Bachevalier, & Mishkin, 1988). Monkeys must gradually learn how the stimuli differ from each other, and performance improves incrementally as training continues. Whereas even large medial temporal lobe lesions spare concurrent discrimination learning (Buffalo, Stefanacci, et al., 1998), the learning of this task is impaired by damage that includes the ventrocaudal neostriatum (Fernandez-Ruiz, Wang, Aigner, & Mishkin, 2001; Teng, Stefanacci, Squire, & Zola, 2000) (Figure 1.5). The neostriatum is part of a corticostriatal system that subserves the gradual learning of habits and stimulus–reward associations (Graybiel, 1995; Mishkin & Petri, 1984).

The simple object discrimination task is quite different from the concurrent discrimination task. When only a single pair of objects must be learned and the objects can be easily distinguished, the discrimination can be quickly acquired by declarative memory. It has often been suggested that discrimination tasks are insensitive to medial temporal lobe lesions (Dore, Thornton, White, & Murray, 1998; Eacott, Gaffan, & Murray, 1994; Nadel & Moscovitch, 1997). However, a distinction needs to be made between rapidly learned discriminations, which are supported by medial temporal lobe structures, and slowly learned discriminations, which are dependent on the neostriatum and insensitive to medial temporal lobe lesions (Figure 1.6) (Fernandez-Ruiz et al., 2001; Squire & Zola-Morgan, 1983; Teng et al., 2000).

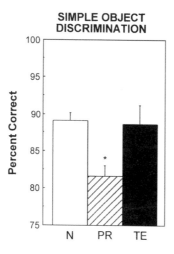
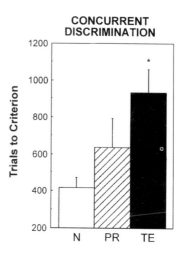

FIGURE 1.5. Performance on the simple object discrimination task (mean of 3 test days) and the concurrent discrimination task (trials to criterion) by 5 monkeys with lesions of the perirhinal cortex (PR), 5 monkeys with lesions of area TE, and 10 normal monkeys (N). Asterisks denote a significant difference between the operated group and normal monkeys ($p < .05$). For concurrent discrimination, there was also a marginally significant difference between the PR and TE groups ($p = .08$). Brackets indicate SEM. Adapted from Buffalo et al. (1999).

One can also ask about the pattern of results observed in monkeys with TE lesions. Why did TE lesions impair concurrent discrimination learning but spare simple object discrimination learning? The suggestion is that intact visual areas upstream from area TE—for example, areas TEO and V4—are sufficient for discrimination between two objects. Because areas TEO and V4 send direct projections to the perirhinal cortex (Suzuki & Amaral, 1994a, 1994b), visual information processed in these areas has access to the medial temporal lobe memory system, even in the absence of area TE. However, these upstream areas are not sufficient to discriminate among the overlapping features of the 16 objects that are used in the 8-pair concurrent discrimination task. Processing these objects requires area TE.

These findings suggest that the perirhinal cortex, like other medial temporal lobe structures, is important for the formation of memory. In contrast, area TE is important for visuoperceptual processing. These findings agree with the observation that large medial temporal lobe lesions in patients, which include damage to the perirhinal cortex, spare the performance of even quite difficult visual discriminations (Stark & Squire, 2000c).

HUMAN EYEBLINK CLASSICAL CONDITIONING

Human eyeblink classical conditioning provides a useful paradigm for exploring the distinction between declarative and nondeclarative forms of memory. In eyeblink classical conditioning, a conditioned stimulus (CS; typically a tone) is presented just prior to an unconditioned stimulus (US; typically a puff of air to the eye). After repeated pairings of the CS and US, subjects begin to blink in response to the CS. The eyeblink response is a learned or conditioned response (CR). The two most commonly studied forms of eyeblink

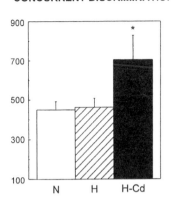

FIGURE 1.6. Acquisition of visual habits is dependent on the integrity of the caudate nucleus. In monkeys, both pattern discrimination (left) and concurrent discrimination (right) tasks are unaffected by hippocampal lesions (H), but are impaired by conjoint hippocampal–caudate lesions (H-Cd). N, 16 normal monkeys; H, 11 monkeys with lesions of the hippocampal region; H-Cd, 7 monkeys with lesions of the hippocampus that also included substantial damage to the tail of the caudate nucleus. Asterisks indicate a significant difference between the operated group and the normal group ($p < .05$). Adapted from Teng, Stefanacci, Squire, and Zola (2000).

classical conditioning are delay conditioning and trace conditioning. In delay conditioning, the CS is presented and remains on until the US is presented. The two stimuli then overlap and coterminate. In trace conditioning, an empty or "trace" interval separates the CS and the US.

Work with rabbits first demonstrated a clear distinction between delay and trace conditioning. The acquisition and retention of delay conditioning require the cerebellum and associated brainstem structures (for a review, see Thompson & Krupa, 1994). No tissue above the level of the midbrain, including the hippocampus, is required for delay conditioning (Mauk & Thompson, 1987). Successful trace conditioning, like delay conditioning, requires the cerebellum (Woodruff-Pak, Lavond, & Thompson, 1985), but trace conditioning differs from delay conditioning in that it also requires the hippocampus (Moyer, Deyo, & Disterhoft, 1990; Solomon, Vander Schaaf, Thompson, & Weisz, 1986). The role of the hippocampus in trace conditioning is time-dependent. When hippocampal lesions were made in rabbits immediately after acquisition, trace conditioning was abolished. In contrast, lesions made 30 days after acquisition had no effect (Kim, Clark, & Thompson, 1995). These findings indicate that trace conditioning shares two important characteristics with declarative memory. First, like declarative memory, trace conditioning requires the hippocampus. Second, in trace conditioning as in other forms of declarative memory, the hippocampus has a time-limited role (Squire, Clark, & Knowlton, 2001).

Trace conditioning appears to require the hippocampus because declarative knowledge of the CS-US relationship must build up and be maintained across many trials. This link between trace conditioning and declarative knowledge was first demonstrated by showing that awareness of the stimulus contingencies is critical for differential trace conditioning. In differential conditioning, the CS+ (e.g., a tone) is followed by the US, and the CS– (e.g., a static noise) is presented alone. Successful differential conditioning occurs when more CRs are elicited by the CS⁺ than by the CS⁻. Because there are several relationships among the stimuli about which a participant can become aware, a variety of questions can be asked about the stimulus contingencies, and a participant's answers to these questions can be compared to differential conditioning performance.

In studies of differential trace and differential delay conditioning, awareness of the stimulus contingencies was found to be a critical factor for successful trace conditioning, but not for successful differential delay conditioning (Clark & Squire, 1998; Manns, Clark, & Squire, in press). Furthermore, amnesic patients with damage that included the hippocampus failed to become aware of the stimulus contingencies and also failed to acquire differential trace conditioning. The same patients were subsequently able to acquire differential delay conditioning as quickly as intact subjects. To clarify the relationship between awareness of the stimulus contingencies and trace conditioning, the level of awareness was manipulated directly (Clark & Squire, 1999). For example, it was found that explaining the stimulus contingencies to individuals before the conditioning session increased awareness and facilitated trace conditioning. Moreover, preventing awareness by engaging participants in a secondary distraction task during the conditioning session reduced awareness and blocked differential trace conditioning. Yet other participants who were given the same distraction task were successful at acquiring differential delay conditioning. Finally, the development of awareness during differential trace conditioning was tracked by using an "online," trial-by-trial measure of awareness (participants were asked to push a button when they believed the US was coming) (Manns, Clark, & Squire, 2000b). Differential trace conditioning was found to emerge approximately in parallel with developing awareness of the stimulus contingencies. These results with differential trace and differential delay conditioning indicate that declarative knowledge, or awareness of the stimulus contingencies, is critical for trace conditioning but not for delay conditioning.

Other studies have indicated that complex stimulus conditions, as well as secondary tasks, can retard differential delay conditioning (Carrillo, Gabrieli, & Disterhoft, 2000; Mayer & Ross, 1969; Ross & Nelson, 1973). In these cases, it is unclear whether awareness of the stimulus contingencies was relevant to the results. For example, in one study of differential delay conditioning (Carrillo et al., 2000), a verbal shadowing task eliminated differential responding in aware and unaware participants alike. Furthermore, the finding that differential delay conditioning was retarded by a distraction task (Carrillo et al., 2000) is not necessarily in conflict with the earlier report that differential delay conditioning succeeded in the face of distraction (Clark & Squire, 1999). The latter study appears to have used a less demanding distraction task (digit monitoring) and an easier conditioning task (tone vs. static noise) than did the former study (verbal shadowing and 1-kHz vs. 5-kHz tones). One possibility is that attention is required when a differential conditioning task is especially difficult, and that in such cases distraction can disrupt performance, whether participants have knowledge of the stimulus contingencies or not.

A different point of view is suggested by a recent report that the success of differential delay conditioning correlated with awareness of the stimulus contingencies as assessed at the end of the conditioning session (Knuttinen, Power, Preston, & Disterhoft, 2001). This finding appears to differ from reports that differential delay conditioning is independent of awareness (Clark & Squire, 1998, 1999). One potentially important difference between the two studies is that different criteria were used to identify and score the CRs. This difference could be important because it can be difficult to identify and discard voluntary eyeblinks, which are distinct from the involuntary, reflexive eyeblinks that are true CRs (Clark & Squire, 2000; Coleman, 1985). If voluntary eye closures were sometimes scored as CRs, then the performance of aware individuals (who would be capable of voluntary eye closures) should be better than the performance of unaware individuals (who would not exhibit voluntary eye closures). For additional discussion of this possibility, see Manns, Clark, and Squire (2001).

The importance of awareness for trace conditioning, but not for delay conditioning, has also been examined in tests of single-cue conditioning. In this case, a single CS⁺ is paired with an airpuff. Reducing awareness by introducing a distraction task impaired single-cue trace conditioning (Manns, Clark, & Squire, 2000a). In another experiment, participants who became aware of the relationship between the CS and the US early in the session conditioned to a greater extent than those who became aware of the relationship later in the session or who never became aware at all. Indeed, awareness of the relationship between the CS and the US during the first 10 conditioning trials predicted the magnitude of single-cue trace conditioning over the entire 120-trial conditioning session (Manns et al., 2000a). Another study of single-cue trace conditioning also found that those individuals designated as "aware" after the session produced more conditioned responses during the first 10 conditioning trials than those designated "unaware" (Woodruff-Pak, 1999).

In contrast to these results for single-cue trace conditioning, awareness was not related to single-cue delay conditioning. Thus, during delay conditioning, participants who became aware of the stimulus contingencies early in the conditioning session conditioned no better than participants who became aware later in the session or did not become aware at all (Manns et al., 2001). Finally, in a different study, participants who conditioned well appeared to be as aware (or unaware) of the stimulus contingencies as participants who conditioned poorly (Papka, Ivry, & Woodruff-Pak, 1997).

These results from single-cue eyeblink conditioning are compatible with previous studies of amnesic patients. First, amnesic patients with hippocampal damage, who would be likely to have difficulty acquiring and retaining awareness of the stimulus contingencies, were impaired at single-cue trace conditioning (McGlinchey-Berroth, Carrillo, Gabrieli, Brawn, & Disterhoft, 1997). Second, amnesic patients performed normally on single-cue delay conditioning (Daum & Ackermann, 1994; Daum, Channon, & Canavan, 1989; Gabrieli et al., 1995).

The distinction between single-cue delay conditioning and single-cue trace conditioning was highlighted in a study of how expectation of the US relates to performance (Clark, Manns, & Squire, 2001). This study was based on a paradigm developed by Perruchet (1985). Participants were first informed that half of the time a tone (the CS) would be followed by an airpuff (the US), and that half of the time the tone would be presented alone. Before each trial, participants rated how strongly they believed that an airpuff would be presented on the next trial. Strings of one, two, three, or four CS-alone trials and one, two, three, or four CS-US trials were presented, such that the probability of a US was independent of string length. Participants exhibited high expectations of the US following strings of CS-alone trials and low expectations of the US following strings of CS-US trials—a phenomenon known as the "gambler's fallacy."

The finding of interest was that expectancy of the airpuff US was positively related to performance in individuals given trace eyeblink conditioning (i.e., greater expectancy of the US was related to a greater probability of CRs). In contrast, expectancy of the US was not related to performance in individuals given delay eyeblink conditioning (Figure 1.7). Instead, delay conditioning was related to the strength of the CS-US association at the time a CS was presented. That is, CR probability was high following a string of CS-US trials, and low following a string of CS-alone trials. This finding suggests that expectation (i.e., awareness) of an imminent US has a different role in trace conditioning than it does in delay conditioning. Table 1.1 summarizes the available findings regarding the role of aware-

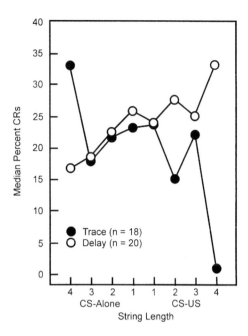

FIGURE 1.7. Median percentage of conditioned responses (CRs) as a function of string length for participants given delay or trace conditioning. String length refers to the number of consecutive trials in which the conditioned stimulus (CS) alone had been presented or both the CS and the unconditioned stimulus (US) had been presented. For the delay group, conditioning performance reflected the recent strength of the CS-US association. That is, participants in the delay group were most likely to emit a CR when they had just experienced a consecutive series of CS-US trials. In contrast, conditioning performance in the trace group paralleled predictions that were made about whether a US would appear on the next trial. That is, participants in the trace group were most likely to emit a CR on trials that they had predicted would include an airpuff (after a string of four CS-alone trials). They were least likely to emit a CR on trials that they had predicted would not include an airpuff (after a string of four CS-US trials). From Clark et al. (2001).

ness in studies of single-cue and differential delay and trace eyeblink classical conditioning. Awareness is important both for single-cue trace conditioning and for differential trace eyeblink classical conditioning.

Taken together, these results indicate that trace conditioning requires an additional level of processing that is not required for delay conditioning. Specifically, trace conditioning (but not delay conditioning) requires the participation of the hippocampus and presumably its interaction with neocortex. Awareness may emerge during trace conditioning because awareness is a typical feature of hippocampus-dependent learning. In this sense, awareness is a reliable indicator of a brain state (a state of interaction between the hippocampus and neocortex) that is conducive to forming and storing declarative memory. Task conditions that reduce awareness disrupt the integrity of this brain state.

Trace conditioning may require declarative knowledge (and awareness) because the trace interval between the CS and US makes it difficult to process the CS-US relationship in an automatic, reflexive way. Whereas the formation of the motor memory in trace conditioning requires the cerebellum, just as in delay conditioning (Woodruff-Pak et al., 1985), trace conditioning also requires the hippocampus (and neocortex), perhaps in order to

TABLE 1.1. Is Awareness Important for Eyeblink Conditioning?

	Delay	Trace
Single-cue	No (Manns, Clark, & Squire, 2001; Papka, Ivry, & Woodruff-Pak, 1997)	Yes (Manns, Clark, & Squire, 2000a; Woodruff-Pak, 1999)
Differential	No (Clark & Squire, 1998, 1999) Yes (Knuttinen et al., 2001)	Yes (Clark & Squire, 1998, 1999; Manns, Clark, & Squire, 2000b; Knuttinen et al., 2001)

Note. The available findings suggest that awareness of the stimulus contingencies is a prerequisite for trace conditioning—both for single-cue conditioning and for differential conditioning. In contrast to the findings for trace conditioning, delay conditioning has usually been found not to require awareness.

represent the stimulus contingencies. If so, then processed information about the CS could be sent to the cerebellum at a time during the trial that is optimal for cerebellar plasticity (i.e., immediately before or during the US). Thus an interesting possibility is that in trace conditioning the cerebellum receives reformatted information from the hippocampus, such that CS information and US information arrive at the cerebellum in temporally overlapping fashion (or in close temporal proximity), such that the cerebellum can use the information (Clark & Squire, 2000).

CONCLUSION

Almost 50 years have passed since the medial temporal lobe was discovered to be important for memory. Since that time, an enormous amount has been learned about the structures within the medial temporal lobe that are important for memory, and about how these structures contribute to memory function. The success of these efforts has been aided by the development of animal models to study both normal memory and memory impairment, and by research focusing on relatively simple memory tasks such as classical conditioning and recognition memory. Perhaps the greatest progress has occurred where it has been possible to move from humans, to monkeys, and even to rodents, using similar concepts and paradigms. It is in these cases that what is being learned about the organization of memory is most likely to be relevant to the human condition.

ACKNOWLEDGMENTS

The work described here was supported by the Medical Research Service of the Department of Veterans Affairs; Grants No. MH24600 and No. MH58933 from the National Institute of Mental Health; and the Metropolitan Life Foundation.

REFERENCES

Aggleton, J. P., & Brown, M. W. (1999). Episodic memory, amnesia, and the hippocampal–anterior thalamic axis. *Behavioral and Brain Sciences, 22,* 425–489.

Aggleton, J. P., Hunt, P. R., & Rawlins, J. N. P. (1986). The effects of hippocampal lesions upon spatial and non-spatial tests of working memory. *Behavioural Brain Research, 19,* 133–146.

Alvarez, P., Zola-Morgan, S., & Squire, L. R. (1995). Damage limited to the hippocampal region produces long-lasting memory impairment in monkeys. *Journal of Neuroscience, 15*, 3796–3807.

Bachevalier, J. (1990). Ontogenetic development of habit and memory formation in primates. *Annals of the New York Academy of Sciences, 608*, 457–474.

Bachevalier, J., Brickson, M., & Hagger, C. (1993). Limbic-dependent recognition memory in monkeys develops early in infancy. *Learning and Memory, 4*, 77–80.

Baddeley, A., Vargha-Khadem, F., & Mishkin, M. (2001). Preserved recognition in a case of developmental amnesia: Implications for the acquisition of semantic memory? *Journal of Cognitive Neuroscience, 13*, 357–369.

Beason-Held, L. L., Rosene, D. L., Killiany, R. J., & Moss, M. B. (1999). Hippocampal formation lesions produce memory impairment in the rhesus monkey. *Hippocampus, 9*, 562–574.

Brown, M. W., & Aggleton, J. P. (2001). Recognition memory: What are the roles of the perirhinal cortex and hippocampus? *Nature Reviews Neuroscience, 2*, 51–61.

Buffalo, E. A., Ramus, S. J., Clark, R. E., Teng, E., Squire, L. R., & Zola, S. M. (1999). Dissociation between the effects of damage to perirhinal cortex and area TE. *Learning and Memory, 6*, 572–599.

Buffalo, E.A., Ramus, S.J., Squire, L.R., & Zola, S.M. (2000). Perception and recognition memory in monkeys following lesions of area TE and perirhinal cortex. *Learning and Memory, 7*, 375–382.

Buffalo, E. A., Reber, P. J., & Squire, L. R. (1998). The human perirhinal cortex and recognition memory. *Hippocampus, 8*, 330–339.

Buffalo, E. A., Stefanacci, L., Squire, L. R., & Zola, S. M. (1998). A reexamination of the concurrent discrimination learning task: The importance of anterior inferotemporal cortex, area TE. *Behavioral Neuroscience, 112*, 3–14.

Carrillo, M. C., Gabrieli, J. D. E., & Disterhoft, J. F. (2000). Selective effects of division of attention on discrimination conditioning. *Psychobiology, 28*, 293–302.

Clark, R. E., Manns, J. R., & Squire, L. R. (2001). Trace and delay eyeblink conditioning: Contrasting phenomena of declarative and nondeclarative memory. *Psychological Science, 12*, 304–308.

Clark, R. E., & Squire, L. R. (1998). Classical conditioning and brain systems: A key role for awareness. *Science, 280*, 77–81.

Clark, R. E. & Squire, L. R. (1999). Human eyeblink classical conditioning: Effects of manipulating awareness of the stimulus contingencies. *Psychological Science, 10*, 14–18.

Clark, R. E., & Squire, L. R. (2000). Awareness and the conditioned eyeblink response. In D. S. Woodruff-Pak & J. E. Steinmetz (Eds.), *Eyeblink classical conditioning: Vol. 1. Applications in humans* (pp. 229–251). Boston: Kluwer.

Clark, R. E., West, A. N., Zola, S. M., & Squire, L. R. (2001). Rats with lesions of the hippocampus are impaired on the delayed nonmatching-to-sample task. *Hippocampus, 11*, 176–186.

Clark, R. E., Zola, S. M., & Squire, L. R. (2000). Impaired recognition memory in rats after damage to the hippocampus. *Journal of Neuroscience, 20*, 451–463.

Coleman, S. R. (1985). The problem of volition and the conditioned reflex: Part I. Conceptual background. *Behaviorism, 13*, 99–124.

Corkin, S. (1984). Lasting consequences of bilateral medial temporal lobectomy: Clinical course and experimental findings in H. M. *Seminars in Neurology, 4*, 249–259.

Corkin, S., Amaral, D. G., Gonzalez, R. G., Johnson, K. A., & Hyman, B. T. (1997). H. M.'s medial temporal lobe lesion: Findings from magnetic resonance imaging. *Journal of Neuroscience, 17*, 3964–3980.

Daum, I., & Ackermann, H. (1994). Dissociation of declarative and nondeclarative memory after bilateral thalamic lesions: A case report. *International Journal of Neuroscience, 75*, 153–165.

Daum, I., Channon, S., & Canavan, A. (1989). Classical conditioning in patients with severe memory problems. *Journal of Neurology, Neurosurgery and Psychiatry, 52*, 47–51.

Dore, F. Y., Thornton, J. A., White, N. M., & Murray, E. A. (1998). Selective hippocampal lesions yield nonspatial memory impairment in rhesus monkeys. *Hippocampus, 4*, 323–329.

Duva, C. A., Floresco, S. B., Wunderlich, G. R., Lao, T. L., Pinel, J. P. J., & Phillips, A. G. (1997). Disruption of spatial but not object-recognition memory by neurotoxic lesions of the dorsal hippocampus in rats. *Behavioral Neuroscience, 111*, 1184–1196.

Eacott, M. J., Gaffan, D., & Murray, E. A. (1994). Preserved recognition memory for small sets, and impaired stimulus identification for large sets, following rhinal cortex ablations in monkeys. *European Journal of Neuroscience, 6*, 1466–1478.

Eichenbaum, H. (1997). Declarative memory: Insights from cognitive neurobiology. *Annual Review of Psychology, 48*, 547–572.

Eichenbaum, H., Dudchenko, P., Wood, E., Shapiro, M., & Tanila, H. (1999). The hippocampus, memory, and place cells: Is it spatial memory or a memory space? *Neuron, 23*, 209–226.

Ennaceur, A. & Delacour, J. (1988). A new one-trial test for neurobiological studies of memory in rats: 1. Behavioural data. *Behavioural Brain Research, 31*, 47–59.

Fernandez-Ruiz, J., Wang, J., Aigner, T., & Mishkin, M. (2001). Visual habit formation in monkeys with neurotoxic lesions of the ventrocaudal neostriatum. *Proceedings of the National Academy of Sciences USA, 98*, 4196–4201.

Finger, S. (1978). *Recovery from brain damage: Research and theory*. New York: Plenum Press.

Fried, I., MacDonald, K. A., & Wilson, C. L. (1997). Single neuron activity in human hippocampus and amygdala during recognition of faces and objects. *Neuron, 18*, 753–765.

Gabrieli, J. D. E., Brewer, J. B., Desmond, J. E., & Glover, G. H. (1997). Separate neural bases of two fundamental memory processes in the human medial temporal lobe. *Science, 11*, 264–266.

Gabrieli, J. D. E., McGlinchey-Berroth, R., Carrillo, M. C., Gluck, M. A., Cermak, L. S., & Disterhoft, J. F. (1995). Intact delay-eyeblink classical conditioning in amnesia. *Behavioral Neuroscience, 109*, 819–827.

Graybiel, A. M. (1995). Building action repertoires: Memory and learning functions of the basal ganglia. *Current Opinion in Neurobiology, 5*, 733–741.

Hampson, R. E., Heyser, C. J., & Deadwyler, S. A. (1993). Hippocampal cell firing correlates of delayed-matching-to-sample performance in the rat. *Behavioral Neuroscience, 107*, 715–739.

Hood, K. L., Postle, B. R., & Corkin, S. (1999). An evaluation of the concurrent discrimination task as a measure of habit learning: Performance of amnesic subjects. *Neuropsychologia, 37*, 1375–1386.

Jarrard, L. E. (1993). On the role of the hippocampus in learning and memory in the rat. *Behavioral and Neural Biology, 60*, 9–26.

Kesner, R. P., Bolland, B. L., & Dakis, M. (1993). Memory for spatial location, motor responses, and objects: Triple dissociation among the hippocampus, caudate nucleus, and extrastriate visual cortex. *Experimental Brain Research, 93*, 462–470.

Kim, J. J., Clark, R. E., & Thompson, R. F. (1995). Hippocampectomy impairs the memory of recently, but not remotely, acquired trace eyeblink conditioned responses. *Behavioral Neuroscience, 109*, 195–203.

Knowlton, B. J., & Squire, L. R. (1995). Remembering and knowing: Two different expressions of declarative memory. *Journal of Experimental Psychology: Learning, Memory, and Cognition, 21*, 699–710.

Knuttinen, M-G., Power, J. M., Preston, A. R., & Disterhoft, J. F. (2001). Awareness in classical differential eyeblink conditioning in young and aging humans. *Behavioral Neuroscience, 115*, 474–757.

Malamut, B. L., Saunders, R. C., & Mishkin, M. (1984). Monkeys with combined amygdalo-hippocampal lesions succeed in object discrimination learning despite 24-hour intertrial intervals. *Behavioral Neuroscience, 98*, 759–769.

Malkova, L., & Mishkin, M. (1997). Memory for the location of objects after separate lesions of the hippocampus and parahippocampal cortex in rhesus monkeys. *Society for Neuroscience Abstracts, 23*, 14.

Manns, J. R., Clark, R. E., & Squire, L. R. (2000a). Awareness predicts the magnitude of single-cue trace eyeblink conditioning. *Hippocampus, 19*, 181–186.

Manns, J. R., Clark, R. E., & Squire, L. R. (2000b). Parallel acquisition of awareness and trace eye-blink classical conditioning. *Learning and Memory, 7*, 267–272.

Manns, J. R., Clark, R. E., & Squire, L. R. (2001). Single-cue delay eyeblink conditioning is unrelated to awareness. *Cognitive, Affective, and Behavioral Neuroscience, 1*, 192–198.

Manns, J. R., Clark, R. E., & Squire, L. R. (in press). Standard delay eyeblink classical conditioning is independent of awareness. *Journal of Experimental Psychology: Animal Behavior Processes.*

Manns, J. R., & Squire, L. R. (1999). Impaired recognition memory on the Doors and People Test after damage limited to the hippocampal region. *Hippocampus, 9*, 495–499.

Manns, J. R., Stark, C. E. L., & Squire, L. R. (2000). The visual paired-comparison task as a measure of declarative memory. *Proceedings of the National Academy of Sciences USA, 97*, 12375–12379.

Mauk, M. D., & Thompson, R. F. (1987). Retention of classically conditioned eyelid responses following acute decerebration. *Brain Research, 403*, 89–95.

Mayer, M. J., & Ross, L. E. (1969). Effects of stimulus complexity, interstimulus interval, and masking task conditions in differential eyelid conditioning. *Journal of Experimental Psychology, 81*, 469–474.

Mayes, A. R. (1988). *Human organic memory disorders.* New York: Cambridge University Press.

McGlinchey-Berroth, R., Carrillo, M. C., Gabrieli J. D. E., Brawn, D. M., & Disterhoft, J. F. (1997). Impaired trace eyeblink conditioning in bilateral, medial-temporal lobe amnesia. *Behavioral Neuroscience, 100*, 873–882.

McKee, R. D., & Squire, L. R. (1993). On the development of declarative memory. *Journal of Experimental Psychology: Learning, Memory, and Cognition, 19*, 397–404.

Mishkin, M. (1978). Memory in monkeys severely impaired by combined but not by separate removal of amygdala and hippocampus. *Nature, 273*, 297–298.

Mishkin, M., Malamut, B., & Bachevalier, J. (1984). Memories and habits: Two neural systems. In G. Lynch, J. L. McGaugh, & N. M. Weinberger (Eds.), *Neurobiology of learning and memory* (pp. 65–77). New York: Guilford Press.

Mishkin, M., & Murray, E. A. (1994). Stimulus recognition. *Current Opinion in Neurobiology, 4*, 200–206.

Mishkin, M., & Petri, H. L. (1984). Memories and habits: Some implications for the analysis of learning and retention. In L. R. Squire & N. Butters (Eds.), *Neuropsychology of memory* (pp. 287–296). New York: Guilford Press.

Mishkin, M., Spiegler, B. J., Saunders, R. C., & Malamut, B. J. (1982). An animal model of global amnesia. In S. Corkin, K. L. Davis, J. H. Growdon, E. Usdin, & R. J. Wurtman (Eds.), *Alzheimer's disease: A report of progress in research* (pp. 235–247). New York: Raven Press.

Moser, E., Moser, M.-B., & Andersen, P. (1993). Spatial learning impairment parallels the magnitude of dorsal hippocampal lesions, but is hardly present following ventral lesions. *Journal of Neuroscience, 13*, 3916–3925.

Moser, M. B., Moser, E. I., Forrest, E., Andersen, P., & Morris, R. G. (1995). Spatial learning with a minislab in the dorsal hippocampus. *Proceedings of the National Academy of Sciences USA, 10*, 9697–9701.

Moyer, J. R., Deyo, R. A., & Disterhoft, J. F. (1990). Hippocampectomy disrupts trace eye-blink conditioning in rabbits. *Behavioral Neuroscience, 104*, 243–252.

Mumby, D. G., Pinel, J. P. J., Kornecook, T. J., Shen, M. J., & Redila, V. A. (1995). Memory deficits following lesions of hippocampus or amygdala in rat: Assessment by an object-memory test battery. *Psychobiology, 23*, 26–36.

Mumby, D. G., Pinel, J. P. J., & Wood, E. R. (1990). Nonrecurring-items delayed nonmatching-to-sample in rats: A new paradigm for testing nonspatial working memory. *Psychobiology, 18*, 321–326.

Mumby, D. G., Wood, E. R., Duva, C. A., Kornecook, T. J., Pinel, J. P. J., & Phillips, A. G. (1996). Ischemia-induced object-recognition deficits in rats are attenuated by hippocampal ablation before or soon after ischemia. *Behavioral Neuroscience, 110*, 266–281.

Mumby, D. G., Wood, E. R., & Pinel, J. P. J. (1992). Object-recognition memory is only mildly impaired in rats with lesions of the hippocampus and amygdala. *Psychobiology, 20*, 18–27.

Murray, E. A., & Bussey, T. J. (2001). Consolidation and the medial temporal lobe revisited: Methodological considerations, *Hippocampus*, *11*, 1–7.

Murray, E. A., & Mishkin, M. (1984). Severe tactual as well as visual memory deficits following combined removal of the amygdala and hippocampus in monkeys. *Journal of Neuroscience*, *4*, 2565–2580.

Murray, E. A., & Mishkin, M. (1998). Object recognition and location memory in monkeys with excitotoxic lesions of the amygdala and hippocampus. *Journal of Neuroscience*, *18*, 6568–6582.

Murray, E. A., & Richmond, B. J. (2001). Role of perirhinal cortex in object perception, memory, and associations. *Current Opinion in Neurobiology*, *11*, 188–193.

Nadel, L., & Moscovitch, M. (1997). Memory consolidation, retrograde amnesia and the hippocampal complex. *Current Opinion in Neurobiology*, *7*, 217–227.

Overman, W. H., Ormsby, G., & Mishkin, M. (1990). Picture recognition vs. picture discrimination learning in monkeys with medial temporal removals. *Experimental Brain Research*, *79*, 18–24.

Papka, M., Ivry, R. B., & Woodruff-Pak, D. S. (1997). Eyeblink classical conditioning and awareness revisited. *Psychological Science*, *8*, 404–408.

Parkinson, J. K., Murray, E. A., & Mishkin, M. A. (1988). A selective mnemonic role for the hippocampus in monkeys: Memory for the location of objects. *Journal of Neuroscience*, *8*, 4159–4167.

Pascalis, O., & Bachevalier, J. (1999). Neonatal aspiration lesions of the hippocampal formation impair visual recognition memory when assessed by paired-comparison task but not by delayed nonmatching-to-sample task. *Hippocampus*, *9*, 609–616.

Perruchet, P. (1985). A pitfall for the expectancy theory of human eyelid conditioning. *Pavlovian Society of Biological Sciences*, *20*, 163–170.

Phillips, R. R., Malmut, B., Bachevalier, J., & Mishkin, M. (1988). Dissociation of the effects of inferior temporal and limbic lesions on object discrimination learning with 24-h intertrial intervals. *Behavioural Brain Research*, *27*, 99–107.

Rampon, C., Ya-Ping, T., Goodhouse, J., Shimizu, E., Kyin, M., & Tsien, J. Z. (2000). Enrichment induces structural changes and recovery from nonspatial memory deficits in CA1 NMDAR1-knockout mice. *Nature Neuroscience*, *3*, 238–244.

Ramus, S. J., Zola-Morgan, S., & Squire, L. R. (1994). Effects of lesions of perirhinal cortex or parahipocampal cortex on memory in monkeys. *Society for Neuroscience Abstracts*, *20*, 1074.

Reed, J. M., & Squire, L. R. (1997). Impaired recognition memory in patients with lesions limited to the hippocampal formation. *Behavioral Neuroscience*, *111*, 667–675.

Rempel-Clower, N. L., Zola, S. M., Squire, L. R., & Amaral, D. G. (1996). Three cases of enduring memory impairment following bilateral damage limited to the hippocampal formation. *Journal of Neuroscience*, *16*, 5233–5255.

Ross, L. E., & Nelson, M. N. (1973). The role of awareness in differential conditioning. *Psychophysiology*, *10*, 91–94.

Rothblat, L. A., & Kromer, L. R. (1991). Object recognition memory in the rat: The role of the hippocampus. *Behavioural Brain Research*, *42*, 25–32.

Schacter, D. L., & Tulving, E. (Eds.). (1994). *Memory systems 1994*. Cambridge, MA: MIT Press.

Schacter, D. L., & Wagner, A. D. (1999). Medial temporal lobe activation in fMRI and PET studies of episodic encoding and retrieval. *Hippocampus*, *9*, 7–24.

Scoville, W. B., & Milner, B. (1957). Loss of recent memory after bilateral hippocampal lesions. *Journal of Neurology, Neurosurgery and Psychiatry*, *20*, 11–21.

Solomon, P. R., Vander Schaaf, E. R., Thompson, R. F., & Weisz, D. J. (1986). Hippocampus and trace conditioning of the rabbit's classically conditioned nictitating membrane response. *Behavioral Neuroscience*, *100*, 729–744.

Squire, L. R. (1992). Memory and the hippocampus: A synthesis from findings with rats, monkeys, and humans. *Psychological Review*, *99*, 195–231.

Squire, L. R., & Butters, N. (Eds.). (1992). *The neuropsychology of memory* (2nd ed.). New York: Guilford Press.

Squire, L. R., Clark, R. E., & Knowlton, B. J. (2001). Retrograde amnesia. *Hippocampus*, *11*, 50–55.

Squire, L. R., & Zola, S. (1998). Episodic memory, semantic memory, and amnesia. *Hippocampus, 8,* 205–211.

Squire, L. R., & Zola-Morgan, S. (1983). The neurology of memory: The case for correspondence between the findings for human and nonhuman primates. In J. A. Deutsch (Ed.), *The physiological basis of memory* (2nd ed., pp. 199–268). New York: Academic Press.

Squire, L. R., & Zola-Morgan, S. (1991). The medial temporal lobe memory system. *Science, 253,* 1380–1386.

Stark, C. E. L., & Squire, L. R. (2000a). fMRI activity in the medial temporal lobe during recognition memory as a function of study–test interval. *Hippocampus, 10,* 329–337.

Stark, C. E. L., & Squire, L. R. (2000b). Recognition memory and familiarity judgments in severe amnesia: No evidence for a contribution of repetition priming. *Behavioral Neuroscience, 114,* 459–467.

Stark, C. E. L., & Squire. L. R. (2000c). Intact visual perceptual discrimination in humans in the absence of perirhinal cortex. *Learning and Memory, 7,* 273–278.

Steele, R. J., & Morris, R. G. (1999). Delay-dependent impairment of a matching-to-place task with chronic and intrahippocampal infusion of the NMDA-antagonist D-AP5. *Hippocampus, 9,* 118–136.

Stefanacci, L., Buffalo, E. A., Schmolck, H., & Squire, L. R. (2000). Profound amnesia after damage to the medial temporal lobe: A neuroanatomical and neuropsychological profile of patient E. P. *Journal of Neuroscience, 20,* 7024–7036.

Suzuki, W. A., & Amaral, D. G. (1994a). Perirhinal and parahippocampal cortices of the macaque monkey: Cortical afferents. *Journal of Comparative Neurology, 350,* 497–533.

Suzuki, W. A., & Amaral, D. G. (1994b). Topographic organization of the reciprocal connections between the monkey entorhinal cortex and the perirhinal and parahippocampal cortices. *Journal of Neuroscience, 14,* 1856–1877.

Suzuki, W. A., & Eichenbaum, H. (2000). The neurophysiology of memory. *Annals of the New York Academy of Sciences, 911,* 175–191.

Suzuki, W. A., Zola-Morgan, S., Squire, L. R., & Amaral, D. G. (1993). Lesions of the perirhinal and parahippocampal cortices in the monkey produce long-lasting memory impairment in the visual and tactual modalities. *Journal of Neuroscience, 13,* 2430–2451.

Teng, E., Stefanacci, L., Squire, L. R., & Zola, S. M. (2000). Contrasting effects on discrimination learning following hippocampal lesions or conjoint hippocampal–caudate lesions in monkeys. *Journal of Neuroscience, 20,* 3853–3863.

Thompson, R. F., & Krupa, D. J. (1994). Organization of memory traces in the mammalian brain. *Annual Review of Neuroscience, 17,* 519–550.

Tulving, E., & Craik, F. I. M. (2000). *The Oxford handbook of memory.* New York: Oxford University Press, Inc.

Tulving, E., & Markowitsch, H. J. (1998). Episodic and declarative memory: Role of the hippocampus. *Hippocampus, 8,* 198–204.

Vargha-Khadem, F., Gadian, D. G., Watkins, K. E., Connelly, A., Van Paesschen, W., & Mishkin, M. (1997). Differential effects of early hippocampal pathology on episodic and semantic memory. *Science, 277,* 376–380.

Wiebe, S. P., & Staubi, U. V. (1999). Dynamic filtering of recognition memory codes in the hippocampus. *Journal of Neuroscience, 19,* 10562–10574.

Wiig, K. A., & Bilkey, D. K. (1995). Lesions of rat perirhinal cortex exacerbate the memory deficit observed following damage to the fimbria-fornix. *Behavioral Neuroscience, 109,* 620–630.

Wood, E. R., Dudchenko, P. A., & Eichenbaum, H. (1999). The global record of memory in hippocampal neuronal activity. *Nature, 397,* 613–616.

Wood, E. R., & Phillips, A. G. (1991). Deficits on a one trial object recognition task by rats with hippocampal CA1 lesions produced by cerebral ischemia. *Neuroscience Research Communications, 9,* 177–182.

Woodruff-Pak, D. S. (1999). New directions for a classical paradigm: Human eyeblink conditioning. *Psychological Science, 10,* 1–3.

Woodruff-Pak, D. S., Lavond, D. G., & Thompson, R. F. (1985). Trace conditioning: Abolished by cerebellar nuclear lesions but not lateral cerebellar cortex aspirations. *Brain Research, 348,* 249–260.

Yonelinas, A. P., Kroll, N. E. A., Dobbins, I., Lazzara M., & Knight, R. T. (1998). Recollection and familiarity deficits in amnesia: Convergence of remember–know, process dissociation, and receiver operating characteristic data. *Neuropsychology, 12,* 323–339.

Zola, S. M., & Squire, L. R. (2001). Relationship between magnitude of damage to the hippocampus and impaired recognition memory in monkeys. *Hippocampus, 11,* 92–98.

Zola, S. M., Squire, L. R., Teng, E., Stefanacci, L., Buffalo, E. A., & Clark, R. E. (2000). Impaired recognition memory in monkeys after damage limited to the hippocampal region. *Journal of Neuroscience, 20,* 451–463.

Zola-Morgan, S., & Squire, L. R. (1984). Preserved learning in monkeys with medial temporal lesions: Sparing of motor and cognitive skills. *Journal of Neuroscience, 4,* 1072–1085.

Zola-Morgan, S., & Squire, L. R. (1985). Medial temporal lesions in monkeys impair memory on a variety of tasks sensitive to human amnesia. *Behavioral Neuroscience, 99,* 22–34.

Zola-Morgan, S., & Squire, L. R. (1986). Memory impairment in monkeys following lesions limited to the hippocampus. *Behavioral Neuroscience, 100,* 155–160.

Zola-Morgan, S., & Squire, L. R. (1993). Neuroanatomy of memory. *Annual Review of Neuroscience, 16,* 547–563.

Zola-Morgan, S., Squire, L. R., & Amaral, D. G. (1986). Human amnesia and the medial temporal region: Enduring memory impairment following a bilateral lesion limited to field CA1 of the hippocampus. *Journal of Neuroscience, 6,* 2950–2967.

Zola-Morgan, S., Squire, L. R., & Amaral, D. G. (1989a). Lesions of the hippocampal formation but not lesions of the fornix or the mammillary nuclei produce long-lasting memory impairment in monkeys. *Journal of Neuroscience, 9,* 898–913.

Zola-Morgan, S., Squire, L. R., & Amaral, D. G. (1989b). Lesions of the amygdala that spare adjacent cortical regions do not impair memory or excerbate the impairment following lesions of the hippocampal formation. *Journal of Neuroscience, 9,* 1922–1936.

Zola-Morgan, S., Squire, L. R., Amaral, D. G., & Suzuki, W. A. (1989). Lesions of perirhinal and parahippocampal cortex that spare the amygdala and hippocampal formation produce severe memory impairment. *Journal of Neuroscience, 9,* 4355–4370.

Zola-Morgan, S., Squire, L. R., Clower, R. P., & Rempel, N. L. (1993). Damage to the perirhinal cortex exacerbates memory impairment following lesions to the hippocampal formation. *Journal of Neuroscience, 13,* 251–265.

Zola-Morgan, S., Squire, L. R., & Mishkin, M. (1982). The neuroanatomy of amnesia: Amygdala–hippocampus versus temporal stem. *Science, 218,* 1337–1339.

Zola-Morgan, S., Squire, L. R., & Ramus, S. J. (1994). Severity of memory impairment in monkeys as a function of locus and extent of damage within the medial temporal lobe memory systems. *Hippocampus, 4,* 483–495.

Zola-Morgan, S., Squire, L. R., Rempel, N. L., Clower, R. P., & Amaral, D. G. (1992). Enduring memory impairment in monkeys after ischemic damage to the hippocampus. *Journal of Neuroscience, 12,* 1582–2596.

2

Exploring the Neural Bases of Complex Memory

ANDREW R. MAYES

Memory for facts or personally experienced episodes, usually referred to as "declarative memory" (Squire, 1992) or "explicit memory" (Graf & Schacter, 1985), involves memory for multiple associations between component pieces of information. In order to stress the importance of this kind of associative complexity and to contrast it with memory that does not require the storage and retrieval of these kinds of factual and episodic association, this form of memory is referred to as "complex memory" in this chapter. Complex memory depends on processing that occurs in the posterior neocortex, the frontal neocortex, and the structures that are damaged in patients who have organic amnesia. These structures include the medial temporal lobes, the midline diencephalon, the basal forebrain, and possibly the ventromedial frontal neocortex. Interactions between neurons in these connected brain regions allow several processes critical for complex memory to be performed. These processes enable facts and episodes to be initially represented; allow what is represented to be at least partially consolidated into long-term memory; permit the strength of this storage to be modulated by various arousal processes around the time of initial encoding; enable the memories thus created to be later rehearsed in various ways and perhaps reorganized; and make it possible for retrieval to occur perhaps many years after a memory was initially laid down.

A neural theory of complex memory must characterize the different processes that mediate it, indicate which brain structures mediate each of these processes, and describe how each process is mediated in detail. Such a theory should (1) indicate how each of the various processes emerges from the pattern of interaction of neurons by using neural network simulations that are faithful to what is known of neural architecture and physiology, as well as the processes underlying complex memory; (2) indicate how these processes trigger and also depend on the synaptic changes that underlie long-term memory storage; and (3) indicate how the whole system of neurons interacts to produce the full range of complex memory behaviors observed in humans. This kind of theoretical account should be able to indicate explicitly the similarities and dissimilarities between putatively distinct kinds of memory, such as episodic memory (Tulving, 1998), semantic memory (Patterson & Hodges, 1995), and priming (Schacter & Buckner, 1998).

It is now possible to pursue these theoretical aims via the use of convergent approaches—that is, lesions and functional imaging of the brain. These approaches have complementary strengths and weaknesses. Lesions are useful in determining whether the normal activity of a brain region is causally necessary for a particular memory process to operate at an intact level. There are clearly limitations on this inference. For example, the region may not itself mediate a specific process, but damage to it may cause a disruption of another connected structure that does mediate this process. Conversely, the brain may reorganize under some conditions following damage, so that atypical structures are able to mediate the process in question. If a fiber tract between two grey matter structures is destroyed, the two structures may still be able to communicate via other, perhaps less direct pathways, so that a process can still be mediated (even if less effectively than before the lesion).

Correlational studies, which measure neural responses when subjects engage in memory processing, do not unequivocally identify the neural activity that causally underlies those processes. However, whereas lesion studies can usually only characterize the functions of one brain structure at a time, functional neuroimaging can tentatively identify the entire system of structures that mediates a specific memory process or set of processes. Through structural equation modeling, it is possible to identify tentatively how a set of connected structures interacts when different memory tasks are being performed. Different imaging methods have different strengths. For example, functional magnetic resonance imaging (fMRI) has good spatial resolution but relatively poor temporal resolution, whereas evoked response potentials (ERPs) have excellent temporal resolution but are very hard to localize spatially. Memory research would benefit from the use of parallel event-related fMRI and ERP studies to attempt to identify neural correlates of processes believed to be mediated neocortically, such as priming, with both spatial and temporal accuracy.

Each approach can be used to help interpret results found with the other. Thus neuroimaging can be used to clarify what a specific lesion has done to a patient. For example, patients with apparently similar lesions can be compared, in order to determine whether the ones with more severe functional deficits show greater disruption of activity in structures outside the lesioned region. Equally, neuroimaging can be used to identify whether a patient shows evidence of having reorganized memory functioning relative to intact individuals, or to show that two apparently disconnected structures can still work together in a coherent manner (using structural equation modeling). Not only can neuroimaging help with the interpretation of the functional effects of lesions, but lesioning can help neuroimaging activations indicate something incidental or causally necessary for the normal performance of a process.

In this chapter, I outline a theoretical position and indicate areas of disagreement or uncertainty, describe some of our work that relates to these issues, and briefly discuss a *possible* way to proceed.

WHAT ARE THE NEURAL BASES OF COMPLEX MEMORY?

Complex information about episodes and facts is represented at different sites primarily within the posterior neocortex. Precisely how this is done is still very poorly understood, but presumably much episodic and some factual information must involve patterned activity at several posterior neocortical sites, each of which represents different components of the encoded information. There will be a considerable overlap between the sites involved in representing facts and episodes, although episodic information is usually likely to contain more sensory information, more reference to spatiotemporal and other contextual features, more reference to experienced emotion, and more reference to self. Episodic information is also likely to contain more components and associations than factual information usually does (i.e., to be more complex). The problem of representation concerns how components are linked together into coherent wholes (e.g., faces or scenes). This problem is not solved, and it remains unclear whether all such associating is done in the same way or whether associations between different kinds of information (e.g., faces and voices) are made in the same way as associations between similar components (e.g., words) or components of single items (e.g., mouths and eyes). However such associating is done, it seems likely that the posterior neocortex is involved in representing complex information at encoding and re-representing it, or some parts of it, at retrieval.

The representation of complex information requires coordination of attention, which determines the components of which the encoder becomes conscious. The frontal neocortex is believed to play a critical role in this coordination, although how many executive processes there are, how they interact with each other, and which frontal regions mediate them remain unresolved (see, e.g., Bechara, Tranel, & Damasio, 2000; Burgess, Veitch, Costello, & Shallice, 2000; Petrides, 2000; Stuss et al., 2000; Stuss, Gallup, & Alexander, 2001). It has become clear, however, that these processes relate closely to working memory and the manipulation of information in the seconds following input (D'Esposito et al., 1995, 1998; Fletcher & Henson, 2001). Executive processes, mediated by the frontal neocortex, are also likely to be involved in searching, reconstructing, and monitoring when subjects try to retrieve complex information intentionally.

Given the pattern of the neocortical inputs to the medial temporal lobes, the hippocampus is in a good position to store an "index," which allows it to associate the components of complex information that are represented in different neocortical regions (see, e.g., Moscovitch, 1995; Teyler & DiScenna, 1986). At retrieval, when some of this information is re-encoded as a cue, the hippocampus is able to reactivate the neocortical regions that were involved in the information's initial representation. There are dissenters from this dominant view. Thus Gray (1982) has argued that the hippocampus is not directly involved in storing factual and episodic information, but that it triggers an attentional orienting response when novel or important inputs are detected. The effect of this would be to enhance storage in posterior neocortical sites where the information is represented. Neocortical storage would be seriously impaired following hippocampal damage, because it would no longer be receiving a tonic up-regulation driven from the hippocampus. It should also show a reduction of phasic modulation in response to particularly interesting or important stimuli, because this depends on the hippocampal mechanism as well.

This equation of posterior neocortex with representation and re-representation, frontal neocortex with coordination during encoding and retrieval, and the medial temporal lobes with consolidation and storage is too simple and requires modification. There are also other points of disagreement that require resolution. First, Murray and Bussey (1999) have argued that the perirhinal cortex may be vital for encoding as well as storing high-level visual object information. This view is consistent with the widely held doctrine that information is stored within the same neurons that represent it (e.g., Gaffan & Hornak, 1997). By extension, one might also argue that the hippocampus may be critical for the encoding of even higher-level associations, such as those that weld visual objects and spatiotemporal context together into a coherent scene. There is no direct evidence supporting either of these possibilities in humans, and some evidence against them (e.g., Buffalo, Reber,

& Squire, 1998; Mayes, Downes, Shogeirat, Hall, & Sagar, 1993). However, tests for high-level perceptual deficits need to be very carefully constructed, so as to prevent patients using their preserved lower-level perceptual processing abilities to solve the perceptual tasks provided. For example, subjects may be able to determine which of several test figures a target figure matches by cross-matching low-level features rather than gestaltic representations of the whole of each figure. It might also be argued that certain frontal neocortical sites may be critical for representing these or similar high-level associations as well, but this will be very hard to examine because of the role of this region in coordinating encoding.

Second, evidence about where storage of specific kinds of information occurs in the brain is surprisingly indirect. Although all neural tissue is probably plastic to some degree, and long-term potentiation (which bears several characteristics indicative of its being a long-term storage process) occurs prominently in the hippocampus (see, e.g., Morris & Frey, 1997), lesion evidence related to amnesia that establishes the medial temporal lobes as a storage site for aspects of episodic and factual information is weak. Further development of stem cell transplantation techniques may, in the future, provide a more direct means of identifying storage sites. Virley and colleagues (1999) have given an example of how this technology might be used to do this. They neurotoxically lesioned the CA1 field of the hippocampus in monkeys that had been trained on a conditional discrimination task. Loss of the ability to show the discrimination following the lesion *indicated* that the memory was hippocampally dependent, as did the finding that learning of new discriminations was severely impaired. However, following either a fetal CA1 or a stem cell transplant, each of which enabled this field of the hippocampus to regenerate in a cytoarchitechonically orderly manner, the animals were able to recall the premorbidly acquired conditional discrimination normally. As the transplant could not have restored any synapses created or adapted to mediate storage, this strongly suggests that the relevant memory was not stored in CA1, although it could have been stored in CA3 or another hippocampal region. If stem cell transplantation can be developed to regenerate cortical regions, it should become possible to determine directly what (if any) information is stored in the medial temporal cortices, as well as various parts of the posterior neocortex and even the frontal neocortex.

Third, there has been recent dissent from the view that episodic and factual information depends on long-term storage in the medial temporal lobes initially, but that with repetition, rehearsal, and time, storage slowly develops in parts of the posterior neocortex so that retrieval no longer needs to use the medial temporal lobes (e.g., Squire & Alvarez, 1995). Instead, although Nadel and Moscovitch (1997) agree that this story applies to the storage of factual information, they argue that episodic memory depends on hippocampal storage for as long as memory lasts. Repetition and rehearsal result in greater redundancy of storage within the hippocampus, but not the slow development of storage within the posterior neocortex. Resolution of this disagreement depends on both lesion evidence and neuroimaging evidence, which are discussed in the next section.

Fourth, whichever of the views described above is nearer the truth, it seems likely that some episodic and factual information is stored in the posterior neocortex as well as the medial temporal lobes *ab initio*. This possibility is supported by evidence that some kinds of perceptual priming depend on storage changes in the posterior neocortex (for reviews, see Mayes & Montaldi, 1999; Schacter & Buckner, 1998; and Wiggs & Martin, 1998). Such priming occurs rapidly, can endure for a year or longer, and probably depends on synaptic changes occurring within the region of the posterior neocortex that represents the relevant information. As complex facts or episodes comprise many new components, it would be very surprising if their storage did not depend on the same highly plastic posterior neocortical system. However, there is growing evidence that those kinds of priming that involve intercomponent associations are disrupted in amnesia (e.g., Chun & Phelps, 1999; Gooding, Mayes, & van Eijk, 2000). These kinds of priming perhaps depend on medial temporal lobe storage. Episodic and factual storage may therefore depend on posterior neocortical storage of intracomponent associations (e.g., to store new faces or objects) and hippocampal storage of intercomponent "indexing" associations.

Further support for this idea that different kinds of episodic and factual information may be rapidly stored in the posterior neocortex as well as the medial temporal lobes comes from recent lesion work of David Gaffan and his colleagues. These workers disconnected the medial temporal lobes and inferior temporal neocortex from the basal forebrain and midbrain by severing the anterior temporal stem and fornix and cutting through the amygdala of monkeys. The animals developed severe amnesia for several memory tasks (Gaffan, Parker, & Easton, 2001). This finding needs confirmation that the effects were on memory rather than on attention or encoding. If it is confirmed, a plausible interpretation would be that inputs from the basal forebrain and midbrain (and probably the amygdala as well) modulate neurons in the medial temporal lobes and posterior neocortex both tonically and phasically so as to regulate storage, and that if this modulation is prevented, these regions cannot store new memories. Interestingly, a companion study in which crossed lesions disconnected the inferior temporal and frontal neocortices from each other produced comparably severe amnesia (Easton & Gaffan, 2001). This suggests that the frontal neocortex may be involved with controlling the storage modulation system.

Fifth, there is disagreement about how distinct the memory functions of different parts of the medial temporal lobes are. More generally, it is still unclear to what extent different sites implicated in amnesia subserve different memory functions. Aggleton and Brown (1999) have argued that the perirhinal cortex and its projection to the dorsomedial thalamus and frontal neocortex are critical for item familiarity memory, whereas the hippocampus and its Papez circuit projections are not needed for familiarity, but are essential for normal recollection. If this is correct, then perirhinal cortex lesions should seriously disrupt item recognition, but although hippocampal lesions should clearly disrupt recall and recollection, they will only mildly impair item recognition. The evidence on the effects of hippocampal lesions is conflicting, however, and apparently similar lesions may have somewhat different effects on item recognition memory. For example, whereas Reed and Squire (1997) found clear item recognition deficits in patients with relatively selective hippocampal lesions, Vargha-Khadem and colleagues (1997) found that three patients with early-onset hippocampal damage showed relative intact item recognition. These latter patients also showed relatively normal memory for semantic information to which there had been repeated exposure over a long period of time, which led Vargha-Khadem and her colleagues to argue that normal hippocampal activity is essential for episodic but not semantic memory. Although the medial temporal lobes probably show some functional heterogeneity, this view, and the postulate that the hippocampus mediates recollection but not familiarity, therefore need more systematic investigation.

Sixth, episodic memory is accompanied by the feeling that what has been retrieved is familiar. The phenomena of *déjà vu* and *jamais vu* are experienced when this feeling occurs or does not occur inappropriately. The mechanism that generates this feeling that one is remembering is not understood. If one imagines that memory for an episode is stored as synaptic changes within the representing neural region, then it seems likely that the stored information will be reactivated more fluently next time some of it is encoded. This enhanced fluency corresponds to priming, and this is not accompanied by a feeling of familiarity, so the mechanism of this feeling remains unexplained. Only two plausible theories exist, and both have problems. Milner (1999) has suggested that an association is formed between the representation of the episode and a brain region (perhaps the hippocampus), which produces a feeling of familiarity. Alternatively, the attributionist account of familiarity can be extended so as to state that in some sense all episodic information is retrieved more fluently, that this is noticed, and that it leads to an attribution of memory (the feeling of memory) being made (Jacoby, Kelley, & Dywan, 1989; Mayes, 2001). Developing an adequate theory of the mechanism of the feeling of memory is important; it will probably resolve the issue of how priming and declarative/explicit memory relate to each other, because a similar feeling of memory usually accompanies the retrieval of semantic memories.

TWO EXAMPLES OF THE USE OF CONVERGENT APPROACHES

If memory storage is transferred from the medial temporal lobes to the posterior neocortex as a result of repetition and rehearsal, retrograde amnesia should show a temporal gradient, with memories acquired earlier in the premorbid period being better preserved. The human literature on retrograde amnesia does not always show such sparing; when it does, gradients are usually decades in length, with only partial sparing of the oldest memories (Hodges, 1995; Mayes, 1988). It seems implausible that any transfer process should last for decades, as this was probably longer than the average lifespan in prehistoric times. More plausibly, transfer, if it exists, might be expected to take weeks, months, or at most a year or so. Such a time scale for transfer is more compatible with what is estimated for animals (see, e.g., Bontempi, Laurent-Demir, Destrade, & Jaffard, 1999). There are patients who show normal memory for facts and episodes out to about a day following learning, who then proceed to forget abnormally fast over a period of weeks or months (see, e.g., Kapur et al., 1996). We have studied one such patient and found that despite usually showing normal memory out to delays of about 1 day, she forgets both factual and episodic memories that have apparently been acquired normally at a pathologically fast rate over the following weeks and months. As a result, she shows severely impaired recall even for information to which she must have been exposed many times over periods ranging from months to many years. This patient has an intact hippocampus, but major bilateral damage in the polar region of the temporal neocortex. It is not implausible to postulate that her initial consolidation of information in the hippocampus is normal, but that she cannot transfer storage to the temporal polar region because it is damaged. This patient and the great majority like her are epileptic, so an alternative interpretation needs to be considered (viz., memories are gradually disrupted by epileptic activity in storage sites).

If storage of episodic and semantic memories transfers in time from the medial temporal lobes to the posterior neocortex, then recalling or recognizing new memories should activate the hippocampus (and perhaps other parts of the medial temporal lobes) more than does recalling or recognizing much older and more practiced memories. It is not clear that neocortical activity for older memories should increase, because the neocortical representing regions should activate even when storage critically depends on the hippocampus. If there is no transfer, but repetition increases the proportion of hippocampal neurons involved in storage, either there should be no change or hippocampal activity should increase. Both Conway and colleagues (1999) and Ryan and colleagues (in press) have found no change in hippocampal activation when older memories were recalled. However, their younger memories ranged from nearly a year to about 4 years in age. We have found similar results in an fMRI study that compared recall of personally relevant routes learned weeks to months earlier and recall of routes well learned 30 years earlier. There was no change in medial temporal lobe activation, but activity did decrease in the left posterior cingulate cortex (Mayes et al., 2000). However, we have also compared recall of overlearned memories of word meanings, map locations, and personal episodic incidents that were acquired between 1 week and a few months prior to scanning with recall of old and very overlearned memories of the same kind. With these, we did find weak evidence that recalling more recently acquired memories did activate parts of the hippocampus more. But even recall of the old factual memories did activate the hippocampus and the parahippocampal cortex more than a low-level baseline. This finding indicates that care must be taken in interpreting the results of such experiments, because medial temporal lobe activation is perhaps being caused by re-encoding as well as retrieval, and the effects of re-encoding may differ depending on the age of the memory retrieved. Future work should try to control for this factor, as well as to compare more recently acquired memories with old, much-practiced memories.

We have extensively tested a patient, Y. R., who lost nearly 50% of her hippocampus in her mid-40s, but whose brain is otherwise fairly intact. On over 40 tests of item recognition, Y. R. performed at a mean level of 0.5 standard deviations below the mean of her control group. This level is slightly, but significantly, below the mean item recognition level of her control subjects. Whether this indicates that her brain damage has caused a very mild item recognition deficit or that her item recognition has not worsened following her damage, but has always been slightly below average, remains uncertain. In contrast to her only slightly below-average item recognition performance, on over 30 recall tests she performed markedly and significantly worse, averaging 3.5 standard deviations below the mean of her control group (see Mayes et al., in press). Y. R. showed an impairment of similar severity on certain tests of associative recognition, which compared studied complexes and foil complexes comprising recombined components. Thus she was impaired at recognizing associations between objects and locations, objects and their temporal order, faces and voices, pictures and sounds, words and their meanings, and animal pictures and occupation names (see, e.g., Mayes et al., 2001; Holdstock et al., in press).

Y. R.'s deficits on these associative recognition tests suggest that she has a particular problem with memory for associations between different kinds of information that are likely to be represented in distinct neocortical regions. As she has shown normal "know" responding levels when given the "remember–know" procedure, the overall pattern of her memory deficits suggests that she has intact familiarity, but impaired recollection and recall. Provided that familiarity memory and recollection/recall are stochastically independent of each other, one would expect her impaired recollection/recall to cause her item recognition to be slightly impaired, which is consistent with her overall item recognition performance. However, if there is a redundancy relationship between familiarity and recollection/recall, then her item recognition should probably be normal; as indicated above, this possibility cannot be ruled out, because her performance lies well within the range of normal variability and because information is lacking on her premorbid memory. Interestingly, Y. R. was also impaired at recalling factual information, whether she had been exposed to this information only briefly or whether she had been exposed to it repeatedly over a period of years. This strongly suggests that her recall deficit involves more than a problem with retrieving item–context associations, which could have been argued if it had been specific to episodic memory.

It is unclear how typical of hippocampal damage Y. R. is, and, relatedly, how good a guide she provides for the normal functions of the hippocampus. It could be that other hippocampal patients with more severe item recognition deficits have undetected damage to other structures that mediate item recognition in intact people. Alternatively, Y. R. could be mediating item recognition with atypical structures. This should be possible to determine by using functional neuroimaging to identify whether Y. R. or patients like her activate unusual brain regions when showing normal item recognition performance. There is, however, preliminary evidence that identifying item familiarity at recognition does not activate the hippocampus (Eldridge, Knowlton, Furmanski, Bookheimer, & Engel, 2000), which suggests that this structure does not normally play a role in this form of memory. The hippocampus is, however, clearly activated during recollection of items (Eldridge et al., 2000). In an event-related fMRI study, however, we have found a suggestion that encoding pictures that are later recognized as familiar is associated with some hippocampal activation, although less than that associated with the encoding of pictures that are later recollected (Montaldi et al., 2000). Unlike Eldridge and colleagues (2000) we did not measure recollection and familiarity in terms of subjects' responses in the remember–know procedure, but instead operationally defined these concepts in terms of whether subjects could or could not identify whether studied pictures had been seen earlier both in the scanner and prior to scanning or only in the scanner. These judgments were almost certainly based on what subjects could recollect from the encoding session in the scanner. This was because during encoding in the scanner, subjects were first asked whether they had seen the to-be-studied picture before and were then asked to thematically categorize it. Subjects were regarded as showing familiarity only if they recognized pictures as having been seen earlier, but did not recollect accurately whether or not they had thought it new or old in the scanner. Our results might mean either of two things: (1) Encoding that later produces only item familiarity still slightly involves the hippocampus; or (2) the subjects we categorized as showing only familiarity were actually recollecting information about the pictures, although this did not help them decide whether or not the pictures had been seen prior to scanning. Further work, using several different procedures to assess familiarity and recollection, is needed to resolve which of these possibilities is correct.

The results of a recent meta-analysis seem to support the possibility that the hippocampus is not involved in item familiarity at all. In this study, Baxter and Murray (2001b) argued that although hippocampal lesions do cause a mild item recognition impairment in monkeys, there is a negative correlation between the extent of hippocampal damage and item recognition deficit severity. Their conclusion is controversial, and more data are clearly desirable to determine whether their main conclusion is valid (Baxter & Murray, 2001a; Zola & Squire, 2001). Nevertheless, if it is correct, it could mean that residual hippocampus disrupts activity in neighboring structures concerned with familiarity memory (e.g., the perirhinal cortex) to a greater degree when there is more of it left, but that the hippocampus itself does not directly contribute to familiarity.

CONCLUSION

Important issues concerning the neural bases of episodic and semantic memory remain unresolved. Resolution will be greatly facilitated by the combined use of lesion and functional neuroimaging approaches. Above all, improved understanding is needed of how the posterior and frontal neocortical regions interact with the regions implicated in amnesia so as to generate the encoding, storage, and retrieval of memories for facts and episodes. Developing this understanding will depend critically on the mutually reinforcing use of lesion and functional neuroimaging approaches.

REFERENCES

Aggleton, J. P., & Brown, M. W. (1999). Episodic memory, amnesia, and the hippocampal–anterior thalamic axis. *Behavioral and Brain Sciences*, 22, 425–489.

Baxter, M. G., & Murray, E. A. (2001a). Effects of hippocampal lesions on delayed nonmatching-to-sample in monkeys: A reply to Zola and Squire. *Hippocampus*, 11, 201–203.

Baxter, M. G., & Murray, E. A. (2001b). Opposite relationship of hippocampal and rhinal cortex damage to delayed nonmatching-to-sample deficits in monkeys. *Hippocampus*, 11, 61–71.

Bechara, A., Tranel, D., & Damasio, H. (2000). Characterization of the decision-making deficit of patients with ventromedial prefrontal cortex lesions. *Brain*, 123, 2189–2202.

Bontempi, B., Laurent-Demir, C., Destrade, C., & Jaffard, R. (1999). Time-dependent reorganization of brain circuitry underlying long-term memory storage. *Nature*, 400, 671–675.

Buffalo, E. A., Reber, P. J., & Squire, L. R. (1998). The human perirhinal cortex and recognition memory. *Hippocampus*, 8, 330–339.

Burgess, P. W., Veitch, E., Costello, A., & Shallice, T. (2000). The cognitive and neuroanatomical correlates of multitasking. *Neuropsychologia*, 38, 848–863.

Chun, M. M., & Phelps, E. A. (1999). Memory deficits for implicit contextual information in amnesic subjects with hippocampal damage. *Nature Neuroscience*, 2, 844–847.

Conway, M. A., Turk, D. J., Miller, S. L., Logan, J., Nebes, R. D., Metzler, C. C. & Becker, J. T. (1999). A positron emission tomography (PET) study of autobiographical memory retrieval. *Memory*, 7, 679–702.

D'Esposito, M., Aguirre, G. K., Zarahn, E., Ballard, D., Shin, R., Lease, J., & Tang, J. (1998). Functional MRI studies of spatial and nonspatial working memory. *Cognitive Brain Research*, 7, 1–13.

D'Esposito, M., Detre, J. A., Alsop, D. C., Shin, R. K., Atlas, S., & Grossman, M. (1995). The neural basis of the central executive system of working memory. *Nature*, 378, 279–281.

Easton, A., & Gaffan, D. (2001). Crossed unilateral lesions of the medial forebrain bundle and either inferior temporal or frontal cortex impair object–reward association learning in rhesus monkeys. *Neuropsychologia*, 39, 71–82.

Eldridge, L. L., Knowlton, B. J., Furmanski, C. S., Bookheimer, S. Y., & Engel, S. A. (2000). Remembering episodes: A selective role for the hippocampus. *Nature Neuroscience*, 3, 1149–1152.

Fletcher, P. C., & Henson, R. N. A. (2001). Frontal lobes and human memory: Insights from functional neuroimaging. *Brain*, 124, 849–881.

Gaffan, D., & Hornak, J. (1997). Amnesia and neglect: Beyond the Delay–Brion system and the Hebb synapse. *Philosophical Transactions of the Royal Society of London, Series B*, 352, 1481–1488.

Gaffan, D., Parker, A., & Easton, A. (2001). Dense amnesia in the monkey after transection of fornix, amygdala and anterior temporal stem. *Neuropsychologia*, 39, 51–70.

Gooding, P. A., Mayes, A. R., & van Eijk, R. (2000). A meta-analysis of indirect memory tests for novel material in organic amnesics. *Neuropsychologia*, 38, 666–676.

Graf, P., & Schacter, D. L. (1985). Implicit and explicit memory for new associations in normal subjects and amnesic patients. *Journal of Experimental Psychology: Learning, Memory, and Cognition*, 11, 501–518.

Gray, J. A. (1982). *The neuropsychology of anxiety*. Oxford: Oxford University Press.

Hodges, J. R. (1995). Retrograde amnesia. In A. D. Baddeley, B. A. Wilson, & F. N. Watts (Eds.), *Handbook of memory disorders* (pp. 81–107). Chichester, England: Wiley.

Holdstock, J. S., Mayes, A. R., Roberts, N., Isaac, C. L., Cezayirli, E., O'Reilly, R. C., & Norman, K. A. (in press). Under what conditions is recognition spared relative to recall following selective hippocampal damage in humans? *Hippocampus*.

Jacoby, L. L., Kelley, C. M., & Dywan, J. (1989). Memory attributions. In H. L. Roediger & F. I. M. Craik (Eds.), *Varieties of memory and consciousness: Essays in honour of Endel Tulving* (pp. 391–422). Hillsdale, NJ: Erlbaum.

Kapur, N., Scholey, K., Moore, E., Barker, S., Brice, S., Thompson, S., Shiel, A., Carn, R., Abbott, P., & Fleming, J. (1996). Long-term retention deficits in two cases of disproportionate retrograde amnesia. *Journal of Cognitive Neuroscience, 8,* 416–434.

Mayes, A. R. (1988). *Human organic memory disorders.* Cambridge, England: Cambridge University Press.

Mayes, A. R. (2001). Aware and unaware memory. Does unaware memory underlie aware memory? In D. McCormack & C. Hoerl (Eds.), *Time and memory: Issues in philosophy and psychology* (pp. 187–212). Oxford: Oxford University Press.

Mayes, A. R., Downes, J. J., Shoqeirat, M., Hall, C., & Sagar, H. J. (1993). Encoding ability is preserved in amnesia. *Neuropsychologia, 31,* 745–759.

Mayes, A. R., Holdstock, J. S., Isaac, C. L., Hunkin, N. M., & Roberts, N. (in press). Relative sparing of item recognition in a patient with adult-onset damage limited to the hippocampus. *Hippocampus.*

Mayes, A. R., Isaac, C. L., Downes, J. J., Holdstock, J. S., Hunkin, N. M., Montaldi, D., MacDonald, C., Cezayirli, E., & Roberts, J. N. (2001). Memory for single items, word pairs, and temporal order of different kinds in a patient with selective hippocampal lesions. *Cognitive Neuropsychology, 18,* 97–123.

Mayes, A. R., Mackay, C. E., Montaldi, D., Downes, J. J., Singh, K. D., & Roberts, N. (2000). Does retrieving decades-old spatial memories activate the medial temporal lobes less than retrieving recently acquired spatial memories? *NeuroImage, 11,* S421.

Mayes, A. R., & Montaldi, D. (1999). The neuroimaging of long-term memory encoding processes. *Memory, 7,* 613–660.

Milner, P. (1999). *The autonomous brain.* Mahwah, NJ: Erlbaum.

Montaldi, D., Mayes, A. R., MacKay, C. E., Singh, K. D., Hankin, N. M., Spencer, T. J., & Roberts, N. M. (2000). Differential activational effects of novelty detection and of associative encoding of pictures producing familiarity or recollection memory: An event-related fMRI study. *NeuroImage, 11,* S423.

Morris, R. G. M., & Frey, U. (1997). Hippocampal synaptic plasticity: Role in spatial learning or the automatic recording of attended experience? *Philosophical Transactions of the Royal Society of London, Series B, 352,* 1489–1503.

Moscovitch, M. (1995). Recovered consciousness: A hypothesis concerning modularity and episodic memory. *Journal of Clinical and Experimental Neuropsychology, 17,* 276–290.

Murray, E. A., & Bussey, T. J. (1999). Perceptual–mnemonic functions of the perirhinal cortex. *Trends in Cognitive Sciences, 3,* 142–151.

Nadel, L., & Moscovitch, M. (1997). Memory consolidation and the hippocampal complex. *Current Opinion in Neurobiology, 7,* 217–227.

Patterson, K., & Hodges, J. R. (1995). Disorders of semantic memory. In A. D. Baddeley, B. A. Wilson, & F. N. Watts (Eds.), *Handbook of memory disorders* (pp. 167–186). Chichester, England: Wiley.

Petrides, M. (2000). Frontal lobes and memory. In F. Boller & J. Grafman (Eds.), *Handbook of neuropsychology* (2nd ed., Vol. 2, pp. 67–84). Amsterdam: Elsevier.

Reed, J. M., & Squire, L. R. (1997). Impaired recognition memory in patients with lesions limited to the hippocampal formation. *Behavioral Neuroscience, 111,* 667–675.

Ryan, L, Nadel, L., Keil, K., Putnam, K., Schnyer, D., Troward, T., & Moscovitch, M. (in press). The hippocampal complex and retrieval of recent and very remote autobiographical memories: Evidenced from functional magnetic resonance imaging in neurologically intact people. *Hippocampus.*

Schacter, D. L., & Buckner, R. L. (1998). Priming and brain. *Neuron, 20,* 185–195.

Squire, L. R. (1992). Memory and the hippocampus: A synthesis from findings with rats, monkeys, and humans. *Psychological Review, 99,* 195–231.

Squire, L. R., & Alvarez, P. (1995). Retrograde amnesia and memory consolidation: A neurobiological perspective. *Current Opinion in Neurobiology, 5,* 169–177.

Stuss, D. T., Gallup, G. G., & Alexander, M. P. (2001). The frontal lobes are necessary for 'theory of mind.' *Brain, 124,* 279–286.

Stuss, D. T., Levine, B., Alexander, M. P., Hong, J., Palumbo, C., Hamer, L., Murphy, K. J., & Izukawa, D. (2000). Wisconsin Card Sorting Test performance in patients with focal frontal and posterior brain damage: Effects of lesion location and test structure on separable cognitive processes. *Neuropsychologia, 38,* 388–402.

Teyler, T. J., & DiScenna, P. (1986). Long-term potentiation. *Annual Review of Neuroscience, 10,* 131–161.

Tulving, E. (1998). Neurocognitive processes of human memory. In C. von Euler, I. Lundberg, & R. Llinas (Eds.), *Basic mechanisms in cognition and language* (pp. 261–281). Amsterdam: Elsevier.

Vargha-Khadem, F., Gadian, D. G., Watkins, K. E., Connelly, A., Van Paesschen, W., & Mishkin, M. (1997). Differential effects of early hippocampal pathology on episodic and semantic memory. *Science, 277,* 376–380.

Virley, D., Ridley, R. M., Sinden, J. D., Kershaw, T. R., Harland, S., Rashid, T., French, S., Sowinski, P., Gray, J. A., Lantos, P. L., & Hodges, H. (1999). Primary CA1 and conditionally immortal MHP36 cell grafts restore conditional discrimination learning and recall in marmosets after excitotoxic lesions of the hippocampal CA1 field. *Brain, 122,* 2321–2335.

Wiggs, C. L., & Martin, A. (1998). Properties and mechanisms of perceptual priming. *Current Opinion in Neurobiology, 8,* 227–233.

Zola, S. M., & Squire, L. R. (2001). Relationship between magnitude of damage to the hippocampus and impaired recognition memory in monkeys. *Hippocampus, 11,* 92–98.

3

Impaired and Preserved Memory Processes in Amnesia

MIEKE VERFAELLIE and MARGARET M. KEANE

After two decades of intensive research on the dissociation between implicit and explicit memory in amnesia, it has become clear that implicit memory tasks do not invariably elicit normal priming in amnesia (Moscovitch, Vriezen, & Gottstein, 1993; Schacter, Chiu, & Ochsner, 1993; Verfaellie & Keane, 2001), and that explicit memory tasks do not elicit uniformly impaired performance (Verfaellie & Treadwell, 1993; Yonelinas, Kroll, Dobbins, Lazzara, & Knight, 1998). For this reason, our approach to the study of amnesia has been to focus on the processes underlying task performance, including processes that may be common to implicit and explicit memory tasks. Our goals in doing so are to better characterize the scope and boundaries of spared and impaired memory in amnesia, and to elucidate the component processes that mediate memory performance in normal cognition. In this chapter, we illustrate this approach and summarize some of our main findings concerning explicit and implicit task performance in amnesia.

ANALYSIS OF COMPONENT PROCESSES CONTRIBUTING TO PERFORMANCE ON EXPLICIT MEMORY TASKS IN AMNESIA

Our characterization of amnesic patients' explicit memory performance has been guided by dual-process models of recognition, which postulate two separate bases for recognition performance: recollection and familiarity (Gardiner, 1988; Jacoby, 1991; Mandler, 1980). "Recollection" refers to a conscious, effortful process in which prior aspects of an experience are retrieved. "Familiarity" is thought to be a subjective feeling that arises when fluent processing of a stimulus is attributed to prior experience with that stimulus. Because amnesic patients' recognition memory can sometimes be surprisingly good (see, e.g., Bowers, Verfaellie, Valenstein, & Heilman, 1988; Johnson & Kim, 1985), we examined whether amnesia might be associated with a relative sparing of familiarity-based recognition.

In one study, we used the process dissociation approach to tease apart the contribution of familiarity and recollection to recognition memory (Verfaellie & Treadwell, 1993).

Subjects performed either an inclusion task in which they endorsed items seen in a first study phase or heard in a second study phase, or an exclusion task in which they endorsed only items seen in the first phase. By comparing performance across these two conditions, we obtained independent estimates of recollection and familiarity. Amnesic patients were severely impaired in recollection. Our initial analysis led us to conclude that familiarity-based recognition was normal in amnesia, but this analysis failed to take into account the fact that amnesic patients endorse more nonstudied words than controls (Verfaellie, 1994). If we take into account this difference in baseline familiarity, a reduction in familiarity-based recognition also becomes apparent in amnesia; importantly, however, this loss is considerably smaller than is the corresponding loss in recollection. Yonelinas and colleagues (1998) considered these data and results from the "remember–know" paradigm (Knowlton & Squire, 1995; Schacter, Verfaellie, & Pradere, 1996), together with new analyses of receiver operating characteristic curves in amnesia. They concluded that all three approaches converge on the notion that the deficit in familiarity in amnesia is less pronounced than the deficit in recollection.

To assess directly whether amnesic patients use perceptual fluency as a basis for familiarity judgments, we performed two experiments (Verfaellie & Cermak, 1999). During the test phase, subjects identified stimuli as they gradually came into view and then made recognition judgments. We reasoned that if subjects used perceptual fluency as a basis of responding, "old" responses should vary as a function of the ease of stimulus identification. In a first experiment, we eliminated the potential contribution of recollection to performance by using a mock subliminal procedure in the study phase. Participants were told that words would be presented very briefly, but in reality no words were presented. Under these conditions, both amnesic patients and controls based their recognition judgments on the fluency with which words were processed. They endorsed as "old" more words that were easy to identify than words that were hard to identify. In a second experiment, words were presented in a study list, so that actual recollection of studied words could also serve as a basis for recognition. Under these conditions, amnesic patients were still influenced by the perceptual fluency of items, but nonamnesic subjects were not. These findings suggest that amnesic patients use a fluency heuristic as a default strategy. Control subjects, in contrast, use this strategy only when no information is available to support recollection.

It is important to point out that in Experiment 2 of the just-described study, effects of perceptual fluency were evident not only in amnesic patients' responses to studied words, but also in their responses to nonstudied words (for similar effects of conceptual fluency, see Rajaram & Geraci, 2000; Whittlesea, 1993). Some have interpreted this as a bias pattern, and have argued therefore that fluency is not the basis of recognition familiarity (e.g., Stark & Squire, 2000). However, this is the pattern we expected: The use of a clarification procedure in this particular paradigm made natural (extraexperimental) variations in fluency salient for both studied and unstudied words in the test phase. We would argue that regardless of its source, fluency of processing gives rise to a sense of familiarity that serves as a basis for recognition performance.

By having subjects perform a perceptual identification task prior to recognition, we exploited differences in perceptual fluency as a source of familiarity. However, in typical recognition tasks in which stimuli are presented in clear view, differences in perceptual fluency may be much less notable, and familiarity may be based largely on the *conceptual* fluency with which stimuli are processed. This reliance on conceptual fluency may explain why familiarity in standard recognition tasks has been dissociated from the processes that mediate perceptual priming (Stark & Squire, 2000; Wagner & Gabrieli, 1998; Wagner, Gabrieli, & Verfaellie, 1997). Importantly, consistent with the emphasis on conceptual fluency as the basis of familiarity, there is no evidence for a dissociation between familiarity-based recognition and conceptual priming.

Implications for Comparing Performance on Recall and Recognition Tasks

Our analysis so far has revealed that amnesic patients have a disproportionate disruption in recollection. But, of note, such a disruption has different consequences for performance on recall and recognition tasks. Whereas familiarity-based processes can serve as a basis for amnesic patients' recognition performance, these processes are largely ineffective in recall tasks, as recall depends primarily on conscious recollection of contextually appropriate information. It follows, therefore, that although both recall and recognition are impaired in amnesia, amnesic patients' recall should be more severely disrupted than their recognition.

Although this prediction appears straightforward, it is difficult to test, because there is no direct way to compare the magnitude of impairment in recall and recognition tasks. Performance across tasks can only be compared indirectly by creating conditions in which recognition memory is equated between an amnesic group and a control group, and then examining whether recall performance is still impaired in the amnesic group. Recognition performance has been equated either by giving amnesic patients additional study time (Hirst et al., 1986; Hirst, Johnson, Phelps, & Volpe, 1988, Exp. 2; Kopelman & Stanhope, 1998) or by testing control subjects at a delay (Haist, Shimamura, & Squire, 1992; Hirst et al., 1988, Exp. 1; Shimamura & Squire, 1988). Perhaps indicative of the complexities inherent in this approach, the results of such studies have been contradictory. Some have reported that when recognition performance was equated between amnesic patients and controls, the patients' recall remained impaired (Hirst et al., 1986, 1988). Others have found that once recognition memory was matched across groups, recall was similar across groups as well (Haist et al., 1992; Kopelman & Stanhope, 1998; MacAndrew, Jones, & Mayes, 1994; Shimamura & Squire, 1988).

In a recent study (Giovanello & Verfaellie, in press), we provided evidence that these contradictory outcomes are attributable at least in part to the different ways in which recognition memory has been equated across groups. In one experiment, both amnesic patients and controls were tested after the same delay, but amnesic patients were given additional study exposures. We hypothesized that even in the face of additional study exposures, the patients' recognition would still be mediated primarily by familiarity—in contrast to that of controls, which would be mediated by recollection as well as by familiarity. This hypothesis was based on a prior study, which demonstrated that additional presentations did not enhance recollection in amnesia in a stem completion task (Cermak, Verfaellie, Sweeney, & Jacoby, 1992). Consistent with our hypothesis, amnesic patients' recall remained impaired, even when recognition was equated (Table 3.1). In a second experiment, recognition memory was equated by giving the amnesic and control groups equal study exposure, but by testing controls after a delay. Because recollection declines more rapidly than does familiarity across a delay (Gardiner & Java, 1991; Hockley & Consoli, 1999; Tulving, 1985), we reasoned that the performance of controls would be mediated mainly by familiarity—as is that of amnesic patients. In accord with this analysis, recall was equivalent across groups under these equating conditions (Table 3.1).

This study highlights the importance of analyzing the performance of control subjects and amnesic patients in terms of underlying processes. When this was done, two appar-

TABLE 3.1. Mean Recall and Recognition Scores for Amnesic Patients and Controls as a Function of Method of Equating Recognition Performance

| | Method of equating | | | |
| | Amnesic patients given additional study | | Controls tested after delay | |
Group	Recall	Recognition	Recall	Recognition
Amnesic	0.12	0.89	0.08	0.76
Control	0.19	0.89	0.11	0.79

Note. Data from Giovanello and Verfaellie (in press).

ently contradictory patterns of performance could both be explained with reference to the notion that amnesic patients have a disproportionate deficit in recollection.

Enhancing the Contribution of Familiarity to Explicit Memory Performance

If amnesic patients have a relative preservation of familiarity-based recognition, the question arises as to whether conditions can be created that enhance patients' reliance on familiarity, thus boosting their recognition performance. We recently explored this possibility by manipulating patients' response criterion in a recognition task (Verfaellie, Giovanello, & Keane, 2001). Our interest in this manipulation arose from a study that compared the performance of patients with ECT-induced amnesia in a high-criterion and a low-criterion condition (Dorfman, Kihlstrom, Cork, & Misiaszek, 1995). In the high-criterion test, patients were encouraged to say yes to a test word only if they were relatively sure it had appeared on the study list. In the low-criterion test, they were told to endorse a test word if it seemed at all familiar. Patients performed significantly better in the low- than in the high-criterion condition—a finding that was attributed to their enhanced reliance on familiarity.

Using a similar manipulation in patients with global amnesia, we did not find that changes in response criterion affected the patients' recognition accuracy (see also Reber & Squire, 1999). However, this manipulation was generally weak, as it failed to induce a shift in response criterion in normal individuals. In a further experiment, response criterion was manipulated indirectly, by giving participants varying information about the alleged proportion of study items in the recognition test (30% vs. 70%). This manipulation was successful: Control subjects showed a shift in response bias, endorsing more items (both studied and nonstudied) in the 70% than in the 30% condition. Critically, in the amnesic group, this manipulation led to enhanced recognition discriminability (Table 3.2). Furthermore, analysis of patients' "remember" and "know" responses indicated that their enhanced discriminability arose from a selective increase in familiarity-based responding. It appears, therefore, that encouraging amnesic patients to rely on their feelings of familiarity can boost their performance.

At present, it remains unclear which manipulations can increase amnesic patients' familiarity-based responding in a recognition memory task. For example, Stark and Squire (2000) used a response deadline to encourage the use of familiarity. They found no evidence to suggest that this manipulation yielded enhanced recognition in four amnesic patients. Further study will be needed to characterize the conditions that can strengthen the contribution of familiarity to amnesic patients' recognition performance.

TABLE 3.2. Proportion of Studied and Unstudied Words Endorsed as Old and d' Scores in the 30% and 70% Criterion Conditions

Group	Studied		Unstudied		d'	
	30%	70%	30%	70%	30%	70%
Amnesic	0.47	0.66	0.24	0.28	0.72	1.02
Control	0.67	0.78	0.05	0.15	2.33	2.14

Note. Data from Verfaellie, Giovanello, and Keane (2001).

ANALYSIS OF PERFORMANCE ON IMPLICIT MEMORY TASKS IN AMNESIA

Scope and Limits of Preserved Priming in Amnesia

Within the domain of implicit memory, it is well established that amnesic patients show normal performance on a wide range of tasks that measure priming for single, familiar items (e.g., words or pictures; Moscovitch et al., 1993; Schacter et al., 1993). It is less clear, however, whether and under what conditions amnesic patients show normal priming for novel associations between normatively unrelated items. The status of such "new-associative" priming effects in amnesia is of particular interest because of its relevance to theories that assign to the hippocampus a critical role in computing arbitrary links between previously unrelated stimuli (Cohen, Poldrack, & Eichenbaum, 1997), and to theories that characterize the core deficit in amnesia as one of binding unrelated pieces of information (Johnson & Chalfonte, 1994; Kroll, Knight, Metcalfe, Wolf, & Tulving, 1996).

We addressed this issue by examining new-associative priming in amnesia in a perceptual identification task (Gabrieli, Keane, Zarella, & Poldrack, 1997), which was modeled on a paradigm first introduced by Graf and Schacter (1985). In the study phase, subjects were asked to read aloud pairs of unrelated words (e.g., "blame–cabin," "storm–merit"). In the test phase, they were asked to identify old word pairs (e.g., "blame–cabin"), recombined word pairs (e.g., "blame–merit"), and new word pairs (e.g., "glory–chart") presented at threshold durations. New-associative priming was reflected by higher identification accuracy for old compared to recombined word pairs. This effect was significant and equivalent in normal and amnesic subjects (Gabrieli et al., 1997), demonstrating that spared priming in amnesia extends to novel word associations.

A similar conclusion was reached by Goshen-Gottstein, Moscovitch, and Melo (2000), who found that amnesic patients showed normal new-associative priming in a lexical decision task. In their study, amnesic patients, like normal subjects, made faster and more accurate lexical decisions to old than to recombined word pairs. Parallel studies in normal cognition suggested that this new-associative priming effect was perceptually based: It was reduced by a study-to-test change in perceptual modality (Goshen-Gottstein & Moscovitch, 1995a), but was unaffected by a level-of-processing manipulation (Goshen-Gottstein & Moscovitch, 1995b).

Not all studies, however, have yielded evidence of implicit memory for new associations in amnesia. Several investigators have reported impaired new-associative priming in a word stem completion task (Cermak, Bleich, & Blackford, 1988; Mayes & Gooding, 1989; Schacter & Graf, 1986b; Shimamura & Squire, 1989). Importantly, however, new-associative priming in stem completion appears to depend upon elaboration of a meaningful link between the words in each pair during the study phase (Schacter & Graf, 1986a), and so may require the establishment of a new *conceptual* association between the words. We hypothesize that the impairment in amnesia is linked to this requirement, and that new-associative priming may be spared in amnesia on tasks that depend upon novel *perceptual* associations (Verfaellie & Keane, 2001).

Interestingly, Paller and Mayes (1994) found that amnesic patients showed impaired new-associative priming in a perceptual identification task in which the words in each pair were presented simultaneously in the study phase but sequentially in the test phase (rather than simultaneously in both phases, as in Gabrieli et al., 1997). Because a change in word pair presentation format from the study to the test phase is likely to disrupt priming of perceptually based associations established in the study phase, the new-associative priming effect in the Paller and Mayes (1994) paradigm may have been based on higher-order (e.g., conceptual) associations between the words in each pair.

Thus, although the evidence is still somewhat limited, the emerging pattern is consistent with the hypothesis that new-associative priming in amnesia is normal for perceptually based associations, but impaired for conceptually based associations (however, see Musen & Squire, 1993). We are currently pursuing this issue in our laboratory by examining priming for new conceptual associations in a broader range of paradigms.

Priming Effects in Amnesia: Implications for Normal Cognition

Evidence about spared and impaired priming effects in amnesia speaks not only to theories about the functions and structures disrupted in amnesia, but also to theories about the cognitive mechanisms underlying implicit memory phenomena in normal cognition. In considering such evidence, we make the assumption that because amnesic patients show normal single-item priming across a wide range of paradigms, task modifications that lead to impaired priming in amnesia likely do so because they induce explicit memory strategies in normal subjects. We have used this reasoning to examine a proposal from Ratcliff and McKoon (1995, 1996, 1997) that priming effects in normal cognition in word and object identification tasks depend upon the operation of a bias mechanism that induces costs as well as benefits in task performance. By this account, recent exposure to stimuli does not increase the efficiency, accuracy, or sensitivity of perceptual identification processes associated with those stimuli (as many theories of priming have assumed); rather, it biases perceptual identification processes toward those stimuli. Thus, according to the bias account, exposure to a word (e.g., "relay") in the study phase of a priming task induces a bias that will enhance subsequent identification of that word, but will harm subsequent identification of orthographically similar words (e.g., "relax"). Ratcliff, McKoon, and their colleagues have provided a wealth of evidence that such costs and benefits are reliably obtained in normal cognition, consistent with the predictions of a bias theory (Ratcliff & McKoon, 1997; Ratcliff, McKoon, & Verwoerd, 1989).

There has been some debate, however, about the extent to which these findings in normal cognition reflect the contribution of explicit rather than implicit memory processes (Light & Kennison, 1996; Schacter & Cooper, 1995). To address this question, we (Keane, Verfaellie, Gabrieli, & Wong, 2000) examined the performance of amnesic patients in the forced-choice perceptual identification paradigm that produced much of the evidence favoring a bias account of priming effects in normal cognition (Ratcliff & McKoon, 1997; Ratcliff et al., 1989). The forced-choice procedure in this paradigm represented a modification of the "standard" perceptual identification task that had previously elicited normal priming in amnesia (Cermak, Talbot, Chandler, & Wolbarst, 1985; Haist, Musen, & Squire, 1991).

The critical stimuli in this experiment were pairs of orthographically similar words (e.g., "relax–relay," "salt–sale"). In the study phase, subjects were exposed to a series of words, including one or neither of the words from each pair. On each trial in the subsequent test phase, a word was flashed briefly on a computer screen and followed by two response alternatives, consisting of the just-flashed word and its orthographic "mate." Subjects were asked to select the choice that matched the just-flashed word. In the "old" condition, the flashed word was identical to a word that had appeared in the study list. In the "lure" condition, the flashed word was the orthographic mate of a word that had appeared in the study list. In the "new" condition, neither the flashed word nor its mate had appeared in the prior study list. Consistent with Ratcliff and McKoon's (1997) results, the control subjects in our experiment identified old words more accurately than new words (a performance benefit), and lure words less accurately than new words (a performance cost). By contrast, the amnesic patients showed the performance benefit, but not the performance cost, in this paradigm. These findings were consistent with the notion that the bias pattern in normal subjects reflected the operation of explicit memory processes that are impaired in amnesia. The performance of amnesic patients in this paradigm (benefits without costs) appeared to be better explained by a sensitivity mechanism.

In a subsequent experiment, we examined costs and benefits in amnesia in a standard perceptual identification task (Keane et al., 2000). We found that the performance benefit in this paradigm (higher accuracy for old compared to new words) was significant and equivalent in amnesic and control subjects. Although there was no cost in terms of accuracy, there was a cost in terms of the proportion of "intrusions" generated in the lure condition compared to the new condition, consistent with Ratcliff and McKoon (1997). That is to say, when subjects misidentified a word, their incorrect response was more likely to be the mate of the flashed word when that mate had appeared in the prior study list than when it had not. This cost was equivalent in normal and amnesic subjects in our experiment. Thus the bias pattern (i.e., benefits coupled with costs) observed in normal subjects in this paradigm does not appear to depend upon explicit memory processes. Together, the findings from these two studies suggest that bias patterns in the forced-choice perceptual identification paradigm depend upon explicit memory processes that are impaired in amnesia, but that bias patterns in the standard paradigm reflect the operation of implicit memory processes that are intact in amnesia.

We have also examined the performance of amnesic patients to address questions about the potential role of explicit memory processes in a different context—namely, that of word stem completion priming. In particular, it has been suggested that cross-modal stem completion priming may reflect contamination by explicit retrieval mechanisms (Jacoby, Toth, & Yonelinas, 1993). Work from Richardson-Klavehn and Gardiner (1996) has clarified this issue, demonstrating that cross-modal stem completion priming reflects *involuntary* (rather than voluntary) retrieval. However, this involuntary retrieval is associated with memorial awareness of the fact that primed completions correspond to previously studied words. One question left unanswered by these findings was whether such conscious memorial awareness plays a causal role in cross-modal stem completion priming (Richardson-Klavehn & Gardiner, 1996; Richardson-Klavehn, Gardiner, & Java, 1994).

In order to address this question, we examined awareness in within- and cross-modality word stem completion in amnesic subjects (Verfaellie, Keane, & Cook, in press). In a study phase, words were presented visually or auditorily; in the subsequent test phase, word stems corresponding to studied and unstudied words were presented visually, and subjects were asked to complete each one with the first word that came to mind. At the conclusion of this task, subjects were asked to circle the completions that they believed had appeared in the prior study phase. Consistent with prior reports (e.g., Graf, Shimamura, & Squire, 1985), we found that priming was greater in the within-modality condition than in the cross-modality condition, and that priming was normal in amnesia both within and across modalities. As expected, normal subjects recognized more of the primed completions as having appeared in the study list than did amnesic patients. Consistent with Richardson-Klavehn and Gardiner (1996), we found that in normal subjects, cross-modal priming was always associated with conscious awareness. By contrast, in amnesic subjects, there was significant cross-modal priming that was not associated with conscious awareness. Thus, although conscious memorial awareness may be associated with cross-modal priming in normal subjects, the data from amnesic patients indicate that it is not a necessary feature of normal cross-modal priming.

Neuroimaging studies have also examined the mechanisms underlying cross-modal priming, and have reopened the possibility that voluntary explicit retrieval mechanisms contribute to the effect. In particular, Schacter, Badgayian, and Alpert (Badgaiyan, Schacter, & Alpert, 2001; Schacter, Badgaiyan, & Alpert, 1999) found that cross-modal stem completion priming in normal subjects was associated with increased activation in right prefrontal cortex. Because this brain region has been implicated in voluntary explicit retrieval (see, e.g., Kapur et al., 1995; Wagner, Desmond, Glover, & Gabrieli, 1998), this finding raised the possibility that such retrieval mechanisms played a key role in the cross-modal priming effect. This possibility appears inconsistent with our finding of normal cross-modal priming in amnesia. However, the method used in the imaging experiments differed from that used in our study. In the imaging study the primed and unprimed stimuli were presented in separate blocks, whereas in our study they were intermixed. In order to address the possibility that the blocked design induced voluntary explicit retrieval in normal subjects, we (Verfaellie et al., in press) administered a blocked version of the paradigm to amnesic and control subjects. Under these conditions, we found normal within-modality priming, but impaired cross-modality priming in amnesia. We interpreted this finding to indicate that the blocked format used in imaging studies induced voluntary retrieval strategies. It should be noted, however, that Badgaiyan and colleagues (2001) have suggested that performance in the imaging studies was associated with involuntary, rather than voluntary, retrieval mechanisms. It is unclear how their interpretation can accommodate our findings in amnesia, unless one assumes that different mechanisms operate in normal individuals and in amnesic patients (Schacter & Badgaiyan, 2001). Further research will be needed to resolve this issue. Nonetheless, our findings of normal cross-modal priming in amnesia in a mixed condition, coupled with impaired cross-modal priming in a blocked condition, suggest that explicit retrieval mechanisms are not necessary for cross-modal priming, but may be recruited under certain conditions.

CONCLUSIONS

Our studies of memory have provided new insights regarding the mechanisms mediating memory performance in amnesia and in normal cognition. At the same time, this work raises further questions about the relationship among the memory processes under investigation. For example, the phenomenon of involuntary conscious memory, which has come to light in the context of behavioral as well as neuroimaging studies, is not yet fully understood. It is intriguing to consider the possible commonality between the memorial awareness that arises involuntarily and the feeling of familiarity that is often experienced in the context of explicit memory tasks. Studies of amnesia may provide fruitful ground to explore the link between these phenomena. More generally, because amnesia lays bare the fault lines among memory processes that operate seamlessly in normal cognition, future studies of amnesic patients may contribute uniquely to our understanding of interactions among memory processes.

ACKNOWLEDGMENTS

Preparation of this chapter was supported by National Institute of Neurological Disorders and Stroke Program Project Grant No. NS26985 and National Institute of Mental Health Grant No. MH57681 to Boston University, and by the Medical Research Service of the VA Healthcare System.

REFERENCES

Badgaiyan, R. D., Schacter, D. L., & Alpert, N. M. (2001). Priming within and across modalities: Exploring the nature of rCBF increases and decreases. *NeuroImage, 13*, 272–282.

Bowers, D., Verfaellie, M., Valenstein, E., & Heilman, K. M. (1988). Impaired acquisition of temporal information in retrosplenial amnesia. *Brain and Cognition, 8*, 47–66.

Cermak, L. S., Bleich, R. P., & Blackford, S. P. (1988). Deficits in the implicit retention of new associations by alcoholic Korsakoff patients. *Brain and Cognition, 7*, 312–323.

Cermak, L. S., Talbot, N., Chandler, K., & Wolbarst, L. R. (1985). The perceptual priming phenomenon in amnesia. *Neuropsychologia, 23*, 615–622.

Cermak, L. S., Verfaellie, M., Sweeney, M., & Jacoby, L. L. (1992). Fluency versus conscious recollection in the word completion performance of amnesic patients. *Brain and Cognition, 20*, 367–377.

Cohen, N. J., Poldrack, R. A., & Eichenbaum, H. (1997). Memory for items and memory for relations in the procedural/declarative memory framework. *Memory, 5*, 131–178.

Dorfman, J., Kihlstrom, J. F., Cork, R. C., & Misiaszek, J. (1995). Priming and recognition in ECT-induced amnesia. *Psychonomic Bulletin and Review, 5*, 244–248.

Gabrieli, J. D. E., Keane, M. M., Zarella, M., & Poldrack, R. A. (1997). Preservation of implicit memory for new associations in global amnesia. *Psychological Science, 8*, 326–329.

Gardiner, J. M. (1988). Functional aspects of recollective experience. *Memory and Cognition, 16*, 309–313.

Gardiner, J. M., & Java, R. J. (1991). Forgetting in recognition memory with and without recollective experience. *Memory and Cognition, 19*, 617–623.

Giovanello, K. S., & Verfaellie, M. (2001). The relationship between recall and recognition in amnesia: Effects of matching recognition between amnesics and controls. *Neuropsychology, 15*, 444–451.

Goshen-Gottstein, Y., & Moscovitch, M. (1995a). Repetition priming for newly formed and preexisting associations: Perceptual and conceptual influences. *Journal of Experimental Psychology: Learning, Memory, and Cognition, 21*, 1229–1248.

Goshen-Gottstein, Y., & Moscovitch, M. (1995b). Repetition priming for newly formed associations are perceptually based: Evidence from shallow encoding and format specificity. *Journal of Experimental Psychology: Learning, Memory, and Cognition, 21*, 1249–1262.

Goshen-Gottstein, Y., Moscovitch, M., & Melo, B. (2000). Intact implicit memory for newly formed verbal associations in amnesic patients following single study trials. *Neuropsychology, 14*, 570–578.

Graf, P., & Schacter, D. L. (1985). Implicit and explicit memory for new associations in normal and amnesic subjects. *Journal of Experimental Psychology: Learning, Memory, and Cognition, 11*, 501–518.

Graf, P., Shimamura, A. P., & Squire, L. R. (1985). Priming across modalities and across category levels: Extending the domain of preserved function in amnesia. *Journal of Experimental Psychology: Learning, Memory, and Cognition, 11*, 385–395.

Haist, F., Musen, G., & Squire, L. (1991). Intact priming of words and nonwords in amnesia. *Psychobiology, 19*, 273–285.

Haist, F., Shimamura, A. P., & Squire, L. R. (1992). On the relationship between recall and recognition memory. *Journal of Experimental Psychology: Learning, Memory, and Cognition, 18*, 691–702.

Hirst, W., Johnson, M. K., Kim, J. K., Phelps, E. A., Risse, G., & Volpe, B. T. (1986). Recognition and recall in amnesics. *Journal of Experimental Psychology: Learning, Memory, and Cognition, 12*, 445–451.

Hirst, W., Johnson, M. K., Phelps, A. E., & Volpe, B. T. (1988). More on recognition and recall in amnesics. *Journal of Experimental Psychology: Learning, Memory, and Cognition, 14*, 758–762.

Hockley, W. A., & Consoli, A. (1999). Familiarity and recollection in item and associative recognition. *Memory and Cognition, 27*, 657–664.

Jacoby, L. L. (1991). A process dissociation framework: Separating automatic from intentional uses of memory. *Journal of Memory and Language, 30*, 513–541.

Jacoby, L. L., Toth, J. P., & Yonelinas, A. P. (1993). Separating conscious and unconscious influences of memory: Measuring recollection. *Journal of Experimental Psychology: General, 122*, 139–154.

Johnson, M. K., & Chalfonte, B. L. (1994). Binding complex memories: The role of reactivation and the hippocampus. In D. L. Schacter & E. Tulving (Eds.), *Memory systems 1994* (pp. 311–350). Cambridge, MA: MIT Press.

Johnson, M. K., & Kim, J. K. (1985). Recognition of pictures by alcoholic Korsakoff patients. *Bulletin of the Psychonomic Society, 23*, 456–458.

Kapur, S., Craik, F. I. M., Jones, C., Brown, G. M., Houle, S., & Tulving, E. (1995). Functional role of the prefrontal cortex in retrieval of memories: A PET study. *NeuroReport, 6*, 1880–1884.

Keane, M. M., Verfaellie, M., Gabrieli, J. D. E., & Wong, B. M. (2000). Bias effects in perceptual identification: A neuropsychological investigation of the role of explicit memory. *Journal of Memory and Language, 43*, 316–334.

Knowlton, B., & Squire, L. (1995). Remembering and knowing: Two different expressions of declarative memory. *Journal of Experimental Psychology: Learning, Memory, and Cognition, 21*, 699–710.

Kopelman, M. D., & Stanhope, N. (1998). Recall and recognition memory in patients with focal frontal, temporal lobe and diencephalic lesions. *Neuropsychologia, 36*, 785–796.

Kroll, N. E. A., Knight, R. T., Metcalfe, J., Wolf, E. S., & Tulving, E. (1996). Conjunction failure as a source of memory illusions. *Journal of Memory and Language, 35*, 176–196.

Light, L. L., & Kennison, R. F. (1996). Guessing strategies, aging, and bias effects in perceptual identification. *Consciousness and Cognition, 5*, 463–499.

MacAndrew, S. B. G., Jones, G. V., & Mayes, A. R. (1994). No selective deficit in recall in amnesia. *Memory, 2*, 241–254.

Mandler, G. (1980). Recognizing: The judgement of previous occurrence. *Psychological Review, 87*, 252–271.

Mayes, A. R., & Gooding, P. (1989). Enhancement of word completion priming in amnesics by cueing with previously novel associates. *Neuropsychologia, 27*, 1057–1072.

Moscovitch, M., Vriezen, E., & Gottstein, J. (1993). Implicit tests of memory in patients with focal lesions or degenerative brain disorders. In H. Spinnler & F. Boller (Eds.), *Handbook of neuropsychology* (Vol. 8, pp. 133–173). Amsterdam: Elsevier.

Musen, G., & Squire, L. R. (1993). On the implicit learning of verbal associations by amnesic patients and normal subjects. *Neuropsychology, 7*, 119–135.

Paller, K. A., & Mayes, A. R. (1994). New-association priming of word identification in normal and amnesic subjects. *Cortex, 30*, 53–73.

Rajaram, S., & Geraci, L. (2000). Conceptual fluency selectively influences knowing. *Journal of Experimental Psychology: Learning, Memory, and Cognition, 26*, 1070–1074.

Ratcliff, R., & McKoon, G. (1995). Bias in the priming of object decisions. *Journal of Experimental Psychology: Learning, Memory, and Cognition, 21*, 754–767.

Ratcliff, R., & McKoon, G. (1996). Bias effects in implicit memory tasks. *Journal of Experimental Psychology: General, 125*, 403–421.

Ratcliff, R., & McKoon, G. (1997). A counter model for implicit priming in perceptual word identification. *Psychological Review, 104*, 319–343.

Ratcliff, R., McKoon, G., & Verwoerd, M. (1989). A bias interpretation of facilitation in perceptual identifiction. *Journal of Experimental Psychology: Learning, Memory, and Cognition, 15*, 378–387.

Reber, P. J., & Squire, L. R. (1999). Relaxing decision criteria does not improve recognition memory in amnesic patients. *Memory and Cognition, 27*, 501–511.

Richardson-Klavehn, A., & Gardiner, J. M. (1996). Cross-modality priming in stem completion reflects conscious memory, but not voluntary memory. *Psychonomic Bulletin and Review, 3*, 238–244.

Richardson-Klavehn, A., Gardiner, J. M., & Java, R. I. (1994). Involuntary conscious memory and the method of opposition. *Memory, 2*, 1–29.

Schacter, D. L., & Badgaiyan, R. D. (2001). Neuroimaging of priming: New perspectives on implicit and explicit memory. *Current Directions in Psychological Science, 10*, 1–4.

Schacter, D. L., Badgaiyan, R. D., & Alpert, N. M. (1999). Visual word stem completion priming within and across modalities: A PET study. *NeuroReport, 10*, 2061–2065.

Schacter, D. L., Chiu, P. C. Y., & Ochsner, K. N. (1993). Implicit memory: A selective review. *Annual Review of Neuroscience, 16*, 159–182.

Schacter, D. L., & Cooper, L. A. (1995). Bias in the priming of object decisions: Logic, assumptions and data. *Journal of Experimental Psychology: Learning, Memory, and Cognition, 21*, 768–776.

Schacter, D. L., & Graf, P. (1986a). Effects of elaborative processing on implicit and explicit memory for new associations. *Journal of Experimental Psychology: Learning, Memory, and Cognition, 12*, 432–444.

Schacter, D. L., & Graf, P. (1986b). Preserved learning in amnesic patients: Perspectives from research on direct priming. *Journal of Clinical and Experimental Neuropsychology, 8*, 727–743.

Schacter, D. L., Verfaellie, M., & Pradere, D. (1996). The neuropsychology of memory illusions: False recall and recognition in amnesic patients. *Journal of Memory and Language, 35*, 319–344.

Shimamura, A. P., & Squire, L. R. (1988). Long-term memory in amnesia: Cued recall, recognition memory and confidence ratings. *Journal of Experimental Psychology: Learning, Memory, and Cognition, 14*, 763–770.

Shimamura, A. P., & Squire, L. R. (1989). Impaired priming of new associations in amnesia. *Journal of Experimental Psychology: Learning, Memory, and Cognition, 15*, 721–728.

Stark, C. E. L., & Squire, L. R. (2000). Recognition memory and familiarity judgments in severe amnesia: No evidence for a contribution of repetition priming. *Behavioral Neuroscience, 114*, 459–467.

Tulving, E. (1985). Memory and consciousness. *Canadian Psychology, 26*, 1–12.

Verfaellie, M. (1994). A re-examination of recognition memory in amnesia: Reply to Roediger and McDermott. *Neuropsychology, 8*, 289–292.

Verfaellie, M., & Cermak, L. S. (1999). Perceptual fluency as a cue for recognition judgments in amnesia. *Neuropsychology, 13*, 198–205.

Verfaellie, M., Giovanello, K. S., & Keane, M. M. (2001). Recognition memory in amnesia: Effects of relaxing response criteria. *Cognitive, Affective and Behavioral Neuroscience, 1*, 3–9.

Verfaellie, M., & Keane, M. M. (2001). Scope and limits of implicit memory in amnesia. In B. De Gelder, E. De Haan, & C. Heywood (Eds.), *Unconscious minds* (pp. 151–162). Oxford: Oxford University Press.

Verfaellie, M., Keane, M. M., & Cook, S. P. (in press). The role of explicit memory processes in cross-modal priming: An investigation of stem completion priming in amnesia. *Cognitive, Affective and Behavioral Neuroscience*.

Verfaellie, M., & Treadwell, J. (1993). Status of recognition memory in amnesia. *Neuropsychology, 7*, 5–13.

Wagner, A. D., Desmond, J. E., Glover, G. H., & Gabrieli, J. D. E. (1998). Prefrontal cortex and recognition memory: Functional-MRI evidence for context-dependent retrieval processes. *Brain*, *121*, 1965–2002.

Wagner, A. D., & Gabrieli, J. D. E. (1998). On the relationship between recognition familiarity and perceptual fluency: Evidence for distinct mnemonic processes. *Acta Psychologica*, *98*, 211–230.

Wagner, A. D., Gabrieli, J. D. E., & Verfaellie, M. (1997). Dissociations between familiarity processes in explicit recognition and implicit perceptual memory. *Journal of Experimental Psychology: Learning, Memory, and Cognition*, *23*, 305–323.

Whittlesea, B. W. A. (1993). Illusions of familiarity. *Journal of Experimental Psychology: Learning, Memory, and Cognition*, *19*, 1235–1253.

Yonelinas, A. P., Kroll, N. E. A., Dobbins, I., Lazzara, M., & Knight, R. T. (1998). Recollection and familiarity deficits in amnesia: Convergence of remember–know, process dissociation, and receiver operating characteristic data. *Neuropsychology*, *12*, 323–339.

4

Anterograde and Retrograde Amnesia Following Frontal Lobe, Temporal Lobe, or Diencephalic Lesions

MICHAEL D. KOPELMAN
and NICOLA STANHOPE

In the second edition of this volume, Kopelman (1992) reviewed his research on patients with Korsakoff's syndrome and Alzheimer dementia, particularly with respect to studies of rates of forgetting and retrograde amnesia (RA). In addition, the extent to which the deficits in these disorders, especially in Alzheimer dementia, might be accounted for in terms of cholinergic depletion was examined. Our more recent research has continued to investigate the pattern and nature of memory deficits in amnesic patients, but has focused particularly upon comparisons of the effects of frontal lobe, diencephalic, and temporal lobe lesions. As the claims for differential patterns of memory deficit in such patients have multiplied, based largely upon single-case studies or small-group investigations of one or another lesion group, it has become increasingly important to carry out a comparative study involving groups of patients with different focal lesions.

The assumptions of such an approach are:

1. Inferences about normal memory functioning can be made from patients with focal pathology. There have long been critics of this approach (Gregory, 1961), and functional neuroimaging in healthy volunteers now provides an alternative. However, the value of lesion studies is beyond question (see the first and second editions of this volume), and they provide important constraints on the interpretation of functional neuroimaging studies, the assumptions and replicability of which have still not been tested to the limits.

2. The approach also assumes that a given cognitive deficit (or deficits) arises from a specific focal lesion, rather than any concomitant disruption of metabolism, perfusion, or structure either "upstream" or "downstream" from the site of principal pathology. Kopelman (2000a) has criticized the readiness with which this assumption is often made, sometimes on rather tenuous evidence; in the present studies, however, quantitative struc-

47

tural MRI and fluoro-deoxyglucose PET findings were available to document the extent and nature of brain pathology/dysfunction.

The investigations described below report findings in a series of comparative studies that examined aspects of anterograde and retrograde memory in patients with frontal lobe, temporal lobe, or diencephalic lesions. The general objectives of these studies were the following:

1. To identify any differences in the pattern of the memory disorder between patients with diencephalic or temporal lobe pathology.
2. To distinguish between the nature of the memory deficits arising from frontal lobe pathology and those resulting from diencephalic/temporal lobe lesions, and also to document the extent of overlap between the effects of frontal lobe versus diencephalic/temporal lobe lesions.
3. To search for correlations between the memory deficits in these patients and quantitative measures of structural or functional disruption in specific brain regions.

PARTICIPANTS

The temporal lobe group ($n = 14$) in these studies included 9 patients with probable or definite (antibody-confirmed) herpes encephalitis, all of whom had CT evidence of temporal lobe damage. It also included 4 patients with hypoxic brain damage. There was 1 patient who had a history of complex partial seizures with bilateral medial temporal lobe atrophy, resulting in memory impairment. The diencephalic group ($n = 15$) consisted of 13 patients who had alcoholic Korsakoff's syndrome and 2 patients who manifested an amnesic syndrome following surgical excision and irradiation of a pituitary adenoma. In the latter 2 patients, the diencephalon was implicated (Guinan, Lowy, Stanhope, Lewis, & Kopelman, 1998). The frontal lobe group ($n = 15$) consisted of 6 patients with focal frontal lesions from various causes (2 bilateral, 3 right-sided, 1 left-sided), as well as 9 patients who were assessed 2 weeks following a bilateral frontal tractotomy. MRI and PET showed extensive frontal changes in these latter patients, although the septal nuclei and other basal forebrain structures were spared. The tractotomy patients were tested 2 weeks following their operation, because Kartsounis, Poynton, Bridges, and Bartlett (1991) had shown that these patients' deficits at this time very closely resembled those exhibited by patients with large frontal lesions, and that the deficits could not be attributed to depression. Twenty controls were also tested.

We and our colleagues (Colchester et al., 2001) have reported that the patients with Korsakoff's syndrome in this sample showed significant atrophy of the thalami on quantitative structural MRI investigation, but no significant atrophy in medial temporal lobe structures. By contrast, the patients with herpes encephalitis showed significant atrophy in the hippocampi and parahippocampal gyri bilaterally, but no significant atrophy in the thalami. The group with hypoxic damage also showed significant atrophy of medial temporal lobe structures, total volume being approximately midway between that of the healthy control group and that of the herpes encephalitis group (Kopelman et al., 2001b). The patients with focal frontal lobe lesions showed significant atrophy in the frontal lobes, but no significant atrophy in either the thalami or medial temporal lobe structures, and this remained true when the frontal tractotomy group was included in the analysis (Colchester et al., 2001; Kopelman et al., 2001b).

ANTEROGRADE MEMORY

One of our initial studies (Kopelman & Stanhope, 1998) investigated the relative impairment of recall memory, compared with recognition memory, across these patient groups. Various authors had described disproportionate impairment in recall memory in patients with frontal lesions (Janowsky, Shimamura, Kritchevsky, & Squire, 1989), whereas others had described individual patients with frontal lobe pathology who showed disproportionate problems in recognition memory (Parkin, Bindschaedler, Harsent, & Metzler, 1996; Schacter, Curran, Galluccio, Milberg, & Bates, 1996). Similarly, Hirst and colleagues (Hirst et al., 1986; Hirst, Johnson, Phelps, & Volpe, 1988) had argued for a disproportionate impairment in recall memory in amnesic patients in general, whereas others (Haist, Shimamura, & Squire, 1992) had produced evidence against this. The issue has become particularly pertinent in the light of claims that hippocampal damage in isolation produces only a recall memory deficit, and perirhinal or parahippocampal damage is required to produce a deficit in recognition memory (Aggleton & Shaw, 1996; Vargha-Khadem et al., 1997; Aggleton & Brown, 1999). Against this, Reed and Squire (1997) have described patients with hippocampal lesions who showed deficits in both recognition and recall memory. A problem with such studies is that they are often confounded by ceiling or floor effects; indeed, it is difficult to avoid these in "matching" performance on either recognition or recall memory tasks.

Our own study (Kopelman & Stanhope, 1998) manipulated exposure times to achieve matching in recognition memory performance, and Figure 4.1 shows that there was no evidence of a recall–recognition discrepancy in any of our groups, relative to controls' performance. This finding also held when performance across the individual etiological groups was examined. The only difference across the groups was that, when the word stimuli were blocked into semantic categories, the patients with frontal lobe lesions were helped to a much greater extent than were the other amnesic patients. This latter result suggested that the frontal lobe group was aided by being provided with an organized structure in the material to be learned. In reviewing the literature, Kopelman (2001) has suggested that disproportionate impairment in recall memory (particularly in hippocampal patients) may simply reflect a mild degree of amnesia, although it has to be acknowledged that (1) there may be differences across individual patients, particularly in those with frontal lobe lesions (compare Janowsky et al., 1989; Parkin et al., 1996; Schacter et al., 1996), and (2) findings may vary according to the delay between stimuli presentation and memory testing (see Kopelman & Stanhope, 1997, and below).

A second study investigated context memory (Kopelman, Stanhope, & Kingsley, 1997). Many investigations have attributed deficits in temporal context memory to frontal lobe pathology (e.g., Butters, Kaszniak, Glisky, Eslinger, & Schacter, 1994; Milner, 1982), whereas others have argued that diencephalic/medial temporal lobe pathology in amnesia can itself produce context memory impairments (Kopelman, 1989; Parkin, Leng, & Hunkin, 1990; Shoqeirat & Mayes, 1991). In particular, Parkin and colleagues (1990; Hunkin, Parkin, & Longmore, 1994) have argued that diencephalic pathology especially affects temporal context memory, whereas medial temporal lobe damage specifically impairs spatial context memory. Our own study (Kopelman, Stanhope, & Kingsley, 1997; Figure 4.2a) showed that diencephalic patients were significantly impaired at temporal context memory; the temporal lobe patients were also impaired, but this just failed to reach significance. By contrast, the temporal lobe patients were significantly impaired at spatial context memory, and patients with right-sided damage performed worse than those with left-sided lesions. On this test, the diencephalic patients showed only a trend toward impairment. However,

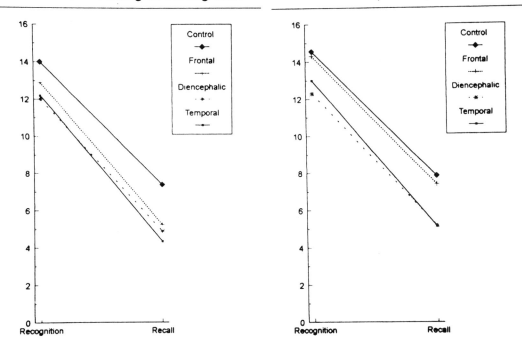

FIGURE 4.1. Recognition and free-recall performance in control, frontal lobe, diencephalic, and temporal lobe patients for (*left*) "matched" samples in which subjects at ceiling levels were excluded, and the groups did not differ significantly in terms of recognition memory scores; (*right*) the total (unselected) samples in each group. From Kopelman and Stanhope (1998). Copyright 1998 by Elsevier Science. Reprinted by permission.

the group × task interaction was not statistically significant. Frontal lobe patients, taken as a group, did not show impairment, but Figure 4.2b shows that patients in whom the pathology invaded the lateral frontocortical margin were very severely impaired at temporal context memory, consistent with an earlier finding by Milner, Corsi, and Lennard (1991). In brief, there was considerable variability in the frontal lobe group, dependent upon the precise site of the lesion.

In parallel with this last study, we also examined frequency judgments—an ability often related to context memory (Stanhope, Guinan, & Kopelman, 1998). On this task, all three patient groups were impaired at estimating how often a series of abstract designs had been presented, relative to healthy controls' performance. It was argued that this impairment in frontal lobe patients might reflect their difficulty in making an organized search in memory for multiple traces of an item, but that the results in temporal lobe patients reflected their "core" memory deficit. In diencephalic patients, the finding may have resulted from the combined effects of a generally poor memory and superimposed frontal pathology.

A major component of our investigations was a study of forgetting rates (Kopelman & Stanhope, 1997). Short-term forgetting over 5 to 15 seconds was investigated using the

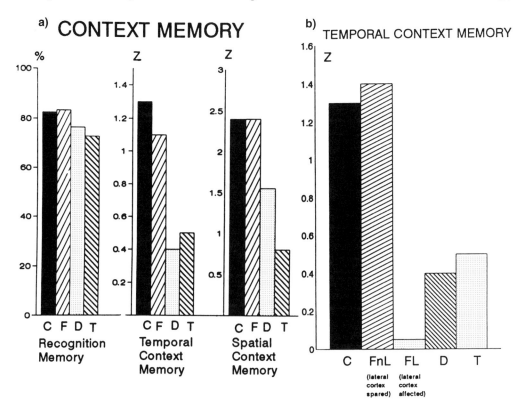

FIGURE 4.2. (a) The performance of the three main lesion groups and healthy controls on (1) recognition memory, (2) temporal context memory (recency judgments), and (3) spatial context memory (position). Z corrects the context scores (the proportion of correctly identified targets for which sequence or position was also correctly given) for differential hit rates (correctly identified true positives in recognition); see Hunkin et al. (1994) and Kopelman et al. (1997). C, healthy controls; F, frontal lobe group; D, diencephalic group; T, temporal lobe group. (b) The performance of the main lesion groups on the temporal context memory task, where the frontal lobe group has been subdivided into 3 patients in whom the lesions penetrated the dorsolateral cortical margin in the frontal lobes, and 12 patients with frontal lesions in whom this region was spared. From Kopelman, Stanhope, and Kingsley (1997). Copyright 1997 by Elsevier Science. Reprinted by permission.

Brown–Peterson test and a visuospatial variant of this. As in earlier studies (Kopelman, 1985, 1991), we found that, if the zero retention delay was discounted, there were no differences in forgetting rates across the patient groups. However, we were particularly interested in examining delays immediately after this point up to about 20 minutes, and in investigating whether there were any difference between recall and recognition memory in this regard; several studies had suggested that there might be a difference, although they were all subject to criticisms. For recognition memory, our investigation showed no differences in forgetting rates for words, pictures, or abstract designs between 1 minute and 10 or 20 minutes. The only group in whom we have found accelerated forgetting on recognition memory testing consists of patients with ECT-related amnesia, in whom there is widespread metabolic disruption (Lewis & Kopelman, 1998; see also Squire, 1981). However, on a recall memory task for pictorial material, diencephalic and temporal lobe patients showed faster forgetting than healthy subjects between 20 seconds and 10 minutes, whereas frontal lobe patients showed only a nonsignificant trend in the same direction (see Figure 4.3). This finding has been replicated in Alzheimer patients (Christensen, Kopelman, Stanhope, Lorentz, & Owen, 1998) and in amnesic patients using verbal material (Green & Kopelman, in press; Isaac & Mayes, 1999a, 1999b). These results suggest that, in addition to amnesic patients' severe impairment in acquiring or learning information, there is a more subtle retention deficit, detectable only on recall memory testing at longer delays.

We also examined patients' own subjective evaluations of their memory (Kopelman, Stanhope, & Guinan, 1998), finding that the frontal lobe and diencephalic patients were particularly impaired. The temporal lobe patients showed significantly better insight into their memory impairment, and across all patients there was a "temporal gradient," such that patients rated their memory for "old" (premorbid) items as better than their memory for "new" (recent) or prospective items (see also Squire & Zouzounis, 1988). As in previous studies, subjective memory evaluations were not correlated with measures of the severity of objective anterograde memory performance. However, there was a consistent pattern of statistically significant (albeit fairly low) correlations between recall of early, remote memories (but *not* more recent memories) and subjective memory evaluations (Table 4.1). In other words, whether the earliest remote or autobiographical memories were

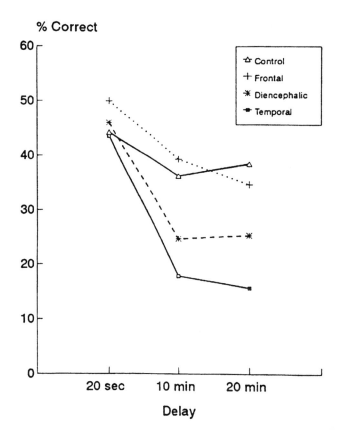

FIGURE 4.3. Recall of pictures of objects—mean percentage correct. From Kopelman, Stanhope, and Kingsley (1997). Copyright 1997 by Elsevier Science. Reprinted by permission.

TABLE 4.1. Correlations between Remote Memories and Old, New, and Prospective Subjective Memory Evaluations

	Old items (10 items)	New items (23 items)	Prospective items (6 items)
News event recall, 1960s	.29*	.21	.31*
News event recognition, 1960s	.35**	.29*	.41**
Autobiographical Memory Interview: Childhood facts	.27*	.25*	.25*
Autobiographical Memory Interview: Childhood incidents	.32*	.34*	.29*

Note. All patients, $n = 44$; news events test, $n = 43$. Adapted from Kopelman, Stanhope, and Guinan (1998). Copyright 1998 by Masson SpA. Adapted by permission.

*$p \le .05$; **$p \le .01$

preserved (or not) seemed to contribute to how subjects evaluated their memory for past, current, and prospective events.

Significant correlations were obtained between MRI measures of critical brain volumes and performance on various anterograde memory tasks (Table 4.2) (Kopelman et al., 2001b). In particular, hippocampal volume showed the strongest and most consistent correlations with test performance, but our measures of medial temporal lobe and thalamic volume also produced statistically significant correlations. Although not shown in this table, total frontal lobe volume correlated significantly with our temporal context memory measure ($r = .42$, $p < .02$), and hippocampal volume with our spatial context memory measure ($r = .60$, $p < .02$). Also of importance (although not shown in the table), there were no significant differences between our hippocampal and parahippocampal measures in terms of the size of their correlations with recall and recognition memory scores, or in terms of verbal versus visual memory (contrast Aggleton & Shaw, 1996, and Kohler et al., 1998).

TABLE 4.2. Anterograde Memory Tasks: Correlations with MRI Measures

	Whole brain	Total temporal	Total medial temporal	Total hippocampal	Total thalamic
GMQ[1]	.41**	.49**	.42**	.63**	.34*
DMQ[2]	.38*	.42**	.36*	.58*	.45**
Word recall	.17	.25	.29	.51*	.24
Word recognition	.21	.22	.35*	.24	.38*
Picture recognition	.24	.31	.41**	.61**	.24
Brown–Peterson					
Verbal	.13	.07	.15	.50*	−.05
Visual					
(Corsi blocks)	.17	.07	.04	.56*	.32*

Note. Adapted from Kopelman et al. (2001b). Copyright by BMJ Publishing Group. Adapted by permission.

[1]General Memory Index (or Quotient) from the Wechsler Memory Scale—Revised (Wechsler, 1987).

[2]Delayed Recall Index from the Wechsler Memory Scale—Revised (Wechsler, 1987).

*$p < .05$, two-tailed; **$p < .01$, two-tailed.

A PET activation study in healthy subjects sought to investigate the particular contributions of medial temporal lobe and frontal lobe structures in learning (Kopelman, Stevens, Foli, & Grasby, 1998). Given that incremental learning from trial to trial is severely impaired in amnesic patients, we predicted that medial temporal lobe activation might be particularly associated with incremental gains in learning. We found that, on a verbal recall task across multiple trials, initial learning activated both the left medial temporal and left frontal regions (Figure 4.4), but that the consolidation or binding of new memories to those already learned seemed to involve two processes: (1) activation in the left medial temporal region during incremental learning, and (2) activation in the right prefrontal–precuneate circuit during the retrieval and reactivation of previously learned material.

In summary, comparison of patient groups with frontal lobe, temporal lobe, and diencephalic lesions showed more overlap in the pattern of their memory deficits than would be predicted from previous single-case or small-group investigations. In particular, the groups resembled one another in terms of their performance on recall and recognition memory tasks and rates of forgetting on recognition memory tests. The groups differed in terms of forgetting rates on recall measures, in that the diencephalic and temporal lobe patients showed faster forgetting than the frontal lobe patients. With respect to subjective memory evaluations, the diencephalic and frontal lobe groups lacked insight, relative to the temporal lobe group. In terms of context memory, patients with lateral frontocortical pathology and those with diencephalic lesions were particularly impaired at a temporal

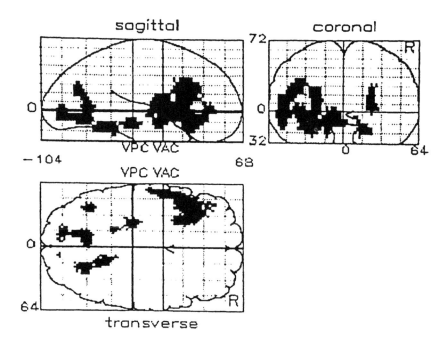

FIGURE 4.4. Foci of activation during initial learning of word lists (novel minus repeated trials). Dark areas indicate increases in regional cerebral blood flow at $p < .001$. There are left frontal and left medial temporal activations. From Kopelman, Stevens, Foli, and Grasby (1998). Copyright 1998 by Oxford University Press. Reprinted by permission.

context task, and patients with temporal lobe lesions showed a nonsignificant trend in the same direction. Performance on the temporal context task correlated significantly with our MRI measure of total frontal volume. Patients with medial temporal lobe or hippocampal pathology, particularly right-sided, showed a significant deficit on our spatial memory measure, and the diencephalic group showed a nonsignificant trend in the same direction. Performance on the spatial context memory task correlated significantly with our MRI measure of total hippocampal volume.

RETROGRADE MEMORY

As in earlier studies of patients with Korsakoff's syndrome or Alzheimer dementia (Kopelman, 1989, 1992, 2000b), one of our major interests was in the pattern and nature of RA across these lesion groups. Measures of autobiographical incident recall, memory for "personal semantic" facts, recall of famous news events, and word completions for the names of famous faces were included in our studies (Kopelman, Stanhope, & Kingsley, 1999).

Across all our measures, patients with Korsakoff's syndrome showed a severe impairment with a characteristically steep temporal gradient (sparing of early memories; see Figure 4.5). By contrast, patients with pathology confined to the diencephalon, resulting from pituitary tumors and their treatment (Guinan et al., 1998), showed intact remote memory across all measures despite substantial anterograde memory impairment. This difference was attributed to the combination of frontal lobe and diencephalic pathology in the Korsakoff patients. Patients with temporal lobe pathology showed a severe impairment across all RA measures, but a flatter temporal gradient than the Korsakoff patients—possibly because the involvement of aspects of semantic memory in herpes encephalitis patients negates the benefit of early or "old" remote memories having adopted a more semantic form (Cermak, 1984). Patients with frontal lobe lesions showed severe impairment in the recall of autobiographical incidents and famous news events, but were relatively spared in the recall of well-rehearsed personal semantic facts; this finding may reflect the greater degree of active or effortful reconstruction that is required in retrieving incidents and news events.

There were other important and interesting findings (Kopelman et al., 1999; Stanhope & Kopelman, 2000). Korsakoff patients' performance did not correlate with either the duration of their amnesia or the length of their drinking history, which means that the findings in that group could not be attributed to a progressive anterograde memory impairment. In general, patients with bilateral frontal pathology performed worse than patients with unilateral frontal lesions. Patients with right frontal lobe or temporal lobe pathology were more impaired than those with left-sided lesions on the news events task, particularly on items in which a famous face was implicated. More particularly, herpes encephalitis patients with right-sided pathology performed particularly badly in the recall of autobiographical incidents, whereas those with unilateral left-sided pathology were particularly impaired at a (famous) name completion task. This latter finding was interpreted as indicating that the right temporal lobe is particularly critical to those processes necessary for the retrieval of past personal memories (such as the conjuring up of appropriate mental imagery), whereas left temporal pathology affects the lexical–semantic labeling of remote memories.

Correlations between retrograde memory measures and quantitative MRI volumes of critical structures (Kopelman et al., 2001a) indicated that widespread neural networks within the temporal and frontal lobes are likely to contribute to both the storage and re-

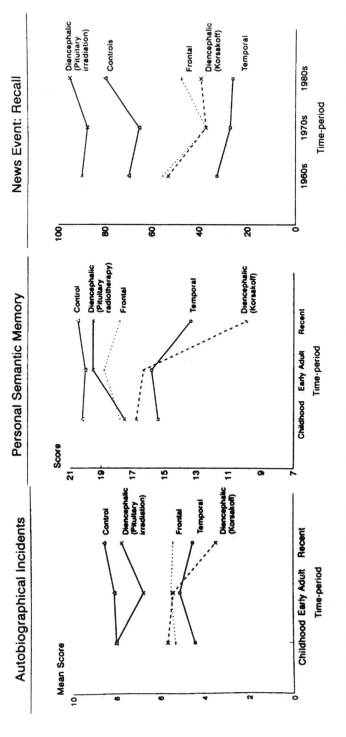

FIGURE 4.5. The performance of healthy controls and lesion groups on three measures of retrograde amnesia—autobiographical incidents and personal semantic memory from the Autobiographical Memory Interview, and a famous news events test. The diencephalic group has been subdivided into 13 patients with alcoholic Korsakoff's syndrome and 2 patients whose diencephalon had been damaged by a pituitary tumor, surgery, and irradiation. From Kopelman, Stanhope, and Kingsley (1999). Copyright 1999 by Elsevier Science. Reprinted by permission.

trieval of "old" or remote memories. The pattern of the correlations differed somewhat across the lesion groups, but multiple-regression analysis indicated that a sizeable proportion of variance in patients' scores on these tasks could be attributed to differences in regional brain volumes. In the diencephalic group, measures of frontal, thalamic, and medial temporal volume accounted for 60% of the variance on the autobiographical and personal semantic memory measures. In the frontal lobe group, these measures accounted for 60% to 68% of the variance. However, in the temporal lobe group, correlations between medial temporal volume and retrograde memory measures were small and nonsignificant. This last observation argues against the "multiple-trace" hypothesis of Nadel and Moscovitch (1997), in which it was predicted that the extent of episodic RA, and the slope of the temporal gradient, would depend critically upon the degree of hippocampal damage.

Further studies have investigated RA in patients with spontaneous confabulation and other forms of false memory (Box, Laing, & Kopelman, 1999; Kopelman, 1999; Kopelman, Ng, & Van Den Brouke, 1997), as well as in patients with psychogenic forms of amnesia (Kopelman, 1995; Kopelman, Christensen, Puffett, & Stanhope, 1994; Kopelman & Morton, 2001). Although a "fugue state" or "functional RA" is rare, psychogenic influences on RA, in the presence of concomitant brain pathology, are probably much more common: in patients with so-called "focal RA," this circumstance can make the interpretation of their disorder very problematic (Kopelman, 2000a). Another difficulty in interpreting "focal RA" is that many of the better described cases had an initially severe anterograde as well as retrograde memory loss, followed by some degree of residual anterograde memory impairment. This situation further confounds the interpretation of this disorder, especially as the types of tasks employed to measure anterograde amnesia and RA have usually differed substantially (Kopelman, 2000a).

In summary, there is evidence that widespread circuits through temporal and frontal neocortex are involved in the storage and retrieval of remote memories, although there is also evidence of more specialized roles within particular brain regions. The findings from the lesion groups have suggested that the frontal lobes may be particularly implicated where remote memory retrieval requires active or effortful reconstruction processes, the right temporal lobe where mental imagery is necessary to conjure up recall of autobiographical or episodic memories, and the left temporal lobe where there is a need for lexical–semantic labeling of remote memories.

CONCLUSIONS

There is more overlap in the effects of frontal lobe, temporal lobe, and diencephalic lesions on memory processes than the literature from single-case and small-group studies would suggest. This is true with respect to both anterograde and retrograde memory. However, there is also evidence of some degree of functional specialization within these brain regions. In anterograde memory, we found that the medial temporal/hippocampal regions were particularly implicated in spatial context memory, whereas the lateral frontocortical region, the diencephalon, and (probably) the temporal lobes were implicated in temporal context memory. There was evidence that the diencephalic and temporal lobe groups manifested faster forgetting on recall measures between approximately 20 seconds and 10 minutes than the frontal lobe patients, but the present studies did not show evidence of any differences between the temporal lobe and diencephalic groups in this regard. Correlational analysis of hippocampal and parahippocampal volumes with recall–recognition measures did not show any significant differences; this would be consistent with the view that it may be relative mildness of amnesia, rather than site of pathology, that results in relative sparing of recognition memory and disproportionate impairment of recall memory. In RA, widespread neural networks have been implicated in the storage and retrieval of remote memories, and multiple-regression analysis of MRI volumes in critical brain regions predicted 60% of the variance in patients' performance on retrograde tasks. However, there was again evidence of some degree of regional specialization, with the frontal lobes playing a critical role in the active reconstruction of old memories, the right temporal lobe in autobiographical recall, and the left temporal lobe in the lexical–semantic labeling of remote memories. Future studies need to examine more closely the possible links between these patterns of regional specialization across the anterograde and retrograde domains.

ACKNOWLEDGMENTS

This work was funded by a Wellcome Trust project grant and by the Special Trustees of St Thomas's Hospital. We are grateful for the help of many collaborators, who were authors on the original papers.

REFERENCES

Aggleton, J. P., & Brown, M. (1999). Episodic memory, amnesia and the hippocampal anterior thalamic axis. *Behavioral and Brain Sciences, 22,* 425–444.

Aggleton, J. P., & Shaw, C. (1996). Amnesia and recognition memory: A re-analysis of psychometric data. *Neuropsychologia, 34,* 51–62.

Box, O., Laing, H., & Kopelman, M. D. (1999). The evolution of spontaneous confabulation, delusional misidentification, and a related delusion in a case of severe head injury. *Neurocase, 5,* 251–262.

Butters, M., Kaszniak, A. W., Gilsky, E. L., Eslinger, P. J., & Schacter, D. L. (1994). Recency discrimination deficits in frontal lobe patients. *Neuropsychology, 8,* 343–353.

Cermak, L. S. (1984). The episodic–semantic distinction in amnesia. In L. R. Squire & N. Butters (Eds.), *Neuropsychology of memory* (pp. 55–62). New York: Guilford Press.

Christensen, H., Kopelman, M. D., Stanhope, N., Lorentz, L., & Owen, P. (1998). Rates of forgetting in Alzheimer dementia. *Neuropsychologia, 36,* 547–557.

Colchester, A., Kingsley, D., Lasserson, D., Kendall, B., Bello, F., Rush, C., Stevens,T., Goodman, G., Heilpern, G., Stanhope, N., & Kopelman, M. D. (2001). Structural MRI volumetric analysis in patients with organic amnesia: I. Methods and findings comparative across diagnostic groups. *Journal of Neurology, Neurosurgery and Psychiatry, 71,* 13–22.

Green, R. E. A., & Kopelman, M. D. (in press). Contribution of context-dependent memory and familiarity judgements to forgetting rates in organic amnesia. *Cortex.*

Gregory, R. L. (1961). The brain as an engineering problem. In W. H. Thorpe & O. L. Zangwill (Eds.), *Current problems in animal behaviour* (pp. 307–330). Cambridge, England: Cambridge University Press.

Guinan, E. M., Lowy, C., Stanhope, N., Lewis, P. D. R., & Kopelman, M. D. (1998). The cognitive effects of pituitary adenomas and their treatments: Two case studies and an investigation of 90 patients. *Journal of Neurology, Neurosurgery and Psychiatry, 65,* 870–876.

Haist, F., Shimamura, A. P., & Squire, L. R. (1992). On the relationship between recall and recognition memory. *Journal of Experimental Psychology: Learning, Memory, and Cognition, 18,* 691–702.

Hirst, W., Johnson, M. K., Kim, J. K., Phelps, E. A., Risse, G., & Volpe, B. T. (1986). Recognition and recall in amnesics. *Journal of Experimental Psychology: Learning, Memory, and Cognition*, *12*, 445–449.

Hirst, W., Johnson, M. K., Phelps, E. A., & Volpe, B. T. (1988). More on recognition and recall in amnesics. *Journal of Experimental Psychology: Learning, Memory, and Cognition*, *14*, 758–762.

Hunkin, N. M., Parkin, A. J., & Longmore, B. E. (1994). Aetiological variation in the amnesic syndrome: Comparisons using the list discrimination task. *Neuropsychologia*, *32*, 819–825.

Isaac, C. L., & Mayes, A. R. (1999a). Rates of forgetting in amnesia: I. Recall and recognition of prose. *Journal of Experimental Psychology: Learning, Memory, and Cognition*, *25*, 963–977.

Isaac, C. L., & Mayes, A. R. (1999b). Rates of forgetting in amnesia: II. Recall and recognition of word lists at different levels of organization. *Journal of Experimental Psychology: Learning, Memory, and Cognition*, *25*, 963–977.

Janowsky, J. S., Shimamura, A. P., Kritchevsky, M., & Squire, L. R. (1989). Cognitive impairment following frontal lobe damage and its relevance to human amnesia. *Behavioral Neuroscience*, *103*, 548–560.

Kartsounis, L. D., Poynton, A., Bridges. P. K., & Bartlett, F. R. (1991). Neuropsychological correlates of stereotactic subcaudate surgery. *Brain*, *114*, 2657–2673.

Kohler, S., Black, S. E., Sinden, M., Szekely, C., Kidron, D., Parker, J. L., Foster, J. K., Moscovitch, M., Winocur, G., Szalai, J. P., & Bronskill, M. J. (1998). Memory impairments associated with hippocampal versus parahippocampal gyrus atrophy: An MR volumetry study in Alzheimer's disease. *Neuropsychologia*, *36*, 901–914.

Kopelman, M. D. (1985). Rates of forgetting in Alzheimer-type dementia and Korsakoff's syndrome. *Neuropsychologia*, *23*, 623–638.

Kopelman, M. D. (1989). Remote and autobiographical memory, temporal context memory, and frontal atrophy in Korsakoff and Alzheimer patients. *Neuropsychologia*, *27*, 437–460.

Kopelman, M. D. (1991). Non-verbal short-term forgetting in the alcoholic Korsakoff syndrome and Alzheimer-type dementia. *Neuropsychologia*, *29*, 737–747.

Kopelman, M. D. (1992). The "new" and the "old": Components of the anterograde and retrograde memory loss in Korsakoff and Alzheimer patients. In L. R. Squire & N. Butters (Eds.), *Neuropsychology of memory* (2nd ed., pp. 130–146). New York: Guilford Press.

Kopelman, M. D. (1995). The assessment of psychogenic amnesia. In A. D. Baddeley, B. A. Wilson, & F. Watts (Eds.), *Handbook of memory disorders* (pp. 427–448). Chichester, England: Wiley.

Kopelman, M. D. (1999). Varieties of false memory. *Cognitive Neuropsychology*, *16*, 197–214.

Kopelman, M. D. (2000a). Focal retrograde amnesia and the attribution of causality: An exceptionally critical review. *Cognitive Neuropsychology*, *17*, 585–621.

Kopelman, M. D. (2000b). The neuropsychology of remote memory. In L. Cermak (Ed.), *Handbook of neuropsychology* (2nd ed., pp. 251–280). Amsterdam: Elsevier.

Kopelman, M. D. (2001). Disorders of memory. *Brain*. Invited review, submitted for publication.

Kopelman, M. D., Christensen, H., Puffett, A., & Stanhope, N. (1994). The great escape: A neuropsychological study of psychogenic amnesia. *Neuropsychologia*, *32*, 675–691.

Kopelman, M. D., Lasserson, D., Kingsley, D., Bello, F., Rush, C., Stanhope, N., Stevens, T., Goodman, G., Heilpern, G., Kendall, B., & Colchester, A. (2001a). *Retrograde amnesia and the volume of critical brain structures*. Manuscript submitted for publication.

Kopelman, M. D., Lasserson, D., Kingsley, D., Bello, F., Rush, C., Stanhope, N., Stevens, T., Goodman, G., Heilpern, G., Kendall, B., & Colchester, A. (2001b). Structural MRI volumetric analysis in patients with organic amnesia: 2. Correlations with anterograde memory and executive tests in 40 patients. *Journal of Neurology, Neurosurgery and Psychiatry*, *71*, 23–28.

Kopelman, M. D., & Morton, J. (2001). Psychogenic amnesia: Functional memory loss. In G. Davies & T. Dalgleish (Eds.), *Recovered memories: The middle ground* (pp. 219–243). Chichester, England: Wiley.

Kopelman, M. D., Ng, N., & Van Den Brouke, O. (1997). Confabulation extending across episodic memory, personal and general semantic memory. *Cognitive Neuropsychology*, *14*, 683–712.

Kopelman, M. D., & Stanhope, N. (1997). Rates of forgetting in organic amnesia following temporal lobe, diencephalic, or frontal lobe lesions. *Neuropsychology, 11,* 343–356.

Kopelman, M. D., & Stanhope, N. (1998). Recall and recognition memory in patients with focal frontal, temporal lobe, and diencephalic lesions. *Neuropsychologia, 36,* 785–796.

Kopelman, M. D., Stanhope, N., & Guinan, E. (1998). Subjective memory evaluations in patients with focal frontal, diencephalic, and temporal lobe lesions. *Cortex, 34,* 191–207.

Kopelman, M. D., Stanhope, N., & Kingsley, D. (1997). Temporal and spatial context memory in patients with focal frontal, temporal lobe, and diencephalic lesions. *Neuropsychologia, 35,* 1533–1545.

Kopelman, M. D., Stanhope, N., & Kingsley, D. (1999). Retrograde amnesia in patients with diencephalic, temporal lobe or frontal lesions. *Neuropsychologia, 37,* 939–958.

Kopelman, M. D., Stevens, T. G., Foli, S., & Grasby, P. (1998). PET activation of the medial temporal lobe in learning. *Brain, 121,* 875–887.

Lewis, P., & Kopelman, M. D. (1998). Rates of forgetting in neuropsychiatric disorders. *Journal of Neurology, Neurosurgery and Psychiatry, 65,* 890–898.

Milner, B. (1982). Some cognitive effects of frontal-lobe lesions in man. *Philosophical Transactions of the Royal Society of London, Series B, 98,* 211–226.

Milner, B., Corsi, P., & Lennard, G. (1991). Frontal-lobe contribution to recency judgements. *Neuropsychologia, 29,* 601–618.

Nadel, L., & Moscovitch, M. (1997). Memory consolidation, retrograde amnesia and the hippocampal formation: A re-evaluation of the evidence and a new model. *Current Opinion in Neurobiology, 7,* 217–227.

Parkin, A. J., Bindschaedler, C., Harsent, L., & Metzler, C. (1996). Pathological false alarm rates following damage to the left frontal cortex. *Brain and Cognition, 32,* 14–27.

Parkin, A. J., Leng, N. R. C., & Hunkin, N. (1990). Differential sensitivity to contextual information in diencephalic and temporal lobe amnesia. *Cortex, 26,* 373–380.

Parkin, A. J., Montaldi, D., Leng, N. R. C., & Hunkin, N. M. (1990). Contextual cueing effects in the remote memory of alcoholic Korsakoff patients and normal subjects. *Quarterly Journal of Experimental Psychology, 42A,* 585–596.

Reed, J. M., & Squire, L. R. (1997). Impaired recognition memory in patients with lesions limited to the hippocampal formation. *Behavioral Neuroscience, 111,* 667–675.

Schacter, D. L., Curran, T., Galluccio, L., Milberg, W. P., & Bates, J. L. (1996). False recognition and the right frontal lobe: A case study. *Neuropsychologia, 34,* 793–808.

Shoqeirat, M. A., & Mayes, A. R. (1991). Disproportionate incidental spatial memory and recall deficits in amnesia. *Neuropsychologia, 29,* 749–770.

Squire, L. R. (1981). Two forms of amnesia: An analysis of forgetting. *Journal of Neuroscience, 1,* 635–640.

Squire, L. R., & Zouzounis, J. A. (1988). Self-ratings of memory dysfunction: Different findings in depression and amnesia. *Journal of Clinical and Experimental Neuropsychology, 10,* 727–738.

Stanhope, N., Guinan, E., & Kopelman, M. D. (1998). Frequency judgements of abstract designs by patients with diencephalic, temporal lobe or frontal lobe lesions. *Neuropsychologia, 36,* 1387–1396.

Stanhope, N., & Kopelman, M. D. (2000). Art and memory: A 7 year follow-up of herpes encephalitis in a professional artist. *Neurocase, 6,* 99–110.

Vargha-Khadem, F., Gadian, D. G., Watkins, K. E., Connelly, A., Van Paesschen, W., & Mishkin, M. (1997). Differential effects of early hippocampal pathology on episodic and semantic memory. *Science, 277,* 376–380.

Wechsler, D. (1987). *Wechsler Memory Scale—Revised.* San Antonio, TX: The Psychological Corporation.

5

Relational Binding Theory and the Role of Consolidation in Memory Retrieval

ARTHUR P. SHIMAMURA

Patients with damage to the medial temporal lobe exhibit a profound and debilitating memory impairment. The characterization of this impairment has significantly advanced our understanding of human memory. The medial temporal lobe comprises the hippocampal complex (hippocampus, dentate gyrus, subiculum) and surrounding neocortical regions (entorhinal cortex, parahippocampal gyrus, perirhinal cortex) (Lavenex & Amaral, 2000; Scoville & Milner, 1957). It is generally acknowledged that damage to the medial temporal lobe produces a significant impairment in new learning capacity (i.e., anterograde amnesia). This impairment affects the ability to retain newly acquired episodic (autobiographical) and semantic (factual) information. Damage to this brain region has little if any effect on perceptual priming or on the retention of simple habits or skills (for reviews, see Gershberg & Shimamura, 1998; Schacter, 1987; Squire, 1987, 1992).

The medial temporal lobe is also associated with impairment in the retrieval of information acquired before the onset of amnesia (i.e., retrograde amnesia). There is less agreement concerning the role of the medial temporal lobe in retrieval. Most would agree that new learning capacity is more affected than retrieval. For example, patient H. M. exhibited a profound anterograde amnesia, but less impairment in retrieving information acquired before his surgery. His retrograde amnesia was time-limited or graded, such that memory for the recent past was more severely affected than memory for the remote past. His good retrieval ability was indicated by the fact that he performed as well as control subjects on a face recognition test of celebrities who became famous prior to his operation (Marslen-Wilson & Teuber, 1974). Yet analyses of retrograde amnesia in other patients with medial temporal lobe damage have led to mixed findings. Controversy exists over the temporal extent of retrograde amnesia, the role of damage outside the medial temporal lobe, and the kind of memory affected (e.g., semantic vs. episodic memory). The aims of this chapter are to address these mixed findings and to reassess the role of the medial temporal lobe in (1) retrieving remote memories and (2) representing episodic and semantic memory.

CONSOLIDATION THEORY

What kind of neural mechanism could account for both severe anterograde amnesia and a time-limited retrograde amnesia? Since the early 1900s, a "consolidation" process has been used to explain this pattern of memory impairment (Burnham, 1903; Muller & Pilzecker, 1900; for reviews, see Glickman, 1961; Squire, 1987). According to consolidation theory, a neural "fixation" process occurs during some time period after a learning event takes place. This process increases the stability or permanence of recently stored information. This process was described cogently by Burnham in 1903:

> The fixing of an impression depends upon a physiological process. It takes time for an impression to become so fixed that it can be reproduced after a long interval; for it to become part of the permanent store of memory considerable time may be necessary. This we may suppose is not merely a process of making a permanent impression upon the nerve cells, but also a process of association, of organization of the new impressions with the old ones. (p. 392)

Burnham's characterization attributed two important features to the notion of consolidation. First, he stated that "considerable time may be necessary" to consolidate a memory trace. Second, he suggested that consolidation is not simply a process of strengthening, but "of organization of the new impressions with the old ones." These two features play an important role in contemporary views of medial temporal lobe function. Various theories have implicated the medial temporal lobe—particularly the hippocampal complex—in the consolidation of new memories in much the same way as Burnham (1903) described (Cohen & Eichenbaum, 1993; Squire, 1992; Squire, Cohen, & Nadel, 1984; Teyler & DiScenna, 1986). Modern views suggest that the hippocampal complex participates in indexing or binding cortical activation associated with new experiences.

The most often cited and best-described theory of medial temporal lobe function was developed by Squire (Squire, 1992; Squire et al., 1984; Squire & Zola, 1998). This view was developed as a way to explain human amnesia, and has had such a substantial impact on the field that it has been described as "the standard model" (Nadel & Moscovitch, 1997). This view has also been implemented in computational models (Alvarez & Squire, 1994; McClelland, McNaughton, & O'Reilly, 1995). As described by Squire and colleagues (1984),

> It is our contention that the neural elements participating in memory storage can undergo reorganization with the passage of time after learning. The most general way to state how this reorganization might occur is to suppose that although some elements are lost through forgetting, those that survive increase their synaptic efficacy. (p. 201)

Later, this characterization gained further support from advances in neuroanatomy and physiology (see Squire, Shimamura, & Amaral, 1989). First, associative plasticity based on N-methyl-D-aspartate (NMDA) receptors provided a neural mechanism for long-term potentiation (LTP). In LTP, rapid and long-lasting binding of neural pathways can be induced in hippocampal tissue. NMDA receptors facilitate the induction of LTP by enacting voltage-regulated (i.e., activity-dependent) channels, which open only when a target neuron has been recently activated. The discovery of NMDA receptors in the CA1 subfield of the hippocampus provided a biophysical mechanism for binding inputs in the hippocampus. A second advance came from neuroanatomical studies of projections to and from the medial temporal lobe (see Insausti, Amaral, & Cowan, 1987; Lavenex & Amaral, 2000). These studies suggested that inputs from diverse polymodal areas in neocortex project to the medial temporal lobe, feed into the hippocampal complex, and send reciprocal projections back to neocortical areas. Such findings led Squire, Shimamura, and Amaral (1989) to make the following conjecture:

> One possibility is that LTP acts as a mechanism for forming and storing conjunctions between two distinct inputs, and that the output of the hippocampal circuitry back to entorhinal cortex signals the forming of this conjunction. . . . In psychological terms, the hippocampus may contribute to the formation of new relationships in long-term memory, such as those formed when associating a stimulus and its spatial/temporal context (thus representing a new event or episode), or when associating facts and the semantic context to which they belong (thus representing a new concept). (p. 221)

THE TEMPORAL EXTENT OF RETROGRADE AMNESIA

Consolidation theory suggests that a fixation process continues to strengthen memory representations during a considerable time after the initial encoding event. If consolidation is halted at some time after learning—that is, before a representation is fully "fixed"—then that memory representation will be fragile and more susceptible to forgetting. If this process is halted very soon after learning, then recently bound memories will be severely affected. Thus consolidation theory suggests a temporal gradient to the pattern of retrograde amnesia, with recent memories more affected than very remote memories. Squire and colleagues (1984) suggested that the medial temporal lobe is critical for this consolidation process to occur. Five properties of this view are as follows:

1. The hippocampal complex acts to bind or associate cortical representations that are activated at any given moment by way of converging inputs into the medial temporal cortex. This binding process is immediate and akin to the neural mechanisms associated with LTP.
2. The binding of cortical representations via the medial temporal lobe increases the probability of these representations being reactivated at a later time.
3. Such reactivations allow for the establishment of cortical–cortical interconnections, which take longer to establish than cortical–hippocampal connections.
4. At some time after the initial encoding event, long-term memories are mediated solely by cortical–cortical interconnections. At this time, the medial temporal lobe—and those cortical–hippocampal connections that supported consolidation—are no longer necessary for retrieval.
5. Consolidation is critical for the binding of new episodic memories and for the binding of new semantic memories.

According to consolidation theory, the medial temporal lobe acts as a rapid binding mechanism that supports the formation and fixation of newly acquired memories. The actual consolidation process involves the formation of cortical–cortical interconnections. Thus the medial temporal lobe acts primarily to bind a representation initially and then to enable reactivation of these representations via cortical–hippocampal connections. In this way, the medial temporal lobe acts as a support system while memory representations are being fixed as stable cortical representations. Thus, at some time after learning, those memories that have been consolidated in cortical representations do not depend upon cortical–hippocampal connections. Studies of retrograde amnesia in patients with damage to the medial temporal lobe have often demonstrated a time-limited or graded retrograde amnesia (for reviews, see Nadel & Moscovitch, 1997; Squire, 1992; Squire & Alvarez, 1995). That is, in many amnesic patients retrograde amnesia occurs, such that recent memories are more affected than very remote memories. The temporal extent of retrograde amnesia has been shown to last from 2 years to many decades (see Rempel-Clower, Zola, Squire, & Amaral, 1996; Squire, 1992; Squire & Alvarez, 1995).

In reviewing studies of retrograde amnesia, Nadel and Moscovitch (1997) noted a rather varied pattern in the extent of retrograde amnesia observed in patients with medial temporal damage. Indeed, reports varied from some patients having rather minor (if any) retrograde amnesia to others having extensive, nongraded retrieval deficits. Findings of long-lasting, nongraded retrograde amnesia led Nadel and Moscovitch to question the validity of extant consolidation theories. In particular, some reports indicated extensive and flat retrograde amnesia lasting for over 30–40 years. Extant consolidation theories would have to assert that the process of consolidation proceeds for an inordinate time period in order to explain such results. Another possibility would be to suggest that disruptions of other brain regions (e.g., frontal lobes, posterior association cortex) are responsible for the pattern of extensive or nongraded retrograde amnesia.

Nadel and Moscovitch (1997) further noted differences in the extent of retrograde amnesia for different forms of memory. Memory for autobiographical episodes was most affected. Such memories assess specific personal events that are associated with a time and place context (e.g., a wedding, birthday, or graduation). Memory for public knowledge, such as public events or famous faces, often exhibited a graded retrograde amnesia and was less impaired than memory for autobiographical episodes. Even less affected was memory for "personal semantics"—that is, personal knowledge not tied to any specific episode (e.g., names of friends, familiar places). Finally, the least observed impairment occurred for overlearned semantic memory (e.g., vocabulary words and factual knowledge learned in school).

MULTIPLE-TRACE THEORY

Based on their review, Nadel and Moscovitch (1997) introduced a new theory of medial temporal lobe function, which they call "multiple-trace" theory. They accept the role of the hippocampal complex in the rapid binding of cortical representations. Their theory also suggests that this binding process increases the probability that representations will be reactivated. That is, they accept properties 1 and 2 of consolidation theory as stated above. However, they make two significant departures from standard consolidation theory. First, they suggest that every reactivation produces a different but related trace in the medial temporal cortex. Thus, as recently bound representations are reactivated, they produce more widespread links within the hippocampal complex. These multiple traces are long-lasting and distributed widely within the hippocampal complex. The forming of multiple traces increases the probability of successful memory retrieval.

A second feature of multiple-trace theory is the manner in which long-term semantic and episodic memories are formed. As stated by Nadel and Moscovitch,

The creation of multiple, related traces facilitates the "extraction" of factual information from an episode and its integration with pre-existing semantic memory stores. Facts about the world (e.g., the Eiffel Tower is in Paris, apples are round, mangoes are a type of fruit, etc.) that are acquired in the context of a specific episode are separated from that episode and ultimately stored independently of it. This process could be viewed as one of the consequences of "consolidation." (p. 223)

According to this view, semantic memories can be ultimately consolidated as cortical representations, but episodic memories are always dependent upon cortical–hippocampal connections. Thus Nadel and Moscovitch (1997) appear to maintain the "standard" view of consolidation with respect to the storage and retrieval of semantic memory and to develop the multiple-trace view for episodic memory, which purportedly always depends on the medial temporal lobe. Nadel and Moscovitch state that any memory that is tied to a time and place context, regardless of its age, will depend upon the medial temporal lobe. Thus they suggest that an amnesic patient will be impaired when asked questions about very remote episodic memories, such as remembering where and when a mango was first tasted.

Aspects of multiple-trace theory were implemented in a computational model (Nadel, Samsonovich, Ryan, & Moscovitch, 2000). This computational model formalized the role of multiple-trace formation with respect to the storage and retrieval of episodic memory. The model assumes that an episodic memory is dependent upon hippocampal–cortical connections that are formed initially and then replicated as multiple traces in the medial temporal lobe. Successful retrieval of an episodic memory is proportional to the number of traces formed for that memory. Several instantiations of the model were analyzed. The ones that successfully simulated findings of retrograde amnesia included a trace replication parameter that minimized replication rate as the memory aged. In essence, multiple-trace theory defines a "consolidation" or "stabilization" process in which memory representations are fixed by increased representation in the medial temporal lobe. It is assumed that stabilization of episodic memory is always dependent upon these multiple traces, though trace formation diminishes with the age of the memory. For semantic memory, it is suggested that at some time after initial trace formation, such memories do not depend upon hippocampal traces. Thus, unlike extant consolidation theories, multiple-trace theory suggests that consolidation or stabilization occurs as increased representation (i.e., multiple traces) in the medial temporal lobe, rather than as increased representation in neocortical regions. Moreover, multiple trace theory suggests that episodic memory retrieval is always dependent upon multiple traces formed in the medial temporal lobe.

Multiple-trace theory has been criticized on several grounds (Graham, 1999; Knowlton & Fanselow, 1998; but see Moscovitch & Nadel, 1998, 1999). Knowlton and Fanselow (1998) argue that temporal gradients in retrograde amnesia are often observed in both human and animal studies, *when damage is limited to the hippocampal complex*. Moreover, they acknowledge the role of the medial temporal lobe in the ability to retrieve information, when task demands require significant online referencing of retrieved information. That is, the act of recollection, particularly when it involves significant search and updating, should place heavy demands on accessing and manipulating information that was just retrieved. It is likely that episodic memory retrieval, such as remembering a childhood birthday party, requires such online processing and manipulation of retrieved fragments of memory. This act should certainly place demands on online executive control, such as those attributed to the prefrontal cortex (see Shimamura, 2000, in press). However, if such retrievals exceed the limits of working memory, then it is likely that the medial temporal lobe participates in facilitating the encoding of these retrieval acts. As such, Knowlton and Fanselow suggest that the medial temporal lobe may be involved in retrieving very remote memories, if task demands impose the need to encode and store information during the act of recollection.

RELATIONAL BINDING THEORY: A NEW ROLE FOR THE MEDIAL TEMPORAL LOBE IN MEMORY RETRIEVAL

A new formulation of consolidation theory, called "relational binding theory," is proposed here. The theory adheres to the five features of consolidation theory delineated above. As such, relational binding theory rejects the two major propositions of multiple-trace theory: (1) that stabilization of a learning event occurs as an increase in memory traces in the hippocampal complex (and not in neocortex), and (2) that the role of the medial temporal lobe is qualitatively different for episodic and semantic memory. Relational binding theory adds a new critical feature. It suggests that the medial temporal lobe, by way of relational binding of cortical–hippocampal connections, *contributes* to the access and retrieval of remote memories.

Consider instances in which a new fact is learned or a new episodic memory is formed. In both cases, learning involves the integration or binding of new information into existing knowledge. During the initial learning event, medial temporal processes bind cortical activations associated with the new memory representation. As explained by extant consolidation theories, the reactivation of cortical–hippocampal connections facilitates the stabilization of cortical networks. Relational binding theory adds to this conceptualization by suggesting that cortical–hippocampal connections that exist at the time of retrieval can be used as associative links to retrieving memories. That is, cortical–hippocampal connections act as shortcuts to retrieval and do not differentiate between "new" and "old" information stored in cortical regions.

Once a cortical–hippocampal connection is established, it can act as a link or bridge. At some time after binding, these connections may decay or may strengthen, depending on the frequency with which they are reactivated. The main point is that these connections not only are critical in reactivating recently bound associations, but also can aid in the retrieval of very remote memories. Retrieval of remote memories is facilitated by hippocampal–cortical connections to the extent that these connections act as efficient retrieval paths. According to this view, hippocampal–cortical connections are *necessary* for the reactivation of recently formed memories, and they also *contribute* to the retrieval of remote memories. By analogy, consider two new communities on opposite sides of a river that are linked by a new bridge. This bridge not only connects these two new communities, but also facilitates interactions between nearby (well-established) communities on opposite sides of the river. That is, the benefit of the bridge is more pervasive than simply linking the two new communities for which it was built. Similarly, the advantage of hippocampal–cortical connections is more pervasive than simply the binding of newly formed memories for which they were established.

Figure 5.1 depicts differences among standard consolidation theory, multiple-trace theory, and relational binding theory with respect to the retrieval of very remote memories. Standard consolidation theory suggests that cortical–hippocampal connections act as a support for the ultimate establishment of cortical–cortical connections. Thus the role of the medial temporal lobe is restricted to supporting or fixing of new representations while cortical–cortical connections are being formed. Retrieval of remote memories—that is, those

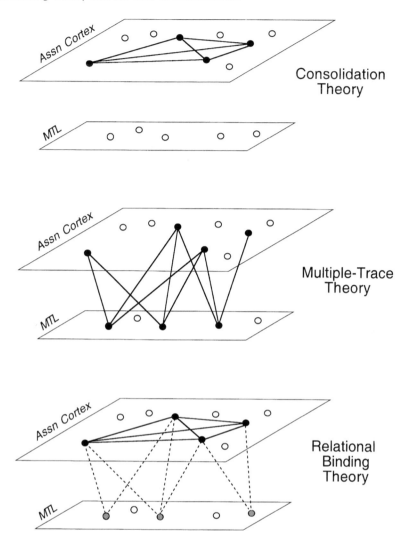

FIGURE 5.1. The role of medial temporal lobe function in retrieval of remote memories, as asserted by consolidation theory, multiple-trace theory, and relational binding theory. For each theory, a diagram represents cortical networks between association cortex (Assn Cortex) and medial temporal lobe (MTL) that are activated during retrieval of remote memories (solid lines and filled circles). According to consolidation theory, remote (i.e., already consolidated) memories are solely represented by cortical–cortical connections, and thus retrieval does not depend upon the medial temporal lobe. According to multiple-trace theory, remote (episodic) memories are established by traces formed in the medial temporal lobe that are always necessary for retrieval. According to relational binding theory, remote memories have been fixed as cortical–cortical connections, but retrieval can be facilitated by connections to the medial temporal lobe that exist during the time of retrieval (dashed lines, shaded circles).

that are presumed "fixed"—do not involve the medial temporal lobe. Multiple-trace theory suggests that stabilization of a memory representation is dependent upon multiple replications of traces within the medial temporal lobe. Thus all remote episodic memories necessarily depend upon these multiple traces. Relational binding theory suggests that the medial temporal lobe can contribute to retrieval of remote memories to the extent that hippocampal–cortical connections act as efficient retrieval paths. Relational binding theory suggests that retrieval of remote memories does not depend upon hippocampal–cortical connections, but it may be facilitated by them. As with standard consolidation theory, it is possible that well-established cortical representations, be they semantic or episodic in nature, may not depend upon the medial temporal lobe for retrieval.

The term "relational binding" characterizes the primary role of the medial temporal lobe. Such representations are relational in that they provide a context within which newly formed neural events are integrated with preexisting memory. "Relational memory" or similar terms have been used previously to indicate the same or similar conceptualizations (Cohen & Eichenbaum, 1993; Shimamura, 1996; see also Paller, 1997; Sutherland & Rudy, 1989; Teyler & DiScenna, 1986; Wickelgren, 1979). The conception has its primary roots in the consolidation view proposed by Squire (1992; Squire et al., 1984; Squire, Shimamura, & Amaral, 1989). In particular, relational binding acts as a support system for the establishment of cortical–cortical connections that are formed by the reactivation of hippocampal–cortical connections.

By contrast, multiple-trace theory suggests that the medial temporal lobe is differently involved for semantic and episodic representations. It is suggested that standard consolidation theory can explain the formation and retrieval of semantic memory, but cannot explain the formation and retrieval of episodic memory. According to relational binding theory, semantic and episodic representations need not be different with respect to medial temporal function. In fact, the distinction between episodic and semantic memory becomes diffuse and less useful when one considers such terms as "personal semantics" or "semanticized episodes." Typical tests of retrograde amnesia, such as tests of public events or famous faces, may be considered "semantic" or "episodic" in nature, presumably as a result of the degree of exposure to such events and celebrities. Rather than suggesting a qualitative difference between semantic and episodic memory, relational binding theory suggests that the primary difference between these two aspects of memories is quantitative. That is, the main difference between "episodic" and "semantic" memory is that semantic representations are typically more often reactivated than episodic representations.

Episodic memory, by definition, is constrained by a momentary experience locked in one place and one time. Thus, in some sense, every episodic memory has its unique spatiotemporal context that cannot be exactly repeated. However, one could reminisce on multiple occasions about a past autobiographical episode, such as the initial experience of tasting a mango. In other instances, aspects or parts of an episodic memory, such as dining at a favorite restaurant, could be represented or associated within multiple experiences. It is argued that the strength of any memory will depend on reactivations of associated representations. To the extent that parts of an episodic memory are reactivated, they will be facilitated by relational binding in the same manner as the consolidation of semantic memories. It is suggested by relational binding theory that a well-established episodic memory could ultimately depend solely on cortical–cortical representations for its retrieval. One could question whether such memory representations are "episodic" or "semantic." Multiple-trace theory, in its adherence to a qualitative difference between semantic and episodic memory, must contend with such a dilemma. Relational binding theory simply suggests that regardless of the type of memory representation, the ultimate formation (i.e., consolidation) of cortical–cortical connections depends upon the frequency with which representations are reactivated.

According to relational binding theory, semantic memory and episodic memory are treated similarly by the medial temporal lobe. These two forms of memory, however, may be represented somewhat differently in the neocortex. Both episodic and semantic memory are likely to be distributed widely in the neocortex. However, there is evidence that semantic memory has greater representation in the left than in the right hemisphere. For example, in patients with frontal–temporal dementia, left temporal damage is often associated with semantic memory impairment, whereas right-hemisphere damage is often associated with visuospatial or episodic memory impairment (Graham, Patterson, & Hodges, 1999; Hodges, Patterson, Oxbury, & Funnell, 1992). As semantic memory is more likely to be tied to verbal–lexical knowledge, and episodic memory is more likely to be tied to spatiovisual knowledge, it is reasonable to suggest some hemispheric laterality in processing semantic and episodic memory. As such, the left medial temporal lobe should be more involved in the consolidation of verbal–semantic memory, whereas the right medial temporal lobe should be more involved in the consolidation of spatial–episodic memory.

Relational binding theory predicts that patients with medial temporal lobe lesions will exhibit deficits on tests of very remote memory to the extent that retrieval can be facilitated by existing hippocampal–cortical connections. Thus, on demanding remote memory tests (such as tests involving the reconstruction of past episodes), patients with medial temporal lobe lesions may exhibit deficits for very remote memories. It is argued, however, that such lesions will always affect recent memories more than remote memories. Thus, with respect to standard views of consolidation theory, the main point is that relational binding theory does not necessarily predict complete preservation of old memories in patients with medial temporal lesions. Various reports suggest that such patients do exhibit remote memory impairment that affects retrieval of information learned at least 10–20 years prior to the onset of amnesia (see Nadel & Moscovitch, 1997; Rempel-Clower et al., 1996; Squire, Haist, & Shimamura, 1989).

Recent neuroimaging findings have suggested that the medial temporal lobe is active during retrieval of remote memories. Stark and Squire (2000) used fMRI to assess medial temporal lobe activity during retrieval after retention intervals of 30 minutes to 1 week. Across these retention intervals, greater medial temporal activity was observed for targets than for foils during tests of recognition memory. In another fMRI task, Ryan and colleagues (2000) asked subjects to recall details of recent events (less than 2 years old) and remote events (at least 20 years old, such as learning to drive or one's wedding day). Medial temporal activation was observed during retrieval of both recent and remote events. These neuroimaging findings suggest that the medial temporal lobe is active during memory retrieval. With respect to relational binding theory, they are consistent with the notion that hippocampal–cortical paths can contribute to retrieval.

By the relatively minor augmentation of traditional consolidation theory, relational binding theory resolves the criticisms of consolidation theory delineated by Nadel and Moscovitch (1997). That is, relational binding theory acknowledges that hippocampal–cortical connections present at the time of retrieval can be used as pathways to memory representations. Thus medial temporal lobe activation—as seen in neuroimaging studies—should occur during attempts to retrieve information. It should remain clear, however, that it is the process of consolidation that is providing these paths. Thus, as with traditional consolidation theory, the primary process associated with medial temporal function is the fixing or strengthening of cortical–cortical representations. With respect to neuropsychological and neuroimaging findings, relational binding theory and multiple-trace theory predict essentially the same general results. Neurobiologically, however, these two theories are diametrically opposed. Relational binding theory suggests that the medial temporal lobe will always be less involved as a memory becomes established. Multiple-trace theory predicts the opposite—that is, as a memory becomes established, its representation in the medial temporal lobe increases.

SUMMARY

In conclusion, extant consolidation theories have been criticized for their difficulty in accounting for long-lasting retrograde amnesia gradients. Multiple-trace theory was proposed as a way to account for impaired retrieval of remote episodic memory. Multiple-trace theory states that episodic memory, unlike semantic memory, is always dependent upon hippocampal–cortical connections, and that the facility of retrieval is based upon multiple traces formed in the hippocampal complex rather than traces formed in the neocortex. Relational binding theory draws on standard consolidation theory, though it differs by suggesting that hippocampal–cortical connections that exist at the time of retrieval can facilitate recollection of very remote memory. Relational binding theory does not depend upon the semantic–episodic distinction. Indeed, it is argued that the semantic–episodic distinction, though useful as a heuristic, loses its usefulness when certain aspects of episodic memory are described as semantic in nature or aspects of semantic memory are described as episodic in nature. Relational binding theory states that declarative memory is based on integrating (i.e., binding) new information with existing representations, regardless of whether representations are semantic or episodic in nature.

REFERENCES

Alvarez, P., & Squire, L. R. (1994). Memory consolidation and the medial temporal lobe: A simple network model. *Proceedings of the National Academy of Sciences USA, 91,* 7041–7045.

Burnham, W. H. (1903). Retroactive amnesia: Illustrative cases and a tentative explanation. *American Journal of Psychology, 14,* 382–396.

Cohen, N. J., & Eichenbaum, H. (Eds.). (1993). *Memory, amnesia, and the hippocampal system.* Cambridge, MA: MIT Press.

Gershberg, F. B., & Shimamura, A. P. (1998). The neuropsychology of human learning and memory. In J. L. Martinez, Jr., & R. P. Kesner, (Eds.), *Neurobiology of learning and memory* (pp. 333–359): San Diego, CA: Academic Press.

Glickman, S. E. (1961). Perseverative neural processes and consolidation of the memory trace. *Psychological Bulletin, 58,* 218–233.

Graham, K. S. (1999). Semantic dementia: A challenge to the multiple-trace theory of memory consolidation. *Trends in Cognitive Sciences, 3,* 85–87.

Graham, K. S., Patterson, K., & Hodges, J. R. (1999). Episodic memory: New insights from the study of semantic dementia. *Current Opinion in Neurobiology, 9,* 245–250.

Hodges, J. R., Patterson, K., Oxbury, S., & Funnell, E. (1992). Semantic dementia: Progressive fluent aphasia with temporal lobe atrophy. *Brain, 115,* 1783–1806.

Insausti, R., Amaral, D. G., & Cowan, W. M. (1987). The entorhinal cortex of the monkey: II. Cortical afferents. *Journal of Comparative Neurology, 264,* 356–395.

Knowlton, B. J., & Fanselow, M. S. (1998). The hippocampus, consolidation and on-line memory. *Current Opinion in Neurobiology, 8,* 293–296.

Lavenex, P., & Amaral, D. G. (2000). Hippocampal–neocortical interaction: A hierarchy of associativity. *Hippocampus, 10,* 420–430.

Marslen-Wilson, W. D., & Teuber, H.-L. (1975). Memory for remote events in anterograde amnesia: Recognition of public figures from news photographs. *Neuropsychologia, 13*, 353–364.

McClelland, J. L., McNaughton, B. L., & O'Reilly, R. C. (1995). Why there are complementary learning systems in the hippocampus and neocortex: Insights from the successes and failures of connectionist models of learning and memory. *Psychological Review, 102*, 419–437.

Moscovitch, M., & Nadel, L. (1998). Consolidation and the hippocampal complex revisited: In defense of the multiple-trace model. *Current Opinion Neurobiology, 8*, 297–300.

Moscovitch, M., & Nadel, L. (1999). Multiple-trace theory and semantic dementia: Response to K. S. Graham (1999). *Trends in Cognitive Sciences, 3*, 87–89.

Muller, G. E., & Pilzecker, A. (1900). Experimentelle Beiträge zur Lehre von Gedachtniss. *Zeitschrift für Psychologie und Physiologie der Sinnersorgans: Erganzungsband, 1*, 1–288.

Nadel, L., & Moscovitch, M. (1997). Memory consolidation, retrograde amnesia and the hippocampal complex. *Current Opinion in Neurobiology, 7*, 431–439.

Nadel, L., Samsonovich, A., Ryan, L., & Moscovitch, M. (2000). Multiple trace theory of human memory: Computational, neuroimaging, and neuropsychological results. *Hippocampus, 10*, 352–368.

Paller, K. A. (1997). Consolidating dispersed neocortical memories: The missing link in amnesia. In A. R. Mayes & J. J. Downes (Eds.), *Theories of organic amnesia* (pp. 73–88). Hove, England: Psychology Press.

Rempel-Clower, N. L., Zola, S. M., Squire, L. R., & Amaral, D. G. (1996). Three cases of enduring memory impairment after bilateral damage limited to the hippocampal formation. *Journal of Neuroscience, 16*, 5233–5255.

Ryan, L., Nadel, L., Keil, T., Putnam, K., Schayer, D., Troward, T., & Moscovitch, M. (2000). Hippocampal activation during retrieval of remote memories. *NeuroImage, 11*, 5396.

Schacter, D. L. (1987). Implicit memory: History and current status. *Journal of Experimental Psychology: Learning, Memory, and Cognition, 13*, 501–518.

Scoville, W. B., & Milner, B. (1957). Loss of recent memory after bilateral hippocampal lesions. *Journal of Neurology, Neurosurgery and Psychiatry, 20*, 11–21.

Shimamura, A. P. (1996). The organization of human memory: A neuropsychological analysis. In K. Ishiawa, J. L. McGaugh, & H. Sakata (Eds.), *Brain processes and memory* (pp. 165–173). Amsterdam: Elsevier.

Shimamura, A. P. (2000). The role of the prefrontal cortex in dynamic filtering. *Psychobiology, 28*, 207–218.

Shimamura, A. P. (in press). Memory retrieval and executive control processes. In D. Stuss & R. T. Knight (Eds.) *The frontal lobes*. New York: Oxford University Press.

Squire, L. R. (1987). *Memory and brain*. New York: Oxford University Press.

Squire, L. R. (1992). Memory and the hippocampus: A synthesis from findings with rats, monkeys, and humans. *Psychological Review, 99*, 195–231.

Squire, L. R., & Alvarez, P. (1995). Retrograde amnesia and memory consolidation: A neurobiological perspective. *Current Opinion in Neurobiology, 5*, 178–183.

Squire, L. R., Cohen, N. J., & Nadel, L. (1984). The medial temporal region and memory consolidation: A new hypothesis. In H. Weingartner & E. S. Parker (Eds.), *Memory consolidation: Psychobiology of cognition* (pp. 185–210). Hillsdale, NJ: Erlbaum.

Squire, L. R., Haist, F., & Shimamura, A. P. (1989). The neurology of memory: Quantitative assessment of retrograde amnesia in two groups of amnesic patients. *Journal of Neuroscience, 9*, 828–839.

Squire, L. R., Shimamura, A. P., & Amaral, D. G. (1989). Memory and the hippocampus. In J. H. Byrne & W. O. Berry (Eds.), *Neural models of plasticity: Experimental and theoretical approaches* (pp. 208–239). San Diego, CA: Academic Press.

Squire, L. R., & Zola, S. M. (1998). Episodic memory, semantic memory, and amnesia. *Hippocampus, 8*, 205–211.

Stark, C. E. L., & Squire, L. R. (2000). fMRI activity in the medial temporal lobe during recognition memory as a function of study–test interval. *Hippocampus, 10*, 329–337.

Sutherland, R. J., & Rudy, J. W. (1989). Configural association theory: The role of the hippocampal formation in learning, memory, and amnesia. *Psychobiology, 17,* 129–144.

Teyler, T. J., & DiScenna, P. (1986). The hippocampal memory indexing theory. *Behavioral Neuroscience, 100,* 147–154.

Wickelgren, W. A. (1979). Chunking and consolidation: A theoretical synthesis of semantic networks, configuring in conditioning, S-R versus cognitive learning, normal forgetting, the amnesic syndrome, and the hippocampal arousal system. *Psychological Review, 86,* 44–60.

6

Cross-Cortical Consolidation as the Core Defect in Amnesia

Prospects for Hypothesis Testing with Neuropsychology and Neuroimaging

KEN A. PALLER

Contemporary methods for monitoring human brain activity during cognition seem poised to power the next stages of advancement in the neuropsychology of memory. An ongoing goal is to map specific cognitive functions to particular brain regions. Beyond mere mapping, however, we must also envision how these functions are coordinated in intricate networks of neural circuits. Many details remain to be elucidated concerning how these networks enable us to accomplish ordinary and extraordinary feats of memory—such as assembling an immense storehouse of knowledge, recalling to mind specific events from many years ago, and maintaining some memories for a lifetime.

Noteworthy neuroscientific insights have been provided by studying many simpler forms of memory. This approach is beneficial, for example, because basic substrates for neural plasticity (e.g., as identified in *Aplysia*) may constitute the building blocks for *all* forms of memory. On the other hand, the neural events supporting *some* forms of memory are fundamentally distinct. Continued investigation of these distinctions may sharpen our abilities to categorize different types of memory. These efforts may simultaneously lead to a more comprehensive understanding of memory and to improvements in our memory classification schemes, which at present tend to rely heavily on behavioral criteria.

DECLARATIVE MEMORY

Observations of preserved and impaired memory in patients with amnesia indicate that the recall and recognition of facts and episodes, or "declarative memory," is dependent on a particular subset of brain regions and can be disrupted selectively. How can we develop a better understanding of this selectivity? Indeed, one might pose this question:

Why is declarative memory different from all other forms of memory?

Here are four answers to this question:

1. Because declarative memory has distinct behavioral characteristics.
2. Because declarative memory has distinct subjective characteristics.
3. Because declarative memory has a distinct cognitive structure.
4. Because declarative memory has distinct neural substrates.

Memory theorists tend to give one or another of these answers greater emphasis, as discussed further below. In any event, determining precisely how each of these criteria map onto the others is an important goal for future research. Toward this end, a useful strategy may be to favor some defining criteria over others. To be more specific about these four sorts of criteria, here are four possible descriptions of the characteristics of declarative memory corresponding to these four answers:

1. Memory performance produced during recall and recognition tests for facts and episodes.
2. Memory that is accompanied by the experience of conscious recollection.
3. Memory that depends on retrieving a conjunction of distinct informational fragments.
4. Memory that requires cross-cortical consolidation (which is mediated by cortico-hippocampal and corticothalamic networks, and which leads to the gradual formation of new coherence ensembles).

Despite widespread agreement about the selectivity of memory deficits in amnesia, a pervasive problem for research in this area is how to arrive at a generally agreed-upon definition for the type of memory that is impaired in amnesia. Although terms such as "explicit memory," "conscious memory," and "aware memory" have been used in this context, sometimes synonymously, here I will rely on the term "declarative memory." One reasonable tactic is to acknowledge that definitions of declarative memory can be allowed to evolve gradually, so that as its unique characteristics become substantiated, they are folded into the definition. The definition can then freely include behavioral, subjective, cognitive, and neural characteristics. On the other hand, there are advantages to the approach of holding to a behavioral definition of declarative memory. The research agenda can then be described as mapping neural, cognitive, and subjective facets of declarative memory onto each other and onto a static behavioral definition.

Figure 6.1 shows a scheme for relating descriptions of declarative memory at different levels. A complete understanding of disorders of declarative memory should describe the three-way connections among the neural dysfunction, the cognitive dysfunction, and the resultant behavioral shortcomings. In the same manner, the neural, cognitive, and behavioral realms must be bridged by a neurocognitive conceptualization of normal declarative memory.

In the coming years, advances in the neuropsychology of memory can be expected from both studies of patients with memory deficits (traditional neuropsychology) and studies of neural events that accompany normal memory phenomena (neuroimaging). Moreover, attempts to combine neuropsychology and neuroimaging should be situated within the context of contemporary theories of memory informed from both psychological and neuroscientific perspectives. In this chapter, I articulate several hypotheses about declarative memory and amnesia, and then consider prospects for future applications of neuroimaging methods to build on the insights from neuropsychology.

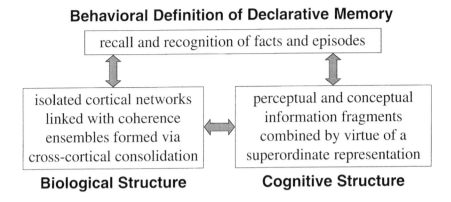

FIGURE 6.1. The three-way theoretical connections among behavior, biology, and cognition that are necessary for a comprehensive understanding of declarative memory. Declarative memory is defined behaviorally, and a neurocognitive theory of declarative memory is depicted in terms of both biological and cognitive structure.

A NEURAL FEATURE OF DECLARATIVE MEMORY: CROSS-CORTICAL CONSOLIDATION

The central hypothesis to be explored here is that *declarative memories characteristically require cross-cortical consolidation*—a process mediated by the confluence of corticothalamic and corticohippocampal networks. The information inherent in personally experienced events and complex facts is stored within a set of distinct zones of the cerebral cortex, each of which is dedicated for processing a specific type of information. Although gaps remain in our ability to describe how information is coded by neuronal connections within and between neocortical zones, it is clear that these zones are specialized for distinct functions. Autobiographical memories are distant reflections of episodes that were originally experienced and understood via information processing in many different neocortical regions. Episodes generally entail a set of attributes (Underwood, 1969), such as a spatial layout of environmental features, sights, sounds, smells, motion, other people, goals, actions, emotional coloring, timing with respect to other events, and so on. Given that major aspects of an episode are represented at distant brain loci, storage of that episode must include new cross-cortical connections. Episodic memory storage depends on a memory trace corresponding to each of these attributes, as well as connections between them. The cortical fragments must be linked together in order for the representation of the episode to survive as a unit to be remembered later.

In short, a memory for an episode inherently has a strong dependence on cross-cortical storage. Whether this applies to memory for facts may depend on how "fact" is defined. When complex information is learned (e.g., factual knowledge about the world expressed as a statement; Shimamura & Squire, 1987), cross-cortical storage may be responsible. On the other hand, when minimal factual knowledge is acquired (e.g., a simple three-word combination; Tulving, Hayman, & Macdonald, 1991), information minimally sufficient to support that learning may be stored within a single neocortical zone responsible for one domain of specialized semantic information. Explicitly stating that this consolidation process is cross-cortical is also important, given that other sorts of consolidation may occur for other sorts of memory and in other brain regions (see, e.g., Brashers-Krug, Shadmehr, & Bizzi, 1996; Gais, Plihal, Wagner, & Born, 2000). Although linking together separate representations in different cortical regions is considered an essential step in the creation of an enduring declarative memory, additional processing at the time of retrieval is also critical. Prefrontal contributions to declarative memory, in particular, come into play here (see, e.g., Knight & Grabowecky, 1995; Shimamura, 1995; Wheeler, Stuss, & Tulving, 1997). Retrieval requirements include conducting a systematic search for stored information, evaluating the products of retrieval and assessing relevance to the task at hand, escaping from the present moment to bring a prior experience to mind, maintaining information in working memory, inhibiting the intrusion of irrelevant information, constructing a scenario within which retrieved information is put together, evaluating the likelihood of different scenarios, and so on.

Establishing long-lasting links between cortical fragments must, of course, be distinguished from establishing analogous but temporary bindings in the present moment, as occurs when an event is experienced. Amnesic patients apparently experience events normally and are able to maintain that information while it stays at the focus of attention (see, e.g., Cave & Squire, 1992). It is in this sense that we claim that encoding can be normal in amnesia. Amnesic patients can form cross-cortical associations temporarily, such that factual or episodic information can be represented and effectively support immediate memory or working memory. The difficulty is in storing that information in an enduring way.

Cross-cortical consolidation proceeds when a set of neuronal ensembles in the neocortex is repeatedly activated, as has been assumed in computational models of consolidation (e.g., McClelland, McNaughton, & O'Reilly, 1995; Murre, 1997; Squire & Alvarez, 1995). A distributed cortical network ultimately represents the remembered information, but it starts out in an unstable form at the time of encoding. The memory generally includes representations of discrete components of an event at multiple levels of relevant perceptual processing streams. Consolidation produces a stable network of distributed cortical representations, but it is not conceptualized here as a passive or automatic process that inevitably runs its course. Rather, consolidation proceeds as the memory is actively used. Components of the network are loosely connected via interposed limbic connections, in such a way that partial information can cue the retrieval of the whole memory (as in "pattern completion"; McClelland et al., 1995; Squire, 1992; Treves & Rolls, 1994). These limbic connections are formed swiftly at encoding so as to unify the distinct cortical components, but the connections are not long-lasting and gradually become less effective with disuse. Importantly, when these connections are used to reactivate the distributed cortical representation for a declarative memory, I have speculated that the process of cross-cortical consolidation is moved forward in a particular way that involves the gradual formation of new neuronal ensembles in the cortex, termed "coherence ensembles" (Paller, 1997).

ANOTHER NEURAL FEATURE OF DECLARATIVE MEMORY: COHERENCE ENSEMBLES

Whenever the network of neocortical neuronal ensembles is activated, one commonly proposed outcome is a strengthening of the corticocortical connections between parts of the network. In contrast, cross-cortical consolidation is here conceptualized as depending on additional neural changes. The network reactivation coincides not only with memory retrieval, but also with associations between that memory and other memories, and with changes to the declarative memory representation in question. The memory may lose some detail, and also gain new meaning in the context of the associations. It may be categorized with other memories. It may also come to be interpreted in a new way in the light of subsequent events. Consolidation proceeds whether or not the individual is intending to memorize or rehearse the memory; it proceeds in conjunction with any associative processing that involves that memory. As the memory takes on additional meaning by taking its place in the context of other stored knowledge, other neurons come to represent this higher-order meaning or thematic information. These other neurons may be located in adjacent portions of the temporal lobe (such as entorhinal cortex or the temporal pole) and perhaps in other areas (such as orbitofrontal cortex, retrosplenial cortex, or posterior cingulate). I refer to these hypothetical neuronal ensembles as "coherence ensembles" (Paller, 1997) because they function to provide coherence to the neocortical fragments that constitute a declarative memory. At the same time, they take over the function of representing the central, superordinate meaning of the memory, including its relationship to other memories and its place within autobiographical and/or general semantic frameworks (akin to "thematic retrieval frameworks"; Hodges & McCarthy, 1995). When coherence ensembles are activated and the gist of the memory is retrieved, their connections enable specifics of the memory to be retrieved. Hippocampal neurons initially participate in this reactivation of a memory, whereas later the newly formed coherence ensembles are sufficient to accomplish this.

Many of the present speculations regarding cross-cortical consolidation and coherence ensembles present prime opportunities to use neuroimaging to seek novel sorts of empirical evidence relevant to these issues. At the same time, this conceptualization of consolidation has much in common with views from many other memory theorists. The memory-indexing theory of Teyler and DiScenna (1986), for example, also suggests that the hippocampus is involved in connecting sets of neocortical ensembles while a cortically based memory is established incrementally. Squire, Cohen, and Nadel (1984) described a consolidation process in which neocortical activity is modified by input from the hippocampal region, leading to neocortical reorganization (see also Damasio, 1989; Eichenbaum, 2000; Halgren, 1984; Marr, 1971; Mesulam, 1998; Milner, 1989; O'Keefe & Nadel, 1978; O'Reilly & Rudy, 2001; Wickelgren, 1979). Nonetheless, one distinctive aspect of the current conceptualization is that new representations, instantiated by neuronal coherence ensembles, are proposed to take over the function of reactivating the array of neocortical loci.

RETROGRADE AMNESIA, ONGOING HIPPOCAMPAL CONTRIBUTIONS, AND SLEEP

What would happen if coherence ensembles were damaged while other medial temporal circuitry was left intact? This condition may constitute a description of damage to critical storage zones leading to focal retrograde amnesia (Kapur, 1993; Markowitsch, 1995; but see Kopelman, 2000). Retrograde impairments could present along with a relatively preserved (though not entirely unaffected) ability to form new declarative memories. This impairment could make old memories inaccessible, because the fragments would be present in the cortex but not connected, so that the episode could no longer be reassembled. Likewise, circumscribed damage to lateral temporal regions may lead to semantic dementia, with remote memories disrupted more than recent memories (Hodges & Graham, 1998). Differential loss of autobiographical versus general semantic information could also be explained if different sorts of coherence ensembles were not randomly scattered about, but functionally clustered in different regions.

Heterogeneity of symptoms in amnesic patients, and dissociations between anterograde and retrograde impairments, may then be explained as follows. A core amnesia with retrograde and anterograde deficits results from brain damage to either corticothalamic or corticohippocampal networks. In severe cases, damage to major portions of the medial temporal region disrupts cross-cortical consolidation entirely and also destroys previously established coherence ensembles. The extent of retrograde impairment depends on the extent to which coherence ensembles are also destroyed. Retrograde memory loss for long time periods results from extensive damage to cortical coherence ensembles. Retrograde deficits are observed in a relatively pure fashion when a subset of established coherence ensembles is damaged, leaving the major machinery for cross-cortical consolidation intact. Other retrieval problems with respect to search, organization, and evaluation emerge and contribute to the memory disorder with additional prefrontal damage.

Whether hippocampal neurons continue to participate after cross-cortical consolidation produces a durable memory remains a question currently under active debate (Nadel & Moscovitch, 1997; Nadel, Samsonovich, Ryan, & Moscovitch, 2000). According to the present view, if an episode continues to be recalled periodically (as is the case for most significant life episodes), new associations will be formed with other events. If a memory is not totally isolated from the rest of an individual's ongoing experiences, it may continue to change rather than remain in a static state. In this sense, cross-cortical consolidation may continue indefinitely. Continued dependence on the hippocampus is determined by the extent to which the fact or episode in question continues to be associatively processed with new information and to evolve accordingly. There may thus be two distinct means for long periods of retrograde amnesia to be produced. One cause would be significant damage to cortical storage zones, and, in particular, to coherence ensembles essential for retrieving declarative memories. The other cause would be prolonged disruption of the hippocampus and related circuitry, so as to disrupt continuing cross-cortical consolidation of remote memories that would otherwise be strengthened through recurring associations with other information (including subsequent episodes of retelling the story to others). As mentioned earlier, deficits in intentional retrieval, such as those produced by frontal damage, could also contribute to failures to consolidate and to retrieve declarative memories. Even in the absence of neurological dysfunction, memories of the contextual details of an episode tend to be difficult to maintain, because they are so heavily based on the singular initial experience of the episode. As time goes by, contextual details of an episode are postulated either to be forgotten or to be represented in the neocortex and linked together with other recallable aspects of the episode by virtue of coherence ensembles. An episodic memory can become thoroughly integrated with other stored information and largely devoid of distinctive contextual detail, and can eventually come to constitute a semantic memory (Cermak, 1984).

Finally, it should be noted that the repeated activation of the neocortical network that is critical for cross-cortical consolidation occurs not only when the memory is retrieved intentionally, but also when it is retrieved unintentionally, and perhaps particularly when retrieval occurs during sleep. Indeed, a high proportion of dreams incorporate recent events of the day or the past several days, such that the consolidation of an episodic memory may progress significantly during the first few nights after the event occurs. Moreover, if dreams provide an opportunity for evaluating possible solutions to ongoing life issues, recent events can be related to long-term goals accordingly. Consolidation will continue to occur to the extent that related events occur on subsequent days. Empirical support for these ideas concerning consolidation during sleep is relatively sparse, although there are several lines of supportive evidence (e.g., Stickgold, 1998; Sutherland & McNaughton, 2000; Winson, 1985).

BEYOND DECLARATIVE MEMORY: QUESTIONS OF DEFINITION

The memory dysfunction in amnesia is not strictly limited to declarative memory. Damage to medial temporal or medial diencephalic brain regions can produce both a deficit in storing declarative memories *and* deficits in certain other types of memory that fall near definitional borders, such as some variations on simple classical conditioning (see, e.g., Gluck, Ermita, Oliver, & Myers, 1997) and some types of new-association priming (see, e.g., Cermak, Bleich, & Blackford, 1988; Paller & Mayes, 1994; Schacter & Graf, 1986; Shimamura & Squire, 1989; but see Gabrieli, Keane, Zarella, & Poldrack, 1997). Some memory phenomena that would normally fall within the category of nondeclarative memory, but that are not preserved in amnesia, should perhaps be reclassified within a new subcategory of nondeclarative memory. The category could be called "nondeclarative memory that depends on neocortical associations."

Would it be a good idea to choose to define new types of memory based on neurobiological criteria instead of behavioral criteria? If so, another possible category would be "cross-cortical consolidation memory," which depends on neocortical associations that require cross-cortical consolidation, and which includes both declarative and nondeclarative varieties. This neural distinction might be the best way to carve nature at the joints. And yet it also risks the danger of circular definitions, given that we don't have an objective marker for cross-cortical consolidation. Future research should pursue this goal. In the meantime, should we continue using current definitions of declarative memory (or explicit memory, conscious memory, or aware memory), or should we define new memory categories in order to cover all the memory abilities impaired in amnesia?

Some researchers have advocated using cognitive criteria to define the type of memory impaired in amnesia. Qualities such as "flexible," "configural," "relational," or "dependent on complex associations" can be emphasized (see, e.g., Cohen & Eichenbaum, 1993; Eichenbaum, 2000; Ryan, Althoff, Whitlow, & Cohen, 2000). But should these attributes be central to the definition of declarative memory? This approach might meet with the same circularity problems as would making the neural criteria central to the definition. Definitions of such terms as "relational" or "flexible" are themselves rather flexible in practice, though operational definitions are possible. Moreover, it is likely that attributes such as "relational" can apply to some memories that are not stored in the cortex and that should be considered nondeclarative, such as some complex motor memories and habits. When a new memory phenomenon is demonstrated via some novel behavioral paradigm, objectively determining whether it depends either on cross-cortical consolidation or on complex associations of some sort may present a challenge.

Until ways to surmount these challenges are well established, it may be best to maintain the behavioral definition of declarative memory as referring to the recall and recognition of facts and episodes, while at the same time hypothesizing neurocognitive reasons for why declarative memory is different from all other types of memory. Cross-cortical consolidation is presumably necessary for normal declarative memory, and it is here hypothesized to be the core defect in amnesia. Importantly, cross-cortical consolidation is also necessary for certain types of associative nondeclarative memory that likewise depend on dispersed neocortical representations.

DECLARATIVE MEMORY AND CONSCIOUS RECOLLECTION

The approach outlined above provides a natural segregation between declarative memory and conscious recollection as follows. "Conscious recollection," the subjective experience of remembering, appears to be contingent on declarative memory, and it tends to happen in concert with the recall and recognition of facts and episodes. Although recollection is central to definitions of aware memory, conscious memory, and explicit memory, it is not formally part of the definition of declarative memory advocated here. Rather, recollection is an additional phenomenon that depends on some of the same neurocognitive substrates as declarative memory. Cross-cortical consolidation is a necessary but not sufficient condition for the conscious recollection of a declarative memory. Cross-cortical consolidation allows a set of isolated cortical networks to become linked together, and once linked in this manner, the composite set of networks corresponds to a declarative memory. This memory can then become accessible to conscious awareness when the distributed cortical representation is reactivated.

Indeed, a central function of corticothalamic connections in declarative memory may be in the temporary activation of the distributed declarative memory. As such, this role may constitute a key difference between the functions of corticothalamic and corticohippocampal networks. Speculatively, the thalamic neurons that are particularly relevant here may be the same neurons characterized neurochemically as calbindin cells that form a so-called "thalamic matrix" (Jones, 1998), given that they are found in all thalamic nuclei and project widely to superficial cortical locations. Medial thalamic connections to multiple cortical regions may be able to support the conscious experience of a remembered event, together with prefrontal networks that support working memory. Medial thalamic damage could thus indirectly disrupt cortical function (Paller et al., 1997). The medial diencephalic contribution to conscious recollection may also entail inhibiting other potential conscious contents, so as to facilitate the conscious retrieval of the memory. Although further evidence is needed on this point, it is conceivable that thalamic control networks are critical for consolidation because they can support both the retrieval and activation of a distributed declarative memory, which thus sets the stage for consolidation to proceed through the action of corticohippocampal networks, as coherence ensembles are formed and strengthened.

NEUROIMAGING AND DECLARATIVE MEMORY

Empirical tests of hypotheses such as those developed above can be expected not only from studies of amnesic patients, but also from monitoring neural activity while memories are normally formed and expressed. In fact, neuroimaging in humans may present fruitful avenues for advancing theories couched at this level. The term "neuroimaging" is used here in the wider sense to refer to techniques that make it possible to observe neural activity or correlated hemodynamic changes, either in specific brain regions or with sufficient temporal resolution to monitor changes in neural activity as cognitive events unfold in time, or both. I place particular emphasis on neurophysiological methods for recording event-related potentials (ERPs), which may be useful for charting the time course of relevant memory processing and ultimately, in conjunction with other neuroimaging measures, for deciphering the dynamics of brain network interactions. Issues that arise in taking this approach apply to multiple methods for monitoring brain activity (e.g., MEG, fMRI, PET, EEG responses in the frequency domain, optical imaging, etc.).

So how can we observe the neural events responsible for forming and remembering declarative memories? One useful step is to make comparisons between declarative memory and other types of memory, in order to search for specific ways in which the neurocognitive structure of declarative memory is distinctive. This approach may not be effective, however, if presumed associations between neural measures and cognitive operations are not valid. Given that our working hypotheses strongly influence how we conceive of the cognitive functions in question, the inaccuracy of our current theories about the component processes of memory may corrupt our observations, and so hamper our ability to test our hypotheses. Fortunately, our understanding of memory can move forward on many fronts simultaneously. For example, better conceptualizations of how information is represented in the cortex may affect how we think about the storage of declarative memories in the cortex (e.g., Mesulam, 1998), which may then lead to corresponding refinements of our views on the component processes of memory.

Observations of neural activity associated with encoding and retrieval are clearly needed to support continuing theoretical progress. Whether these observations can be connected to current theories, and to future theories, may depend on the extent to which valid and specific associations are made between the neural measures and discrete cognitive events. Memory functions, however, can be difficult to isolate. Encoding and retrieval, in particular, do not occur *only* when an experimenter instructs a subject to store or recall information, respectively. So how can neural measures extracted from the EEG be tightly associated with the neurocognitive events responsible for declarative memory?

To start to answer this question, we may first note that differential EEG responses to remembered items in recognition tests, as compared to responses to new items, constitute a robust electrophysiological phenomenon tied to declarative memory (see reviews by Friedman & Johnson, 2000; Mecklinger, 2000; Paller, 2000; Rugg & Wilding, 2000). ERPs recorded at the time of retrieval differ systematically between old and new items in both explicit and implicit memory tests. Presumably, these "ERP repetition effects" reflect several cognitive events potentially related to memory retrieval. Given the foregoing discussion, it is clearly appropriate to determine the extent to which observed neural activity specifically reflects component processes of declarative memory.

In my laboratory, we have used several methods for gaining this specificity. Contrasts between responses to test items associated with different levels of memory performance have been particularly informative. In several experiments, two types of studied words gave rise to perceptual priming effects of the same magnitude, but provoked very different levels of recognition accuracy. We inferred that the contrast could be recast in terms of high and low recollection, such that corresponding ERP differences could be interpreted as electrophysiological correlates of recollecting declarative memories, devoid of any confounding influence related to perceptual priming (Gonsalves & Paller, 2000a; Paller & Kutas, 1992; Paller, Kutas, & McIsaac, 1995; see also Paller, Bozic, Ranganath, Grabowecky, & Yamada, 1999, for similar effects with faces).

A variation on the same basic strategy was used in other experiments, such that conditions were set up to provide a contrast between words associated with similar levels of recognition but systematically different levels of perceptual priming. As a result, brain potentials were linked to neural events underlying perceptual priming restricted to the level of visual word form (Paller & Gross, 1998; Paller, Kutas, & McIsaac, 1998). These electrophysiological correlates of visual word-form priming were most prominent at occipital scalp locations and occurred at a latency slightly earlier than that typically found for electrophysiological correlates of visual word recollection (Figure 6.2). Neuroimaging studies using PET and fMRI suggest that perceptual priming may result from decreased neural activity following percep-

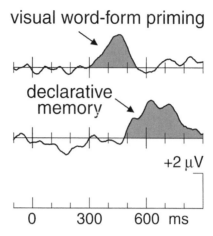

FIGURE 6.2. Brain potentials specifically associated with declarative memory and one type of nondeclarative memory, priming of visual word form. The upper waveform was computed by subtracting brain potentials elicited by words previously viewed forward or backward; priming was greater in the former than in the latter condition. Data from Paller and Gross (1998). The lower waveform was computed by subtracting brain potentials elicited by words previously studied with emphasis on visual imagery versus orthographic processing; recollection was stronger in the former than in the latter condition. Data from Paller and Kutas (1992).

tual learning (Schacter & Buckner, 1998; Wiggs & Martin, 1998). Furthermore, MEG evidence concerning the timing of repetition-related changes implicates top-down influences on earlier cortical regions, rather than effects on initial stages of sensory information processing (Dale et al., 2000). Electrophysiological correlates of perceptual priming can also be revealed in recordings from single neurons in monkey visual cortex. In particular, some neurons in ventral temporal areas tend to show reduced responses during stimulus repetition—a phenomenon termed "repetition suppression" (Desimone, 1996). Combining results from these different methods may lead to a better understanding of priming, as well as a better understanding of how priming is different from declarative memory.

In addition, however, we will also need more thorough evaluations of neural correlates of recollection that will allow us to decompose the various steps that lead to recollection. Many neuroimaging studies have tackled these questions—for example, by manipulating the type of information that subjects retrieve during a recognition test (e.g., Johnson, Kounios, & Noble, 1997; Ranganath, Johnson, & D'Esposito, 2000; Ranganath & Paller, 1999, 2000; Wilding, 2000). However, much controversy currently surrounds our ability to empirically separate retrieval success, retrieval effort, and other processes relevant for retrieval (see review by Rugg & Wilding, 2000).

Memory research using ERPs has not only focused on the retrieval phase, but also on neural events that take place at the time of encoding. Many studies have shown that both hemodynamic and electrophysiological measures can be predictive of later declarative memory performance (for review, see Wagner, Koutstaal, & Schacter, 1999). These effects are sometimes termed "Dm" as a shorthand for neural _d_ifferences based on later _m_emory performance (Paller, Kutas, & Mayes, 1987). In a recent example of this sort of work, ERPs were recorded in response to pictures of common objects and to corresponding words presented during a study phase (Gonsalves & Paller, 2000b). When the words were shown, subjects were instructed to generate a visual image of the object. For half of the words, a picture of that object was never presented. Nevertheless, subjects later claimed to remember some of the non-presented pictures that were only imagined; these can be considered "false memories" or "source-monitoring errors" (Johnson, Hashtroudi, & Lindsay, 1993; Schacter, Norman, & Koutstaal, 1998). As shown in Figure 6.3, ERPs in response to words differed according to whether the items would later be falsely remembered or not. These ERP differences were interpreted as reflections of visual imagery generated in response to the words, given that similar ERPs in a prior experiment were shown to vary systematically as a function of the extent to which visual imagery was engaged (Gonsalves & Paller, 2000a). Other ERPs in response to pictures also differed systematically in amplitude according to whether the picture would be accurately recognized later. Neural activity observed at encoding thus influenced the outcome of later recognition testing, both for accurate and for false memories. Furthermore, similar ERPs were also recorded during retrieval, and the amplitude of these ERPs was larger for accurate picture memories than for false memories, suggesting that visual imagery was less vivid for false memories.

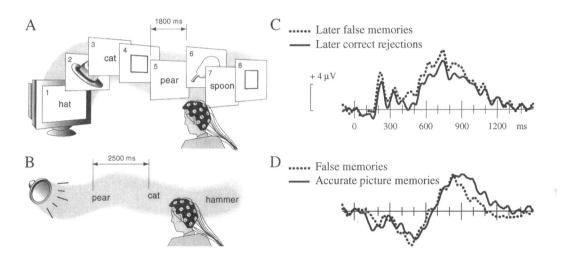

FIGURE 6.3. Behavioral paradigm and electrophysiological results from an investigation of false memories (Gonsalves & Paller, 2000b). (A) In the study phase, subjects viewed a series of words and were required to make a size judgment for each one ("Is the object larger or smaller than the video monitor?"). Half of the words were followed by a color image of the corresponding object, and half were followed by an empty rectangle. (B) In the test phase, subjects listened to a series of words and were required to decide whether the corresponding image had been viewed during the study phase. When a subject claimed to remember seeing a picture that was only imagined, these trials were designated "false memories." (C) ERPs recorded to words in the study phase (from the midline occipital scalp location) differed at 600–900 milliseconds according to whether a false memory occurred in the test phase for that item. (D) Midline occipital ERPs recorded to auditory words in the test phase differed at 900–1,200 milliseconds according to whether that trial constituted an accurate memory or a false memory. These potentials were interpreted as indications of visual imagery that was recapitulated at retrieval for pictures either perceived in the study phase or, to a lesser extent, imagined in the study phase. A and B are from de Schipper, S. (2000, December 2). Sterke verbeelding: Valse herinnering blijkt uit hersengolven [Strong imagination: False memory is evident from brainwaves]. *NRC Handelsblad*, p. 47. Copyright 2000 by *NRC Handelsblad*. Adapted by permission. Data in C and D from Gonsalves and Paller (2000b).

Thus it is possible to monitor relevant neural activity both at encoding and at retrieval using ERPs. Yet, as stated above, the core defect in amnesia is postulated to be at storage rather than at encoding or retrieval. How should future theory-driven research attempt to promote advances in our understanding of consolidation? According to the views expressed above, storage and retrieval are intertwined, because cross-cortical consolidation entails retrieval. Therefore, one way to study consolidation would be to observe neural activity during a retrieval event wherein associations are made and the memory in question is strengthened. It may also be helpful if distinct cortical networks can be monitored as consolidation proceeds. The configuration of cortical networks involved in an episodic memory might be expected to change over time in ways that implicate storage processes. For example, informative differences may emerge if comparisons can be made between declarative memories that are matched in strength but systematically differ in only the number of distinct types of information linked together to form the memory. There are also many open questions regarding the role of the hippocampus and whether this role changes over the lifetime of a memory. If hippocampal contributions decrease over time, one might expect that new activity corresponding to the formation of coherence ensembles might emerge in other brain locations. Although there is not currently an abundance of evidence that can be brought to bear on these and many other related questions about human memory, approaches utilizing scalp and intracranial ERP recordings and fMRI time series analyses do hold promise for clarifying these issues. The further addition of deactivation studies using transcranial magnetic stimulation may also be useful.

Finally, a coming together of neuropsychology and neuroimaging can also be expected in studies with patients suffering from memory disorders (e.g., Eustache, Desgranges, Aupee, Guillery, & Baron, 2000; Olichney et al., 2000). Structural neuroimaging in patients tells only part of the story, in that the pattern of cognitive deficits must be related not only to sites of structural damage but also to distant neural dysfunction that results from the structural damage. Patients with alcoholic Korsakoff's syndrome, for example, have patterns of glucose hypometabolism that suggest cortical dysfunction secondary to thalamic damage (Paller et al., 1997). Future neuroimaging research may thus be able to reveal other indications of impaired cross-cortical consolidation.

In conclusion, theory-driven research into the neurocognitive structure of human memory can receive support from neuropsychological studies of amnesic patients and from neuroimaging studies in healthy and memory-impaired populations. The combination of neuropsychology and neuroimaging will certainly produce new perspectives on neurobiological hypotheses about declarative memory. Previously it may have appeared that some speculations couched at the level of neural networks—as exemplified by groups of temporarily connected neuronal ensembles, unitized representations in discrete cortical zones, a linking process for dispersed neocortical representations based on corticothalamic and corticohippocampal networks, and the concept of coherence ensembles—were hypotheses about human memory that could not easily be addressed in humans. Now, due to methodological advances in cognitive neuroscience, we can more easily envision how hypotheses like these can be put to proper empirical test using a range of techniques for studying the human brain.

ACKNOWLEDGMENTS

Research funding from the National Institute of Neurological Disorders and Stroke is gratefully acknowledged. I also wish to thank Paul Reber, Marcia Grabowecky, Marsel Mesulam, Dan Schacter, and Larry Squire for their support and helpful discussion.

REFERENCES

Brashers-Krug, T., Shadmehr, R., & Bizzi, E. (1996). Consolidation in human motor memory. *Nature, 382,* 252–255.

Cave, C. B., & Squire, L. R. (1992). Intact verbal and nonverbal short-term memory following damage to the human hippocampus. *Hippocampus, 2,* 151–163.

Cermak, L. S. (1984). The episodic–semantic distinction in amnesia. In L. R. Squire & N. Butters (Eds.), *Neuropsychology of memory* (pp. 55–62). New York: Guilford Press.

Cermak, L. S., Bleich, R. P., & Blackford, S. P. (1988). Deficits in the implicit retention of new associations by alcoholic Korsakoff patients. *Brain and Cognition, 7,* 145–156.

Cohen, N. J., & Eichenbaum, H. (1993). *Memory, amnesia, and the hippocampal system.* Cambridge, MA: MIT Press.

Dale, A. M., Liu, A. K., Fischl, B. R., Buckner, R. L., Belliveau, J. W., Lewine, J. D., & Halgren, E. (2000). Dynamic statistical parametric mapping: Combining fMRI and MEG for high-resolution imaging of cortical activity. *Neuron, 26,* 55–67.

Damasio, A. R. (1989). Time-locked multiregional retroactivation: A systems-level proposal for the neural substrates of recall and recognition. *Cognition, 33,* 25–62.

Desimone, R. (1996). Neural mechanisms for visual memory and their role in attention. *Proceedings of the National Academy of Sciences USA, 93,* 13494–13499.

Eichenbaum, H. (2000). A cortical–hippocampal system for declarative memory. *Nature Reviews Neuroscience, 1,* 41–50.

Eustache, F., Desgranges, B., Aupee, A. M., Guillery, B., & Baron, J. C. (2000). Functional neuroanatomy of amnesia: Positron emission tomography studies. *Microscopy Research and Technique, 51,* 94–100.

Friedman, D., & Johnson, R., Jr. (2000). Event-related potential (ERP) studies of memory encoding and retrieval: A selective review. *Microscopy Research and Technique, 51,* 6–28.

Gabrieli, J. D. E., Keane, M. M., Zarella, M. M., & Poldrack, R. A. (1997). Preservation of implicit memory for new associations in global amnesia. *Psychological Science, 8,* 326–329.

Gais, S., Plihal, W., Wagner, U., & Born, J. (2000). Early sleep triggers memory for early visual discrimination skills. *Nature Neuroscience, 3,* 1335–1339.

Gluck, M. A., Ermita, B. R., Oliver, L. M., & Myers, C. E. (1997). Extending models of hippocampal function in animal conditioning to human amnesia. *Memory, 5,* 179–212.

Gonsalves, B., & Paller, K. A. (2000a). Brain potentials associated with recollective processing of spoken words. *Memory and Cognition, 28,* 321–330.

Gonsalves, B., & Paller, K. A. (2000b). Neural events that underlie remembering something that never happened. *Nature Neuroscience, 3,* 1316–1321.

Halgren, E. (1984). Human hippocampal and amygdala recording and stimulation: Evidence for a neural model of recent memory. In L. R. Squire & N. Butters (Eds.), *Neuropsychology of memory* (pp. 165–182). New York: Guilford Press.

Hodges, J. R., & Graham, K. S. (1998). A reversal of the temporal gradient for famous person knowledge in semantic dementia: Implications for the neural organisation of long-term memory. *Neuropsychologia, 36,* 803–825.

Hodges, J. R., & McCarthy, R. A. (1995). Loss of remote memory: A cognitive neuropsychological perspective. *Current Opinion in Neurobiology, 5,* 178–183.

Johnson, M. K., Hashtroudi, S., & Lindsay, D. S. (1993). Source monitoring. *Psychological Bulletin, 114,* 3–28.

Johnson, M. K., Kounios, J., & Nolde, S. F. (1997). Electrophysiological brain activity and memory source monitoring. *NeuroReport, 8,* 1317–1320.

Jones, E. G. (1998). Viewpoint: The core and matrix of thalamic organization. *Neuroscience, 85,* 331–345.

Kapur, N. (1993). Focal retrograde amnesia in neurological disease: A critical review. *Cortex, 29,* 217–234.

Knight, R. T., & Grabowecky, M. (1995). Escape from linear time: Prefrontal cortex and conscious experience. In M. S. Gazzaniga (Ed.), *The cognitive neurosciences* (pp. 1357–1371). Cambridge, MA: MIT Press.

Kopelman, M. D. (2000). Focal retrograde amnesia and the attribution of causality: An exceptionally critical review. *Cognitive Neuropsychology, 17,* 585–621.

Markowitsch, H. J. (1995). Which brain regions are critically involved in the retrieval of old episodic memory? *Brain Research Reviews, 21,* 117–127.

Marr, D. (1971). Simple memory: A theory for archicortex. *Philosophical Transactions of the Royal Society of London, Series B, 262,* 23–81.

McClelland, J. L., McNaughton, B. L., & O'Reilly, R. C. (1995). Why there are complementary learning systems in the hippocampus and neocortex: Insights from the successes and failures of connectionist models of learning and memory. *Psychological Review, 102,* 419–457.

Mecklinger, A. (2000). Interfacing mind and brain: A neurocognitive model of recognition memory. *Psychophysiology, 37,* 565–582.

Mesulam, M.-M. (1998). From sensation to cognition. *Brain, 121,* 1013–1052.

Milner, P. M. (1989). A cell assembly theory of hippocampal amnesia. *Neuropsychologia, 27,* 23–30.

Murre, J. M. (1997). Implicit and explicit memory in amnesia: Some explanations and predictions by the TraceLink model. *Memory, 5,* 213–232.

Nadel, L., & Moscovitch, M. (1997). Memory consolidation, retrograde amnesia and the hippocampal complex. *Current Opinion in Neurobiology, 7,* 217–227.

Nadel, L., Samsonovich, A., Ryan, L., & Moscovitch, M. (2000). Multiple trace theory of human memory: Computational, neuroimaging, and neuropsychological results. *Hippocampus, 10,* 352–368.

O'Keefe, J., & Nadel, L. (1978). *The hippocampus as a cognitive map.* Oxford: Clarendon Press.

Olichney, J. M., Van Petten, C., Paller, K. A., Salmon, D. P., Iragui, V. J., & Kutas, M. (2000). Word repetition in amnesia: Electrophysiological measures of impaired and spared memory. *Brain, 123,* 1948–1963.

O'Reilly, R. C., & Rudy, J. W. (2001). Conjunctive representations in learning and memory: Principles of cortical and hippocampal function. *Psychological Review, 108,* 311–345.

Paller, K. A. (1997). Consolidating dispersed neocortical memories: The missing link in amnesia. *Memory, 5,* 73–88.

Paller, K. A. (2000). Neural measures of conscious and unconscious memory. *Behavioural Neurology, 12,* 127–141.

Paller, K. A., Acharya, A., Richardson, B. C., Plaisant, O., Shimamura, A. P., Reed, B. R., & Jagust, W. J. (1997). Functional neuroimaging of cortical dysfunction in alcoholic Korsakoff's syndrome. *Journal of Cognitive Neuroscience, 9,* 277–293.

Paller, K. A., Bozic, V. S., Ranganath, C., Grabowecky, M., & Yamada, S. (1999). Brain waves following remembered faces index conscious recollection. *Cognitive Brain Research, 7,* 519–531.

Paller, K. A., & Gross, M. (1998). Brain potentials associated with perceptual priming versus explicit remembering during the repetition of visual word-form. *Neuropsychologia, 36,* 559–571.

Paller, K. A., & Kutas, M. (1992). Brain potentials during memory retrieval provide neurophysiological support for the distinction between conscious recollection and priming. *Journal of Cognitive Neuroscience, 4,* 375–391.

Paller, K. A., Kutas, M., & Mayes, A. R. (1987). Neural correlates of encoding in an incidental learning paradigm. *Electroencephalography and Clinical Neurophysiology, 67,* 360–371.

Paller, K. A., Kutas, M., & McIsaac, H. K. (1995). Monitoring conscious recollection via the electrical activity of the brain. *Psychological Science, 6,* 107–111.

Paller, K. A., Kutas, M., & McIsaac, H. K. (1998). An electrophysiological measure of priming of visual word-form. *Consciousness and Cognition, 7,* 54–66.

Paller, K. A., & Mayes, A. R. (1994). New-association priming of word identification in normal and amnesic subjects. *Cortex, 30,* 53–73.

Ranganath, C., & Paller, K. A. (1999). Frontal brain potentials during recognition are modulated by requirements to retrieve perceptual detail. *Neuron, 22,* 605–613.

Ranganath, C., & Paller, K. A. (2000). Neural correlates of memory retrieval and evaluation. *Cognitive Brain Research*, *9*, 209–222.

Ranganath, C., Johnson, M. K., & D'Esposito, M. (2000). Left anterior prefrontal activation increases with demands to recall specific perceptual information. *Journal of Neuroscience*, *20*, RC108.

Rugg, M. D., & Wilding, E. L. (2000). Retrieval processing and episodic memory. *Trends in Cognitive Sciences*, *4*, 108–115.

Ryan, J. D., Althoff, R. R., Whitlow, S., & Cohen, N. J. (2000). Amnesia is a deficit in relational memory. *Psychological Science*, *11*, 454–461.

Schacter, D. L., & Buckner, R. L. (1998). Priming and the brain. *Neuron*, *20*, 185–195.

Schacter, D. L., & Graf, P. (1986). Preserved learning in amnesic patients: Perspectives from research on direct priming. *Journal of Clinical and Experimental Neuropsychology*, *8*, 727–743.

Schacter, D. L., Norman, K. A., & Koutstaal, W. (1998). The cognitive neuroscience of constructive memory. *Annual Review of Psychology*, *49*, 289–318.

Shimamura, A. P. (1995). Memory and frontal lobe function. In M. S. Gazzaniga (Ed.), *The cognitive neurosciences* (pp. 803–813). Cambridge, MA: MIT Press.

Shimamura, A. P., & Squire, L. R. (1987). A neuropsychological study of fact memory and source amnesia. *Journal of Experimental Psychology: Learning, Memory, and Cognition*, *13*, 464–473.

Shimamura, A. P., & Squire, L. R. (1989). Impaired priming of new associations in amnesia. *Journal of Experimental Psychology: Learning, Memory, and Cognition*, *15*, 721–728.

Squire, L. R. (1992). Memory and the hippocampus: A synthesis from findings with rats, monkeys, and humans. *Psychological Review*, *99*, 195–231.

Squire, L. R., & Alvarez, P. (1995). Retrograde amnesia and memory consolidation: A neurobiological perspective. *Current Opinion in Neurobiology*, *5*, 169–177.

Squire, L. R., Cohen, N. J., & Nadel, L. (1984). The medial temporal region and memory consolidation: A new hypothesis. In H. Weingartner & E. Parder (Eds.), *Memory consolidation* (pp. 185–210). Hillsdale, NJ: Erlbaum.

Stickgold, R. (1998). Sleep: Off-line memory reprocessing. *Trends in Cognitive Sciences*, *2*, 484–492.

Sutherland, G. R., & McNaughton, B. (2000). Memory trace reactivation in hippocampal and neocortical neuronal ensembles. *Current Opinion in Neurobiology*, *10*, 180–186.

Teyler, T. J., & DiScenna, P. (1986). The hippocampal memory indexing theory. *Behavioral Neuroscience*, *100*, 147–154.

Treves, A., & Rolls, E. T. (1994). Computational analysis of the role of the hippocampus in memory. *Hippocampus*, *4*, 374–391.

Tulving, E., Hayman, C. A., & Macdonald, C. A. (1991). Long-lasting perceptual priming and semantic learning in amnesia: A case experiment. *Journal of Experimental Psychology: Learning, Memory, and Cognition*, *7*, 595–617.

Underwood, B. J. (1969). Attributes of memory. *Psychological Review*, *76*, 559–573.

Wagner, A. D., Koutstaal, W., & Schacter, D. L. (1999). When encoding yields remembering: Insights from event-related neuroimaging. *Philosophical Transactions of the Royal Society of London, Series B*, *354*, 1307–1324.

Wheeler, M. A., Stuss, D. T., & Tulving, E. (1997). Toward a theory of episodic memory: The frontal lobes and autonoetic consciousness. *Psychological Bulletin*, *121*, 331–354.

Wickelgren, W. A. (1979). Chunking and consolidation: A theoretical synthesis of semantic networks, configuring in conditioning, S-R versus cognitive learning, normal forgetting, the amnesic syndrome, and the hippocampal arousal system. *Psychological Review*, *86*, 44–60.

Wiggs, C. L., & Martin, A. (1998). Properties and mechanisms of perceptual priming. *Current Opinion in Neurobiology*, *8*, 227–233.

Wilding, E. L. (2000). In what way does the parietal ERP old/new effect index recollection? *International Journal of Psychophysiology*, *35*, 81–87.

Winson, J. (1985). *Brain and psyche: The biology of the unconscious*. Garden City, NY: Doubleday/Anchor.

7

Developmental Amnesia

A Challenge to Current Models?

ALAN BADDELEY

When Elizabeth Warrington retired from her clinical post, her colleagues organized a festschrift, inviting a number of her collaborators to take part and give papers on the areas of their collaboration. I was invited to talk about amnesia, which placed me in a dilemma. On the one hand, I was delighted to be asked. The study of amnesia has had, and continues to have, a huge influence on my approach to human memory. My interest in neuropsychology can be traced back to a conversation with Elizabeth in which I argued that it was very unlikely that neuropsychological patients would be obliging enough to have their lesions in areas that are relevant to our theories. She invited me to see a "pure" amnesic patient, N. T. This led to a very rapid conversion on my part, to a very fruitful series of collaborations (e.g., Baddeley & Warrington, 1970; Warrington & Baddeley, 1974), and to a continuing interest in amnesia.

On the other hand, although I continue to follow the amnesia literature, I myself had not worked on the amnesic syndrome for some years. The basic reason for my lack of activity was simple: I could not think of any worthwhile experiments. I was convinced that great progress had been made and that important questions remained. However, it was not clear how they could be answered, at least by a cognitive psychologist like myself. Reflecting on my dilemma, I decided that it might nonetheless be useful to present my rather downbeat view of the field, in the hope that it might generate some productive disagreement. What was my view?

I was, and still am, in no doubt that the study of amnesia has made a major contribution to our understanding of human memory. Although theorists differ on whether they prefer to talk about structures, systems, or processes, I would argue that the distinction between long-term memory (LTM) and short-term memory (STM) or working memory (WM) has been massively influenced by neuropsychological evidence, and that the distinction remains a valuable one. Similarly, a distinction between declarative or episodic memory, and a range of nondeclarative implicit learning and memory systems, represents a real theoretical advance (Squire, 1992). Beyond this, various important issues remain to be resolved. On these points I tended to opt for what appeared to be the simplest interpretation, using this as a null hypothesis, which later or more complex approaches would need to displace.

The distinction between semantic and episodic memory is a good example. The distinction has indubitably been a valuable one, but the evidence for separate systems is less convincing (Squire & Zola, 1998). Amnesic patients do typically have preserved semantic memory for material before their acquired memory loss, but then they may also have well-preserved early memories of an apparently episodic nature, allowing them to recollect specific episodes in rich detail (Wilson & Baddeley, 1988). The most parsimonious interpretation would seem to be that semantic memory represents the accumulation of many episodes, acquired across many contexts, and hence decontextualized. This potentially allows rapid decontextualized retrieval rather than recollection, but does not necessarily imply a separate storage system (Baddeley, 1984).

Attempts to explain the amnesic syndrome in terms of the failure of cognitive processes have continued to be proposed, as alternatives to a more neurobiological interpretation such as consolidation—a process that appears to give the cognitive psychologists rather less scope for investigation. Interpretations in terms of proactive interference (Warrington & Weiskrantz, 1970) and levels of processing (Cermak & Reale, 1978) were proposed, but ran into difficulties from later experimental results (Meudell, Mayes, & Neary, 1980; Warrington & Weizkrantz, 1978). A third influential theory of amnesia attributed it to the failure to encode or store contextual cues adequately (e.g., Winocur & Kinsbourne, 1978). This approach is, however, open to the argument that contextual associations, although extremely important in allowing subsequent recall of a specific event, are no different from other novel associations. In this view, impaired contextual coding is simply another instance of a more basic mnemonic binding deficit, which in turn is attributable to failure of consolidation—a lack of "mnemonic glue." Rejection of this interpretation requires clear evidence that the contextual deficit is disproportionate in amnesic patients when other variables such as degree and nature of learning are taken into account; this is a methodologically difficult task (Mayes, 1988; Mayes, Mendell, & Som, 1981).

The third area in which progress seems to have been very slow is in making a good case for different types of amnesia. It is of course clear that poor memory may result from more general processing deficits, such as the dysexecutive syndrome that may result from frontal lobe damage (Baddeley & Wilson, 1988; Shallice, 1988). Within the amnesic syndrome itself, however, attempts to demonstrate clear subtypes have proved somewhat problematic. Colleagues in the neuropsychology of language, with its numerous varieties of aphasia and dyslexia, seem to regard this as a sign of lack of sophistication on the part of those of us in memory research. My response to this slur is to suggest that memory systems are much more basic and fundamental in evolutionary terms than the myriad of Johnny-come-lately processes involved in language and reading, and hence more monolithic and unitary (and important!). I had to admit, however, that a little more fractionation might be fruitful in tackling the remaining problems.

Unsuccessful earlier attempts at subtyping have included, for example, the suggestion of differential rates of forgetting as a function of area of lesion (e.g., Parkin, 1992). However, in general, amnesic patients appear to forget at a normal rate (Kopelman, 1985), and although one hears occasional clinical reports of particularly rapid forgetting, evidence for a separate subgroup does not at present appear to be strong.

A related issue involving some controversy is that of the respective role in amnesia of recall and recognition. Huppert and Piercy (1979) and Hirst and colleagues (1986) both proposed that amnesic patients show greater recall than recognition deficits. However, such studies suffer from the problem of equating recall and recognition in level of difficulty (see Baddeley, Vargha-Khadem, & Mishkin, 2001; Shallice, 1988), with later studies such as that of Haiste, Shimamura, and Squire (1992) suggesting that recall and recognition are equally impaired in amnesia. A somewhat more cogent case for a relative preservation of recognition in a small subset of amnesic patients has been made by Aggleton and colleagues (Aggleton & Brown, 1999; Aggleton & Shaw, 1997), who argue that recognition memory may be preserved when damage is limited to the hippocampus. However, their conclusions, based on the post hoc analysis of a large number of cases, inevitably introduce the possibility of some form of inadvertent bias. Moreover, Reed and Squire (1997), reporting data from a group of amnesic patients whose damage is principally limited to the hippocampus, find clear evidence of impaired recognition memory.

The conclusion of my invited review of amnesia was therefore somewhat staid. I made a clear distinction between LTM and WM, and between an explicit memory system and a series of implicit memory systems that were themselves certainly dissociable. For the rest, I opted for the Scottish judicial term of "not proven," with the simplest set of assumptions being these: (1) that semantic memory represents an accumulation of episodes; (2) that the amnesic syndrome is unitary; and (3) that it reflects a problem at the neurobiological level (lack of "mnemonic glue") rather than at a cognitive processing level. I took comfort from the fact that Larry Squire, who is far more closely in touch with this area than I am, appeared to hold a broadly similar view (Squire, Knowlton, & Musen, 1993). I gave my talk, and escaped the question time relatively unscathed. Then, a week or two later, I was invited by Faraneh Vargha-Khadem to see a young patient whom she thought I might find interesting.

The young man in question, Jon, was one of a group of three described by Vargha-Khadem and colleagues (1997). He appeared to have been amnesic from an early age, probably as a result of anoxia associated with prematurity, resulting in a reduction of about 50% in hippocampal volume, with comparatively little damage outside this system (Gadian et al., 2000). Despite impaired performance on standardized memory tests, and a degree of everyday memory deficit that has made it difficult for him to obtain and keep a job, Jon has developed above-average intelligence and apparently normal language and knowledge of the world. There was, however, a suggestion that he and the other two cases might possibly have relatively preserved recognition memory.

We had, in fact, just developed a test that claimed equally sensitive measures of both recall and recognition for visual and verbal materials (Baddeley, Emslie, & Nimmo-Smith, 1994). Although we had found the test to be sensitive to overall memory deficits resulting from Alzheimer's disease, schizophrenia, and normal aging (Baddeley, 1996), and to be sensitive to the visual–verbal memory difference in cases of left and right hemispherectomy (Morris, Abrahams, Baddeley, & Polkey, 1995), I had yet to find an individual who showed a clear recall–recognition difference. I therefore readily accepted the invitation to test Jon.

The test, which is known as the Doors and People Test (Baddeley et al., 1994), measures visual recognition memory by presenting a sequence of 12 colored photographs of doors, each accompanied by a spoken label such as "church door" and "barn door." This is followed by 12 test sets, each comprising 4 pictures, all of which fit the assigned label, hence minimizing the role of verbal coding. A second sequence of harder pictures is then presented and tested. Verbal recognition involves presenting a series of 12 names, then testing with 12 sets of 4, where level of difficulty is determined by the degree of similarity between the name and the distractors (e.g., "John Wilkins," tested by presenting "John Wilkes," "John Wilkinson," "John Wilkins," and "John Wilkie"). Again, a further 12 items are presented and tested. Verbal recall is tested by presenting the names and photographs of four individuals—a postman, a minister, a newspaper boy, and a doctor. Recall of the names is then cued by occupation, and up to three further trials are given. The visual recall task involves presenting four crosses that differ in their overall shape, the decoration at the crux, and the decoration at the end of the arms. The subjects are required to copy and then recall by drawing. Again, a further three trials are given. Both learning tasks are subsequently retested after a filled delay. The test is standardized against a normal population, allowing scaled scores to be calculated. It provides a set of standardized measures—namely, recall and recognition, and visual and verbal memory, together with subsidiary measures of rate of learning and delayed recall. Jon and two control subjects were tested on this task. Their results are shown in Figure 7.1.

It is clear that while Jon's recall performance is impaired, his recognition memory is normal, as compared either to the general population or to the two control subjects. Jon's impaired recall is consistent with his performance on the Rivermead Behavioural Memory Test and the California Verbal Learning Test (Baddeley et al., 2001). We went on to test his performance on a range of other recognition tests, including a rapid cumulative recognition test devised by Shepard and Teghtsoonian (1961), and two forced-choice recognition tests on which Reed and Squire (1997) found marked impairment in their hippocampal amnesic patients, who also proved to be impaired on the recognition component of the Doors and People Test (Manns & Squire, 1999). Jon performed at a normal level on all these tests of recognition.

We then attempted to test memory under conditions that begin to approach those under which semantic memory is typically acquired. This required a test involving complex real-world information, presented both visually and auditorily, preferably with several presentations distributed across days. To test this, we took advantage of videos based on newsreels from a period before Jon was born (hence unfamiliar, though meaningful). Subjects were shown 40-minute videos of newsreels from 1937 and 1957, and subsequently tested by

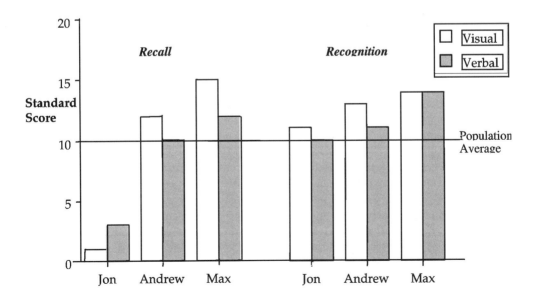

FIGURE 7.1. Performance of Jon and two control subjects on the Doors and People Test of visual and verbal recall and recognition. Data from Baddeley, Vargha-Khadem, and Mishkin (2001).

cued recall or recognition. One newsreel was presented only once, while the other was shown four times over a 2-day period. After a single presentation, Jon's recognition was comparable to that of the controls, but his recall was impaired; after four presentations, his recall improved to the level of the controls.

The fact that distributed, repeated presentation markedly improved Jon's recall performance reinforces the evidence derived from conversing with Jon, in suggesting that it is not the capacity to recall per se that is absent. Our result also hints at an answer to the paradox of why Jon appears to have good semantic memory despite his apparent amnesia. However, we have yet to work out exactly what aspect of our newsreel study allowed recall performance to improve so clearly.

Vargha-Khadem and Mishkin (in press) report on a growing body of patients with developmental amnesia who broadly resemble Jon, although typically showing more extensive damage and a greater degree of intellectual impairment. It will be important to study the recall–recognition performance of such cases, together with the degree of preservation of semantic memory, before drawing firm conclusions. Furthermore, new adult cases of preserved recognition with impaired recall are beginning to appear (Holdstock et al., 2000). It will be interesting to see to what extent such cases show an ongoing capacity for upgrading semantic memory under conditions such as our video study. It would, in addition, be desirable for such a study to be performed on classic amnesic patients. It is conceivable that they would show the degree of improved recall shown by Jon following distributed practice, although this seems unlikely, as existing literature suggests that densely amnesic patients do not update their semantic memory (Gabrieli, Cohen, & Corkin, 1988) or do so to a very limited extent (Kitchener, Hodges, & McCarthy, 1998).

To return to Jon, however, how can his pattern of symptoms be explained? First of all, it is important to note that his deficit is not one of recall per se, since he can recall semantic information, or indeed events from his life. What he seems to lack is the capacity to recollect, to perform the task which Tulving (1985) refers to as crucial to episodic memory—namely, reinvoking the experience remembered, which allows the rememberer to "travel backward in time." We had great difficulty in getting Jon to understand this concept of "remembering," in the sense of recollecting information associated with an event. He could tell us how he had traveled to the clinic that day, but could not provide any specific detail that would allow that journey to be differentiated from any other. When we tested his verbal recognition using the "remember–know" procedure (Gardiner & Java, 1993), he used the "remember" category quite frequently. However, when asked to elaborate subsequently, he replied that he imagined the presentation of the relevant word on a card, and categorized the vivid images as "remembered" and the less vivid as "known"— a response suggesting the use of a fluency heuristic rather than episodic recollection. We suspected that Jon does not understand the concept of remembering because he lacks the recollective experience, but we could not be absolutely sure that on this occasion he was not simply failing to understand our explanation of "remember."

Fortunately, Düzel, Vargha-Khadem, Heinze, and Mishkin (2001) throw further light on the issue in a study of the electrophysiological activity associated with "remember" and "know" responses. Whereas normal subjects show different electrophysiological signatures associated with these two judgments, Jon's recognition performance is associated only with the "know" signature. Subsequent work by Maguire (in press) probed long-term autobiographical memories in Jon and control subjects, using fMRI to study the process of recollecting such events. She was able to identify one or two events for which Jon appeared to have recollective experience, as measured by the presence of contextual information from experiencing the event. These few cases appeared to evoke the excitatory pattern associated with recollection, suggesting that Jon is in principle capable of remembering in the sense implied by Tulving (1985), but that this very rarely occurs.

Let us assume for the present that other cases like Jon will be identified, and that developmental amnesia can be established as a general syndrome rather than a striking single case. What would the implications be? First of all, Jon's case suggests that there are indeed different varieties of amnesia, with provisional evidence suggesting that intact hippocampal function may not be necessary for good recognition. This clearly leaves a large number of questions at the neuroanatomical level. For example, why do the hippocampal patients of Reed and Squire (1997) and Manns and Squire (1999) clearly show a recognition memory deficit, while Jon and the various patients described by Aggleton and Brown (1999) and by Holdstock and colleagues (2000) do not? One possibility is that recognition impairment may reflect some form of damage that does not show up on current structural MRI; this clearly requires further investigation.

A second issue concerns the relationship between recall and recognition. The existence of two contributions to recognition performance has been acknowledged at least since the publication of Mandler's (1980) article. One might, however, expect that in the absence of one of these two components, Jon's performance would be poorer than it is. Two possibilities suggest themselves here. One is that someone with Jon's intelligence and sophistication as a subject would have performed in the above-average range if it were not for the absence of recollection. Another possibility, however, is that more than two sources of information may contribute to recognition performance. One of these may be the recollective component that Tulving (1985) regards as essential for episodic remembering; this appears to be absent in both Jon and other amnesic patients. A second may reflect an implicit system, possibly based on priming, that is preserved in both Jon and classic amnesic patients. A third component may be assumed to be preserved in Jon but not in most amnesic subjects. This, of course, raises the question of what might constitute this third type of memory.

Another way of conceptualizing the problem is in terms of different sets of cues, rather than different basic systems. In this view, recognition memory reflects a mnemonic decision based on a range of available evidence, which comes from the interpretation of three (or possibly many more) cues or sources of information. The increasing acceptance of phenomenological judgments (as in the case of the "remember–know" procedure), together with the use of electrophysiological neuroradiological methods to cross-validate such methods, may potentially lead to the discovery and analysis of a much richer array of such cues. For the present, however, we need to move forward cautiously in order to avoid some of the problems encountered by the overreliance on introspection in the early years of the 20th century, which led to the growth of behaviorism.

What are the implications of our results for the understanding of semantic memory? The fact that Jon has developed an apparently normal semantic memory despite serious episodic memory limitations might seem to argue for separate systems (Tulving & Markovitch, 1998). However, given that Jon's recognition memory and semantic memory performance is normal despite the absence of episodic memory, this would seem to point to a less central role for episodic memory than I, at least, had previously assumed. Episodic memory, although undoubtedly a useful cue in locating episodes in time and space, would not, in this view, appear to be the most salient problem encountered in the classic amnesic syndrome. The assumption of an additional store, or of multiple cues rather than separate systems, thus appears to offer a possible alternative to a simple semantic–episodic structural dichotomy. Such assumptions are worth further exploration.

An important further possibility, however, is that the crucial difference between Jon and the classic amnesic patient is in the timing of his insult. Perhaps if the problem occurs early enough in life, then neural plasticity will allow compensatory processes to develop, leading to preserved recognition memory and/or preserved semantic development. This is a tempting hypothesis, which is currently being investigated by Vargha-Khadem and her colleagues by comparing children who have acquired their amnesia at different ages. So far, however, there is little support for the idea that age of acquisition of the deficit has the predicted effect (Vargha-Khadem & Mishkin, in press); still, this is likely to remain a very active research area. Another way of tackling the same problem is to look at the capacity to update semantic memory in patients with impaired recall and preserved recognition who have acquired their amnesia as adults. It would be desirable to test them both via naturalistic methods such as studying recently developed vocabulary (Gabrieli et al., 1988), and via experimental methods such as that used in our news video study.

The observation that spaced repetition enhances Jon's recall capacity also invites further investigation. Simple verbal repetition does not appear to lead to learning, as indicated by Jon's list-learning performance on the California Verbal Learning Test; is the crucial factor the spacing, the nature of the material, its manner of encoding, or an interaction between these variables? This question is particularly relevant to the practical problem of optimizing educational methods for children with developmental amnesia, and for memory rehabilitation more generally.

In conclusion, studying Jon has substantially challenged my own view of the nature and implications of amnesia. Our results need to be replicated, and their range and typicality need to be explored in both children and adults. Only then will it become clear to just what extent our results challenge existing views on the nature and development of human memory.

ACKNOWLEDGMENTS

The speculations described within this chapter have benefited from many discussions with Faraneh Vargha-Khadem and Mort Mishkin, and from the comments of various anonymous referees on our joint paper. The support of Medical Research Council Grant No. G9423916 is gratefully acknowledged.

REFERENCES

Aggleton, J. P., & Brown, M. W. (1999). Episodic memory, amnesia and the hippocampal–anterior thalamic axis. *Behavioral and Brain Sciences, 22,* 425–490.

Aggleton, J. P., & Shaw, C. (1996). Amnesia and recognition memory: A re-analysis of psychometric data. *Neuropsychologia, 34,* 51–62.

Baddeley, A. D. (1984). Neuropsychological evidence and the semantic episodic distinction: Commentary on Tulving. *Behavioral and Brain Sciences, 7,* 238–239.

Baddeley, A. D. (1996). Applying the psychology of memory to clinical problems. In D. Herrmann, M. Johnson, C. McEvoy, C. Hertzog, P. Hertel, & M. Johnson (Eds.), *Basic and applied memory research* (pp. 195–219). Mahwah, NJ: Erlbaum.

Baddeley, A. D., Emslie, H., & Nimmo-Smith, I. (1994). *Doors and People: A test of visual and verbal recall and recognition.* Bury St. Edmunds, England: Thames Valley Test Company.

Baddeley, A. D., Vargha-Khadem, F., & Mishkin, M. (2001). Preserved recognition in a case of developmental amnesia: Implications for the acquisition of semantic memory? *Journal of Cognitive Neuroscience, 13,* 357–369.

Baddeley, A. D., & Warrington, E. K. (1970). Amnesia and the distinction between long- and short-term memory. *Journal of Verbal Learning and Verbal Behavior, 9,* 176–189.

Baddeley, A. D., & Wilson, B. A. (1988). Frontal amnesia and the dysexecutive syndrome. *Brain and Cognition, 7*, 212–230.

Cermak, L. S., & Reale, L. (1978). Depth of processing and retention of words by alcoholic Korsakoff patients. *Journal of Experimental Psychology: Human Learning and Memory, 4*, 165–174.

Düzel, E., Vargha-Khadem, F., Heinze, H. J., & Mishkin, M. (2001). ERP evidence for recognition without episodic recollection in a patient with early hippocampal pathology. *Proceedings of the National Academy of Sciences USA, 92*, 8101–8106.

Gabrieli, J. D. E., Cohen, N. J., & Corkin, S. (1988). The impaired learning of semantic knowledge following bilateral medial temporal-lobe resection. *Brain and Cognition, 7*, 157–177.

Gadian, D. G., Aicardi, J., Watkins, K. E., Porter, D. A., Mishkin, M., & Vargha-Khadem, F. (2000). Developmental amnesia associated with early hypoxic–ischaemic injury. *Brain, 123*, 499–507.

Gardiner, J. M., & Java, R. J. (1993). Recognising and remembering. In A. F. Collins, S. E. Gathercole, M. A. Conway, & P. E. Morris (Eds.), *Theories of memory* (pp. 163–188). Hove, England: Erlbaum.

Haiste, F., Shimamura, A. P., & Squire, L. R. (1992). On the relationship between recall and recognition memory. *Journal of Experimental Psychology: Learning, Memory, and Cognition, 18*, 691–702.

Hirst, W., Johnson, M. K., Kim, J. K., Phelps, E. A., Risse, G., & Volpe, B. T. (1986). Recognition and recall in amnesics. *Journal of Experimental Psychology, 12*, 445–451.

Holdstock, J. S., Mayes, A. R., Cezayirli, E., Isaac, C. L., Aggleton, J. P., & Roberts, N. (2000). A comparison of egocentric and allocentric spatial memory in a patient with selective hippocampal damage. *Neuropsychologia, 38*, 410–425.

Huppert, F. A., & Piercy, M. (1979). Normal and abnormal forgetting in amnesia: Effect of locus of lesion. *Cortex, 15*, 385–390.

Kitchener, E. G., Hodges, J. R., & McCarthy, R. (1998). Acquisition of post-morbid vocabulary and semantic facts in the absence of episodic memory. *Brain, 121*, 1313–1327.

Kopelman, M. D. (1985). Rates of forgetting in Alzheimer-type dementias and Korsakoff's syndrome. *Neuropsychologia, 23*, 623–638.

Mandler, G. (1980). Recognising: The judgement of previous occurrence. *Psychological Review, 87*, 252–271.

Manns, J. R., & Squire, L. R. (1999). Impaired recognition memory on the Doors and People Test after damage limited to the hippocampal region. *Hippocampus, 9*, 495–499.

Maguire, E. (in press). Neuroimaging studies of episodic memory. *Philosophical Transactions of the Royal Society of London, Series B.*

Mayes, A. (1988). *Human organic memory disorders.* Cambridge, England: Cambridge University Press.

Mayes, A., Meudell, P. R., & Som, S. (1981). Further similarities between amnesia and normal attenuated memory: Effects with paired-associate learning and context shifts. *Neuropsychologia, 19*, 655–664.

Meudell, P. R., Mayes, A., & Neary, D. (1980). Orienting task effects on the recognition of humorous material in amnesic and normal subjects. *Journal of Clinical Neuropsychology, 2*, 1–14.

Morris, R. G., Abrahams, S., Baddeley, A. D., & Polkey, C. E. (1995). Doors and People: Visual and verbal memory following unilateral temporal lobectomy. *Neuropsychology, 9*, 464–469.

Parkin, A. J. (1992). Functional significance of etiological factors in human amnesia. In L. R. Squire & N. Butters (Eds.), *Neuropsychology of memory* (2nd ed., pp. 122–129). New York: Guilford Press.

Reed, J. M., & Squire, L. R. (1997). Impaired recognition memory in patients with lesions limited to the hippocampal formation. *Behavioral Neuroscience, 111*, 667–675.

Shallice, T. (1988). *From neuropsychology to mental structure.* Cambridge, England: Cambridge University Press

Shepard, R. N., & Teghtsoonian, M. (1961). Retention of information under conditions approaching a steady state. *Journal of Experimental Psychology, 62*, 302–309.

Squire, L. R. (1992). Declarative and non-declarative memory: Multiple brain systems supporting learning and memory. *Journal of Cognitive Neuroscience, 4,* 232–243.

Squire, L. R., Knowlton, B., & Musen, G. (1993). The structure and organisation of memory. *Annual Review of Psychology, 44,* 453–495.

Squire, L. R., & Zola, S. M. (1998). Episodic memory, semantic memory and amnesia. *Hippocampus, 8,* 205–211.

Tulving, E. (1985). Memory and consciousness. *Canadian Psychologist, 26,* 1–12.

Tulving, E., & Markovitch, H. L. (1998). Episodic and declarative memory: The role of the hippocampus. *Hippocampus, 8,* 198–204.

Vargha-Khadem, F., Gadian, D. G., Watkins, K. E., Connelly, A., Van Paesschen, W., & Mishkin, M. (1997). Differential effects of early hippocampal pathology on episodic and semantic memory. *Science, 277,* 376–380.

Vargha-Khadem, F., & Mishkin, M. (in press). Dissociations in cognitive memory: The syndrome of developmental amnesia. *Philosophical Transactions of the Royal Society of London, Series B.*

Warrington, E. K., & Weiskrantz, L. (1970). Amnesic syndrome: Consolidation or retrieval? *Nature, 226,* 628–630.

Warrington, E. K., & Weiskrantz, L. (1978). Further analyses of the prior learning effect in amnesic patients. *Neuropsychologia, 16,* 169–176.

Warrington, E. K., & Baddeley, A. D. (1974). Amnesia and memory for visual location. *Neuropsychologia, 12,* 257–263.

Wilson, B. A., & Baddeley, A. D. (1988). Semantic, episodic and autobiographical memory in a post-meningitic amnesic patient. *Brain and Cognition, 8,* 31–46.

Winocur, G., & Kinsbourne, M. (1978). Contextual cueing as an aid to Korsakoff amnesics. *Neuropsychologia, 16,* 671–682.

8

Impact of Temporal Lobe Amnesia, Aging, and Awareness on Human Eyeblink Conditioning

JOHN F. DISTERHOFT, MARIA C. CARRILLO,
CATHERINE B. FORTIER, JOHN D. E. GABRIELI,
M-GRACE KNUTTINEN, REGINA McGLINCHEY-BERROTH,
ALISON PRESTON, and CRAIG WEISS

Eyeblink conditioning is an associative learning task that was developed in the early 20th century by experimental psychologists as a tool for understanding the laws of learning in humans. A tone, light, or somatosensory conditioned stimulus (CS) precedes the presentation of the unconditioned stimulus (US), currently a puff of air to the cornea. After a number of pairings, eyeblink conditioned responses (CRs) occur to the CS prior to the presentation of the US. This task was studied extensively in humans and has a large historical literature (e.g., Cason, 1922; Telford & Anderson, 1932).

The recent resurgence in the study of eyeblink conditioning originated in the work of Isidore Gormezano, who adapted eyeblink conditioning in the rabbit as a technique for addressing issues concerning "voluntary responding" that had been raised in the human eyeblink conditioning literature (Gormezano, 1966). The problem he was addressing was how to determine whether a subject made a CR because of associative learning that had occurred, or because the subject realized consciously that the CS preceded the US and was responding in a conscious or voluntary way and as soon as possible after the CS onset. The issue, then, was whether the eyeblinks that were being studied were evidence of associative learning or rather of eyelid movements to CS presentation that were determined mainly by reaction time. Gormezano reasoned that an experimental animal would not have any reason to make voluntary responses in this experimental situation. Accordingly, the laws of learning could be explored without contamination by voluntary responding. Gormezano selected the rabbit as his experimental animal, because rabbits are easily restrained and have large eyes that facilitate measurement of the CR and the unconditioned response (UR). He and his colleagues demonstrated that rabbits acquired high levels of eyeblink conditioning, had very regular and relatively rapid acquisition curves, and showed low levels of pseudoconditioning or sensitization when the tone and puff were presented in an unpaired fashion (Gormezano & Schneiderman, 1962; Gormezano & Kehoe, 1983).

Richard Thompson and his colleagues began using the eyeblink conditioning behavioral model in the rabbit in combination with multiple-neuron recording in the hippocampus, in studies aimed at defining the neurobiological substrates of associative learning (Thompson et al., 1976). Shortly after, we began to use this behavioral task in rabbits in combination with single-neuron recording (Disterhoft, Kwan, & Lo, 1977). Work analyzing the neural substrates of this task from our laboratories, as well as from many others over the years, has now made eyeblink conditioning the most thoroughly studied and best-understood task for exploring the neural substrates of associative learning (Gormezano, Prokasy, & Thompson, 1987; Woodruff-Pak & Steinmetz, 2000a, 2000b). We and others have used multiple- and single-neuron *in vivo* neurophysiological recording, lesions, neuro-anatomical tract tracing, and biophysical measurements in brain slices to understand the neural systems mediating this task in animals, as well as some of the mechanisms by which conditioning occurs.

In brief, the sensory input systems by which the CS and US enter the brain, as well as some of the changes that occur there during learning, have been characterized (Disterhoft, Quinn, & Weiss, 1987). Also, the final output pathway from the accessory abducens nucleus, which controls nictitating membrane extension, has been visualized and physiologically characterized during and after learning (Disterhoft, Quinn, Weiss, & Shipley, 1985). In addition, cerebellar circuitry and associated brainstem circuitry have been identified as critically involved in the acquisition and retention of CRs but not URs in short-delay conditioning, where the CS and US overlap temporally (Thompson, 1986, 1990). The hippocampus has been identified as essential for successful acquisition of the more difficult trace conditioning paradigm, where a stimulus-free "trace" period intervenes between CS offset and US onset (Moyer, Deyo, & Disterhoft, 1990; Solomon, Vander Schaaf, Thompson, & Weisz, 1986). The hippocampus is also essential for two-tone discrimination reversal conditioning (Berger & Orr, 1983). Finally, aged animals have been found to show greater impairments in trace conditioning than in delay conditioning (Knuttinen, Gamelli, Weiss, Power, & Disterhoft, 2001; Solomon & Groccia-Ellison, 1996; Thompson, Moyer, & Disterhoft, 1996).

We recently began a series of studies in humans to determine whether similar brain systems and mechanisms are engaged during acquisition of eyeblink conditioning in humans as in other mammals. The goal of this approach is initially to determine how well the animal data can be used to predict human performance during the task. As our understanding of the similarities in substrates across species improves, it should be possible to use the animal models more advantageously for focused experiments (e.g., tests of proposed treatments for Alzheimer's disease and for treatments to facilitate recovery from stroke), as well as for studies that aim for a deeper understanding of the mechanisms by which learning occurs in the human brain.

DELAY AND TRACE CONDITIONING

Our initial study in humans explored the status of delay eyeblink conditioning in patients with medial temporal lobe amnesia (Gabrieli et al., 1995). We compared well-characterized patients who had spared intellectual and attentional abilities, but severely impaired memory for verbal and nonverbal material, with control subjects matched for age, level of education, and intelligence. We observed no differences between the amnesic patients and control subjects in total number of CRs, in acquisition or extinction rate, or in the latencies and amplitudes of the CRs (Figure 8.1). These data were precisely what could be predicted from animal studies demonstrating that acquisition of delay eyeblink conditioning is unimpaired in hippocampectomized animals (Akase, Alkon, & Disterhoft, 1989; Schmaltz & Theios, 1972).

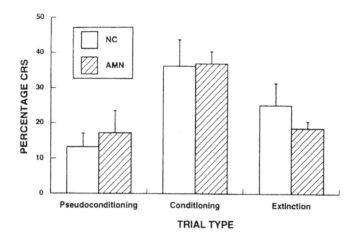

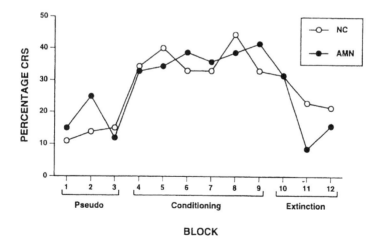

FIGURE 8.1. *Top:* Mean percentage of CRs for seven normal control (NC) and seven amnesic (AMN) participants in pseudoconditioning (unpaired tones), conditioning (tones paired with airpuffs), and extinction (tone alone) trials. *Bottom:* Mean percentage of CRs for the same participants shown by blocks in pseudoconditioning (Pseudo; 5 tones per block), conditioning (10 tones per block), and extinction (10 tones per block) trials. From Gabrieli et al. (1995). Copyright 1995 by the American Psychological Association. Reprinted by permission.

We then carried out a second study in a group of patients with alcoholic Korsakoff's amnesia, using the same delay conditioning parameters as in our study of the temporal lobe patients (McGlinchey-Berroth et al., 1995). Individuals who were recovering from chronic alcoholism, and healthy normal subjects, constituted the control groups. This study demonstrated that delay conditioning is not intact in all amnesic groups. In fact, the Korsakoff patients showed essentially no eyeblink conditioning, while the recovering alcoholic individuals showed some acquisition but were impaired with respect to the controls. This severe impairment occurred in the Korsakoff patients, although their delayed recollection of verbal and visual material was as impaired as that of the group with temporal lobe amnesia. We attributed the eyeblink conditioning deficit in the two alcoholic groups to the fact that chronic alcohol abuse is known to cause cerebellar degeneration. It has been well established that cerebellar damage impairs or blocks delay eyeblink conditioning, depending upon the size and location of the lesions (Thompson & Kim, 1996). We conclude that hippocampal/temporal lobe damage sufficient to cause severe amnesia does not affect delay eyeblink conditioning in human subjects, as predicted from the hippocampal lesion studies in experimental animals.

Trace eyeblink conditioning, in which a stimulus-free trace interval intervenes between the CS and US, is dependent on the hippocampus in the rabbit (Moyer et al., 1990; Solomon et al., 1986) and the rat (Weiss, Bouwmeester, Power, & Disterhoft, 1999). In our studies, we have routinely demonstrated that animals unable to exhibit trace conditioning due to hippocampal damage are unimpaired in their capacity for delay conditioning. Some aspect of the temporal demands of the trace conditioning paradigm appears to require the involvement of the hippocampus in order for successful acquisition to occur. This is true not only for eyeblink conditioning in the rabbit and rat, but also for fear conditioning in these species; that is, trace fear conditioning is impaired, whereas delay fear conditioning is intact (McEchron, Bouwmeester, Tseng, Weiss, & Disterhoft, 1998; McEchron, Tseng, & Disterhoft, 2000).

We sought to test the generalizability of this finding in humans, using trace eyeblink conditioning (McGlinchey-Berroth et al., 1997). Each subject was conditioned and extinguished with three trace intervals—500, 750, and 1,000 milliseconds (msec). We again compared well-characterized amnesic patients who had preserved intellectual and attentional function, but severely impaired delayed recall and recognition performance, with control subjects matched for age, education, and intellectual ability (five of the amnesic patients and their five controls had participated in the Gabrieli et al. [1995] delay-conditioning study). Participants were trained sequentially at the three trace intervals, from shortest to longest, with at least a 2-week period intervening between training sessions.

Compared to their matched control subjects, the amnesic patients were impaired in their acquisition of trace eyeblink CRs at each of the three trace intervals (Figure 8.2). These differences occurred in the absence of any differences between the amnesic patients and controls in CR onset latency or CR and UR amplitude, though the peak CR latency for the amnesic patients was about 50 msec shorter than that of the controls. The patients and controls also exhibited equivalent extinction in the 500- and 750-msec trace interval paradigm, the only trace intervals at which the patients showed significant (but impaired) acquisition.

Our findings in the trace eyeblink conditioning task in human amnesic patients are convergent with, although not precisely the same as, our findings with rabbits and rats. Hippocampectomized rabbits and rats show essentially no acquisition in trace eyeblink conditioning, even following extensive conditioning. The amnesic patients were impaired in the 500-msec and 750-msec trace interval conditions relative to their matched controls,

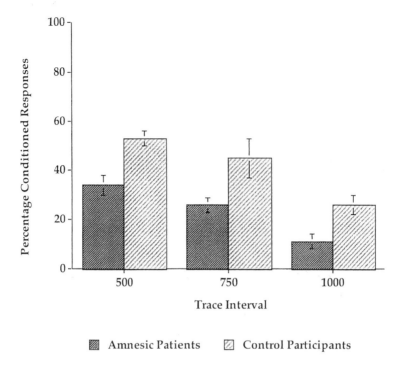

FIGURE 8.2. Mean percentage of CRs for amnesic patients and control participants as a function of trace interval. Note the impairment in the amnesic patients at each trace interval. From McGlinchey-Berroth et al. (1997). Copyright 1997 by the American Psychological Association. Reprinted by permission.

although, unlike the animals, they did exhibit some acquisition at these trace intervals. The 1,000-msec trace interval was especially sensitive to temporal lobe damage in the patients. In addition, Woodruff-Pak (1993) demonstrated that the medial temporal lobe amnesia patient H. M. and another such patient were able to acquire and retain trace eyeblink conditioning, although they did so relatively slowly. There are several possible explanations for the divergent effects between the humans and animals. First, it is unlikely that the humans had complete hippocampal lesions comparable to those in the experimental animals (although the entorhinal cortex is almost completely absent in H. M.; Corkin, Amaral, Gonzalez, Johnson, & Hyman, 1997). Second, the acquisition that did occur in the trace conditioning paradigm may well have been mediated and retained by whatever brain system was involved in the unimpaired acquisition of the delay conditioning paradigm. Note that H. M. showed successful retention of trace eyeblink conditioning 2 years after his initial training. Possible candidates for mediating the task, with or without some residual hippocampus, are the cerebellar–brainstem system and/or the interconnected basal ganglia.

AWARENESS AND ATTENTION

The relation of attention and awareness to eyeblink conditioning has a long history (Cole, 1939; Grant, 1939, 1973). A recent study by Clark and Squire (1998) brought this issue to the fore within the context of the neurobiological substrates of eyeblink conditioning, as well as its broader theoretical implications. Clark and Squire showed that patients with medial temporal lobe amnesia were able to acquire delay discrimination eyeblink conditioning (tone vs. white noise), although they had no awareness of stimulus relationships in a posttraining questionnaire. In contrast, the amnesic patients were unable to acquire the trace discrimination eyeblink conditioning task, and of course showed no awareness of stimulus contingencies. The especially interesting findings were that some of the control subjects were also unable to acquire the delay and trace discrimination tasks. In the case of delay conditioning, there was no relationship between the ability to acquire the task and awareness of the stimulus contingencies. However, all subjects able to acquire the trace discrimination conditioning task were aware of the stimulus contingencies. Thus Clark and Squire suggested that trace eyeblink conditioning may be an associative task that requires declarative memory. This raises the possibility that analyses of the neurobiological substrates of declarative learning may be carried out in animal models with trace conditioning.

We have discussed previously some of the issues raised in this study (LeBar & Disterhoft, 1998). First, it should be noted that the impaired performance of amnesic patients in trace discrimination learning was as expected, given our studies of single-cue trace eyeblink conditioning. This finding confirmed the notion that trace conditioning is dependent on the hippocampus. However, we suggested that the conclusion regarding the declarative nature of trace eyeblink conditioning should be accepted with caution. The discrimination paradigm adds a complexity to the training situation not present in single-cue delay and trace conditioning studies. This complexity could involve aspects of cognition or awareness. It seemed possible not only that trace conditioning is declarative, but also that discriminative eyeblink conditioning, whether delay or trace, may have this feature as well. Subsequent studies have demonstrated that acquisition of single-cue trace conditioning (Manns, Clark, & Squire, 2000a; Woodruff-Pak, 1999), but not of delay conditioning (Manns, Clark, & Squire, 2001), is related to subject awareness of stimulus contingencies. We have therefore explored the relation of awareness with acquisition of two-tone discriminative delay and trace conditioning. Moreover, the subjects in Clark and Squire's study were elderly amnesic patients and age-matched controls. The age of the subjects could have affected their performance in the training tasks, as well as their ability to respond accurately to a posttraining questionnaire probing awareness of the stimulus and reinforcement contingencies. We have addressed this possibility empirically. Finally, we suggested that parallel brain systems could be involved in mediating the temporal aspect of the trace discrimination task and the awareness component; that is, awareness could be mediated by different brain systems than the system(s) supporting trace conditioning itself. This concept is in agreement with the suggestion that awareness is a result of hippocampal–neocortical interactions during acquisition of trace conditioning (Clark & Squire, 1998; Manns, Clark, & Squire, 2000a, 2000b). Thus awareness may be a natural concomitant of hippocampus-dependent memory, rather than a requirement of it (Eichenbaum, 1999). We have carried out several studies that are relevant to these general issues.

Our initial study examined the contribution of attention to eyeblink conditioning in the delay, trace, delay discrimination, and delay discrimination reversal paradigms (Carrillo, Gabrieli, & Disterhoft, 2000). Young adult subjects were trained in the single-cue or two-cue discrimination tasks while concurrently experiencing one of three levels of distraction: full attention (no distraction); concurrently watching a silent movie; or concurrently performing a verbal shadowing task (repeating back the words to the first chapter of a horror novel read over a tape recorder). Our initial hypothesis was that single-cue delay conditioning would probably not be affected by any of the distraction conditions, whereas single-cue trace conditioning would be affected, especially by the verbal shadowing task. To our surprise, we found that neither single-cue delay nor single-cue trace conditioning was affected by any of the distraction tasks, even the rather difficult verbal shadowing task. In contrast, we observed a graded effect of the distraction tasks on the two-tone delay discrimination task (Figure 8.3). The subjects in the full-attention condition demonstrated the largest amount of discrimination; those experiencing the silent movie were intermediate in their level of discrimination between the CS$^+$ and CS$^-$; and the subjects experiencing the verbal shadowing task showed no acquisition to either the CS$^+$ or the CS$^-$, and of course no discrimination. During discrimination reversal, only the full-attention group successfully reversed the discrimination and, by the end of the training, showed a good separation between the new CS$^+$ and CS$^-$. Awareness was evaluated by a posttraining interview in which subjects were asked to relate the purpose of the experiment. The only group that had a significant number of unaware subjects was the verbal shadowing group (6 of 16). A separate analysis of the acquisition rates for the aware and unaware subjects in the verbal shadowing group showed no difference in performance between the two subgroups. All subjects, whether aware or unaware, were unable to acquire the two-tone delay eyeblink discrimination task. This finding suggests that level of awareness was not related to lack of performance in this delay discrimination conditioning task. Given the dramatic effects of division of attention on the two-tone delay discrimination and reversal task, we did not extend these studies to the two-tone trace discrimination paradigm.

Our overall conclusion from this study is that attention has surprisingly little effect on single-cue trace and delay conditioning, but clearly has an effect on the ability of subjects to perform even delay discrimination conditioning. Because there was a major effect of division of attention on the two-cue discrimination task but not the single-cue tasks, we suggested that the discrimination per se required a substantial degree of attention. Also, because division of attention affected neither delay nor trace single-cue conditioning, it seems likely that the neural system mediating this attention should be separate from the cerebellum, which is critical for delay conditioning, and from the hippocampus, which is critical for trace conditioning. Although attention and awareness are not precisely the same construct, the hypothesis that parallel brain systems mediate conditioning and attention is similar to the hypothesis for awareness and conditioning discussed above. Our finding of the effects of dividing attention on delay discrimination conditioning differs somewhat from that of Clark and Squire (1999), who observed that a concurrent digit task affected delay discrimination conditioning no more than a silent movie task, but disrupted trace discrimination conditioning much more than the silent movie task did. The distraction tasks and the discrimination tasks were not the same in the different studies, and it may be the case that a more demanding distraction task (e.g., shadowing) combined with a more difficult discrimination (e.g., two tones) will be more disruptive than the digit task in combination with an easier tone–white noise discrimination.

We recently completed a study designed to explore the issues of awareness in delay and trace discrimination eyeblink conditioning in young and aging subjects (Knuttinen, Power, Preston, & Disterhoft, 2001). The purpose of our study was to evaluate the potential impact of age and of the delay versus trace eyeblink discrimination task on awareness and conditioning performance. The subjects watched a silent movie, Charlie Chaplin's *The Gold Rush*, during the training session, and were told that they would be questioned about it afterward. The subjects were given a questionnaire after the training session (the same one used by Clark & Squire, 1998) to test their knowledge of the movie's content and of the stimulus and reinforcement contingencies. Behavioral acquisition and discrimination between the CS$^+$ and CS$^-$ were clear on a subject-by-subject basis in both the delay and trace discrimination eyeblink conditioning paradigms (Figure 8.4). The major findings of

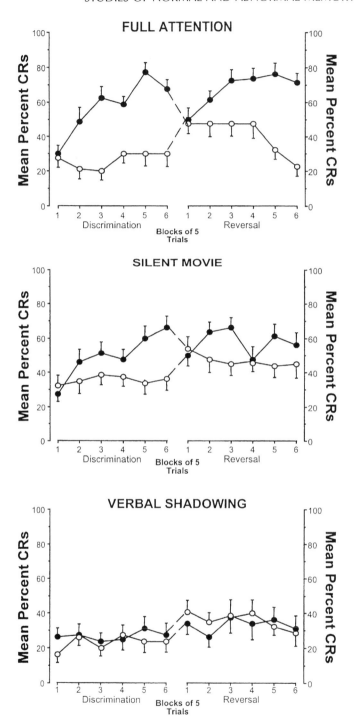

FIGURE 8.3. Discrimination and discrimination reversal in young controls under three attention conditions: full attention, silent movie, and verbal shadowing. Filled circles, CS+; open circles, CS−. From Carrillo, Gabrieli, and Disterhoft (2000). Copyright 2000 by Psychonomic Society Publications. Reprinted by permission.

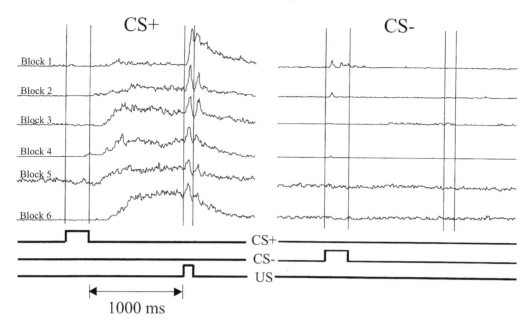

FIGURE 8.4. Development of the CR to the CS⁺ over the course of training within a single conditioning session in the 1,000-msec trace. Each conditioning block consisted of 20 trials. Depicted here are averaged responses of these 10 CS⁺ and 10 CS⁻ trials. *Left:* The increasingly developing CR, over the course of six trial blocks. Early in training, a small response was given to the CS⁺, which subsequently increased in amplitude and latency of the peak response. *Right:* In a similar yet opposite fashion, initial responses were made to the CS⁻, which slowly disappeared as the training session continued. From Knuttinen, Power, Preston, and Disterhoft (2001). Copyright 2001 by the American Psychological Association. Reprinted by permission.

our study were straightforward. Both the young and aged subjects in the delay and trace discrimination conditions showed a very high level of knowledge of the movie content. In addition, there were subgroups of subjects who were aware of the stimulus contingencies in both the delay and trace discrimination eyeblink conditioning groups. Importantly, the aware subjects showed the highest level of conditioning in both the delay and trace discrimination conditioning groups and in both the young adult and older adult groups. Finally, performance of the young and aged subjects was comparable in the delay discrimination paradigm, but the aged subjects were clearly inferior to the young subjects in the trace conditioning paradigm, especially at the 1,000-msec trace interval (Figure 8.5).

Our study confirmed previous studies with animals indicating that trace conditioning, but not delay conditioning, is impaired with aging (Graves & Solomon, 1985; Knuttinen, Power, et al., 2001; Solomon & Groccia-Ellison, 1996; Thompson et al., 1996). An earlier study had reported impaired acquisition in delay conditioning in aging humans (Woodruff-Pak & Thompson, 1988). However, that study used shorter CS-US intervals than our study, and aged individuals appear to have difficulty eliciting CRs rapidly (Woodruff-Pak & Papka, 1996). Our study also confirmed previous findings that awareness of stimulus contingencies is correlated with successful acquisition of trace single-cue (Manns et al., 2000a, 2000b, 2001; Woodruff-Pak, 1999) and trace discrimination (Clark

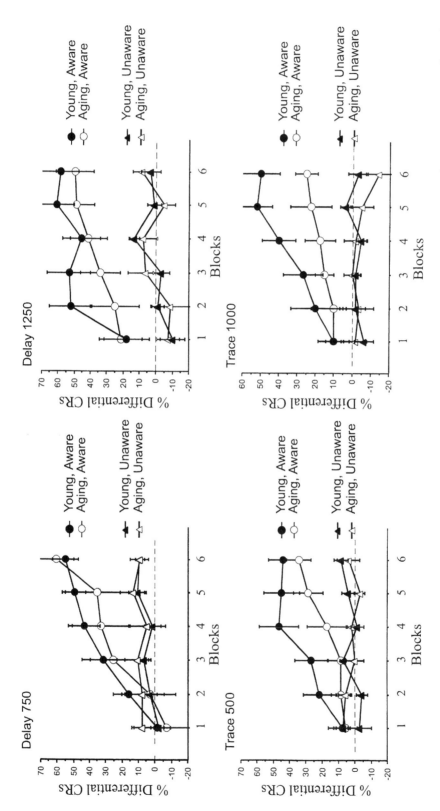

FIGURE 8.5. Percentage of differential eyeblink CRs for each block of 20 trials (% CRs to the CS⁺ minus % CRs to the CS⁻). *Upper panels:* Both young aware and aging aware subjects attained a level of at least 50% differential CRs in the 750-msec delay and 1,250-msec delay paradigms, compared to only 10% differential CRs in the unaware groups. *Lower panels:* Young and aging aware subjects increased their percentage of differential CRs across the conditioning session in the 500-msec trace and 1,000-msec trace paradigms. The young subjects learned better than the aging subjects in the 500-msec trace and especially the 1,000-msec trace paradigm. From Knuttinen, Power, Preston, and Disterhoft (2001). Copyright 2001 by the American Psychological Association. Reprinted by permission.

& Squire, 1998) eyeblink conditioning. Our data indicate that the fact that Clark and Squire used aging subjects in their original study apparently did not affect the pattern of their results relating awareness to acquisition of trace eyeblink conditioning. We did find that more young subjects than aging subjects were aware of the stimulus contingencies in the post hoc questionnaire. However, in agreement with older studies (Cole, 1939; Grant, 1939, 1973; Ross & Nelson, 1973) and in disagreement with more recent work (Clark & Squire, 1998, 1999; Daum, Channon, Polkey, & Gray, 1991 [for conditional delay discrimination conditioning]; and Manns et al., 2001 [for single-cue delay conditioning]), we found that awareness was also correlated with acquisition for delay discrimination eyeblink conditioning. Our data suggest to us that the discriminative aspect of the eyeblink conditioning paradigm, rather than the trace versus delay aspect, may be associated with declarative memory in nonamnesic subjects evaluated with a post hoc questionnaire. However, the studies done recently and cited above are not unanimous on this point. As a matter of fact, our study (Knuttinen, Power, et al., 2001) is unique in the finding that successful acquisition of delay discrimination eyeblink conditioning is associated with awareness of the stimulus contingencies in intact subjects. It should also be noted that we found in our study of the effects of division of attention on delay discrimination and discrimination reversal eyeblink conditioning that subjects in the verbal shadowing group were unable to acquire or reverse the discrimination, whether they were aware or unaware of the stimulus contingencies (Carrillo et al., 2000). It is not clear where this observation fits in relation to the other studies addressing the relation of awareness and delay conditioning, as this subgroup of subjects was unable to acquire the task.

Manns and colleagues (2001) suggest that the difference between our most recent study and theirs may lie in our definition of CRs. We excluded responses with latencies shorter than 100 msec after CS onset—a criterion that we have used in all of our human eyeblink conditioning studies to date, and that was designed to eliminate alpha responses and short-latency voluntary responses (Gormezano, 1966). Manns and colleagues used a 1,250-msec CS-US interstimulus interval in their single-cue delay eyeblink training paradigm, and excluded as voluntary responses any eyeblinks that began before 500 msec prior to US onset (750 msec after CS onset in their study). Manns and colleagues suggest that the different criteria used for inclusion of a response as a CR may have led to the discrepancy in findings regarding the relation of awareness to success in acquisition of delay eyeblink conditioning. As the review that they cite notes, it has been very difficult to eliminate voluntary responders from human eyeblink studies (Coleman & Webster, 1988; see also Gormezano, 1966). And, as Manns and colleagues note, the average responses illustrated in Figure 8.4 (from Knuttinen, Power, et al., 2001) do not meet their latency criterion for a CR. But we should point out that this figure illustrates average EMG responses for blocks of 10 trials, not an individual CR. In addition, Figure 8.3 illustrates responses for a trace conditioning subject, where our data clearly converge with Clark and Squire (1998) and Manns and colleagues (2000a, 2000b) in indicating that awareness is related to successful acquisition. The very reasonable possibility that response definition in delay conditioning has led to the discrepancy in our findings as regards the relation of awareness to acquisition of delay eyeblink conditioning will no doubt be determined in future studies that compare results using our groups' two alternative methods for inclusion of a response as a CR or non-CR.

We might note an interesting "sidebar" to this discussion of potential discrepancies in studies addressing the relation of awareness to acquisition. Gormezano (1966) began using animals to study behavioral and neural mechanisms of eyeblink conditioning as a way to finesse the issue of voluntary responders in his human studies. It seems obvious that we don't have to worry about voluntary responding in rabbits, rats, cats, or mice. Experimental psychologists and behavioral neuroscientists have now studied eyeblink conditioning in animal models extensively for four decades, and have certainly made progress in outlining the neural circuits mediating this associatively learned response. We have also begun to understand some of the cellular and subcellular alterations that underlie eyeblink conditioning. We are now in a position to redirect a portion of our experiments back to humans, in an attempt to delineate brain circuits in humans that may mediate this well-defined associative task. But among the important features of human cognitive function are conscious awareness and the ability to perform voluntary responses. So the issue of voluntary responding has returned as an unavoidable issue in these studies. And we obviously will have to pay special attention to this vexing issue of voluntary responders. We are fortunate to be in a stronger position now than 40 years ago to use physiological and imaging tools (e.g., evoked potentials and PET or fMRI imaging) in combination with careful behavioral evaluation to address these issues. We may be able to use this opportunity to cast more direct light on the brain mechanisms of awareness, leading presumably to voluntary responding, during this period of renewed interest in the study of human eyeblink conditioning.

EFFECTS OF LESIONS ON DISCRIMINATION AND DISCRIMINATION REVERSAL EYEBLINK CONDITIONING

We have carried out three studies exploring discrimination conditioning in humans with brain lesions. The first was aimed at determining the potential parallel between the human and rabbit in terms of the effect of hippocampal/temporal lobe lesions on delay discrimination and discrimination reversal eyeblink conditioning (Carrillo et al., in press). We studied eight patients with medial temporal lobe amnesia who were impaired in recall tests, but had preserved intellectual and attentional function, and their demographically matched controls. Our findings generally agreed with those observed previously in rabbits (Berger & Orr, 1983) and in human amnesic patients regarding the initial discrimination (Clark & Squire, 1998). Both the patients with temporal lobe amnesia and their matched controls showed discrimination between the CS+ and CS− during the initial training trials, but the amnesic patients showed CRs to both the CSs after the reversal occurred. The amnesic pattern of responses was precisely that demonstrated by the hippocampally lesioned rabbits of Berger and Orr. The amnesic subjects did not exhibit the flexibility that the controls did and inhibit responses to the new CS− (Cohen & Eichenbaum, 1993). Awareness was not related to the ability of the amnesic patients to acquire the initial delay discrimination response; that is, they acquired the initial discrimination, regardless of their posttraining verbal reports of awareness of stimulus contingencies. This finding for amnesic subjects is in agreement with previous studies (Clark & Squire, 1998; Daum et al., 1991).

For a second study, we used a temporal delay eyeblink discrimination task modeled after one developed in the rabbit by Mauk and Ruiz (1992). One of two tones was paired with an airpuff after a relatively short CS-US interval (350 msec), and the other was paired with the airpuff after a longer interval (750 msec). Patients with temporal lobe amnesia were impaired in this task (McGlinchey-Berroth, Brawn, & Disterhoft, 1999). They showed shorter latency CRs to the longer tone than controls did, as well as more "nonadaptive CRs" that ended earlier than in controls and did not overlap the UR. They also showed fewer CRs overall during acquisition and showed less extinction (i.e., more CRs during extinction training). Our data suggest a role of the hippocampal system in controlling the precise timing of conditioned eyeblinks within the context of the temporal discrimination task, as well as in controlling both the acquisition and extinction of CRs within this context.

The third study involved a patient with almost complete cerebellar cortical atrophy but with marked sparing of the dentate nucleus (Fortier, Disterhoft, & McGlinchey-Berroth, 2000). Our original intention was to use the temporal delay discrimination task described above with this patient. When we trained her in the temporal discrimination task, she showed complete lack of acquisition (i.e., no responses to either the CS+ or CS-). She showed the same failure to respond to either CS in a simpler two-tone delay discrimination task. We then trained her on single-cue trace conditioning, which she acquired and extinguished similarly to her normal controls. The same was true for single-cue delay conditioning. What was striking was her complete inability to acquire either the temporal delay discrimination task or a simpler two-tone delay discrimination task. These data suggest that the cerebellar cortex is required for discrimination eyeblink conditioning, even though it is not required for either single-cue delay or trace eyeblink conditioning. These striking observations were made in experiments done with a single subject who presented with a very unusual clinical syndrome, so they should be interpreted with appropriate caution. But they certainly suggest that the cerebellar cortex is uniquely involved in discrimination as compared to single-cue eyeblink conditioning.

CONCLUSIONS

Our behavioral studies thus far indicate that the neurobiological circuitry mediating eyeblink conditioning in the human brain is similar or identical to that used in the experimental animals that have been studied. Delay and two-tone delay discrimination conditioning are intact in humans with medial temporal lobe amnesia. Trace conditioning, especially with a long stimulus-free trace interval, and discrimination reversal are impaired in humans with medial temporal lobe amnesia. Both individuals with alcoholic Korsakoff's syndrome and nonamnesic individuals recovering from alcoholism, who have damage to their cerebellar cortex as a result of long-term alcohol abuse, are impaired in delay conditioning. Trace discrimination conditioning, but not delay discrimination conditioning, is impaired in aged participants. All of these findings are consistent with what would have been predicted from the animal literature.

Our findings for discrimination conditioning are also providing insights that were not initially predictable from the animal work. Our experiments suggest that including a discrimination component to the eyeblink conditioning task adds a higher-level cognitive or awareness component that may be mediated in parallel to the temporal lobe system required for trace conditioning. For example, neither the distraction of a silent movie nor verbal shadowing affected acquisition of single-cue delay or single-cue trace conditioning. Yet both distraction tasks impaired the acquisition and especially the reversal of two-tone delay discrimination conditioning. In our studies, acquisition of both delay and trace eyeblink discrimination conditioning were correlated with awareness of stimulus contingencies, in both young and aged nonamnesic participants. Thus, in intact subjects who can be evaluated with a post hoc questionnaire, acquisition of both delay and trace discrimination versions of eyeblink conditioning are associated with awareness of stimulus contingencies. Our findings therefore suggest that both of these tasks, as well as single-cue trace conditioning (Manns et al., 2000a; Woodruff-Pak, 1999), have declarative components, as originally was suggested for trace discrimination eyeblink conditioning by Clark and Squire (1998). As discussed above, our findings regarding the relation of awareness to acquisition of delay discrimination conditioning are at variance with other recent studies addressing this issue. There is the possibility, to be empirically explored, that this variance can be explained by differences in the criteria applied for defining an eyeblink as a CR. Finally, in a case study of a woman with severe cerebellar cortical deterioration but apparently intact cerebellar deep nuclei, we observed successful acquisition of trace and delay single-cue eyeblink conditioning, but no capacity for acquisition of delay discriminative eyeblink conditioning. This series of studies indicates that there is something special about the discrimination task, whether trace or delay. Not as much animal work has been done with discrimination paradigms, especially those requiring reversals, because animals take a long time to acquire them. Humans, presumably because of their superior cognitive ability, learn discriminations and reversals relatively quickly. Thus these kinds of higher-order tasks seem especially interesting to explore in human subjects.

We have begun a series of imaging studies that may allow us to identify the unique neural substrates of different higher-order conditioning tasks. For example, the different substrates of delay as compared to trace eyeblink conditioning, as well as the unique region(s) activated in subjects who are aware as opposed to those who are unaware, may be delineated with imaging techniques. In an initial PET study, in which young adult participants were trained in the scanner, we showed activation of the cerebellar cortex, temporal lobe, caudate, and frontal cortex (among other regions), which changed along with behavioral acquisition of the delay eyeblink task (Blaxton et al., 1996). In more recent fMRI studies of delay eyeblink conditioning in young adult subjects, we have found activity in regions that we anticipated from animal studies would be activated during acquisition of the eyeblink CR (e.g., the cerebellar cortex, temporal lobe, frontal cortex, anterior cingulate, and frontal cortex) (Knuttinen et al., 2000; Preston et al., 2000). As yet, we have not explored higher-order conditioning tasks with brain imaging. Such studies are an obvious next step and should lead to a deeper appreciation of the neural systems engaged during acquisition and consolidation of these behavioral tasks. If we can determine the region(s) importantly involved in, for example, trace eyeblink conditioning in the human brain, we can focus our efforts on studying mechanisms of associative learning in animal models with confidence that we are analyzing the substrates of declarative memory. The general approach of combining brain imaging with eyeblink conditioning holds promise for gaining insight into the neural mechanisms of eyeblink conditioning in the human brain, as well as for further exploring the parallels between humans and other mammals.

ACKNOWLEDGMENT

Preparation of this chapter was supported by National Institutes of Health Grants No. R03 AG16031 (to John F. Disterhoft) and No. P50 NS26985 (to Regina McGlinchey-Berroth).

REFERENCES

Akase, E., Alkon, D. L., & Disterhoft, J. F. (1989). Hippocampal lesions impair memory of short-delay conditioned eyeblink in rabbits. *Behavioral Neuroscience, 103,* 935–943.

Berger, T. W., & Orr, W. B. (1983). Hippocampectomy selectively disrupts discrimination reversal conditioning of the rabbit nictitating membrane response. *Behavioral Brain Research, 8,* 49–68.

Blaxton, T. A., Zeffiro, T., Gabrieli, J., Bookheimer, S. Y., Carrillo, M., Theodore, W., & Disterhoft, J. F. (1996). Changes in cerebral blood flow during eyeblink conditioning in humans. *Journal of Neuroscience, 16,* 4032–4040.

Carrillo, M. C., Gabrieli, J. D. E., & Disterhoft, J. F. (2000). Selective effects of division of attention upon discrimination conditioning. *Psychobiology, 28,* 293–302.

Carrillo, M. C., Gabrieli, J. D. E., Hopkins, R. O., McGlinchey-Berroth, R., Fortier, C. B., Kesner, R. P., & Disterhoft, J. F. (in press). Spared discrimination and impaired reversal eyeblink conditioning in patients with temporal lobe amnesia. *Behavioral Neuroscience, 115.*

Cason, H. (1922). The conditioned eyelid reaction. *Journal of Experimental Psychology, 5,* 153–195.

Clark, R. E., & Squire, L. R. (1998). Classical conditioning and brain systems: The role of awareness. *Science, 280,* 77–81.

Clark, R. E., & Squire, L. R. (1999). Human eyeblink classical conditioning: Effects of manipulating awareness of the stimulus contingencies. *Psychological Science, 10,* 14–18.

Cohen, N. J., & Eichenbaum, H. (Eds.). (1993). *Memory, amnesia, and the hippocampal system.* Cambridge, MA: MIT Press.

Cole, L. E. (1939). A comparison of factors of practice and knowledge of experimental procedure in conditioning the eyelid response of human subjects. *Journal of General Psychology, 20,* 349–373.

Coleman, S. R., & Webster, S. (1988). The problem of volition and the conditioned reflex. Part II. Voluntary-responding subjects, 1951–1980. *Behaviorism, 16,* 17–49.

Corkin, S., Amaral, D. G., Gonzalez, R. G., Johnson, K. A., & Hyman, B. T. (1997). H. M.'s medial temporal lobe lesion: Findings from magnetic resonance imaging. *Journal of Neuroscience, 17,* 3964–3979.

Daum, I., Channon, S., Polkey, C. E., & Gray, J. A. (1991). Classical conditioning after temporal lobe lesions in man: Impairment in conditional discrimination. *Behavioral Neuroscience, 105,* 396–408.

Disterhoft, J. F., Kwan, H. H., & Lo, W. D. (1977). Nictitating membrane conditioning to tone in the immobilized albino rabbit. *Brain Research, 137,* 127–143.

Disterhoft, J. F., Quinn, K. J., & Weiss, C. (1987). Analyses of the auditory input and motor output pathways in rabbit nictitating membrane conditioning. In I. Gormezano, W. F. Prokasy, & R. F. Thompson (Eds.), *Classical conditioning* (pp. 93–116). Hillsdale, NJ: Erlbaum.

Disterhoft, J. F., Quinn, K. J., Weiss, C., & Shipley, M. T. (1985). Accessory abducens nucleus and conditioned eye retraction/nictitating membrane extension in rabbit. *Journal of Neuroscience, 5,* 941–950.

Eichenbaum, H. (1999). Conscious awareness, memory and the hippocampus. *Nature Neuroscience, 2,* 775–776.

Fortier, C. B., Disterhoft, J. F., & McGlinchey-Berroth, R. (2000). Cerebellar cortical degeneration disrupts discrimination learning but not delay or trace classical eyeblink conditioning. *Neuropsychology, 14,* 537–550.

Gabrieli, J. D. E., McGlinchey-Berroth, R., Carrillo, M. C., Gluck, M. A., Cermak, L. S., & Disterhoft, J. F. (1995). Intact delay-eyeblink conditioning in amnesia. *Behavioral Neuroscience, 109,* 819–827.

Gormezano, I. (1966). Classical conditioning. In J. B. Sidowski (Ed.), *Experimental methods and instrumentation in psychology* (pp. 385–420). New York: McGraw-Hill.

Gormezano, I., & Kehoe, E. J. (1983). Twenty years of classical conditioning research with the rabbit. *Progress in Psychobiology and Physiological Psychology, 10,* 198–275.

Gormezano, I., Prokasy, W. F., & Thompson, R. F. (Eds.). (1987). *Classical conditioning.* Hillsdale, NJ: Erlbaum.

Gormezano, I., & Schneiderman, N. (1962). Nictitating membrane: Classical conditioning and extinction in the albino rabbit. *Science, 138,* 33–34.

Grant, D. A. (1939). The influence of attitude on the conditioned eyelid response. *Journal of Experimental Psychology, 25,* 333–346.

Grant, D. A. (1973). Cognitive factors in eyelid conditioning. *Psychophysiology, 10,* 75–81.

Graves, C. A., & Solomon, P. R. (1985). Age-related disruption of trace but not delay classical conditioning of the rabbit's nictitating membrane response. *Behavioral Neuroscience, 99,* 88–96.

Knuttinen, M-G., Gamelli, A. E., Weiss, C., Power, J. M., & Disterhoft, J. F. (2001). Age-related effects on learning eyeblink conditioning in the Fisher 344 x Brown Norway F1 hybrid rat. *Neurobiology of Aging, 22,* 1–8.

Knuttinen, M-G., Power, J. M., Preston, A. R., & Disterhoft, J. F. (2001). Awareness in classical differential eyeblink conditioning in young and aging humans. *Behavioral Neuroscience, 115,* 747–757.

Knuttinen, M-G., Weiss, C., Parrish, T. B., LaBar, K. S., Gitelman, D. R., Power, J. M., Mesulam, M.-M., & Disterhoft, J. F. (2000). Event-related fMRI of delay eyeblink conditioning. *NeuroImage, 11,* 416.

LaBar, K. S., & Disterhoft, J. F. (1998). Conditioning, awareness, and the hippocampus. *Hippocampus, 8,* 620–626.

Manns, J. R., Clark, R. E., & Squire, L. R. (2000a). Awareness predicts the magnitude of single-cue trace eyeblink conditioning. *Hippocampus, 10,* 181–186.

Manns, J. R., Clark, R. E., & Squire, L. R. (2000b). Parallel acquisition of awareness and trace eyeblink classical conditioning. *Learning and Memory, 7,* 267–272.

Manns, J. R., Clark, R. E., & Squire, L. R. (2001). Single-cue eyeblink conditioning is unrelated to awareness. *Cognitive, Affective and Behavioral Neuroscience, 2,* 192–198.

Mauk, M. D., & Ruiz, B. P. (1992). Learning-dependent timing of Pavlovian eyelid responses: Differential conditioning using multiple interstimulus intervals. *Behavioral Neuroscience, 106*(4), 666–681.

McEchron, M. D., Bouwmeester, H., Tseng, W., Weiss, C., & Disterhoft, J. F. (1998). Hippocampectomy disrupts auditory trace fear conditioning and contextual fear conditioning in the rat. *Hippocampus, 8,* 638–646.

McEchron, M. D., Tseng, W., & Disterhoft, J. F. (2000). Neurotoxic lesions of the dorsal hippocampus disrupt auditory-cued trace heart rate (fear) conditioning in rabbit. *Hippocampus, 10,* 739–751.

McGlinchey-Berroth, R., Brawn, C., & Disterhoft, J. F. (1999). Temporal discrimination learning in severe amnesics reveals an alteration in the timing of eyeblink conditioned responses. *Behavioral Neuroscience, 113,* 10–18.

McGlinchey-Berroth, R., Carrillo, M. C., Brawn, C. M., Gabrieli, J. D. E., Cermak, L. S., & Disterhoft, J. F. (1997). Impaired trace eyeblink conditioning in medial temporal lobe amnesia. *Behavioral Neuroscience, 111,* 873–882.

McGlinchey-Berroth, R., Cermak, L. S., Carrillo, M. C., Armfield, S., Gabrieli, J. D. E., & Disterhoft, J. F. (1995). Impaired delay eyeblink conditioning in amnesic Korsakoff's patients and recovered alcoholics. *Alcoholism: Clinical and Experimental Research, 19,* 1127–1132.

Moyer, J. R., Deyo, R. A., & Disterhoft, J. F. (1990). Hippocampectomy disrupts trace eye-blink conditioning in rabbits. *Behavioral Neuroscience, 104,* 242–252.

Preston, A. R., Knuttinen, M-G., Christoff, K., Glover, G. H., Gabrieli, J. D. E., & Disterhoft, J. F. (2000). The neural basis of classical eyeblink conditioning: An event-related fMRI study. *Society for Neuroscience Abstracts, 26,* 709.

Ross, L. E., & Nelson, M. N. (1973). The role of awareness in differential conditioning. *Psychophysiology, 10,* 91–94.

Schmaltz, L. W., & Theios, J. (1972). Acquisition and extinction of a classically conditioned response in hippocampectomized rabbits (*Oryctolagus cuniculus*). *Journal of Comparative and Physiological Psychology, 79,* 328–333.

Solomon, P. R., & Groccia-Ellison, M. E. (1996). Classic conditioning in aged rabbits: Delay, trace, and long-delay conditioning. *Behavioral Neuroscience, 110,* 427–435.

Solomon, P. R., Vander Schaaf, E., Thompson, R. F., & Weisz, D. J. (1986). Hippocampus and trace conditioning of the rabbit's classically conditioned nictitating membrane response. *Behavioral Neuroscience, 100,* 729–744.

Telford, C. W., & Anderson, B. O. (1932). The normal wink reflex: Its facilitation and inhibition. *Journal of Experimental Psychology, 15,* 235–266.

Thompson, L. T., Moyer, J. R., Jr., & Disterhoft, J. F. (1996). Trace eyeblink conditioning in rabbits demonstrates heterogeneity of learning ability both between and within age groups. *Neurobiology of Aging, 17,* 619–629.

Thompson, R. F. (1986). The neurobiology of learning and memory. *Science, 233,* 941–947.

Thompson, R. F. (1990). Neural mechanisms of classical conditioning in mammals. *Philosophical Transactions of the Royal Society of London, Series B, 329,* 161–170.

Thompson, R. F., Berger, T. W., Cegavske, C. F., Patterson, M. M., Roemer, R. A., Teyler, T. J., & Young, R. A. (1976). A search for the engram. *American Psychologist, 31,* 209–227.

Thompson, R. F., & Kim, J. J. (1996). Memory systems in the brain and localization of a memory. *Proceedings of the National Academy of Sciences, USA, 93,* 13438–13444.

Weiss, C., Bouwmeester, H., Power, J. M., & Disterhoft, J. F. (1999). Hippocampal lesions prevent trace eyeblink conditioning in the freely moving rat. *Behavioral Brain Research, 99*(2), 123–132.

Woodruff-Pak, D. S. (1993). Eyeblink classical conditioning in H. M.: Delay and trace paradigms. *Behavioral Neuroscience, 107*(6), 911–925.

Woodruff-Pak, D. S. (1999). New directions for a classical paradigm: Human eyeblink conditioning. *Psychological Science, 10,* 1–3.

Woodruff-Pak, D. S., & Papka, M. (1996). Alzheimer's disease and eyeblink conditioning: 750 ms trace vs. 400 ms delay paradigm. *Neurobiology of Aging, 17*(3), 397–404.

Woodruff-Pak, D. S., & Steinmetz, J. E. (Eds.). (2000a). *Eyeblink classical conditioning: Vol. 1. Human applications.* Boston: Kluwer.

Woodruff-Pak, D. S., & Steinmetz, J. E. (Eds.). (2000b). *Eyeblink classical conditioning: Vol. 2. Animal models.* Boston: Kluwer.

Woodruff-Pak, D. S., & Thompson, R. F. (1988). Classical conditioning of the eyeblink response in the delay paradigm in adults aged 18–83 years. *Psychology and Aging, 3,* 219–229.

9

Memory Illusions in Amnesic Patients

Findings and Implications

DANIEL L. SCHACTER, MIEKE VERFAELLIE, and WILMA KOUTSTAAL

Studies of patients with organic amnesia have contributed enormously to understanding the neuropsychology of memory. Scoville and Milner's (1957) pioneering observations concerning the effects of bilateral medial temporal lobe (MTL) removal in patient H. M. convincingly revealed the key role of the MTL in establishing new memories of day-to-day experiences. Later studies of H. M. and many other amnesic patients revealed dramatic dissociations between impaired explicit or declarative memory and preserved implicit or nondeclarative memory (cf. Schacter, 1987; Squire, 1992). These dissociations have played a critical role in shaping the view that memory consists of multiple forms or systems (see, e.g., Cohen & Eichenbaum, 1993; Schacter & Tulving, 1994; Squire & Zola-Morgan, 1991).

Research concerning amnesic patients has been rather less influential in the analysis of constructive aspects of memory—the errors, distortions, and illusions that sometimes characterize memory in the laboratory and in everyday life (Bartlett, 1932; Loftus, 1979; Neisser, 1967; Schacter, 1999b, 2001). Studies of confabulation in amnesic patients have led to ideas and hypotheses about mechanisms involved in memory monitoring and verification processes (e.g., Burgess & Shallice, 1996; Dalla Barba, 1993; Johnson, 1991; Moscovitch, 1989, 1995; Schacter, Norman, & Koutstaal, 1998; Schnider & Ptak, 1999), but apart from a focus on this question, students of amnesia have been largely mute concerning errors, illusions, and related constructive aspects of memory.

During the past few years, the situation has begun to change. A number of research groups have begun to focus on illusory or false memories in amnesic patients, attempting to use these observations to gain insight into the basic memory processes that underlie such errors. Cognitive psychologists generally agree that memory errors and illusions can provide revealing insights into the operation of basic memory processes (e.g., Jacoby, Kelley, & Dywan, 1989; Johnson, Hashtroudi, & Lindsay, 1993; Roediger, 1996; Schacter, 1996), and a similar consensus seems to be emerging in neuropsychology (see, e.g., Parkin, 1997; Rapcsak, Nielsen, Glisky, & Kaszniak, Chapter 10, this volume; and the papers in Schacter,

1999a). The purpose of this chapter is to review some of our own and others' work that has explored illusory memories in amnesic patients, and to consider several key empirical and theoretical issues that these studies have raised. We focus primarily on the phenomenon of "false recognition," which occurs when an individual mistakenly claims that a novel item or event is familiar. We first review recent studies that examine the nature and basis of false recognition in amnesic patients, and then turn to some unresolved questions and issues that require attention in future research.

FALSE RECOGNITION OF WORDS

Within experimental psychology, Underwood (1965) provided an early and influential demonstration of false recognition. He used a continuous-recognition paradigm in which words were presented and subjects made "old–new" decisions about each one. Some of the words were repeated; others were preceded by semantically, associatively, or physically similar words, or by entirely new words. Subjects responded "old" to the related words at a somewhat higher rate than to entirely unrelated new words, thereby documenting the occurrence of false recognition.

The first experimental study of false recognition in amnesic patients, reported by Cermak, Butters, and Gerrein (1973), employed a procedure similar to that introduced by Underwood (1965): a continuous-recognition paradigm in which new and old words were intermixed, and subjects responded "old" or "new" to each test item. New words were preceded by a single homophone, associate, or synonym. Six amnesic patients with Korsakoff's syndrome and six matched controls participated in the study. The amnesic patients showed a higher level of false recognition than did controls to both homophones and associates; neither amnesic patients nor controls in this experiment showed significant false recognition to synonyms.

Amnesic patients also recognized fewer of the words that had been presented previously. Cermak and colleagues (1973) argued that decreased true recognition and increased false recognition on the part of the amnesic patients reflected poor semantic encoding of target words: The patients did not encode deeply enough to remember words that were actually presented, or to reject new words that were related to previously exposed items.

To our knowledge, no studies followed up on the Cermak and colleagues (1973) results; in fact, we are unable to identify any studies reported during the next two decades that specifically focused on false recognition in amnesic patients. We initiated a series of such studies during the mid-1990s. We were inspired in part by striking results from a paradigm initially developed by Deese (1959), and later revived and modified by Roediger and McDermott (1995), which yields surprisingly high levels of false recognition in healthy young participants with intact brain function. In the Deese/Roediger–McDermott or "DRM" paradigm, participants study a list of associated words that all converge on a nonpresented "theme word," and are then tested for studied words, the nonstudied theme word, and other nonstudied words that are unrelated to the target item. For instance, participants might study a list of words such as "candy," "sour," "bitter," "good," "taste," "tooth," "nice," "honey," "soda," "chocolate," "heart," "cake," "eat," and "pie," which all converge on the nonpresented theme word "sweet." Roediger and McDermott (1995) found that participants claimed to recognize nonpresented theme words such as "sweet" about as often as they claimed to recognize words that actually appeared on the study lists (such as "taste"), falsely recognizing approximately 80% of the theme words—much higher than the relatively modest rates of false recognition reported by Underwood (1965). Participants expressed high confidence in their false-recognition responses and often claimed to possess specific recollections of having encountered the word. These results were soon confirmed and extended by others (e.g., Mather, Henkel, & Johnson, 1997; Norman & Schacter, 1997; Payne, Elie, Blackwell, & Neuschatz, 1996; Robinson & Roediger, 1997). Although there has been some debate regarding the nature and implications of this robust false-recognition effect (cf. Miller & Wolford, 1999; Roediger & McDermott, 1999; Wixted & Stretch, 2000), the existence and reliability of the effect have been firmly established.

Our main motivation in extending the DRM paradigm to amnesic patients was to gain insight into the brain mechanisms underlying this memory illusion. We (Schacter, Verfaellie, & Pradere, 1996) exposed 12 amnesic patients (6 patients with Korsakoff's syndrome, 5 patients with MTL damage resulting from anoxia or encephalitis, and 1 patient with thalamic damage) and matched controls to lists of semantic associates (e.g., "candy," "sour," "sugar," "bitter," "good," "taste," etc.). Participants were later tested with previously studied words (e.g., "taste"), theme words that were semantically related to previously presented words (e.g., "sweet"), and new words that were unrelated to previously studied ones (e.g., "point").

As expected from previous studies of recognition memory in amnesia (e.g., Haist, Shimamura, & Squire, 1992), amnesic patients had difficulty distinguishing between previously studied words and unrelated new items: They attained fewer hits to old words, and made more false alarms to new unrelated words, than did matched controls. More importantly, the amnesic patients also showed significantly lower levels of false recognition to the nonpresented theme words than did the controls (who showed the expected high levels of false recognition to the theme words). Reduced or "impaired" false recognition was observed both in the amnesic patients with Korsakoff's syndrome and the mixed-etiology amnesic group that consisted primarily of patients with MTL damage. More recently, Melo, Winocur. and Moscovitch (1999) have replicated these findings in amnesic patients with mixed etiologies involving damage to MTL, diencephalic, or frontal lobe structures.

To assess the generality of our results beyond the DRM paradigm, we (Schacter, Verfaellie, & Anes, 1997) attempted to replicate the finding of reduced false recognition for semantic associates in amnesic patients with a new set of semantically related words. We also sought to determine whether the effect is restricted to the semantic domain, or extends to perceptual false recognition. It has been argued that perceptually based memory processes are preserved in amnesic patients, whereas conceptually or semantically based processes are impaired (e.g., Blaxton, 1989, 1995; see also Wagner, Gabrieli, & Verfaellie, 1997). From this perspective, amnesic patients might show "preserved" false recognition (i.e., false-positive responding rates similar to those shown by controls) after studying perceptually related materials.

To test this hypothesis, we (Schacter, Verfaellie, & Anes, 1997) used materials based on the experiments of Shiffrin, Huber, and Marinelli (1995). Shiffrin and colleagues found that when college students studied lists of words, such as "fade," "fame," "fake," "mate," "late," "date," and "rate," they later showed false recognition to perceptually related words, such as "fate." We adapted their paradigm for use with amnesic patients. Results of two experiments were largely similar to the earlier ones (Schacter, Verfaellie, & Pradere, 1996). Both patients with MTL damage and patients with Korsakoff's syndrome exhibited impaired true recognition of studied words in the semantic and perceptual conditions. More important, they also showed reduced false recognition for new words, whether they were semantically or perceptually related to previously studied words (for a summary of false-recognition results from our two studies, see Table 9.1).

TABLE 9.1. False Recognition of Words by Amnesic Patients and Matched Controls in Experiments by Schacter, Verfaellie, and Pradere (1996) and Schacter, Verfaellie, and Anes (1997)

Type of materials	Amnesic patients	Matched controls
Semantic associates	.16	.57
Conceptually related	.16	.24
Perceptually related	.12	.40

Note. Data concerning semantic associates from Schacter, Verfaellie, and Pradere (1996); data concerning conceptually and perceptually related words from Schacter, Verfaellie, and Anes (1997). The table displays corrected false-recognition scores in which false alarms to unrelated new words are subtracted from false alarms to related new words. Data from Schacter, Verfaellie, and Pradere are averaged across conditions in which either a free-recall test or an arithmetic test preceded the recognition test.

There was one difference worth noting between the results of our two studies. In the Schacter, Verfaellie, and Pradere (1996) study, amnesic patients showed reduced false recognition on two different measures: (1) the absolute proportion of "old" responses to nonpresented theme words; and (2) a corrected false-recognition measure in which the proportion of false alarms to unrelated new words is subtracted from the proportion of false alarms to theme words. The latter measure is an important one, because amnesic patients sometimes exhibit a bias to respond "old" to unrelated new words, reflecting the fact that they have great difficulty distinguishing between old and new items. Because such a tendency could inflate estimates of false recognition to related theme words, it is important to use corrected false-recognition measures (or signal detection analyses) that take into account such a response bias. In the Schacter, Verfaellie, and Anes (1997) study, amnesic patients showed a heightened tendency to respond "old" to new words that were not perceptually or conceptually related to previously studied ones. As a consequence, the overall proportion of "old" responses to semantically or perceptually related new words did not differ significantly between amnesic patients and controls. Instead, reduced false-recognition to semantically or perceptually related new words was evident only in corrected false-recognition measures that took account of this bias. Nonetheless, we (Schacter, Verfaellie, & Anes, 1997) concluded from these data that amnesic patients showed deficient retention of what we termed "conceptual gist" and "perceptual gist"—information about the shared semantic or perceptual features of studied information that underlies false-recognition responses (cf. Brainerd & Reyna, 1998; Reyna & Brainerd, 1995; Schacter, Norman, & Koutstaal, 1998).

The findings from the foregoing studies suggest that the MTL/diencephalic structures that are damaged in amnesic patients play a role in storing and/or retrieving the semantic or perceptual information that supports false recognition in normal controls. However, these findings contrast sharply with the results discussed earlier from Cermak and colleagues (1973), where amnesic patients showed increased, rather than decreased, false recognition. What accounts for the contrasting pattern of results? In both of our studies, we suggested that when numerous associates are presented for study, as in the DRM paradigm or the related procedures used in the Schacter, Verfaellie, and Anes (1997) study, normal controls establish a well-organized representation of the general semantic or perceptual features of the list—that is, the conceptual or perceptual gist. When this gist representation is matched by a new theme word, normal controls experience a strong sense of familiarity or recollection that results in a powerful false-recognition effect. Amnesic patients, by contrast, encode or retain less gist information and thus show reduced levels of false recognition. Likewise, control subjects can use the potent gist representation to reject new words that are unrelated to, or clearly incongruent with, the perceptual or conceptual gist of studied items, whereas amnesic patients cannot.

Different factors may be operating when only a single related item precedes a new word, as in the study by Cermak and colleagues (1973). Under these conditions, controls should establish a much weaker gist representation than when numerous associates are studied (for particularly clear evidence relating increased category size to increased gist memory in normal controls, see Brainerd & Reyna, 1998, Exp. 3). An equally important factor is that healthy controls can use their intact explicit memory abilities to counter or suppress any familiarity that may be elicited by a related new word. For instance, a healthy control who encounters the nonstudied word "table," and can recollect having previously studied the associate "chair," can use this information to avoid making a false-recognition response. In contrast, amnesic patients are less able to use explicit recollection to suppress whatever weak sense of familiarity might be elicited by a new related word. In this scenario, amnesic patients can exhibit increased levels of false recognition compared with control subjects.

Based on this analysis, we (Schacter, Verfaellie, & Pradere, 1996) suggested that it should be possible to show higher or lower levels of false recognition in amnesic patients compared with controls by creating conditions that are more or less conducive to using explicit recollection to suppress false recognition. We (Schacter, Verfaellie, Anes, & Racine, 1998) tested this idea by repeatedly presenting amnesic patients and matched controls with the same study lists of DRM semantic associates, and testing them with lists composed of previously studied words, semantically related lures, and unrelated lures. We hypothesized that with repeated study and testing of the same lists, normal controls would show increasing explicit recollection of previously presented words, and would use this memory to reduce false alarms to related words that were not presented (see, e.g., McDermott, 1996). By contrast, we hypothesized a contrasting pattern of results in amnesic patients. Based on the data discussed so far, we expected that amnesic patients would continue to show reduced levels of both true and false recognition compared to controls on the first study–test trial. We also expected that with repetition of study–test lists, amnesic patients would continue to show impaired levels of veridical recognition memory compared to controls, although they should show some increases in true recognition across trials.

The key prediction involved levels of false recognition to nonstudied theme words as a function of repetition. We hypothesized that amnesic patients, in contrast to controls, would be unable to use explicit recollection to reduce false recognition across trials. On the contrary, their false recognition might even increase as a function of repetition. Consider that with repetition of study list associates, the theme or gist of the study list should become increasingly accessible. If, as we suggested, the recognition performance of amnesic patients in the DRM paradigm is based largely on a degraded representation of semantic or conceptual gist, and if that representation benefits from repetition, then amnesic patients might show enhanced false recognition across trials. Thus we predicted an interaction between groups and trials for false recognition of related lures: Reduced false recognition in amnesic patients on the first trials should be greatly attenuated, and possibly eliminated or even reversed over the course of multiple study–test trials.

Consider also that with repetition of study list associates, the theme or gist of the study lists should become increasingly accessible. If, as we suggested, the recognition performance of amnesic patients in the DRM paradigm is based largely on a degraded representation of semantic or conceptual gist, and if that representation benefits from repetition, then amnesic patients might even show increased false recognition across trials.

Results were generally consistent with these predictions. Amnesic patients showed reduced levels of corrected false recognition on the first test trial, thus replicating previous results. With repetition, false recognition of theme words in healthy controls declined significantly. In contrast, amnesic patients with MTL damage did not reduce their false-recognition responses with repetition; they showed a flat or fluctuating pattern across trials. Patients with Korsakoff's syndrome actually showed a significant *increase* in false recognition across trials. Although the reasons for the differing patterns in the amnesic group are not entirely clear, it is possible that problems resulting from frontal lobe dysfunction, often observed in Korsakoff patients, made it especially difficult for them to suppress the growing influence of semantic gist across trials (see Schacter, Verfaellie, Anes, & Racine, 1998, for a more detailed discussion). Consistent with this view, in more recent work using the same paradigm in patients with Alzheimer's disease—who are often characterized by both MTL and frontal dysfunction—Budson, Daffner, Desikan, and Schacter (2000) have documented a similar pattern of increasing false recognition across trials.

These results support the analysis we put forward in an attempt to resolve the apparent discrepancy between Cermak and colleagues' (1973) finding of increased false recognition in amnesic patients for lures that were related to only a single study item and our findings (Schacter, Verfaellie, & Anes, 1997; Schacter, Verfaellie, & Pradere, 1996) of decreased false recognition in amnesic patients for lures that were related to multiple study items. When experimental conditions allow or encourage the use of explicit recollection to counter or suppress false-recognition responses—as in Cermak and colleagues' experiment, or in the five-repetition condition of the Schacter, Verfaellie, and colleagues (1998) study—healthy controls can do so to a much greater extent than can amnesic patients. By contrast, when experimental conditions promote the development of powerful gist representations in normal controls, but work against the use of explicit recollection to counter them—as in the Schacter, Verfaellie, and Pradere (1996) and Schacter, Verfaellie, and Anes (1997) experiments—amnesic patients show reduced false recognition. These observations lead us to conceptualize false recognition as the outcome of a kind of competition between two opposing forces: conceptual or perceptual gist, which fuels the development of illusory memories, and explicit recollection of specific information, which can help to keep in check the undue influence of gist representations.

FALSE RECOGNITION OF PROTOTYPES AND PICTURES

Though the foregoing analysis seems to capture well the main features of extant data concerning false recognition in amnesic patients, it is not entirely straightforward. One problem concerns our suggestion that gist information (see, e.g., Brainerd & Reyna, 1998; Payne et al., 1996), or overreliance on shared semantic or perceptual features (Schacter, Norman, & Koutstaal, 1998), is primarily responsible for false recognition in the DRM and related paradigms. Though this is a plausible suggestion, other interpretations are also possible. For instance, false recognition in the DRM procedure may be a consequence of "implicit associative responses" (Underwood, 1965) that occur when participants are exposed to lists of semantic associates during the study phase of the experiment. When studying a list of semantic associates, participants may activate or even consciously generate the non-presented lure word (i.e., "sweet"). On a later memory test, false recognition may occur because participants experience a type of source confusion, mistakenly remembering that they heard or saw the theme word that they themselves have generated (Roediger, Balota, & Watson, 2001; Roediger & McDermott, 1995). From this perspective, amnesic patients may be less likely to generate the theme word at the time of study, and therefore show reduced false recognition. Alternatively, amnesic patients may generate the theme word as frequently as control subjects, but later forget this generated item, just as they forget other individual items that actually appeared on the list. Therefore, reduced false recognition may occur because amnesic patients are not as susceptible as controls to source confusions from internally generated items. In short, reduced false recognition in amnesic patients may not be attributable to degraded gist representations, as we have suggested, but rather to impaired memory for specific, individual items.

To address this issue, and also to expand the generality of our research, we have conducted two sets of experiments involving false recognition of pictorial materials. We made use of paradigms in which false recognition is unlikely to result from generating specific items at study, and hence can be more confidently attributed to the influence of gist representations than in the DRM procedure.

In the first such experiment, we (Koutstaal, Schacter, Verfaellie, Brenner, & Jackson, 1999) examined true and false recognition of novel abstract patterns. Each pattern was a complex, multifeatured shape constructed from a particular prototype. Eighteen different prototypes were used. Individual shapes were manipulated so as to generate a metric of "transformational distance"—the degree of perceptual similarity between a particular item and its prototype, as determined by the number and magnitude of perceptual changes made to particular attributes of each prototype. Thus there were 18 different categories of abstract shapes, each defined relative to a particular prototype. Within each category, 3 different transformational distances were used: near, middle, and far distortions of the prototype. This manipulation was crossed with a manipulation of category size: Participants studied either 1, 3, 6, or 9 shapes from a particular category.

During the study phase, participants rated the complexity of each shape. On a subsequent recognition test, participants made "old–new" decisions about studied and nonstudied shapes from each transformational distance (near, middle, and far), about the prototype from each category (which had never been presented) and also about novel shapes that were unrelated to the previously studied categories.

We reasoned that during the study phase of the experiment, it was highly unlikely that patients or controls would generate a nonpresented prototype or distortion, in the same sense that they might generate a word such as "sweet" in the DRM paradigm. However, previous studies had already shown that normal subjects exhibit high levels of false recognition to nonpresented prototypes of dot patterns (e.g., Posner & Keele, 1968), and we expected to observe similar effects in our controls. The key question was whether amnesic patients would exhibit reduced false recognition of prototypes.

The general answer to this question was "yes." Reduced or "impaired" false recognition of prototypes was more evident in the mixed-etiology amnesic group consisting primarily of patients with MTL damage than in the Korsakoff group (mainly because the alcoholic control patients to whom we compared the patients with Korsakoff's syndrome showed unusually high levels of false recognition even to unrelated new items). Amnesic patients also tended to show reduced false recognition of nonprototypical items in the conditions that encouraged the development of robust gist representations in healthy controls: with near and middle distortions of the prototypes, and following the study of large categories (see Figure 9.1). To the extent that participants are unlikely to generate these novel items during the study phase, these results support our claim that reduced false recognition in amnesic patients is attributable to the influence of a degraded gist representation, rather than to poor memory for a specific item generated during the study phase.

We also found that under conditions that did not promote the development of powerful gist representations in control subjects, such as the far transformational distance or small category size, there was little or no false-recognition "impairment" in the amnesic group (Figure 9.1). This latter finding fits well with our preceding analysis of differences between the early results of Cermak and colleagues (1973) and our later results with the DRM semantic-associates approach and related procedures (Schacter, Verfaellie, & Anes, 1997; Schacter, Verfaellie, & Pradere, 1996; Schacter, Verfaellie, et al., 1998). When experimental conditions favor the development of robust gist representations that cannot be easily countered by explicit recollection, amnesic patients are likely to show reduced false recognition. But when experimental conditions result in weaker gist representations that can be countered with explicit recollection, controls can suppress their false-recognition responses, but amnesic patients cannot. These contrasting processes can reduce, eliminate, or even reverse the differences between amnesic patients and controls that are observed in "strong-gist" conditions.

Note, however, that these findings were obtained in an experimental paradigm that relies almost exclusively on perceptual memory processes. It is thus unclear whether the principal conclusions we have drawn from this experiment also apply to conditions in which semantic or conceptual factors play a role—as in our previous studies with the DRM and related procedures. To examine the issue, we (Koutstaal, Verfaellie, & Schacter, 2001) used a para-

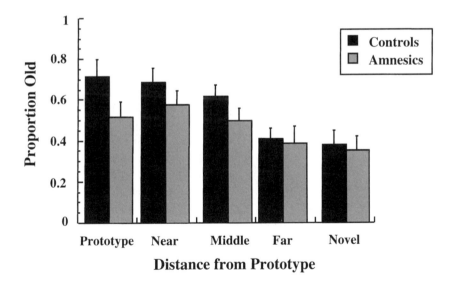

FIGURE 9.1. False recognition of visual patterns by amnesic patients and matched controls in an experiment by our group (Koutstaal, Schacter, Verfaellie, Brenner, & Jackson, 1999). In this experiment, participants studied complex, multifeatured shapes that were each constructed from a particular prototype. There were 18 different categories of shapes, each defined relative to a particular prototype. Within each category, three different transformational distances were used: near, middle, and far distortions of the prototype. The data in the figure show the proportions of "old responses" (false alarms) to the prototype, each of the three types of distortions, and novel items that were not related to a prototype. See text for further explanation.

digm involving categorized pictures that draws on both perceptual and conceptual memory processes. Initially developed (Koutstaal & Schacter, 1997) to examine age-related differences in false recognition, the procedure involves presenting participants with detailed colored pictures of common objects, such as cats or teapots, and varying the size of each category (ranging from 18 different exemplars to only a single exemplar). Participants are later given an "old–new" recognition test consisting of studied pictures, related lure items consisting of nonstudied pictures from previously studied categories, and nonstudied pictures that are unrelated to studied categories. Because the related lures are detailed pictures that participants have not seen prior to the experiment, it is highly unlikely that participants generate specific representations of those pictures at the time of study (just as we have argued for the abstract-shapes paradigm discussed above). Thus false recognition in the paradigm we used probably reflects the influence of general or gist-based similarity—both perceptual and conceptual—between related lure pictures and previously studied pictures.

Based on our previous results, we predicted reduced or impaired false recognition of related lures in amnesic patients following the study of a large number of categorically related pictures. An initial experiment provided evidence of trends in this direction, but the tendency toward reduced false recognition in the amnesic group did not attain statistical significance. We suspected that the relatively weak effects might have been attributable to the use of item-specific recollection by control subjects to suppress false-recognition responses. Accordingly, we carried out an additional experiment designed to minimize such influences. This experiment yielded strong evidence for reduced false recognition of related lures from large categories in amnesic patients (for further details and qualifications, see Koutstaal et al., 2001). These results thus extend the findings of the Koutstaal and colleagues (1999) study beyond the domain of purely perceptual memory processes into the domain of conceptual memory. They also further confirm that amnesic patients show reduced false recognition under conditions where memory for gist, rather than source confusions regarding individual items, is the primary determinant of illusory memory.

One final observation from the latter experiments should be noted. Although our emphasis here has been on establishing the conditions under which amnesic patients show impaired memory for the perceptual or conceptual gist of studied items, a further question one might ask concerns *the relative magnitude* of their impairment in gist-based memory versus their impairment in the explicit recollection of item-specific information. To address this question, one might contrast in both amnesic patients and controls the level of false recognition of related lures with the level of veridical recognition for related targets. However, the usefulness of this comparison is to some extent vitiated by the possibility that the same general similarity or gist information that contributes to false-recognition responses might *also* help to support veridical recognition for related list items. The inclusion of a manipulation of category size in the experiments using categorized pictures (Koutstaal et al., 2001) enabled us to examine the extent of impairment of gist-based versus item-specific memory in amnesic patients while circumventing this difficulty. Rates of false recognition for category lures that were related to a large number of study items provided an index of gist memory, whereas rates of veridical recognition for targets that were unrelated to any of the other list items (one-of-a-kind or single-item categories) provided an index of item-specific memory. A comparison of these two measures showed that although (as noted above) gist memory in amnesic patients was significantly impaired relative to gist memory in controls, the impairment in item-specific memory was even greater. Stated differently, although amnesic patients showed reduced "memory" for items that were similar to but not actually identical to items that they had studied, this deficit in gist memory was not as pronounced as the deficit they demonstrated for actually studied items when those items were unrelated to any of the other items they had encountered.

This finding underscores an important point regarding the nature of the impairment of gist memory in amnesia. Under conditions that foster the formation and retention of robust gist representations among control participants, patients with amnesia show reduced false recognition. Nonetheless, the rates of false recognition shown by amnesic patients under these same conditions are also usually elevated above the level found for entirely unrelated "new" items. Relative to controls with intact memory and intact brain function, amnesic patients show a partial—and less efficient—ability to extract, retain, and retrieve information concerning the conceptual or perceptual gist of studied items, rather than an *absence* of an ability to benefit from such information.

Several factors may contribute to the differential levels of impairment shown by amnesic patients for gist information relative to item-specific information. Memory for gist and item-specific information may depend on qualitatively different underlying processes (see, e.g., Reyna & Brainerd, 1995), with the latter more impaired than the former in amnesic patients. Alternatively, remembering item-specific information may be in some sense more difficult than remembering gist information. Given their generally impaired explicit or declarative memory capacities, the greater difficulty associated with remembering item-specific information may have a disproportionately large impact on the performance of amnesic patients compared with controls.

In either scenario, two possibly related findings merit consideration. First, research by Verfaellie and Cermak (1994) using a rather different approach (Watkins & Kerkar, 1985) suggested that whereas amnesic patients may show especially impaired memory for specific occurrences, memory for repeated occurrences may be "superadditive": Recall of twice-presented items was higher than would be expected on the basis of recall of one of two (different) once-presented items. However, a particular feature concerning these items (color) was less likely to be recalled than was the color of the once-presented items. Second, recent work examining the relative impairment of recollection versus familiarity in amnesia has suggested that although both components are impaired (Knowlton & Squire, 1995), recollection is particularly adversely affected (Yonelinas, Kroll, Dobbins, Lazzara, & Knight, 1998). The comparison of veridical recognition for one-of-a-kind target items versus false recognition of many-exemplar lure items may partially map onto a similar distinction, with successful recognition of one-of-a-kind targets especially (albeit not exclusively or entirely) drawing on recollection, and incorrect identification of many-of-a-kind lures drawing especially on familiarity. Again, questions concerning whether these differences reflect qualitatively distinct underlying processes or quantitative variations in difficulty remain to be addressed in future studies.

UNRESOLVED ISSUES AND FUTURE DIRECTIONS

The main lesson from our studies of false recognition in amnesic patients is relatively clear and consistent: Under conditions that favor the development of strong gist representations, and that work against using explicit recollection to suppress such representations, amnesic patients show reduced false recognition compared to healthy controls. Nonetheless, there remain a number of issues and puzzles that require examination and clarification.

First, though we have focused on false recognition, data from the DRM procedure also exist concerning free recall. As shown initially by Deese (1959), and later by Roediger and McDermott (1995) and others (e.g., Read, 1996), participants frequently intrude nonpresented theme words such as "sweet" during a free-recall test. In our initial study using the DRM procedure, we found that amnesic patients intruded the theme word in free recall about as often as control subjects did (Schacter, Verfaellie, & Pradere, 1996). Moreover, because amnesic patients recalled fewer studied items than controls, when expressed as a proportion of correctly recalled items, amnesic patients actually showed relatively *greater* false recall than did controls. Although these false-recall data are apparently in conflict with our results on false recognition, one further finding is critical to interpreting these data: Amnesic patients also made many more intrusions of unrelated words than did the controls. When these intrusions were taken into account, amnesic patients actually intruded a smaller proportion of theme words than did controls. Still, control subjects produced more studied words than theme words on the free-recall test, whereas amnesic patients showed the opposite effect.

Taken together, these findings suggest that amnesic patients have little or no access to specific information about studied items; their recall performance appeared to rely nearly exclusively on degraded gist memory. These considerations may help to make some sense of free-recall data reported by Melo and colleagues (1999), who found that amnesic patients with MTL/diencephalic damage (*n* = 4) intruded more theme words on a free-recall test than did controls (these same patients showed reduced false recognition of theme words on a subsequent recognition test). Contrary to the results of the Schacter, Verfaellie, and Pradere (1996) study, these patients did not, as a group, show heightened intrusions of unrelated words (although one of the four patients did show this effect). Though it is unclear why Melo and colleagues found greater intrusion of theme words in amnesic patients than controls, and we did not (differences in the relative severity of amnesia or other characteristics of patients in the two experiments could have played a role), both studies agree on one important finding: Amnesic patients produce a higher proportion of theme words than list words on a free-recall task, whereas normal controls show the opposite pattern. Thus it seems clear that patients tend to rely more on gist information during recall than do controls. Further research with free-recall tests is needed to characterize the extent to which such information is preserved or degraded.

A second issue that requires further research concerns the relation between our finding of reduced false recognition of prototypes and other forms of gist information in amnesia, and previous reports that amnesic patients show normal acquisition of prototypes in category-learning experiments (e.g., Knowlton & Squire, 1993). If amnesic patients can learn new categorical information, as expressed by their ability to correctly classify prototypes on the basis of recent learning, why do they not falsely recognize prototypes to the same extent as control subjects do? Early evidence reported by Kolodny (1994) in the context of a category-learning study suggested that amnesics falsely recognize prototypes even more often than control subjects. However, as we have noted elsewhere (Koutstaal et al., 1999), Kolodny did not report data concerning amnesic patients' false alarms to unrelated lure items. If amnesic patients showed elevated false-alarm rates to unrelated lures, this bias in responding could account for their apparent "preservation" of false recognition to prototypes. Stated slightly differently, amnesic patients in this experiment might well have shown reduced false recognition if Kolodny had used corrected false-recognition measures (on which we have relied) that take account of general tendencies to respond "old" to both unrelated and related new items.

Another possible explanation of preserved category learning and reduced false recognition of prototypes in amnesia is that category-learning experiments use indirect or implicit tests to assess classification of prototypes (Knowlton & Squire, 1993), whereas experiments examining false recognition in amnesia have relied exclusively on direct or explicit tests. It is well known that implicit and explicit tests can tap different types of memory processes or representations (cf. Jacoby, 1991; Roediger, 1990; Schacter, Chiu, & Ochsner, 1993; Squire, 1992), and this could be the source of differences between false-recognition and category-learning experiments (Kitchener & Squire, 2000; Koutstaal et al., 1999). One way to examine this issue would be to alter recognition test instructions so that they do not require patients to make "old–new" judgments about specific list items. For example, Brainerd and Reyna (1998; see also Schacter, Cendan, Dodson, & Clifford, in press) used test instructions in a study with the DRM materials that required subjects to respond "old" when a test probe fit a previously studied theme, regardless of whether the specific item had appeared previously. If amnesic patients do indeed possess intact gist representations, but fail to gain access to them on recognition tests, then patients may endorse nonstudied theme words as often as controls do when tested with instructions that require only memory for the theme or gist of previously studied lists. We are currently examining this possibility experimentally.

Note that Kitchener and Squire (2000) have recently reported that amnesic patients showed impaired prototype classification on a category-learning task that used verbal stimuli; prior demonstrations of preserved category-learning had all made use of non-verbal stimuli. If verbal category learning is impaired in amnesic patients, and this deficit reflects an impoverished gist representation, then there may be no conflict at all with our repeated finding of reduced false recognition of verbal materials by amnesic patients in the DRM paradigm (Schacter, Verfaellie, & Anes, 1997; Schacter, Verfaellie, & Pradere, 1996; Schacter, Verfaellie, et al., 1998). Yet this interpretation still leaves open the question of why we found reduced false recognition of prototypes with nonverbal materials (Koutstaal et al., 1999). As Kitchener and Squire (2000) note, in addition to task differences (category classification vs. "old–new" recognition), the contrasting findings could result from another important procedural difference in category-learning and false-recognition studies. Successful category-learning studies typically involve training on only a single category, whereas we have exposed amnesic patients to multiple categories. Further research will be required to examine directly this and other possible sources of the observed differences.

Finally, we have noted earlier that an important goal in studying false recognition in amnesic patients is to gain insight into the brain mechanisms of memory illusions. In addition to studies of amnesic patients, we and others are pursuing complementary approaches to this basic issue. For instance, several neuroimaging studies provide evidence for MTL activation during false recognition (Cabeza, Rao, Wagner, Mayer, & Schacter, 2001; Schacter, Buckner, Koutstaal, Dale, & Rosen, 1997; Schacter, Reiman, et al., 1996). This evidence converges nicely with our findings of reduced false recognition in amnesic patients with MTL damage. Recent electrophysiological evidence has begun to delineate the ways in which true and false recognition differ (Curran, Schacter, Johnson, & Spinks, 2001; Gonsalves & Paller, 2000; Fabiani, Stadler, & Wessels, 2000). Other studies have revealed increased false recognition in patients with damage to specific regions of the frontal lobes (e.g., Parkin, Ward, Bindschaedler, Squires, & Powell, 1999; Rapcsak et al., Chapter 10, this volume; Rapcsak, Reminger, Glisky, Kaszniak, & Comer, 1999; Schacter, Curran, Galluccio, Milberg, & Bates, 1996). When the results from these different approaches are combined, we are optimistic that the study of memory illusions, distortions, and other constructive aspects of remembering that have long intrigued cognitive psychologists will make an increasingly important contribution to the neuropsychology of memory.

ACKNOWLEDGMENTS

Preparation of this chapter was supported by Grant No. NS26985 from the National Institute of Neurological Disorders and Stroke, Grant No. AG08441 from the National Institute on Aging, and Grant No. MH57681 from the National Institute of Mental Health. We thank Steve Prince for his assistance.

REFERENCES

Bartlett, F. C. (1932). *Remembering*. Cambridge, England: Cambridge University Press.

Blaxton, T. A. (1989). Investigating dissociations among memory measures: Support for a transfer-appropriate processing framework. *Journal of Experimental Psychology: Learning, Memory, and Cognition, 15,* 657–668.

Blaxton, T. A. (1995). A process-based view of memory. *Journal of the International Neuropsychological Society, 1,* 112–114.

Brainerd, C. J., & Reyna, C. F. (1998). When things that were never experienced are easier to "remember" than things that were. *Psychological Science, 9,* 484–489.

Budson, A. E., Daffner, K. R., Desikan, R., & Schacter, F. L. (2000). When false recognition is unopposed by true recognition: Gist-based memory distortion in Alzheimer's disease. *Neuropsychology, 14,* 277–287.

Burgess, P. W., & Shallice, T. (1996). Confabulation and the control of recollection. *Memory, 4,* 359–411.

Cabeza, R., Rao, S. M., Wagner, A. D., Mayer, A. R., & Schacter, D. L. (2001). Can medial temporal lobe regions distinguish true from false?: An event-related fMRI study of veridical and illusory recognition memory. *Proceedings of the National Academy of Sciences USA, 98,* 4805–4810.

Cermak, L. S., Butters, N., & Gerrein, J. (1973). The extent of the verbal encoding ability of Korsakoff patients. *Neuropsychologia, 11,* 85–94.

Cohen, N. J., & Eichenbaum, H. (1993). *Memory, amnesia, and the hippocampal system.* Cambridge, MA: MIT Press.

Curran, T., Schacter, D. L. Johnson, M. K., & Spinks, R. (2001). Brain potentials reflect behavioral differences in true and false recognition. *Journal of Cognitive Neuroscience, 13,* 201–216.

Dalla Barba, G. (1993). Confabulation: Knowledge and recollective experience. *Cognitive Neuropsychology, 10,* 1–20.

Deese, J. (1959). On the prediction of occurrence of particular verbal intrusions in immediate recall. *Journal of Experimental Psychology, 58,* 17–22.

Fabiani, M., Stadler, M. A., & Wessels, P. M. (2000). True but not false memories produce a sensory signature in human lateralized brain potentials. *Journal of Cognitive Neuroscience, 12,* 941–949.

Gonsalves, B., & Paller, K. A. (2000). Neural events that underlie remembering something that never happened. *Nature Neuroscience, 3,* 1316–1321.

Haist, F., Shimamura, A. P., & Squire, L. R. (1992). On the relationship between recall and recognition memory. *Journal of Experimental Psychology: Learning, Memory, and Cognition, 18,* 691–702.

Jacoby, L. L. (1991). A process dissociation framework: Separating automatic from intentional uses of memory. *Journal of Memory and Language, 30,* 513–541.

Jacoby, L. L., Kelley, C. M., & Dywan, J. (1989). Memory attributions. In H. L. Roediger III & F. I. M. Craik (Eds.), *Varieties of memory and consciousness: Essays in honour of Endel Tulving* (pp. 391–422). Hillsdale, NJ: Erlbaum.

Johnson, M. K. (1991). Reality monitoring: Evidence from confabulation in organic brain disease patients. In G. P. Prigatano & D. L. Schacter (Eds.), *Awareness of deficit after brain injury: Clinical and theoretical issues* (pp. 176–197). New York: Oxford University Press.

Johnson, M. K., Hashtroudi, S., & Lindsay, D. S. (1993). Source monitoring. *Psychological Bulletin, 114*, 3–28.

Kitchener, E. G., & Squire, L. R. (2000). Impaired verbal category learning in amnesia. *Behavioral Neuroscience, 114*, 907–911.

Knowlton, B. J., & Squire, L. R. (1993). The learning of categories: Parallel brain systems for item memory and category level knowledge. *Science, 262*, 1747–1749.

Knowlton, B. J., & Squire, L. R. (1995). Remembering and knowing: Two different expressions of declarative memory. *Journal of Experimental Psychology: Learning, Memory and Cognition, 21*, 699–710.

Kolodny, J. A. (1994). Memory processes in classification learning: An investigation of amnesic performance in categorization of dot patterns and artistic styles. *Psychological Science, 5*, 164–169.

Koutstaal, W., & Schacter, D. L. (1997). Gist-based false recognition of pictures in older and younger adults. *Journal of Memory and Language, 37*, 555–583.

Koutstaal, W., Schacter, D. L., Verfaellie, M., Brenner, C. J., & Jackson, E. M. (1999). Percfeptually based false recognition of novel objects in amnesia: Effects of category size and similarity to category prototypes. *Cognitive Neuropsychology, 16*(3, 4, 5), 317–341.

Koutstaal, W., Verfaellie, M., & Schacter, D. L. (2001). Recognizing identical vs. similar categorically related common objects: Further evidence for degraded gist-representations in amnesia. *Neuropsychology*, 268–289.

Loftus, E. F. (1979). *Eyewitness testimony*. Cambridge, MA: Harvard University Press.

Mather, M., Henkel, L. A., & Johnson, M. K. (1997). Evaluating characteristics of false memories: Remember/know judgments and memory characteristics questionnaire compared. *Memory and Cognition, 25*, 826–837.

McDermott, K. B. (1996). The persistence of false memories in list recall. *Journal of Memory and Language, 35*, 212–230.

Melo, B., Winocur, G., & Moscovitch, M. (1999). False recall and false recognition: An examination of the effects of selective and combined lesions to the medial temporal lobe/diencephalon and frontal lobe structures. *Cognitive Neuropsychology, 16*, 343–359.

Miller, M. B., & Wolford, G. L. (1999). Theoretical commentary: The role of criterion shift in false memory. *Psychological Review, 106*, 398–405.

Moscovitch, M. (1989). Confabulation and the frontal systems: Strategic versus associative retrieval in neuropsychological theories of memory. In H. L. Roediger III & F. I. M. Craik (Eds.), *Varieties of memory and consciousness: Essays in honour of Endel Tulving* (pp. 133–160). Hillsdale, NJ: Erlbaum.

Moscovitch, M. (1995). Confabulation. In D. L. Schacter, J. T. Coyle, G. D. Fischbach, M.-M. Mesulam, & L. E. Sullivan (Eds.), *Memory distortion: How minds, brains, and societies reconstruct the past* (pp. 226–254). Cambridge, MA: Harvard University Press.

Neisser, U. (1967). *Cognitive psychology*. New York: Appleton-Century-Crofts.

Norman, K. A., & Schacter, D. L. (1997). False recognition in young and older adults: Exploring the characteristics of illusory memories. *Memory and Cognition, 25*, 838–848.

Parkin, A. J. (1997). The neuropsychology of false memory. *Learning and Individual Differences, 9*, 341–357.

Parkin, A. J., Ward, J., Bindschaedler, C., Squires, E. J., & Powell, G. (1999). False recognition following frontal lobe damage: The role of encoding factors. *Cognitive Neuropsychology, 16*, 243–265.

Payne, D. G., Elie, C. J., Blackwell, J. M., & Neuschatz, J. S. (1996). Memory illusions: Recalling, recognizing, and recollecting events that never occurred. *Journal of Memory and Language, 35*, 261–285.

Posner, M. I., & Keele, S. W. (1968). On the genesis of abstract ideas. *Journal of Experimental Psychology, 77*, 353–363.

Rapcsak, S. Z., Reminger, S. L., Glisky, E. L., Kazniak, A. W., & Corner, J. F. (1999). Neuropsychological mechanisms of false facial recognition following frontal lobe damage. *Cognitive Neuropsychology, 16*, 267–292.

Reyna, V. F., & Brainerd, C. J. (1995). Fuzzy-trace theory: An interim synthesis. *Learning and Individual Differences, 7*, 1–75.

Read, J. D. (1996). From a passing thought to a false memory in 2 minutes: Confusing real and illusory events. *Psychonomic Bulletin and Review, 3*, 105–111.

Robinson, K. J., & Roediger, H. L., III. (1997). Associative processes in false recall and false recognition. *Psychological Science, 8*, 231–237.

Roediger, H. L., III. (1990). Implicit memory: Retention without remembering. *American Psychologist, 45*, 1043–1056.

Roediger, H. L., III. (1996). Memory illusions. *Journal of Memory and Language, 35*, 76–100.

Roediger, H. L., III, Balota, D. A., & Watson, J. M. (2001). Spreading activation and the arousal of false memories. In H. L. Roediger III, J. S. Nairne, I. Neath, & A. M. Surprenant (Eds.), *The nature of remembering: Essays in honor of Robert G. Crowder* (pp. 95–115) Washington, DC: American Psychological Association Press.

Roediger, H. L., III, & McDermott, K. B. (1995). Creating false memories: Remembering words not presented in lists. *Journal of Experimental Psychology: Learning, Memory, and Cognition, 21*, 803–814.

Roediger, H. L., III, & McDermott, K. B. (1999). False alarms about false memories. *Psychological Review, 106*, 406–410.

Schacter, D. L. (1987). Memory, amnesia, and frontal lobe dysfunction. *Psychobiology, 15*, 21–36.

Schacter, D. L. (1996). *Searching for memory: The brain, the mind, and the past.* New York: Basic Books.

Schacter, D. L. (Ed.). (1999a). *The cognitive neuropsychology of false memories.* Hove, England: Psychology press.

Schacter, D. L. (1999b). The seven sins of memory: Insights from psychology and cognitive neuroscience. *American Psychologist, 54*(3), 182–203.

Schacter, D. L. (2001). *The seven sins of memory: How the mind forgets and remembers.* Boston: Houghton Mifflin.

Schacter, D. L., Buckner, R. L., Koutstaal, W., Dale, A. M., & Rosen, B. R. (1997). Late onset of anterior prefrontal activity during retrieval of veridical and illusory memories: An event-related fMRI study. *NeuroImage, 6*, 259–269.

Schacter, D. L., Cendan, D. L., Dodson, C. S., & Clifford, E. R. (in press). Retrieval conditions and false recognition: Testing the distinctiveness heuristic. *Psychonomic Bulletin and Review.*

Schacter, D. L., Chiu, C. Y. P., & Ochsner, K. N. (1993). Implicit memory: A selective review. *Annual Review of Neuroscience, 16I*, 159–182.

Schacter, D. L., Curran, T., Galluccio, L., Milberg, W., & Bates, J. (1996). False recognition and the right frontal lobe: A case study. *Neuropsychologia, 34*, 793–808.

Schacter, D. L., Norman, K. A., & Koutstaal, W. (1998). The cognitive neuroscience of constructive memory. *Annual Review of Psychology, 49*, 289–318.

Schacter, D. L., Reiman, E., Curran, T., Yun, L. S., Bandy, D., McDermott, K. B., & Roediger, H. L., III. (1996). Neuroanatomical correlates of veridical and illusory recognition memory: Evidence from positron emission tomography. *Neuron, 17*, 267–274.

Schacter, D. L., & Tulving, E. (Eds.). (1994). *Memory systems 1994.* Cambridge, MA: MIT Press.

Schacter, D. L., Verfaellie, M., & Anes, M. D. (1997). Illusory memories in amnesic patients: Conceptual and perceptual false recognition. *Neuropsychology, 11*, 331–342.

Schacter, D. L., Verfaellie, M., Anes, M. D., & Racine, C. (1998). When true recognition suppresses false recognition: Evidence from amnesic patients. *Journal of Cognitive Neuroscience, 10*, 668–679.

Schacter, D. L., Verfaellie, M., & Pradere, D. (1996). The neuropsychology of memory illusions: False recall and recognition in amnesic patients. *Journal of Memory and Language, 35*, 319–334.

Schnider, A., & Ptak, R. (1999). Spontaneous confabulators fail to suppress currently irrelevant memory traces. *Nature Neuroscience, 2*, 677–681.

Scoville, W. B., & Milner, B. (1957). Loss of recent memory after bilateral hippocampal lesions. *Journal of Neurology, Neurosurgery and Psychiatry, 20*, 11–21.

Shiffrin, R. M., Huber, D. E., & Marinelli, K. (1995). Effects of category length and strength on familiarity in recognition. *Journal of Experimental Psychology: Learning, Memory, and Cognition, 21*, 267–287.

Squire, L. R. (1992). Memory and the hippocampus: A synthesis from findings with rats, monkeys, and humans. *Psychological Review, 99*, 195–231.

Squire, L. R., & Zola-Morgan, M. (1991). The medial temporal lobe memory system. *Science, 253*, 1380–1386.

Underwood, B. J. (1965). False recognition produced by implicit verbal responses. *Journal of Experimental Psychology, 70*, 122–129.

Verfaellie, M., & Cermak, L. S. (1994). Acquisition of generic memory in amnesia. *Cortex, 30*, 293–303.

Wagner, A. D., Gabrieli, J. D. E., & Verfaellie, M. (1997). Dissociations between familiarity processes in explicit–recognition and implicit–perceptual memory. *Journal of Experimental Psychology: Learning, Memory, and Cognition, 23*, 305–232.

Watkins, M. J. & Kerkar, S. P. (1985). Recall of a twice-presented item without recall of either presentation: Generic memory for events. *Journal of Memory and Language, 24*, 666–678.

Wixted, J. T., & Stretch, V. (2000). The case against a criterion-shift account of false memory. *Psychological Review, 107*, 368–376.

Yonelinas, A. P., Kroll, N. E., Dobbins, I., Lazzara, M., & Knight, R. T. (1998). Recollection and familiarity deficits in amnesia: Convergence of remember–know, process dissociation, and receiver operating characteristic data. *Neuropsychology, 12*, 323–339.

10

The Neuropsychology
of False Facial Recognition

STEVEN Z. RAPCSAK, LIS NIELSEN,
ELIZABETH L. GLISKY,
and ALFRED W. KASZNIAK

Neurological disorders of face recognition have been the subject of scientific inquiry for more than a century (Benton, 1990). For much of this time, researchers have focused their attention on investigating the behavioral and neural basis of the dramatic face memory loss that is the hallmark of prosopagnosia (Damasio, Damasio, & Van Hoesen, 1982; De Renzi, Perani, Carlesimo, Silveri, & Fazio, 1994; Meadows, 1974; Sergent & Signoret, 1992). However, recent advances in the cognitive neuroscience of memory illusions (for reviews, see Schacter, 1995; Schacter, Norman, & Koutstaal, 1998) have prompted a more systematic exploration of the neuropsychological mechanisms and anatomical correlates of false facial recognition (Rapcsak, Polster, Comer, & Rubens, 1994; Rapcsak, Polster, Glisky, & Comer, 1996; Rapcsak et al., 1998; Rapcsak, Reminger, Glisky, Kaszniak, & Comer, 1999; Young, Flude, Hay, & Ellis, 1993; Ward et al., 1999). Collectively, these efforts have led to a growing appreciation of the fact that face recognition is not merely the automatic product of a direct match between the face cue and representations of faces stored in memory. Instead, remembering faces is more appropriately viewed as a dynamic and constructive process that requires an interaction between the face memory system and executive systems involved in the strategic control of conscious recollection.

"False facial recognition" may be defined operationally as a type of memory distortion in which patients mistakenly believe that novel faces are familiar. Such misattributions of familiarity may give rise to false alarms in episodic face memory experiments, but they can also be demonstrated by simply asking patients to decide whether they have ever seen a particular face before (Rapcsak et al., 1994, 1996, 1998, 1999). From a cognitive perspective, false recognition provides an interesting contrast to the loss of facial familiarity that characterizes the memory impairment of individuals with prosopagnosia. In addition to the notable differences in clinical presentation, the two types of face memory disorder also seem to have different neuroanatomical substrates. Specifically, prosopagnosia is typi-

130

cally associated with right ventromedial temporal lobe damage, whereas some of the most striking cases of false facial recognition have been observed following damage to the right prefrontal cortex (Rapcsak et al., 1994, 1996, 1998, 1999).

This chapter provides an overview of our recent studies of false facial recognition in patients with right frontal lobe lesions. In particular, we describe a series of experiments designed to elucidate the cognitive deficits responsible for memory illusions within the anterograde and retrograde domains of face memory. To distinguish patterns of memory impairment attributable to the breakdown of executive control and monitoring operations from those that arise as a result of direct damage to the face memory storage system, we contrast the performance of patients with frontal lobe damage to that of patients with right temporal lobe lesions.

ANTEROGRADE FACE MEMORY EXPERIMENTS

In Experiment 1, we examined the relationship between false recognition and face memory loss. Participants included 9 patients with right frontal lobe lesions (mean age = 64.7 years), 9 patients with right ventromedial temporal lobe damage (mean age = 62.9 years), and 24 normal controls (mean age = 61.3 years). Preliminary assessment of face memory with the Warrington Recognition Memory Test (WRMT) revealed that both patient groups were impaired relative to controls (mean = 44.30), with temporal lobe patients obtaining lower scores (mean = 31.56) than frontal lobe patients (mean = 37.89). The defective performance of frontal lobe and temporal lobe patients on this relatively easy forced-choice test of recognition memory suggested that both groups had difficulty encoding distinctive memory representations for novel faces. Not surprisingly, the anterograde face memory deficit was most severe in patients with right temporal lobe damage.

In order to assess susceptibility to false recognition, the three experimental groups were administered single-probe "yes–no" tests of face recognition memory. In the study phase, faces from a college yearbook were presented on a computer screen. There were four different versions of this test, distinguished by the number of faces to be remembered: 32, 24, 16, and 8. In the test phase, target faces were mixed randomly with an equal number of distractor faces selected from the same yearbook. Participants were asked to respond "yes" if the picture was of a face that they had seen in the study phase, and "no" if the picture was of a face not presented before. Hit and false-alarm rates combined across the four sets of faces are shown in Figure 10.1. Formal analyses indicated that temporal lobe patients had lower hit rates (mean = .59) than either frontal lobe patients (mean = .85) or controls (mean = .88). There were no differences in hits between the frontal and control groups. By contrast, frontal lobe patients had higher false-alarm rates (mean = .46) than either temporal lobe patients (mean = .27) or normal controls (mean = .12). Temporal lobe patients also produced more false alarms than controls did.

To obtain a more precise index of memory accuracy and detect possible differences in response bias, we calculated the discrimination and bias measures derived from the two-high-threshold model of recognition memory (Snodgrass & Corwin, 1988). The Discrimination Index (Pr) is a corrected memory accuracy score computed by the formula $H - FA$, where H = hit rate and FA = false-alarm rate.[1] The Bias Index (Br), which reflects the tendency to say "yes" to an item when an individual is in the uncertain state (i.e., when dis-

---

[1] In calculating hit and false-alarm rates, we applied the correction formula recommended by Snodgrass and Corwin (1988).

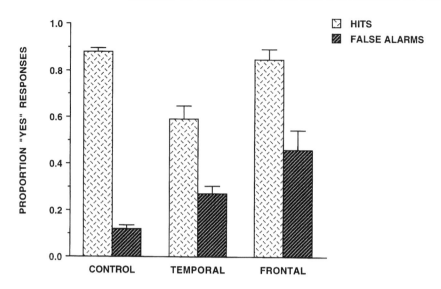

FIGURE 10.1. Hit and false-alarm rates in Experiment 1.

crimination is less than optimal because the information in memory is insufficient to de-termine whether an item is "old" or "new"), is computed as $FA/(1 - Pr)$. A Br value of .5 indicates a neutral bias; values less than .5 are consistent with a conservative bias; and values greater than .5 suggest a liberal bias. Analyses conducted on the derived measures revealed that discrimination scores were lower in frontal lobe patients (mean = .37) and temporal lobe patients (mean = .30) than in normal controls (mean = .72). However, dis-crimination scores were not significantly different for the two patient groups. Examina-tion of the response bias data indicated that frontal lobe patients had a more liberal bias (mean = .71) than either temporal lobe patients (mean = .41) or controls (mean = .50). There were no differences between temporal lobe patients and normal controls on the bias measure.

The main conclusion to be drawn from Experiment 1 is that false facial recognition in anterograde tests is not simply the result of poor memory for the study faces. Temporal lobe patients produced the lowest hit rates of all participants, and they also obtained the worst face memory scores on the WRMT. Nevertheless, frontal lobe patients surpassed temporal lobe patients in false alarms by a significant margin. Based on these findings, we suggest that an adequate explanation of false recognition is not to be found in the severity of the face memory loss per se, but rather in the decision strategy adopted under condi-tions of reduced memory discrimination. Critical support for this hypothesis comes from the observation that despite similar memory discrimination scores, frontal lobe patients showed an abnormally liberal response bias, whereas temporal lobe patients (if anything) demonstrated a slightly conservative bias.

It has been proposed that both familiarity and recollection can serve as the basis for rec-ognition memory decisions (Jacoby & Dallas, 1981; Mandler, 1980). Whereas familiarity-based judgments are relatively automatic, recollection frequently entails an effortful and strategic memory search to retrieve specific contextual information linking the test item to the study episode. As a result, item-specific recollection depends heavily on an accurate and detailed mental representation of the study context (Norman & Schacter, 1996). When high-quality item-specific information is unavailable, however, individuals may respond on the basis of general or "gist" memory for the study episode (Brainerd, Reyna, & Kneer, 1995). The gist representation preserves categorical information about what study items had in common, but it cannot accurately discriminate between targets and similar distractors. According to "fuzzy-trace" theory (Brainerd et al., 1995), hits in recognition experiments are driven primarily by item-specific memory, whereas gist memory is the principal source of false alarms. It has also been demonstrated that by relying consistently on specific recollection to support a positive recognition decision, normal individuals can oppose the influence of general or gist-based familiarity and thereby suppress false recognition (Jacoby, 1991; Multhaup, 1995; Schacter, Israel, & Racine, 1999).

As noted earlier, it is likely that frontal lobe patients had difficulty encoding detailed item-specific memory representations for study faces in the anterograde memory experiments. However, it seems reasonable to assume that they had relatively preserved gist memory for the study episode. For instance, patients probably remembered that they saw pictures of young people on the computer screen, while retaining impoverished memory representations for the individual faces presented. Overreliance on gist memory can explain both the inflated hit rates and the pathologically high false-alarm rates documented in frontal lobe patients (cf. Schacter, Curran, Galluccio, Milberg, & Bates, 1996; Curran, Schacter, Norman, & Galluccio, 1997), since both target faces and distractors would be consistent with this type of generic description of the study episode. It is possible, however, that in addition to (or instead of) impoverished encoding, frontal lobe patients were impaired in their ability to initiate and conduct a strategic memory search to retrieve critical item-specific contextual information. Furthermore, the striking failure of these patients to realize that the absence of specific recollection is inconsistent with a positive recognition decision suggests a breakdown of monitoring and criterion-setting functions. Specifically, it appears that instead of carefully evaluating memory traces evoked by test items for attributes considered diagnostic of the study episode, frontal lobe patients adopted lenient decision criteria and accepted gist-based familiarity as conclusive evidence of prior occurrence. By the same token, the lower hit and false-alarm rates observed in patients with right temporal lobe damage suggest that strategic monitoring and decision functions in these individuals may have been relatively preserved. As a result, temporal lobe patients were more likely to realize that their inability to retrieve specific contextual information about test items was incompatible with a positive recognition decision. It is also possible, however, that temporal lobe patients retained a less robust gist representation of the study episode. Lower levels of gist-based familiarity with test items would render these patients less vulnerable to memory illusions.

In Experiment 2, we examined the influence of gist memory on false recognition by using both gist-consistent and gist-inconsistent distractor items. Participants included four right frontal lobe patients who produced particularly high false-alarm rates in Experiment 1, five patients with right temporal lobe damage, and five normal controls. In the study phase, participants viewed a series of 32 white male faces on a computer screen. In the test phase, target faces were mixed randomly with 16 new white male faces (gist-consistent distractors) and 8 nonwhite male and 8 white female faces (gist-inconsistent distractors). Test instructions were the same as in Experiment 1. Hit and false-alarm rates from Experiment 2 are shown in Table 10.1. For comparison, we have also included data for the same individuals from the 32-item recognition test in Experiment 1, where no obvious category differences existed between target faces and distractors. It is apparent that the inclusion of gist-inconsistent distractors resulted in a reduction of false-alarm rates in all three experimental groups. The actual proportion of gist-consistent versus gist-inconsistent false alarms

TABLE 10.1. Hit and False-Alarm Rates from the 32-Item Face Memory Tests in Experiments 1 and 2

	Experiment 1 (noncategorized distractors)		Experiment 2 (categorized distractors)	
	Hits	False alarms	Hits	False alarms
Controls	.81	.22	.81	.11
Temporal lobe patients	.56	.42	.51	.27
Frontal lobe patients	.91	.76	.90	.37

is shown in Figure 10.2. Additional analysis of this data indicated that the vast majority of false-recognition errors in controls (94%) and in frontal lobe patients (81%) occurred to gist-consistent distractors. By contrast, gist-consistent errors accounted for a relatively smaller portion of false alarms in patients with temporal lobe damage (63%).

The results of Experiment 2 demonstrate that gist memory is the primary source of false alarms both in normal controls and in patients with right frontal lobe lesions. The critical difference is of course that normal individuals can use item-specific recollection to oppose the influence of gist memory on recognition decisions, whereas frontal lobe patients apparently cannot. On the other hand, the influence of gist memory appears to be somewhat attenuated in patients with right temporal lobe lesions, consistent with the hypothesis that in addition to item-specific memory impairment, these patients have difficulty encoding general or categorical information about study items. These findings, as well as other reports of reduced gist-based false recognition in amnesic patients (Koutstaal, Schacter, Verfaellie, Brenner, & Jackson, 1999; Schacter, Verfaellie, & Anes, 1997; Schacter, Verfaellie, Anes, & Racine, 1998; Schacter, Verfaellie, & Pradere, 1996), suggest that medial temporal lobe structures are important for encoding both the specific information that

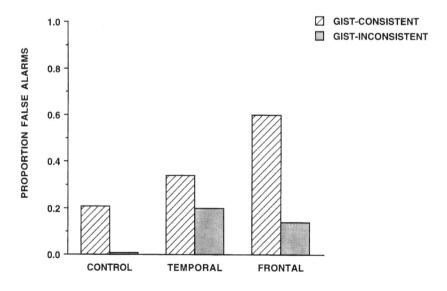

FIGURE 10.2. Proportion of gist-consistent versus gist-inconsistent false alarms in Experiment 2.

supports veridical recognition and the gist representation that may give rise to memory illusions.

RETROGRADE FACE MEMORY EXPERIMENTS

The main objective of the experiments described in this section was to determine whether the cognitive deficits identified in frontal lobe patients in anterograde memory tests also contributed to false recognition within the retrograde domain. Assessing false facial recognition by using retrograde memory paradigms also offers certain advantages. First, the demands imposed by these tests are similar to what people must do in real-life situations—that is, determine both the familiarity and the actual identity of a person, based on his or her facial appearance. Second, the performance of frontal lobe patients in retrograde tests is less likely to be influenced by defective encoding or memory storage, because the relevant information in most cases will have been acquired years before the onset of the neurological deficit. As a result, retrograde tests provide an opportunity to examine the impact of executive dysfunction on the recovery of information from a relatively preserved memory storage system.

Participants in Experiment 3 were the same as in Experiment 1. Stimuli consisted of 32 famous faces (i.e., entertainers and politicians who became famous in the time period between the 1930s and the 1980s) and 32 unfamiliar faces that were considered to have a "celebrity-type" appearance. Faces were presented in random order on a computer screen for "yes–no" familiarity decisions. Participants were instructed to call a face familiar if they thought that they had seen that particular individual before, either in person or through the mass media. After completion of the test, the same famous faces were presented again, and participants were asked to identify these individuals. Hit and false-alarm rates from the familiarity decision test are shown in Figure 10.3. Formal analyses indicated that temporal lobe patients had lower hit rates (mean = .55) than either frontal lobe patients (mean = .86) or controls (mean = .92). Frontal lobe patients and controls did not differ in terms

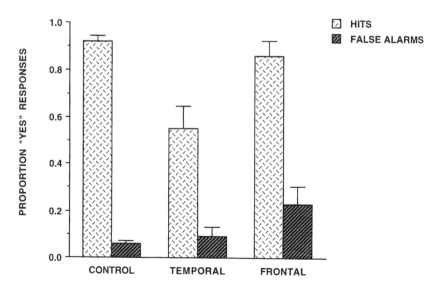

FIGURE 10.3. Hit and false-alarm rates in Experiment 3.

of hits to famous faces. By contrast, frontal lobe patients produced more false alarms to unfamiliar faces (mean = .23) than normal controls did (mean = .06). The difference in false alarms between frontal lobe and temporal lobe patients (mean = .09) approached significance. However, there were no differences in false alarms between temporal lobe patients and controls. Additional analyses revealed that temporal lobe patients correctly identified a smaller proportion of the famous face stimuli (mean = .49) than frontal lobe patients (mean = .74) or controls (mean = .86), whereas the latter two groups did not differ from each other.

The findings of Experiment 3 provide further support for the hypothesis that false facial recognition is not simply the result of face memory loss. Temporal lobe patients had much more severe retrograde face memory impairment than frontal lobe patients, but it was again the frontal lobe group that produced the greatest number of false-recognition errors. We note, however, that the propensity for false recognition was generally stronger in anterograde tests than in the retrograde test. In fact, some frontal lobe patients who obtained pathologically high false-alarm rates in anterograde tests performed entirely within the normal range in the retrograde memory paradigm. To explain this dissociation, we suggest that frontal lobe patients produced more false-recognition errors in anterograde tests because impoverished item-specific memory for the study faces made it particularly difficult to discriminate between targets and similar distractors. As a result, anterograde tests placed greater demands on strategic frontal memory retrieval, monitoring, and decision functions than the retrograde test, in which preserved access to detailed memory representations for highly familiar famous faces made it relatively easy to distinguish targets from foils. Consistent with the hypothesis that "weak" memory representations require more effortful and strategic processing, a recent functional imaging study demonstrated greater right prefrontal activation when normal individuals made "yes–no" recognition decisions about novel faces that they were exposed to only 60 seconds prior to scanning, compared to faces that were thoroughly learned a week earlier with additional practice on the day before the study (Wiser et al., 2000).

To account for memory illusions in retrograde tests, we propose that recognition decisions within the retrograde domain of face memory can also be made on the basis of specific recollection or by relying on general or "gist" memory. Specific recollection involves not only the activation of a stored face memory representation for a familiar individual, but also the retrieval of pertinent biographical information that provides the appropriate context for the sense of familiarity and thus results in person identification. By contrast, the gist component of retrograde face memory contains information about the structural characteristics of faces in general. This type of gist representation may correspond to abstract facial prototypes extracted from the multitude of faces encountered in everyday life (Cabeza, Bruce, Kato, & Oda, 1999; Light, Kayra-Stuart, & Hollander, 1979; Valentine & Bruce, 1986; Valentine & Ferrara, 1991). Novel faces that resemble the prototype may evoke a compelling sense of familiarity and therefore give rise to memory illusions. Consistent with this hypothesis, "typical" faces or faces that match certain occupational stereotypes (e.g., "actress-type" faces) are more likely to induce false-recognition errors in face memory experiments (Bartlett, Hurry, & Thorley, 1984; Klatzky, Martin, & Kane, 1982; Light et al., 1979; Vokey & Read, 1992). However, because general or gist-based facial familiarity is by definition context-free, normal individuals can suppress false recognition by requiring that specific recollection accompany a positive memory decision. As a result, normal controls in Experiment 3 were able to reject most unfamiliar faces by realizing that the inability to retrieve specific contextual information must mean that the face is novel, even though it may have appeared familiar at first. On the other hand, our findings suggest that patients with right frontal lobe damage made recognition decisions by relying on general facial familiarity without attempting to engage in effortful context retrieval. As discussed before, the failure of these patients to interpret the absence of specific recollection as being inconsistent with a positive recognition decision implies an additional impairment of monitoring and criterion-setting functions. Although the lower false-alarm rates of temporal lobe patients are consistent with the notion that executive control and monitoring operations in these individuals were relatively preserved, it is also possible that right temporal lobe lesions compromised both the specific and the general components of face memory. As noted earlier, a reduction in gist-based facial familiarity would decrease the risk of false recognition. In fact, severe damage to both components of face memory might explain why patients with dense prosopagnosia typically report that all faces look completely unfamiliar.

If our hypothesis that reliance on context recollection provides an effective mechanism for suppressing false recognition is correct, then we might be able to reduce false alarms in frontal lobe patients by requiring that they adopt stringent decision criteria and endorse faces only when they have access to identity-specific biographical information. This prediction was tested in three patients with right frontal lobe damage who produced especially high false-alarm rates in Experiment 3. Stimuli for Experiment 4 included the 32 famous faces from Experiment 3, along with a new set of 32 unfamiliar faces. Faces were presented in random order on a computer screen for "yes–no" familiarity decisions. Unlike in Experiment 3, participants were specifically instructed to call faces familiar only if they could remember both the occupation and the name of the person. Hit and false-alarm rates from Experiments 3 and 4 are shown in Figure 10.4. It is readily apparent that by encouraging patients to rely on specific recollection to support a positive recognition decision, we were able to reduce and in fact almost completely eliminate false-recognition errors. These findings suggest that although frontal lobe patients do not spontaneously engage in effortful memory retrieval and monitoring operations, it may be possible to train these

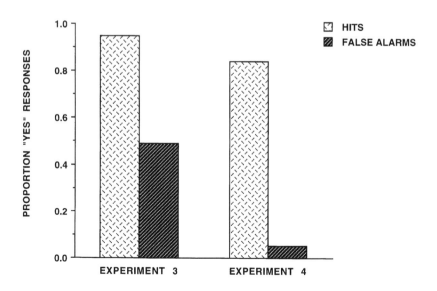

FIGURE 10.4. Hit and false-alarm rates of three frontal lobe patients in Experiments 3 and 4.

individuals to use conscious recollection rather than familiarity as the appropriate basis for recognition decisions.

CONCLUSIONS

Evidence from functional imaging studies suggests that face memory is mediated by a distributed neural system that includes the inferotemporal cortex, medial temporal lobe, and prefrontal cortex (Courtney, Ungerleider, Keil, & Haxby, 1997; Grady et al., 1995; Haxby et al., 1996; Kelley et al., 1988; McDermott, Buckner, Petersen, Kelley, & Sanders, 1999). Our findings demonstrate that damage to the temporal versus frontal components of this network may result in different types of face memory impairment. The memory disorder of our patients with right temporal lobe lesions was characterized by marked anterograde and retrograde face memory loss. These observations are consistent with the well-established role of right temporal lobe structures in the encoding, storage, and retrieval of face memory information. By comparison, the memory deficit of our patients with damage to the right prefrontal cortex was relatively mild and was mostly apparent in anterograde or episodic memory tests. Furthermore, the performance of the frontal lobe patients was influenced by the format of the recognition test. Frontal lobe patients performed significantly better than temporal lobe patients on a forced-choice test of face recognition memory (the WRMT), in which simple comparisons of differences in facial familiarity may have been sufficient to distinguish targets from distractors. However, the advantage of the frontal lobe group was no longer apparent in single-probe "yes–no" recognition tests, which place greater demands on strategic context retrieval, monitoring, and criterion-setting functions (Nolde, Johnson, & Raye, 1998; Norman & Schacter, 1996; Parkin, Yeomans, & Bindschaedler, 1994). These findings are consistent with the notion that frontal lobe damage primarily interferes with cognitive operations that support conscious recollection, while leaving familiarity-based recognition processes relatively intact.

As we have seen, defective item-specific recollection carries with it the risk of false recognition, because patients cannot effectively oppose the influence of undifferentiated familiarity on recognition decisions. Specifically, we propose that without access to detailed contextual information, our frontal lobe patients did not have a reliable mechanism for discriminating between familiarity based on memory for specific faces and familiarity based on memory for faces in general. Memory illusions were a direct result of the confusion between these two different sources of familiarity and reflected the tendency to mistake general knowledge for memories of specific events (cf. Curran et al., 1997; Jacoby, Kelley, & Dywan, 1989; Johnson & Raye, 2000). Based on these observations, we suggest that the primary role of the prefrontal cortex in face memory is to promote the encoding and retrieval of contextual information critical for attributing facial familiarity to a specific source. Closely related executive functions include the monitoring and verification of the information retrieved from memory in response to the facial cue. Of course, effortful context recollection and extensive source monitoring are not usually necessary when we are dealing with highly familiar faces in everyday life. In fact, the recognition of frequently encountered faces probably requires only limited frontal lobe participation and may be accomplished by relying primarily on the routine operations of the temporal lobe face memory system. However, frontal executive memory functions assume a more critical role under conditions of uncertainty, when the face cue does not automatically elicit relevant contextual information and the source of familiarity is left unspecified (e.g., when we are not sure whether a familiar-looking face is somebody we know). In these situations, the prefrontal cortex is responsible for implementing strategic cognitive operations necessary to boost item-specific recollection, while at the same time reducing the influence of undifferentiated familiarity on recognition decisions and thus protecting against memory illusions. In this sense, the executive control and monitoring functions performed by the prefrontal cortex serve to improve memory accuracy by increasing the signal-to-noise ratio within the face memory system.

Our account of false facial recognition has several features in common with other theoretical models that have implicated defective strategic recollection and source-monitoring failure in the pathogenesis of memory distortions (Johnson, Hashtroudi, & Lindsay, 1993; Moscovitch, 1995; Schacter, Norman, & Koutstaal, 1998). Our findings are also consistent with other reports of increased false recognition following frontal lobe damage (Delbecq-Derouesné, Beauvois, & Shallice, 1990; Parkin, Bindschaedler, Harsent, & Metzler, 1996; Schacter, Curran, et al., 1996; Swick & Knight, 1999). It is clear, however, that the neuropsychological model outlined in this chapter will require further refinements and modifications. For instance, functional imaging studies have provided evidence that different episodic memory operations are mediated by distinct regions within the prefrontal cortex (for reviews, see Petrides, 1996; Owen, 1997; Wagner, 1999). In particular, it has been proposed that the ventrolateral prefrontal cortex is involved in the strategic encoding and retrieval of information initially processed in posterior cortical areas. Consistent with this hypothesis, levels of activation within ventrolateral frontal lobe regions predict whether items will be remembered or forgotten in recognition memory experiments (Brewer, Zhao, Desmond, Glover, & Gabrieli, 1998; Wagner et al., 1998). By contrast, the dorsolateral and anterior prefrontal cortex may be involved in high-level executive and control functions that include the monitoring and verification of the information retrieved from long-term memory. As a result of this regional specialization, patterns of memory impairment in patients with prefrontal damage may vary, depending on lesion size and location. For example, selective damage to the right ventrolateral prefrontal cortex may be associated with defective item recognition in face memory tests. However, additional damage to the dorsolateral and/or anterior prefrontal regions involved in monitoring and control operations would be required to produce prominent memory distortions. Unfortunately, the small sample size and the considerable variability of lesion location in our patients prevent us from drawing any firm conclusions about the specific contribution of different frontal regions to memory. We note, however, that patients with pervasive false recognition generally had lesions encompassing several subdivisions of lateral and anterior prefrontal cortex. Furthermore, some of our patients had evidence of ventromedial frontal lobe involvement. The role of orbitofrontal cortex in executive memory functions is also supported by studies of patients with confabulation (Benson et al., 1996; Moscovitch, 1995).

Regional specialization for different memory operations may also exist within temporal lobe memory systems. For instance, it has been proposed that recollection versus familiarity-based recognition processes are supported by distinct medial temporal lobe areas (Aggleton & Saunders, 1997; Gabrieli et al., 1997). Selective damage to temporal lobe structures critical for recollection may increase the risk of false recognition, because patients would have difficulty opposing the influence of general or gist-based familiarity on recognition decisions (cf. Budson, Daffner, Desikan, & Schacter, 2000; Schacter, Verfaellie, et al., 1998). Defective item-specific recollection may have particularly devastating consequences for performance in episodic "yes–no" face recognition memory experiments, where the normally high degree of structural similarity between targets and distractors makes it difficult to respond on the basis of familiarity alone. On the other hand, susceptibility to false recognition is expected to be reduced in patients with more extensive temporal lobe damage that has compromised not only the areas important for specific recollection, but also the neural structures that support the familiarity-based component of recognition memory. Although these comments are speculative, we offer them to emphasize the need for future research on the relationship between lesion location and face memory impairment, and to underscore the fact that a comprehensive model of face recognition will require a more complete understanding of the dynamic interaction between different frontal and temporal cortical systems in memory.

ACKNOWLEDGMENT

This work was supported by the Cummings Endowment Fund to the Department of Neurology at the University of Arizona.

REFERENCES

Aggleton, J. P., & Saunders, R. C. (1997). The relationship between temporal lobe and diencephalic structures implicated in anterograde amnesia. *Memory, 5*, 49–71.

Bartlett, J. C., Hurry, S., & Thorley, W. (1984). Typicality and familiarity of faces. *Memory and Cognition, 12*, 219–228.

Benson, D. F., Djenderedjian, A., Miller, B. L., Pachana, N. A., Chang, L., Itti, L., Eng, G. E., & Mena, I. (1996). Neural basis of confabulation. *Neurology, 46*, 1239–1243.

Benton, A. (1990). Facial recognition 1990. *Cortex, 26*, 491–499.

Brainerd, C. J., Reyna, V. F., & Kneer, R. (1995). False recognition reversal: When similarity is distinctive. *Journal of Memory and Language, 34*, 157–185.

Brewer, J. B., Zhao, Z., Desmond, J. E., Glover, G. H., & Gabrieli, J. D. E. (1998). Making memories: Brain activity that predicts how well visual experience will be remembered. *Science, 281*, 1185–1187.

Budson, A. E., Daffner, K. R., Desikan, R., & Schacter, D. L. (2000). When false recognition is unopposed by true recognition: Gist-based memory distortion in Alzheimer's disease. *Neuropsychology, 14*, 277–287.

Cabeza, R., Bruce, V., Kato, T., & Oda, M. (1999). The prototype effect in face recognition: Extensions and limits. *Memory and Cognition, 27*, 139–151.

Courtney, S. M., Ungerleider, L. G., Keil, K., & Haxby, J. V. (1997). Transient and sustained activity in a distributed neural system for human working memory. *Nature, 386*, 608–611.

Curran, T., Schacter, D. L., Norman, K. A., & Galluccio, L. (1997). False recognition after a right frontal lobe infarction: Memory for general and specific information. *Neuropsychologia, 35*, 1035–1049.

Damasio, A. R., Damasio, H., & Van Hoesen, G. W. (1982). Prosopagnosia: Anatomic basis and behavioral mechanisms. *Neurology, 32*, 331–341.

Delbecq-Derouesné, J., Beauvois, M. F., & Shallice, T. (1990). Preserved recall versus impaired recognition: A case study. *Brain, 113*, 1045–1074.

De Renzi, E., Perani, D., Carlesimo, G. A., Silveri, M. C., & Fazio, F. (1994). Prosopagnosia can be associated with damage confined to the right hemisphere: An MRI and PET study and a review of the literature. *Neuropsychologia, 32*, 893–902.

Gabrieli, J. D. E., Brewer, J. B., Desmond, J. E., & Glover, G. H. (1997). Separate neural bases of two fundamental memory processes in the human medial temporal lobe. *Science, 276*, 264–266.

Grady, C. L., Macintosh, R. A., Horwitz, B., Maisog, J. M., Ungerleider, L. G., Mentis, M. J., Pietrini, P., Schapiro, M. B., & Haxby, J. V. (1995). Age-related reductions in human recognition memory due to impaired encoding. *Science, 269*, 218–221.

Haxby, J. V., Ungerleider, L. G., Horwitz, B., Maisog, J. M., Rapoport, S. I., & Grady, C. L. (1996). Face encoding and recognition in the human brain. *Proceedings of the National Academy of Sciences USA, 93,* 922–927.

Jacoby, L. L. (1991). A process dissociation framework: Separating automatic from intentional uses of memory. *Journal of Memory and Language, 30,* 513–541.

Jacoby, L. L., & Dallas, M. (1981). On the relationship between autobiographical memory and perceptual learning. *Journal of Experimental Psychology: General, 3,* 306–340.

Jacoby, L. L., Kelley, C. M., & Dywan, J. (1989). Memory attributions. In H. L. Roediger & F. I. M. Craik (Eds.), *Varieties of memory and consciousness: Essays in honor of Endel Tulving* (pp. 391–422). Hillsdale, NJ: Erlbaum.

Johnson, M. K., Hashtroudi, S., & Lindsay, D. S. (1993). Source monitoring. *Psychological Bulletin, 114,* 3–28.

Johnson, M. K., & Raye, C. L. (2000). Cognitive and brain mechanisms of false memories and beliefs. In D. L. Schacter & E. Scarry (Eds.), *Memory, brain, and belief* (pp. 35–86). Cambridge, MA: Harvard University Press.

Kelley, W. M., Miezin, F. M., McDermott, K. B., Buckner, R. L., Raichle, M. E., Cohen, N. J., Ollinger, J. M., Akbudak, E., Conturo, T. E., Snyder, A. Z., & Petersen, S. E. (1998). Hemispheric specialization in human frontal cortex and medial temporal lobe for verbal and nonverbal memory encoding. *Neuron, 20,* 927–936.

Klatzky, R. L., Martin, G. L., & Kane, R. A. (1982). Semantic interpretation effects on memory for faces. *Memory and Cognition, 10,* 195–206.

Koutstaal, W., Schacter, D. L., Verfaellie, M., Brenner, C., & Jackson, E. M. (1999). Perceptually-based false recognition of novel objects in amnesia: Effects of category size and similarity to category prototypes. *Cognitive Neuropsychology, 16,* 317–341.

Light, L. L., Kayra-Stuart, F., & Hollander, S. (1979). Recognition memory for typical and unusual faces. *Journal of Experimental Psychology: Human Learning and Memory, 5,* 212–228.

Mandler, G. (1980). Recognizing: The judgment of previous occurrence. *Psychological Review, 87,* 252–271.

McDermott, K. B., Buckner, R. L., Petersen, S. E., Kelley, W. M., & Sanders, A. L. (1999). Set- and code-specific activation in the frontal cortex: An fMRI study of encoding and retrieval of faces and words. *Journal of Cognitive Neuroscience, 11,* 631–640.

Meadows, J. C. (1974). The anatomical basis of prosopagnosia. *Journal of Neurology, Neurosurgery and Psychiatry, 37,* 489–501.

Moscovitch, M. (1995). Confabulation. In D. L. Schacter (Ed.), *Memory distortion: How minds, brains, and societies reconstruct the past* (pp. 226–251). Cambridge, MA: Harvard University Press.

Multhaup, K. S. (1995). Aging, source, and decision criteria: When false fame errors do and do not occur. *Psychology and Aging, 10,* 492–497.

Nolde, S. F., Johnson, M. K., & Raye, C. L. (1998). The role of prefrontal cortex during tests of episodic memory. *Trends in Cognitive Sciences, 2,* 399–406.

Norman, K. A., & Schacter, D. L. (1996). Implicit memory, explicit memory, and false recollection: A cognitive neuroscience perspective. In L. M. Reder (Ed.), *Implicit memory and metacognition* (pp. 229–257). Mahwah, NJ: Erlbaum.

Owen, A. M. (1997). The functional organization of working memory processes within human lateral frontal cortex: The contribution of functional neuroimaging. *European Journal of Neuroscience, 9,* 1329–1339.

Parkin, A. J., Bindschaedler, C., Harsent, L., & Metzler, C. (1996). Pathological false alarm rates following damage to the left frontal cortex. *Brain and Cognition, 32,* 14–27.

Parkin, A. J., Yeomans, J., & Bindschaedler, C. (1994). Further characterization of the executive memory impairment following frontal lobe lesions. *Brain and Cognition, 26,* 23–42.

Petrides, M. (1996). Specialized systems for the processing of mnemonic information within the primate frontal cortex. *Philosophical Transactions of the Royal Society of London, Series B, 351,* 1455–1462.

Rapcsak, S. Z., Polster, M. R., Comer, J. S., & Rubens, A. B. (1994). False recognition and misidentification of faces following right hemisphere damage. *Cortex, 30,* 565–583.

Rapcsak, S. Z., Polster, M. R., Glisky, M. L., & Comer, J. S. (1996). False recognition of unfamiliar faces following right hemisphere damage: Neuropsychological and anatomical observations. *Cortex, 32,* 593–611.

Rapcsak, S. Z., Kaszniak, A. W., Reminger, S. L., Glisky, M. L., Glisky, E. L., & Comer, J. F. (1998). Dissociation between verbal and autonomic measures of memory following frontal lobe damage. *Neurology, 50,* 1258–1265.

Rapcsak, S. Z., Reminger, S. L., Glisky, E. L., Kaszniak, A. W., & Comer, J. F. (1999). Neuropsychological mechanisms of false facial recognition following frontal lobe damage. *Cognitive Neuropsychology, 16,* 267–292.

Schacter, D. L. (1995). Memory distortion: History and current status. In D. L. Schacter (Ed.), *Memory distortion: How minds, brains, and societies reconstruct the past* (pp. 1–43). Cambridge, MA: Harvard University Press.

Schacter, D. L., Curran, T., Galluccio, L., Milberg, W. P., & Bates, J. F. (1996). False recognition and the right frontal lobe: A case study. *Neuropsychologia, 34,* 793–808.

Schacter, D. L., Israel, L., & Racine, C. (1999). Suppressing false recognition in younger and older adults: The distinctiveness heuristic. *Journal of Memory and Language, 40,* 1–24.

Schacter, D. L., Norman, K. A., & Koutstaal, W. (1998). The cognitive neuroscience of constructive memory. *Annual Review of Psychology, 49,* 289–318.

Schacter, D. L., Verfaellie, M., & Anes, M. D. (1997). Illusory memories in amnesic patients: Conceptual and perceptual false recognition. *Neuropsychology, 11,* 331–342.

Schacter, D. L., Verfaellie, M., Anes, M. D., & Racine, C. (1998). When true recognition suppresses false recognition: Evidence from amnesic patients. *Journal of Cognitive Neuroscience, 10,* 668–679.

Schacter, D. L., Verfaellie, M., & Pradere, D. (1996). The neuropsychology of memory illusions: False recall and recognition in amnesic patients. *Journal of Memory and Language, 35,* 319–334.

Sergent, J., & Signoret, J.-L. (1992). Varieties of functional deficits in prosopagnosia. *Cerebral Cortex, 2,* 375–388.

Snodgrass, J. G., & Corwin, J. (1988). Pragmatics of measuring recognition memory: Applications to dementia and amnesia. *Journal of Experimental Psychology: General, 117,* 34–50.

Swick, D., & Knight, R. T. (1999). Contributions of prefrontal cortex to recognition memory: Electrophysiological and behavioral evidence. *Neuropsychology, 13,* 155–170.

Valentine, T., & Bruce, V. (1986). The effects of distinctiveness in recognizing and classifying faces. *Perception, 15,* 525–535.

Valentine, T., & Ferrara, A. (1991). Typicality in categorization, recognition and identification: Evidence from face recognition. *British Journal of Psychology, 82,* 87–102.

Vokey, J. R., & Read, J. D. (1992). Familiarity, memorability, and the effect of typicality on the recognition of faces. *Memory and Cognition, 20,* 291–302.

Wagner, A. D. (1999). Working memory contributions to human learning and remembering. *Neuron, 22,* 19–22.

Wagner, A. D., Schacter, D. L., Rotte, M., Koutstall, W., Maril, A., Dale, A. M., Rosen, B. R., & Buckner, R. L. (1998). Building memories: Remembering and forgetting of verbal experiences as predicted by brain activity. *Science, 281,* 1188–1191.

Ward, J., Parkin, A. J., Powel, G., Squires, E. J., Townshend, J., & Bradley, V. (1999). False recognition of unfamiliar people: "Seeing film stars everywhere." *Cognitive Neuropsychology, 16,* 293–315.

Wiser, A. K., Andreasen, N. C., O'Leary, D. S., Crespo-Facorro, B., Boles-Ponto, L. L., Watkins, G. L., & Hichwa, R. D. (2000). Novel vs. well-learned memory for faces: A positron emission tomography study. *Journal of Cognitive Neuroscience, 12,* 255–266.

Young, A. W., Flude, B. M., Hay, D. C., & Ellis, A. W. (1993). Impaired discrimination of familiar from unfamiliar faces. *Cortex, 29,* 65–75.

11

The Role of the Basal Ganglia in Learning and Memory

BARBARA J. KNOWLTON

Textbooks in neuroscience generally discuss the basal ganglia as a component of the motor system. The strongest support for this idea comes from the study of patients with basal ganglia disorders, in which disorders or controlled movement are pronounced. Patients with Huntington's disease exhibit involuntary writhing and jerking movements, whereas patients with Parkinson's disease exhibit muscular rigidity, tremor, slowness, and difficulty initiating movement. However, the fact that these patients exhibit cognitive deficits as well suggests that the basal ganglia also play a role in abilities that are not directly motor.

The anatomical connections of the basal ganglia are consistent with a role in influencing the pyramidal motor system. The caudate and putamen receive projections from virtually all cortical regions. These projections are organized in an anterior-to-posterior fashion, with projections from the frontal cortex terminating in the head of the caudate and putamen (neostriatum), and projections from the occipital lobe terminating in the tail of the caudate. The primary output of the basal ganglia is through the internal globus pallidus, which projects to thalamic nuclei and brainstem motor nuclei. The thalamic target nuclei include the ventral anterior and ventrolateral nuclei, which project to the primary and supplementary motor cortices. Thus the basal ganglia are in a position to influence the pyramidal motor system, based on input from diverse cortical regions including the motor cortex itself. However, the mediodorsal nucleus of the thalamus is also targeted by the globus pallidus, and this nucleus projects to regions in the frontal lobe that play a role in cognitive functions that are nonmotor. The basal ganglia are thus intimately interconnected with almost all frontal lobe regions.

The relationship between the frontal lobes and the basal ganglia has been characterized in terms of loops from the frontal cortex to the striatum, the globus pallidus, and the thalamus, and then back to the frontal cortex. Five distinct loops have been identified, each appearing to be relatively anatomically segregated from the others at all levels of the circuit (Alexander, DeLong, & Strick, 1986). The motor circuit originates in the supplementary motor cortex, and the oculomotor circuit originates in the frontal eye fields. The other three circuits have been thought to be involved in cognition and emotion, and to originate in the dorsolateral, orbitofrontal, and cingulate cortices (Mega & Cummings, 1994). Thus there is overwhelming evidence based on neuroanatomy alone that the basal ganglia play a role in cognition.

Findings from neuropsychological patients suggest that these cognitive circuits are functionally important. Patients with Huntington's disease or Parkinson's disease often exhibit deficits in executive function, as well as cognitive slowing and mood disorders consistent with frontal lobe involvement (Brandt & Butters, 1986; Brown & Marsden, 1988; Taylor, Saint-Cyr, & Lang, 1986). In Huntington's disease, degeneration occurs within the neostriatum; in Parkinson's disease, degeneration occurs in the substantia nigra, a major input to the neostriatum. Although patients with Huntington's disease exhibit more profound cognitive deficits (dementia is one clinical characteristic of the disease), and the two patient groups have quite different motor abnormalities, both groups show deficits on tests of frontal lobe function, such as the Wisconsin Card Sorting Test and measures of verbal fluency.

Patients with basal ganglia disorders also exhibit impairments in declarative memory that are consistent with frontal lobe dysfunction (Butters, Wolfe, Granholm, & Martone, 1986; Taylor, Saint-Cyr, & Lang, 1990). For example, these patients exhibit deficits in recall that are disproportionate to their recognition abilities, and they show decreased use of clustering strategies in recall. These patient groups have shown deficits in nondeclarative memory tasks as well. Early demonstrations of this occurred in the domain of motor skill learning. For example, patients with Huntington's disease were found to be impaired relative to control participants in the rotary-pursuit learning task (Gabrieli, Stebbins, Singh, Willingham, & Goetz, 1997; Heindel, Butters, & Salmon, 1988). Patients with Parkinson's disease have also been found to exhibit deficits in motor learning (Haaland, Harrington, O'Brien, & Hermanowicz, 1997; Schugens, Breitenstein, Ackermann, & Daum, 1998; Soliveri, Brown, Jahanshahi, Caraceni, & Marsden, 1997). Plasticity in motor cortical regions appears to be a substrate for motor skill learning, so the basal ganglia may play a minor role in some cases when learning relies on cortical systems.

Motor skill learning is one of the classic preserved abilities both in amnesic patients and in patients with Alzheimer's disease (Dick, Nielson, Beth, Shankle, & Cotman, 1995; Tranel, Damasio, Damasio & Brandt, 1994). Thus the performance of patients with basal ganglia damage and patients with medial temporal lobe damage may be doubly dissociated from each other on measures of motor skill learning and recognition.

The interpretation of problems with motor skill learning in these patients is complicated by the fact that their motor performance is severely impaired relative to that of control subjects. Because baseline performance is often not equated, it can be difficult to compare learning for the two groups. However, deficits in these patients have also been observed in a number of other nondeclarative learning tasks that do not directly involve the performance of motor skills. In one study, patients with Huntington's disease were impaired at demonstrating the normal influence of recent stimuli when making weight judgments (Heindel, Salmon, & Butters, 1991). Normal subjects will tend to judge weights as being heavier if they have been previously exposed to lighter weights, and they will judge weights as lighter if they have previous experience with heavy weights. This biasing effect does not depend on declarative memory for lifting the biasing weights, because amnesic patients show this effect to the same extent as controls (Benzing & Squire, 1989). This biasing effect may be due to a mismatch between the actual weight and the motor program used to lift the weight that has been formulated based on recent experience with other weights. Patients with Huntington's disease may not incorporate this experience in reformulating the motor program used to lift the weights, and thus may be insensitive to biasing.

Patients with Huntington's disease also appear to have difficulty with perceptual–motor learning tasks that are learned normally by amnesic patients and patients with Alzheimer's disease. These include prism adaptation, in which subjects learn to decrease visually guided reaching error when wearing prism goggles (Paulsen, Butters, Salmon, Heindel, & Swenson, 1993). Learning this skill relies on the interface between the visual and motor systems. Other evidence suggests that patients with Huntington's disease or Parkinson's disease have difficulty learning to read mirror-reversed text (Koenig, Thomas-Anterion, & Laurent, 1999; Martone, Butters, Payne, Becker, & Sax, 1984). Although this skill probably depends on learning specific transformed letter identities, learning to scan the stimuli appropriately may also play a role.

One skill learning task that has been studied extensively with basal ganglia patients is the serial reaction time task. In this task, subjects see a stimulus move from location to location on a screen, and their task is to press a key corresponding to that location as quickly as possible. Unbeknownst to the subjects, the stimuli do not appear randomly, but rather appear according to a specific sequence. It can be shown that the reaction times of both normal subjects and amnesic patients benefit from the sequence, because if the stimuli are abruptly switched to a random sequence, there is a slowing of performance that is identical for the two groups (Nissen & Bullemer, 1987; Reber & Squire, 1994). Patients with Huntington's disease are impaired at this implicit sequence-learning task (Knopman & Nissen, 1991; Willingham & Koroshetz, 1993). Patients with Parkinson's disease have also been reported to show deficits, although these deficits may be apparent only when extensive training is used (see Figure 11.1) (Doyon et al., 1997; Ferraro, Balota, & Connor, 1993; Helmuth, Mayr, & Daum, 2000; Jackson, Jackson, Harrison, Henderson, & Kennard, 1995; Pascual-Leone et al., 1993; Sommer, Grafman, Clark, & Hallett, 1999).

Performance in the serial reaction time task is generally measured as the time required to press a key in response to a stimulus. In that sense, it is a motor learning task. However, it appears that the sequence information that is learned is more abstract than a series of movements. Instead, subjects learn a series of response locations, as indicated by the finding that there is excellent transfer of sequence learning to a new set of motor effectors, but poor transfer when new response locations are mapped onto the training sequence (Willingham, 1999; Willingham, Wells, Farrell, & Stemwedel, 2000). The fact that patients with basal ganglia disorders are impaired in sequence learning suggests that their impairment involves the implicit learning of information that is not specific to a motor response. The successive response locations gradually become associated with each other as a result of practice. Thus one important element of the type of learning that is dependent on the basal ganglia may be this gradual learning of associations. Deficits in motor skill learning in patients with basal ganglia disorders have also been interpreted in this way. Performance of motor actions depends on the learning of a sequence of components, and one component becomes associated with the subsequent component through practice. Fluid performance of the motor skill would result from a tight association between each component and its subsequent component through plasticity in the basal ganglia system (Graybiel, 1995). The contents of motor skill learning are quite inaccessible to declarative knowledge. Likewise, although the elements of a spatial sequence may be correctly recognized by some subjects, this knowledge is not necessary for improvement in performance as measured by reaction times.

The idea that patients with basal ganglia disorders may have an impairment in implicit associative learning has found support in work with experimental animals. Damage to the caudate nucleus in rats results in deficits in the "win–stay" radial-arm maze task, in which rats learn to traverse maze arms in which a cue is present in order to receive a food

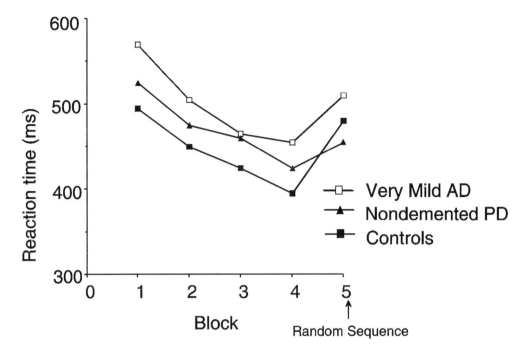

FIGURE 11.1. Patients with very mild Alzheimer's disease (AD), nondemented patients with Parkinson's disease (PD), and normal control subjects all showed improvement across blocks in the serial reaction time task when a fixed, 10-item sequence of locations was used. The PD patients appeared to have acquired less sequence-specific information than the other groups, because they showed a smaller reaction time increase when the sequence was switched to a random presentation of locations. Data from Ferraro, Balota, and Connor (1993).

reward (McDonald & White, 1994; Packard, Hirsh, & White, 1989). Performance on this same task is unaffected by lesions of the hippocampus or related structures. Rats appear to learn stimulus–response (S-R) associations in this task. That is, rather than learning an association between the cue and the food reinforcer, rats appear to learn to associate the cue with the arm entry response (Sage & Knowlton, 2000). The role of the food reinforcer is simply to strengthen this connection during training. This type of learning has historically been referred to as "habit learning" (see Mishkin & Petrie, 1984, for a review). Several researchers have suggested that other tasks that have been shown to be dependent on the caudate nucleus in experimental animals, such as some forms of discrimination learning, are also examples of habit learning (Battig, Rosvold, & Mishkin, 1962; Packard & McGaugh, 1992; Teng, Stefanacci, Squire, & Zola, 2000).

These studies of habit learning in experimental animals raise the question of whether there is a similar learning system in humans that is also dependent on the basal ganglia. This question cannot be answered in the obvious way of giving the same tests to humans that have been used with experimental animals, because humans appear to learn most discrimination tasks in a few trials using declarative memory, and not in the gradual manner that is typical in animals (Squire, Zola-Morgan, & Chen, 1988). One area in which the habit-learning system may be operating in humans is in the learning of categories in which the membership rules are not easy to verbalize, and thus are not easy to discern through hypothesis testing or memory for specific trials. One example is a task in which the subject must classify intersecting lines into two categories (Figure 11.2). Category membership can be defined by a linear (and thus easily verbalizable) relationship between the horizontal and vertical lines. Learning this type of classification problem appears to be intact in patients with Parkinson's disease, and may depend on the integrity of frontal lobe function (Maddox & Filoteo, in press). In contrast, when category membership is defined by a nonlinear relationship between horizontal and vertical line lengths, amnesic patients appear to learn to categorize these stimuli as well as normal subjects do, whereas patients with Parkinson's disease exhibit impaired performance (Filoteo, Maddox, & Davis, 2001; Maddox & Filoteo, in press).

It is important to note that patients with Parkinson's disease and Huntington's disease do not have a global deficit in implicit category learning. These patients appear to perform normally on tasks in which subjects are presented with a set of stimuli that belong

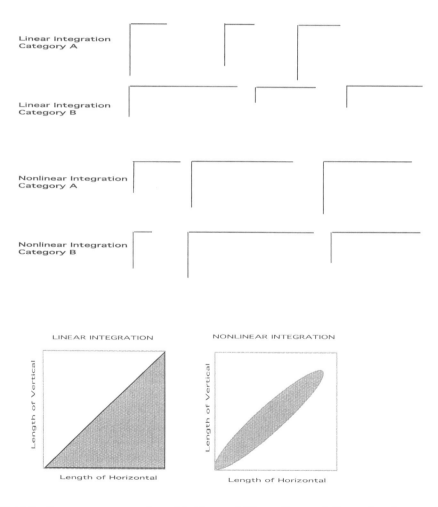

FIGURE 11.2. Category structures from Maddox and Filoteo (in press). Examples of categories defined by a linear categorization rule (vertical length greater or less than horizontal length; diagram on the left) and a nonlinear categorization rule (diagram on the right). In both cases, the shaded area in the diagrams refers to members of category A.

in one category (such as dot patterns or letter strings), and then are asked to classify whether or not new stimuli are part of the same category or not (Knowlton et al., 1996; Reber & Squire, 1999). In these tasks, the subjects receive no feedback during training and do not classify the items into two different categories. Thus subjects do not need to learn associations in these tasks; rather, they can respond based on the fact that items similar to the trained category can be processed more efficiently than dissimilar items, due to perceptual fluency's resulting from exposure to items during training. This type of learning may have a locus in cortical areas involved in perception, and thus should not be greatly affected by disorders of the basal ganglia. Neuroimaging data support a cortical locus for this type of category learning (Reber, Stark, & Squire, 1998).

Another strategy for developing habit-learning tasks in humans has been to use probabilistic associations between cues and correct responses. In such a task, declarative memory for each individual trial is not useful. Rather, correct responding can result from gradually building up an association across multiple trials. This gradual associative learning is thought to be characteristic of the caudate-dependent habit-learning tasks studied in animals. In a "weather prediction" version of the probabilistic classification task, the stimuli are cards with geometric shapes. On each trial, one to three cards appear, and the subject must guess whether the outcome will be sunny or rainy weather. Each card is associated with one of the two outcomes 60–85% of the time. Although subjects often feel as if they are guessing, they gradually learn to select the most associated outcome for each combination across trials. Amnesic patients perform as well as controls on this task, demonstrating that declarative memory of the cue–outcome associations is not necessary for normal performance (Knowlton, Squire, & Gluck, 1994). In contrast, patients with Huntington's disease and Parkinson's disease exhibit impaired learning on this task (Knowlton, Mangels, & Squire, 1996; Knowlton et al., 1996). The contrasting performance of patients with medial temporal lobe damage and patients with basal ganglia disorders on this task is reminiscent of the findings in habit-learning tasks used in animals. Moreover, the double dissociation between the performance of amnesic patients and patients with Parkinson's disease on the probabilistic classification task and a declarative memory questionnaire about the study episode establishes that these two forms of learning are dependent on distinct systems.

In the probabilistic classification task, it is not the case that the cue–outcome associations are fundamentally inaccessible to declarative memory. In fact, with extended training, individuals with intact memory are able to acquire declarative, flexible knowledge of the structure of the task (Reber, Knowlton, & Squire, 1996). The pattern of neuropsychological data is consistent with the finding that declarative learning can eventually influence performance on this task. With more than about 100 trials of training, control subjects begin to outperform amnesic patients, and patients with Parkinson's disease who have intact declarative memory begin to catch up to the level of control subjects.

Evidence from functional neuroimaging is consistent with neostriatal involvement in skill-learning and habit-learning tasks. The neostriatum is generally activated during performance of the serial reaction time task when there is an implicitly learned sequence, compared to blocks of trials in which locations are presented randomly (Peigneux et al., 2000; Rauch et al., 1997). Learning in the probabilistic classification task is also associated with activation in the caudate nucleus (Poldrack, Prabhakaran, Seger, & Gabrieli, 1999). This activation occurs early in training, and is accompanied by a decrease in medial temporal lobe activation. These findings suggest the intriguing possibility that the declarative and habit-learning systems may be mutually inhibitory. The medial temporal lobe memory system appears to be specialized for rapid learning of information about individual trials, whereas the neostriatal habit system appears to be specialized for gradual learning across many trials. Thus the two systems may occasionally be in conflict, if the response based on an implicitly learned habit differs from a response based on declarative learning about a recent episode. (See Ashby, Alfonso-Reese, Turken, & Waldron, 1998, for a computational model of basal ganglia function in which competition between implicit and declarative rule learning is a critical feature.)

A clear example of such conflict has been demonstrated in rats tested in a plus-shaped maze. Animals start from one arm of the maze and food is placed at the end of an arm 90 degrees from the start arm. Rats quickly learn the location of the reward in the maze. On transfer trials from the opposite start arm, they enter the same arm that had been reinforced (thus turning in the direction opposite from the direction they had turned during training). However, with extended training, the rats appear to respond based on an S-R habit. That is, when starting from the opposite end of the maze, they continue to make a turn in the same direction as they had during training. If a local anesthetic is injected into the caudate nucleus after extended training, rats will again respond based on memory for location and will turn in the opposite direction when started from the opposite end of the maze (Packard & McGaugh, 1996). Thus, with extended training, the S-R habit appears to overwhelm the more rapidly learned spatial memory, but the spatial memory can be "unmasked" if neostriatal function is compromised.

It is important to note that there are significant differences between the probabilistic classification task and the maze tasks used to measure habit learning in rats. In the case of the tasks used in animals, habit learning is evident only after many trials, and its control over behavior increases with extended training. However, for the probabilistic classification task, extended training appears to allow subjects to develop declarative representations that exert some control over behavior. This may be due to the way human subjects approach the task; subjects are likely to be motivated to acquire conscious knowledge of the task structure, and the probabilistic task structure makes this more difficult until later in training.

Another potential difference between the habit-learning tasks used in experimental animals and the probabilistic learning task studied with humans is the extent to which learning consists of an S-R association. In the win–stay task, for example, rats appear to learn an association between a cue and a motor response (running down an arm). In the probabilistic classification task, what is learned is not a specific motor response, but rather a tendency to react in a particular way to a cue. Subjects may still be learning S-R associations, but the response is a more abstract tendency to make a particular choice given a cue, independently of the motor response selected.

Another cognitive domain in which patients with Parkinson's disease have deficits is in switching between tasks. For example, these patients have difficulty with the Wisconsin Card Sorting Test, in which the subject must shift from sorting cards along one dimension (i.e., color) to another (i.e., shape). One study showed that patients with Parkinson's disease had greater difficulty shifting set when subjects were switched to sorting along a dimension that had been present previously (and thus was subject to learned irrelevance; Owen et al., 1993). For example, they had difficulty shifting from sorting to color to sorting to shape if differences in shape had been present in the previous sorting trials. Medicated patients with Parkinson's disease performed much better if the irrelevant dimension in the previous sorting trials was not present after the switch. Thus there was no impairment if the stimuli that were being sorted according to color differed in terms of number and not shape, and then differed in terms of shape and color after the switch to the shape-sorting task.

In another study, patients and control subjects were asked to switch between a color-naming and a shape-naming task. Reaction time suffered more for the patients than it did for controls when they switched tasks than when they performed the same task a second time. The presence of an irrelevant dimension (such as differences in color during the shape-naming task or differences in shape during the color-naming task) also slowed their performance compared to controls (Hayes, Davidson, Keele, & Rafal, 1998).

These deficits in set shifting may be related to the deficits in habit formation discussed previously. Sorting or naming based on a given dimension could be viewed as performance of an S-R habit. Putting a card with yellow circles into the "yellow" pile, or saying "yellow" in response to a stimulus, is based on an association between the cue and the appropriate response. These associations may be maintained in short-term memory, and thus they differ from skills and habits that are stored in long-term memory and are later retrieved. Nevertheless, the basal ganglia may be important in the online production of these S-R behaviors. If the links between the stimulus and the response are tenuous, switching between them may be more difficult. Although these behaviors may be produced by cortical systems, the basal ganglia may allow these S-R associations to be produced more fluently in an automatic fashion.

This question naturally arises: To what extent do deficits in habit learning or implicit category learning have a negative impact on the everyday lives of patients with basal ganglia disorders? The types of tasks that have been used in the laboratory to demonstrate deficits in these patients are generally quite unlike anything encountered in daily life. However, it seems likely that these implicit learning deficits are clinically significant. Although rigidity, tremor, and slowness of movement are the most debilitating symptoms of Parkinson's disease, these patients also exhbit bradyphrenia, or slowness of thought, under many circumstances (Hanes, Pantelis, Andrewes, & Chiu, 1996; Pate & Margolin, 1994). This slowness may arise because the basal ganglia are important for performing tasks automatically. Patients must therefore perform in a deliberate fashion tasks that would ordinarily be performed by habit.

To put memory systems in an evolutionary context, it has been argued that the pressures arising from managing increasingly complex social networks have played the primary role in shaping human cognition (Dunbar, 2000; Tomasello, 2000). The everyday cognitive problem that the basal ganglia learning system may be specialized to solve is the acquisition of the ability to use nonverbal information to make automatic social inferences. Nonverbal communication has been shown to have a major influence on one's inferences about social situations. Our knowledge and ability to decode and generate nonverbal social cues are implicit, for the most part. For example, we are almost totally unaware of the information that leads us to feel that other people do or do not like us, based on their verbal tone and "body language." Learning to read (and perhaps produce) these cues presumably arises gradually from social experience throughout life. The basal ganglia may be the site where these nonverbal cues become linked with appropriate responses (Lieberman, 2000). There are several studies suggesting that patients with Parkinson's disease are impaired in decoding nonverbal communication, such as prosody (Benke, Bosch, & Andree, 1998; Speedie, Brake, Folstein, Bowers, & Heilman, 1990). Indeed, the depression that commonly occurs with basal ganglia disorders may even be exacerbated by the impaired processing of the positive regard shown by others.

The study of the basal ganglia in implicit learning may prove to be an area of convergence among neuropsychology, behavioral neuroscience, and the emerging field of social-cognitive neuroscience. Links have already been made between the effects of basal ganglia damage in humans and experimental animals. The suggestion that the cognitive processes that depend on the basal ganglia are critical in the domain of social behavior is an intriguing possibility. The basal ganglia may turn out to play a much greater role in human mental activity than previously thought.

REFERENCES

Alexander, G. E., DeLong, M. R., & Strick, P. L. (1986). Parallel organization of functionally segregated circuits linking basal ganglia and cortex. *Annual Review of Neuroscience, 9,* 357–381.

Ashby, F. G., Alfonso-Reese, L. A., Turken, A. U., & Waldron, E. M. (1998). A neuropsychological theory of multiple systems in category learning. *Psychological Review, 105,* 442–481.

Battig, K., Rosvold, H. E. & Mishkin, M. (1962). Comparison of the effects of frontal and caudate lesions on discrimination learning in monkeys. *Journal of Comparative and Physiological Psychology, 55,* 458–463.

Benke, T., Bosch, S., & Andree, B. (1996). A study of emotional processing in Parkinson's disease. *Brain and Cognition, 38,* 36–52.

Benzing, W. C., & Squire, L. R. (1989). Preserved learning and memory in amnesia: Intact adaptation-level effects and learning of stereoscopic depth. *Behavioral Neuroscience, 103,* 538–547.

Brandt, J., & Butters, N. (1986). The neuropsychology of Huntington's disease. *Trends in Neurosciences, 9,* 118–120.

Brown, R. G., & Marsden, C. D. (1990). Cognitive function in Parkinson's disease: From description to theory, *Trends in Neurosciences, 13,* 21–29.

Butters, N., Wolfe, J., Granholm, E., & Martone, M. (1986). An assessment of verbal recall, recognition and fluency abilities in patients with Huntington's disease. *Cortex, 22,* 11–32.

Dick, M. B., Nielson, K. A., Beth, R. E., Shankle, W. R., & Cotman, C. W. (1995). Acquisition and long-term retention of a fine motor skill in Alzheimer's disease. *Brain and Cognition, 29,* 294–306.

Doyon, J., Gaudreau, D., Laforce, R., Castonguay, M., Bedard, P. J., Bedard, F., & Bouchard, J. P. (1997). Role of the striatum, cerebellum, and frontal lobes in the learning of a visuomotor sequence. *Brain and Cognition, 34,* 218–245.

Dunbar, R. I. M. (2000). Causal reasoning, mental rehearsal, and the evolution of primate cognition. In C. Heyes & L. Huber (Eds.), *The evolution of cognition* (pp. 205–219). Cambridge, MA: MIT Press.

Ferraro, F. R, Balota, D. A., & Connor, L. T. (1993). Implicit memory and the formation of new associations in nondemented Parkinson's disease individuals and individuals with senile dementia of the Alzheimer's type: A serial reaction time (SRT) investigation. *Brain and Cognition, 21,* 163–180.

Filoteo, J. V., Maddox, W. T., & Davis, J. D. (2001). Quantitative modelling of category learning in amnesic patients. *Journal of the International Neuropsychological Society, 7,* 1–19.

Gabrieli, J. D. E., Stebbins, G. T., Singh, J., Willingham, D. B., & Goetz, C. G. (1997). Intact mirror-tracing and impaired rotary-pursuit skill learning in patients with Huntington's disease: Evidence for dissociable memory systems in skill learning. *Neuropsychology, 11,* 272–281.

Graybiel, A. M. (1995). Building action repertoires: Memory and learning functions of the basal ganglia. *Current Opinion in Neurobiology, 5,* 733–741.

Haaland, K. Y., Harrington, D. L., O'Brien, S., & Hermanowicz, N. (1997). Cognitive–motor learning in Parkinson's disease. *Neuropsychology, 11,* 180–186.

Hanes, K. R., Pantelis, C., Andrewes, D. G., & Chiu, E. (1996). Bradyphrenia in Parkinson's disease, Huntington's disease, and schizophrenia. *Cognitive Neuropsychiatry, 1,* 165–170.

Hayes, A. E., Davidson, M. C., Keele, S. W., & Rafal, R. D. (1998). Toward a functional analysis of the basal ganglia. *Journal of Cognitive Neuroscience, 10,* 178–198.

Heindel, W. C. Butters, N., & Salmon, D. P. (1988). Impaired learning of a motor skill in patients with Huntington's disease. *Behavioral Neuroscience, 102,* 141–147.

Heindel, W. C., Salmon, D. P., & Butters, N. (1991). The biasing of weight judgments in Alzheimer's and Huntington's disease: A priming or programming phenomenon? *Journal of Clinical and Experimental Neuropsychology, 13,* 189–203.

Helmuth, L. L., Mayr, U., & Daum, I. (2000). Sequence learning in Parkinson's disease: A comparison of spatial-attention and number-response sequences. *Neuropsychologia, 38,* 1443–1451.

Jackson, G. M., Jackson, S. R., Harrison, J., Henderson, L., & Kennard, C. (1995). Serial reaction time learning and Parkinson's disease: Evidence for a procedural learning deficit. *Neuropsychologia, 33,* 577–593.

Knopman, D., & Nissen, M. J. (1991). Procedural learning is impaired in Huntington's disease: Evidence from the serial reaction time task. *Neuropsychologia, 29,* 245–254.

Knowlton, B. J., Mangels, J. A., & Squire, L. R. (1996). A neostriatal habit learning system in humans. *Science, 273,* 1399–1402.

Knowlton, B. J., Squire, L. R., & Gluck, M. A. (1994). Probabilistic classification learning in amnesia. *Learning and Memory, 1,* 106–120.

Knowlton, B. J., Squire, L. R., Paulsen, J. S., Swerdlow, N. R., Swenson, M., & Butters, N. (1996). Dissociations within nondecorative memory in Huntington's disease. *Neuropsychologia, 10,* 538–548.

Koenig, O., Thomas-Anterion, C., & Laurent, B. (1999). Procedural learning in Parkinson's disease: Intact and impaired cognitive components. *Neuropsychologia, 37,* 1103–1109.

Lieberman, M. D. (2000). Intuition: A social cognitive neuroscience approach. *Psychological Bulletin, 126,* 109–137.

Maddox, W. T., & Filoteo, J. V. (in press). Striatal contributions to category learning: Quantitative modeling of simple linear and complex nonlinear rule learning in patients with Parkinson's disease. *Journal of the International Neuropsychological Society.*

Martone, M., Butters, N., Payne, M., Becker, J. T., & Sax, D. S. (1984). Dissociations between skill learning and verbal recognition in amnesia and dementia. *Archives of Neurology, 41,* 965–970.

McDonald, R. J., & White, N. M. (1994). Parallel information processing in the water maze: Evidence for independent memory systems involving dorsal striatum and hippocampus. *Behavioral and Neural Biology, 61,* 260–270.

Mega, M. S., & Cummings, J. L. (1994). Frontal–subcortical circuits and neuropsychiatric disorders. *Journal of Neuropsychiatry and Clinical Neurosciences, 6,* 358–370.

Nissen, M. J., & Bullemer, P. (1987). Attentional requirements of learning: Evidence from performance measures. *Cognitive Psychology, 19,* 1–32.

Owen, A. M., Roberts, A. C., Hodges, J. R., Summers, B. A., Polkey, C. E., & Robbins, T. W. (1993). Contrasting mechanisms of impaired attentional shifting in patients with frontal lobe damage or Parkinson's disease. *Brain, 116,* 1159–1175.

Packard, M. G., Hirsh, R., & White, N. M. (1989). Differential effects of fornix and caudate nucleus lesions on two radial maze tasks: Evidence for multiple memory systems. *Journal of Neuroscience, 9,* 1465–1472.

Packard, M. G., & McGaugh, J. L. (1996). Inactivation of hippocampus or caudate nucleus with lidocaine differentially affects expression of place and response learning. *Neurobiology of Learning and Memory, 65,* 65–72.

Pascual-Leone, A., Grafman, J., Clark, K., Stewart, M., Massaquoi, S., Lou, J. S., & Hallet, M. (1993). Procedural learning in Parkinson's disease and cerebellar degeneration. *Annals of Neurology, 34,* 594–602.

Pate, D. S. & Margolin, D. I. (1994). Cognitive slowing in Parkinson's and Alzheimer's patients: Distinguishing bradyphrenia from dementia. *Neurology, 44,* 669–674.

Paulsen, J. S., Butters, N., Salmon, D. P., Heindel, W. C., & Swenson, M. R. (1993). Prism adaptation in Alzheimer's and Huntington's disease. *Neuropsychology, 7,* 73–81.

Peigneux, P., Maquet, P., Meulemans, T., Destrebecqz, A., Laurys, S., Degueldre, C., Delfiore, G., Aerts, J., Luxen, A., Franck, G., Van Der Linden, M., & Cleeremans, A. (2000). Sriatum forever, despite sequence learning variability: A random effect analysis of PET data. *Human Brain Mapping, 10,* 179–194.

Poldrack, R. A., Prabhakaran, V., Seger, C. A., & Gabrieli, J. D. E. (1999). Striatal activation during acquisition of a cognitive skill. *Neuropsychology, 13,* 564–574.

Rauch, S. L., Whalen, P. J., Savage, C. R., Curran, T., Kendrick, A., Brown, H. D., Bush, G., Breiter, H. C., & Rosen, B. R. (1997). Striatal recruitment during an implicit sequence learning task as measured by functional magnetic resonance imaging. *Human Brain Mapping, 5,* 124–132.

Reber, P. J., Knowlton, B. J., & Squire, L. R. (1996). Dissociable properties of memory systems: Difference in the flexibility of declarative and nondeclarative knowledge. *Behavioral Neuroscience, 110,* 861–871.

Reber, P. J., & Squire, L. R. (1994). Parallel brain systems for learning with and without awareness. *Learning and Memory, 1,* 217–229.

Reber, P. J., & Squire, L. R. (1999). Intact learning of artificial grammars and intact category learning by patients with Parkinson's disease. *Behavioral Neuroscience, 113,* 235–242.

Reber, P. J., Stark, C. E. L., & Squire, L. R. (1998). Contrasting cortical activity associated with category memory and recognition memory. *Learning and Memory, 5,* 420–428.

Sage, J. R., & Knowlton, B. J. (2000). Effects of US devaluation on win–stay and win–shift radial arm maze performance in rats. *Behavioral Neuroscience, 114,* 295–306.

Schugens, M. M., Breitenstein, C., Ackermann, H., & Daum, I. (1998). Role of the striatum and the cerebellum in motor skill acquisition. *Behavioural Neurology, 11,* 149–157.

Soliveri, P., Brown, R. G., Jahanshahi, M., Caraceni, T., & Marsden, C. D. (1997). Learning manual pursuit tracking skills in patients with Parkinson's disease. *Brain, 120,* 1325–1337.

Sommer, M., Grafman, J., Clark, K., & Hallett, M. (1999). Learning in Parkinson's disease: Eyeblink conditioning, declarative learning and procedural learning. *Journal of Neurology, Neurosurgery and Psychiatry, 67,* 27–34.

Speedie, L. J., Brake, N., Folstein, S. E., Bowers, D., & Heilman, K. M. (1990). Comprehension of prosody in Huntington's disease. *Journal of Neurology, Neurosurgery and Psychiatry, 53,* 607–610.

Squire, L. R., Zola-Morgan, S., & Chen, K. S. (1988). Human amnesia and animal models of amnesia: Performance of amnesic patients on tests designed for the monkey. *Behavioral Neuroscience, 102,* 210–221.

Taylor, A. E., Saint-Cyr, J. A., & Lang, A. E. (1986). Frontal lobe dysfunction in Parkinson's disease; The cortical focus of neostriatal outflow. *Brain, 109,* 279–292.

Taylor, A. E., Saint-Cyr, J. A., & Lang, A. E. (1990). Memory and learning in early Parkinson's disease: Evidence for a frontal lobe syndrome. *Brain and Cognition, 13,* 211–232.

Teng, E., Stefanacci, L., Squire, L. R., & Zola, S. M. (2000). Contrasting effects on discrimination learning after hippocampal lesions and conjoint hippocampal–caudate lesions in monkeys. *Journal of Neuroscience, 20,* 3853–3863.

Tomasello, M. (2000). Two hypotheses about primate cognition. In C. Heyes & L. Huber (Eds.), *The evolution of cognition* (pp. 165–183). Cambridge, MA: MIT Press.

Tranel, D., Damasio, A. R., Damasio, H., & Brandt, J. P. (1994). Sensorimotor skill learning in amnesia: Additional evidence for the neural basis of nondeclarative memory. *Learning and Memory, 1,* 165–179.

Willingham, D. B. (1999). The neural basis of motor-skill learning. *Current Directions in Psychological Science, 8,* 178–182.

Willingham, D. B. & Koroshetz, W. J. (1993). Evidence for dissociable motor skills in Huntington's disease patients. *Psychobiology, 21,* 173–182.

Willingham, D. B., Wells, L. A., Farrell, J. M., & Stemwedel, M. E. (2000). Implicit motor sequence learning is represented in response locations. *Memory and Cognition, 28,* 366–375.

12

Electrophysiological Studies of Retrieval Processing

MICHAEL D. RUGG, JANE E. HERRON, and ALEXA M. MORCOM

This chapter describes one approach to the investigation of intentional memory retrieval. The approach involves the use of an online measure of brain activity—event-related potentials (ERPs)—to permit the neural correlates of different retrieval processes to be characterized in terms of their timing, sensitivity to experimental manipulations, and intracerebral origins. Different classes of retrieval process are studied in the context of a theoretical framework in which these processes can be operationalized through specific experimental manipulations. We focus here on the approach as it has been applied to "yes–no" recognition memory, currently the most commonly employed memory test in studies of this kind.

RECOGNITION MEMORY

One way in which a positive recognition judgment is supported is through retrieval of the study event that included the test item. This form of memory—"episodic retrieval" or "recollection"—is thought to involve an interaction between a retrieval cue (self-generated or provided by the environment) and a memory trace (Tulving, 1983), and leads to the reconstruction of aspects of the episode represented in the trace. The retrieval of episodic information provides the rememberer both with the knowledge that a recognition test item corresponds to a recently experienced event, and with contextual information about the event (such as where and when it was experienced). Whether or not an episodic retrieval attempt is successful is influenced by numerous factors—not least, how the event was initially encoded into memory (Craik & Lockhart, 1972). Also important, however, are the cues available and the processes engaged during the retrieval attempt. The importance of retrieval cues and their processing is emphasized in such principles as "transfer-appropriate processing" (Morris, Bransford, & Franks, 1977) and "encoding specificity" (Tulving & Thomson, 1973), which propose, broadly speaking, that memory performance is a function of the degree to which cognitive operations engaged at encoding are recapitulated at retrieval.

According to "dual-process" theories of recognition memory (e.g., Mandler, 1980), recognition judgments can also be supported through an acontextual sense of familiarity. This form of memory is held to be dissociable from recollection on phenomenal (see, e.g., Gardiner & Java, 1993), functional (see, e.g., Jacoby & Kelley, 1992), and neurological (see, e.g., Aggleton & Brown, 1999) grounds. Although dual-process theories of recognition memory can muster a variety of sources of experimental support, they have not gone unchallenged. In particular, it has been argued that much of the behavioral evidence held to support dual-process models can be interpreted within a single-process framework, on the assumption that familiarity and recollection differ merely with respect to the "strength" and the specificity of information retrieved (e.g., Donaldson, 1996; Mulligan & Hirshman, 1997). We return to this issue later (see "Postretrieval Processes," below).

THE ERP METHOD

As already noted, the studies we describe below all employed an electrophysiological method—ERPs—to measure neural activity associated with different kinds of retrieval process. An ERP waveform represents the average time-locked electrical activity elicited by a particular class of experimental item (Kutas & Dale, 1997). Because their temporal resolution is on the order of milliseconds, ERPs are well suited to addressing questions about the time course of the neural correlates of item-related cognitive processes. A major drawback of the method, however, is that there are no general solutions for the localization of the sources of ERP activity. This drawback does not compromise the assessment of whether stimuli from different experimental conditions engage distinct neural populations as such assessments can be made perfectly adequately on the basis of contrasts of ERP scalp distributions (Kutas & Dale, 1997; Rugg & Coles, 1995). It does, however, impose severe limitations on the strength of the neuroanatomical conclusions that can be drawn.

RETRIEVAL PROCESSING

The theoretical perspective encompassing the studies reported below came out of a review of studies of the neural correlates of retrieval processing by Rugg and Wilding (2000). Rugg and Wilding have attempted to provide a framework within which ERP and other neuroimaging studies of episodic retrieval could be interpreted. They argue (see also Burgess & Shallice, 1996) that it is useful to distinguish between processes that operate on a retrieval cue in the course of an attempt to retrieve information from memory ("preretrieval processes") and processes that operate on the products of a retrieval attempt ("postretrieval processes"). They identify three kinds of preretrieval processes that have been proposed on the basis of ERP and neuroimaging findings. The first of these is retrieval "mode," a notion introduced by Tulving (1983). According to Tulving's original conception, retrieval mode is a cognitive state that causes events to be processed as episodic retrieval cues rather than as mere inputs from the environment, and is a prerequisite for successful episodic retrieval. More recently, it has been proposed that retrieval mode also supports the phenomenal experience of "reliving the past" ("autonoetic" remembering) that forms part of episodic retrieval (Wheeler, Stuss, & Tulving, 1997).

Another class of preretrieval processes identified by Rugg and Wilding (2000) is associated with retrieval "effort" (Schacter, Alpert, Savage, Rauch, & Albert, 1996). Effort refers to the mobilization of processing and attentional resources in service of a retrieval attempt, and covaries with the difficulty of the retrieval task and the motivation of the rememberer. A final class of preretrieval processes has been termed retrieval "orientation" (Rugg, Allan, & Birch, 2000). Orientation refers to the way in which a retrieval cue is processed to meet the demands of a given retrieval task; for example, the same cues may be processed differently, according to whether memory is probed for pictorial or verbal information (see "Retrieval Effort and Orientation," below).

According to Rugg and Wilding (2000), mode, effort, and orientation all represent retrieval processes that underlie the use of a cue in a retrieval attempt, and are engaged regardless of whether the attempt is successful. Indeed, Rugg and Wilding have argued that when one is investigating the neural correlates of effort and orientation, it is desirable to restrict analysis to neural activity elicited by retrieval cues bearing no relation to items from a preceding study phase (e.g., "new" items in a recognition memory test), on the assumption that these cues, unlike those eliciting successful retrieval, will fully engage preretrieval processes but will engage postretrieval processes to a limited degree only.

Postretrieval processes are associated with the recovery and representation of retrieved information, and with its subsequent evaluation. According to Rugg and Wilding (2000), the neural correlates of postretrieval processes can be identified by contrasting the activity elicited by retrieval cues associated with successful versus unsuccessful retrieval. This proposal—which in effect operationalizes postretrieval processing in terms of retrieval "success"—neglects the fact that even when a retrieval attempt is unsuccessful, postretrieval and executive processes of some kind are required to monitor the outcome of the attempt and to initiate an appropriate course of action (e.g., to iterate the memory search, respond "no," etc.). To our knowledge, however, no ERP studies have so far attempted to dissociate the neural correlates of success from the correlates of these other kinds of postretrieval operation (see Henson, Rugg, Shallice, & Dolan, 2000, and Rugg, Fletcher, et al., 1998, for examples of two neuroimaging studies reporting findings relevant to this distinction).

ERP STUDIES OF RETRIEVAL PROCESSING

In the following sections, we give examples of studies that have used ERPs to identify the neural correlates of different retrieval processes and to begin to characterize their temporal and functional properties.

Retrieval Mode

As noted above, retrieval mode is held to be a cognitive state that both biases the processing of stimulus events and supports autonoetic remembering. Tulving and colleagues have long championed the view that the neural correlates of retrieval mode are revealed by contrasting the neural activity associated with performance of episodic retrieval tasks (such as yes–no recognition) with activity associated with nonepisodic tasks (such as semantic judgment) (e.g., Wheeler et al., 1997). They have argued that the activation of the right anterior prefrontal cortex frequently observed for such contrasts in functional neuroimaging studies indicates that this region plays a key role in supporting retrieval mode (but see Rugg & Wilding, 2000). Using ERPs, Düzel and colleagues (1999) have reported data consistent with the proposal. To permit investigation of slow, temporally sustained ERP effects, Düzel and colleagues recorded direct-current potentials while subjects were presented with a series of short word lists and cued at the beginning of each list to perform either a recognition memory or a semantic judgment on the constituent words. Relative to the semantic task, the cue to perform the recognition task elicited a sustained positive shift that began prior to the presentation of the first word and showed an anterior right frontal scalp maximum.

We (Morcom & Rugg, 2001) followed up Düzel and colleagues' (1999) findings, using a trial-by-trial cueing procedure to induce "episodic" or "semantic" task sets. Subjects first studied a list of visually presented words. In a subsequent test session, these words were presented along with an equal number of new ones. A cue appeared 1.5 seconds before each test word and signaled on a random basis whether the word should be subjected to a recognition or a semantic ("animate–inanimate") judgment. Of interest were the ERP waveforms elicited by the different cues; if the cue to make a recognition judgment leads to adoption of retrieval mode, one would expect to see its putative neural signature—right frontal positivity, according to Düzel and colleagues—in the interval between the cue and the test item.

The results of the study are shown in Figure 12.1. The waveforms are separated according to whether the cue signaled a switch from one task to the other, signaled the same task as on a preceding switch trial, or signaled the same task as that performed for the past two or more trials. The rationale for this separation was based both on the observation of Düzel and colleagues (1999) that their putative correlate of retrieval mode did not develop fully until the first item or two had been presented, and on findings from the "task-switching" literature suggesting that task sets can take several trials to develop (Allport & Wylie, 2000). As can be seen from Figure 12.1, waveforms elicited by the two task cues

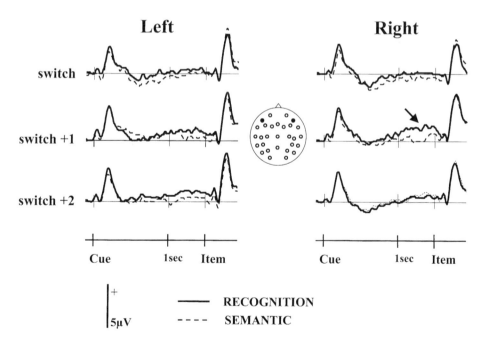

FIGURE 12.1. Grand-average waveforms ($n = 20$). ERPs elicited by cues signaling an upcoming recognition versus semantic judgment are shown for left and right frontal electrodes (locations as indicated in figure). "switch," trials on which a task switch was signaled; "switch + 1," trials immediately following a switch; "switch + 2," all other trials. Arrow shows the enhanced right frontal positivity elicited on switch + 1 trials for the recognition task. Data from Morcom and Rugg (2001).

differed little on switch trials or on trials preceded by two or more trials of the same type. On the trial immediately following a switch, however, ERPs elicited by cues signaling a recognition judgment were more positive than those signaling the semantic task, and this difference was greater over the right than the left frontal scalp—an asymmetry in the same direction as that reported by Düzel and colleagues. Unlike in Düzel and colleagues' study, however, these ERP set effects did not show a sharp maximum over the right frontal scalp; as shown in Figure 12.2, the effects were diffusely distributed, with a general tendency to be greater over the right than the left hemisphere.

These findings are consistent with the idea that recognition memory and semantic judgment engage different task sets. Our tentative explanation for the finding that ERPs differentiated these sets predominantly on trials immediately following a task switch is that the adoption of a set takes time and, as suggested by Düzel and colleagues (1999; see also Rogers & Monsell, 1995), may require presentation of a relevant test item. Thus it is not the switch trial, but the one subsequent to it, on which a cue is most effective in inducing the appropriate set. Once adopted, however, a set is maintained until the next switch trial, and hence differences between sets are no longer manifest in neural activity locked to the prestimulus cue.

Do these findings support the broader notion of episodic retrieval mode? Certainly they are consistent with that notion, although less clearly indicative of a selective role for the right prefrontal cortex than are the findings of Düzel and colleagues (1999). The reasons for the disparity between our and Düzel and colleagues' findings are unclear. They could reflect differences due to block versus trial-wise task switching, or to any of the several other procedural differences between the studies. In any case, the validity of the retrieval mode notion will depend on how generalizable findings such as those reported by Düzel and colleagues and ourselves turn out to be. Crucially, similar results need to be demonstrated when other pairs of tasks that differ in their episodic retrieval demands are contrasted.

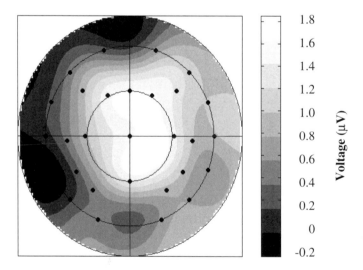

FIGURE 12.2. Scalp distribution of the difference between ERPs elicited by cues signaling an upcoming recognition versus semantic judgment on the trial following a task switch. Distribution shown for 1,000–1,500 msec postcue latency interval. Data from Morcom and Rugg (2001).

Retrieval Effort and Orientation

The neural correlates of retrieval effort and orientation are operationalized in terms of item-related activity elicited by retrieval cues when there is minimal confounding with the correlates of retrieval success (see "Retrieval Processing," above). Rugg and Wilding (2000) have proposed that correlates of effort may be investigated by manipulating task difficulty while holding study task and retrieval cues constant—the assumption being that the more difficult the retrieval task, the greater the effort expended (see, e.g., Buckner, Koutstaal, Schacter, Wagner, & Rosen, 1998). Rugg and Wilding have further proposed that the neural correlates of orientation may be revealed by contrasting activity elicited by physically identical retrieval cues when these are employed to probe memory for different kinds of information. As they note, in many ERP and neuroimaging studies difficulty and the nature of the sought-for information have been confounded, making it impossible to determine whether effort and orientation can be fractionated. Findings from two ERP studies in which this confound was avoided suggest that different retrieval orientations are neurally dissociable (Johnson, Kounios, & Nolde, 1997; Wilding, 1999). The crucial conditions in both studies involved ERPs elicited during tests of source memory. In Johnson and colleagues (1997), retrieval orientation was varied by a manipulation of study task; in Wilding (1999), it was varied by the requirement to recover information about different attributes of study episodes. In each case, ERPs elicited by unstudied items varied with orientation, despite there being little difference in the difficulty of the retrieval tasks. These studies do not, however, speak to the question of whether effort and orientation are independent, and their findings relate only to tasks in which there is an explicit requirement to retrieve contextual (source) information about a test item.

Robb and Rugg (in press) addressed these issues in a study in which difficulty and the form of the sought-for information were varied orthogonally. ERPs were obtained during four separate tests of recognition memory. Orientation was manipulated by varying study material: The study phases preceding two of the tests employed pictures, whereas the study phases preceding the other two tests employed words. Effort was manipulated by using a combination of the variables of length of study list and study–test interval to vary the ease with which recognition decisions could be made. Analysis of behavioral performance showed that the effects of the material and difficulty manipulations were both significant, but that there was little or no interaction between the two manipulations.

The ERP waveforms elicited by new test items in this study are shown in Figure 12.3. As was the case for the behavioral measures, the effects of the difficulty and material manipulations did not interact; in fact, the ERP modulations associated with these variables barely overlapped in time. Effects of difficulty were small, confined to the first 200–250 milliseconds (msec) poststimulus, and emerged at the moment of stimulus onset at central and parietal electrode sites. Since the waveforms were aligned on a prestimulus baseline, the very early onset of the effects almost certainly indicates that they actually began before the stimuli were presented, suggesting that difficulty modulated prestimulus preparatory or anticipatory processing in addition to any influence it may have had on the processing of the test items. The effect of study material on ERPs were much more striking. As is evident in Figure 12.3, the effect took the form of a sustained vertex–maximum difference, beginning at about 250 msec, between the ERPs elicited by the test words probing for different kinds of encoded information. The magnitude, scalp distribution, and time course of this effect were unaffected by the difficulty manipulation.

These findings suggest that retrieval effort and retrieval orientation—at least as operationalized by the manipulations employed here—have distinct neural and functional bases.

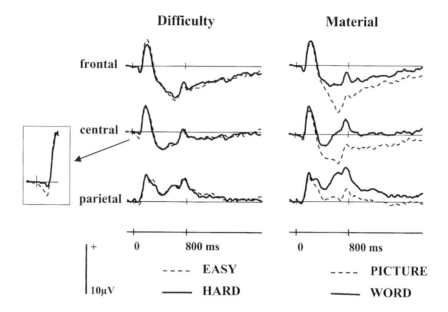

FIGURE 12.3. Grand-average waveforms (*n* = 19). In each column, ERPs are shown from midline frontal, central, and parietal scalp locations. *Left:* Waveforms collapsed across the study material manipulation and overlaid according to test difficulty. Small effects of difficulty can be seen from stimulus onset until about 200 msec poststimulus (see insert). *Right:* Waveforms collapsed over difficulty and overlaid according to study material. Data from Robb and Rugg (2001).

Thus differing retrieval demands can have marked effects on the processing of physically identical retrieval cues, independent of the effort required to use the cues to probe memory. The findings highlight the fact that people are able to exert control over how they process a retrieval cue, perhaps in an attempt to optimize the cue's effectiveness by deriving from it information compatible with that being probed for. To the extent that this suggestion is correct, the findings suggest that people are able to vary the processing of retrieval cues in accordance with the transfer-appropriate processing principle (see "Recognition Memory," above).

Postretrieval Processes

As noted earlier (see "Retrieval Processing," above), virtually all ERP studies of recognition memory examining the neural correlates of what we here call postretrieval processing have confounded such processing with retrieval success, operationalized by the contrast between activity elicited by correctly classified "old" and "new" test items. It was the employment of this contrast that marked the first use of ERPs to study memory retrieval (Sanquist, Rohrbaugh, Syndulko, & Lindsley, 1980), and the results of the numerous subsequent studies have been the subject of comprehensive reviews (e.g., Friedman & Johnson, 2000; Rugg, 1995). A key finding from these studies is that, relative to the ERPs elicited by correctly classified new items, ERPs to items correctly judged as old show a characteristic positive-going shift. This shift—sometimes referred to as the "left parietal old–new effect"—begins at about 450 msec poststimulus, has a duration of about 500 msec, and (as its name implies) is usually maximal over the left parietal scalp. A substantial body of evidence suggests that the effect is a correlate of episodic retrieval (recollection), rather than the mere reflection of a positive recognition response (Rugg & Allan, 2000).

Whereas the left parietal effect appears to be a good candidate for an electrophysiological correlate of successful episodic retrieval, it is less certain whether there exists a correlate for familiarity, the other proposed basis of recognition memory (see "Recognition Memory," above). Early attempts to identify a neural correlate of familiarity met with no success: Old–new effects associated with recognition in the apparent absence of episodic retrieval (defined by the failure to specify the source of a recognized test item) were found to be smaller than the effects elicited by recollected items, but not to differ from them in any qualitative way (e.g., Wilding & Rugg, 1996). These findings are more consistent with the notion of familiarity as an attenuated or impoverished form of recollection than with the concept of familiarity as an independent form of memory.

A different conclusion is reached from more recent work where the probability that a recognition judgment would be based primarily on familiarity was manipulated directly. Rugg, Mark, and colleagues (1998) employed a study task in which depth of processing (semantic vs. alphabetic judgments) was cued on a trial-by-trial basis. Performance on a subsequent recognition memory test was considerably higher for deeply than for shallowly studied words. Mirroring this finding, the left parietal effect elicited by correctly recognized deeply studied words was markedly greater than that elicited by recognized shallowly studied items (see Figure 12.4), consistent with the widely accepted idea that episodic memory is facilitated by semantic relative to nonsemantic encoding tasks (Craik & Lockhart, 1972). As can be seen in Figure 12.4, however, the ERPs also showed an earlier, frontally distributed old–new effect that did not differentiate between words subjected to semantic versus nonsemantic encoding. Furthermore, as depicted in the insert, this effect was absent for old items that were incorrectly classified as new, suggesting that it reflects a process contributing to a positive recognition judgment. In light of behavioral findings suggesting that familiarity-based recognition is less sensitive to depth-of-processing manipulations than is recognition based on recollection (Yonelinas, Kroll, Dobbins, Lazzara, & Knight, 1998), Rugg, Mark, and colleagues (1998) proposed that the frontal effect is an electrophysiological correlate of familiarity.

If Rugg, Mark, and colleagues' (1998) interpretation of the functional significance of their frontal old–new effect is correct, the effect should be elicited by other classes of items that receive positive recognition judgments on the basis of their familiarity. One such class are new items incorrectly classified as old (i.e., "false alarms"). According to dual-process models, false alarms principally occur when the familiarity of a new item exceeds the criterion for a positive recognition judgment and is not opposed by the recollection that the item did not appear at study (Jacoby & Kelley, 1972). We therefore investigated whether false alarms are associated with a frontal old–new ERP effect. To obtain a high false-alarm rate in the absence of an excessively liberal response criterion, we employed a two-phase study procedure. In phase 1, a set of words was presented in a shallow encoding task (alphabetic judgment). In phase 2—the study phase proper— half of these words, along with an equal number of new items, were presented in a deep encoding task (sentence generation). At test, subjects were presented with words that had been seen in both study phases, words that had been seen in phase 1 only, words that had been seen in phase 2 only, and new words. The instructions were to respond

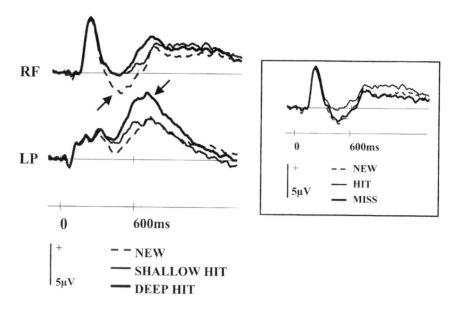

FIGURE 12.4. Grand-average waveforms ($n = 30$) depicting some of the findings of Rugg, Mark, et al. (1998). The main figure depicts waveforms from right frontal (RF) and left parietal (LP) electrodes elicited by correctly classified new words, and correctly classified old words that had been subjected to deep or shallow study (hits). The frontal and left parietal old–new effects are indicated with arrows. The insert illustrates frontal waveforms elicited by new words, and correctly (hits) and incorrectly (misses) classified shallowly studied words. The frontal old–new effect is absent for the incorrectly classified items. Data from Rugg, Mark, et al. (1998).

"old" to any item presented in phase 2, and "new" to all other items. The rationale was that words presented only in phase 1 would receive a boost to their familiarity but little or no episodic encoding, leading subsequently to a high false-alarm rate, and consequently enough trials to form reliable ERPs. This expectation was met, in that the phase 1 items gave rise to markedly higher false-alarm rates that those shown for the first time at test (42% vs. 23%). The relevant ERPs are shown in Figure 12.5, where it can be seen that, relative to correctly rejected phase 1 items, phase 1 words attracting a false alarm elicited a early frontal old–new effect comparable in size to the effect elicited by items presented in both the study phases and correctly endorsed as old. By contrast, a parietal effect was evident only for correctly classified old words. On the assumption that false alarms occurred because familiarity was high and unopposed by recollection, the findings are consistent with the view that early frontal old–new effects and later parietal effects are correlates of familiarity and recollection, respectively.

The findings described above suggest that the neural correlates of recollection and familiarity can be dissociated in terms of their functional, temporal, and neuroanatomical characteristics. Together with similar results from other laboratories (Curran, 2000; Mecklinger, 2000), the findings lend strong support to dual-process models of recognition memory; they indicate that with respect to recognition memory at least, retrieval "success," as manifested in positive recognition judgments, can be based on at least two different kinds of retrieved information.

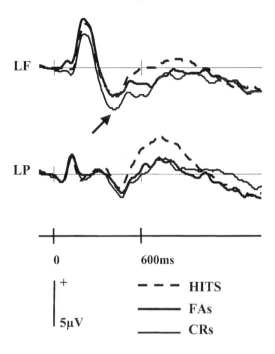

FIGURE 12.5. Grand-average waveforms (*n* = 17). Hits, ERPs elicited by words shown in both study phases and correctly judged as old; FAs, words studied in phase 1 only and incorrectly judged as old; CRs, words studied in phase 1 only and correctly judged as new. Early frontal old–new effect common to hits and false alarms is indicated by the arrow.

CONCLUDING COMMENTS

The findings presented in this chapter were chosen to illustrate how a noninvasive measure of brain activity—ERPs—can be employed to address questions about the processes engaged during intentional memory retrieval. The findings suggest that in broad terms at least, the theoretical framework outlined by Rugg and Wilding (2000) may be useful for identifying and characterizing different retrieval processes at the level of their neural correlates. Of course, the studies described here represent only a tiny fraction of those needed to achieve these aims, which require investigation of a much greater range of encoding conditions, materials, and memory tests.

There is no reason in principle why the approach outlined here cannot be employed with other methods for studying brain activity noninvasively, the most appropriate perhaps being event-related functional magnetic resonance imaging (D'Esposito, Zarahn, & Aguirre, 1999). Such studies, which to date have focused almost exclusively on retrieval success (Rugg & Henson, in press), will permit the neural systems supporting different pre- and postretrieval processes to be localized with considerably more precision than is possible with ERPs. Together with the development of methods to integrate electrophysiological and hemodynamic data (Kutas & Dale, 1997), this raises the exciting prospect of a specification of both the temporal dynamics and the neural bases of retrieval processing.

ACKNOWLEDGMENT

We and our research are supported by the Wellcome Trust.

REFERENCES

Allport, A., & Wylie, G. (2000). Task-switching, stimulus-response bindings, and negative priming. In S. Monsell & J. Driver (Eds.), *Attention and performance XVIII* (pp. 35–70). Cambridge, MA: MIT Press.

Aggleton, J. P., & Brown, M. W. (1999). Episodic memory, amnesia, and the hippocampal–anterior thalamic axis. *Behavioral and Brain Sciences, 22,* 425–444.

Buckner, R. L., Koutstaal, W., Schacter, D. L., Wagner, A. D., & Rosen, B. R. (1998). Functional–anatomic study of episodic retrieval using fMRI: I. Retrieval effort versus retrieval success. *NeuroImage, 7,* 151–162.

Burgess, P. W., & Shallice, T. (1996). Confabulation and the control of recollection. *Memory, 4,* 359–411.

Craik, F. I. M., & Lockhart, R. S. (1972). Levels of processing: A framework for memory research. *Journal of Verbal Learning and Verbal Behavior, 11,* 671–684.

Curran, T. (2000). Brain potentials of recollection and familiarity. *Memory and Cognition, 28,* 923–938.

D'Esposito, M., Zarahn, E., & Aguirre, G. K. (1999). Event-related functional MRI: Implications for cognitive psychology. *Psychological Bulletin, 125,* 155–164.

Donaldson, W. (1996). The role of decision processes in remembering and knowing. *Memory and Cognition, 24,* 523–533.

Düzel, E., Cabeza, R., Picton, T. W., Yonelinas, A. P., Schleich, H., Heinze, H., & Tulving, E. (1999). Task-related and item-related brain processes of memory retrieval. *Proceedings of the National Academy of Sciences USA, 96,* 1794–1799.

Friedman, D., & Johnson, R. (2000). Event-related potential (ERP) studies of memory encoding and retrieval: A selective review. *Microscopy Research and Technique, 51,* 6–28.

Gardiner, J. M., & Java, R. I. (1993). Recognising and remembering. In A. Collins, M. A. Conway, S. E. Gathercole, & P. E. Morris (Eds.), *Theories of memory* (pp. 163–188). Hillsdale, NJ: Erlbaum.

Henson, R. N. A., Rugg, M. D., Shallice, T., & Dolan, R. J. (2000). Confidence in recognition memory for words: Dissociating right prefrontal roles in episodic retrieval. *Journal of Cognitive Neuroscience, 12,* 913–923.

Jacoby, L. L., & Kelley, C. (1992). Unconscious influences of memory: Dissociations and automaticity. In A. D. Milner & M. D. Rugg (Eds.), *The neuropsychology of consciousness* (pp. 201–234). London: Academic Press.

Johnson, M. K., Kounios, J., & Nolde, S. F. (1997). Electrophysiological brain activity and memory source monitoring. *NeuroReport, 8,* 1317–1320.

Kutas, M., & Dale, A. (1997). Electrical and magnetic readings of mental functions. In M. D. Rugg (Ed.), *Cognitive neuroscience* (pp. 169–242). Hove, England: Psychology Press.

Mandler, G. (1980). Recognizing: The judgment of previous occurrence. *Psychological Review, 87,* 252–271.

Mecklinger, A. (2000). Interfacing mind and brain: A neurocognitive model of recognition memory. *Psychophysiology, 37,* 565–583.

Morcom, A. M., & Rugg, M. D. (2001). *Getting ready to remember: The neural correlates of task set during recognition memory.* Manuscript submitted for publication.

Morris, C. D., Bransford, J. D., & Franks, J. J. (1977). Levels of processing versus transfer appropriate processing. *Journal of Verbal Learning and Verbal Behavior, 16,* 519–533.

Mulligan, N. W., & Hirshman, E. (1997). Measuring the bases of recognition memory: An investigation of the process–dissociation framework. *Journal of Experimental Psychology: Learning, Memory, and Cognition, 23,* 280–304.

Robb, W. G. K., & Rugg, M. D. (in press). Electrophysiological dissociation of retrieval orientation and retrieval effort. *Psychonomic Bulletin and Review.*

Rogers, R. D., & Monsell, S. (1995). Costs of a predictable switch between simple cognitive tasks. *Journal of Experimental Psychology: General, 124*(2), 207–231.

Rugg, M. D. (1995). ERP studies of memory. In M. D. Rugg & M. G. H. Coles (Eds.), *Electrophysiology of mind, event-related brain potentials and cognition* (pp. 132–170). Oxford: Oxford University Press.

Rugg, M. D., & Allan, K. (2000). Memory retrieval: An electrophysiological perspective. In M. S. Gazzaniga (Ed.), *The new cognitive neurosciences* (2nd ed., pp. 805–816). Cambridge, MA: MIT Press.

Rugg, M. D., Allan, K., & Birch, C. S. (2000). Electrophysiological evidence for the modulation of retrieval orientation by depth of study processing. *Journal of Cognitive Neuroscience, 12,* 664–678.

Rugg, M. D., & Coles, M. G. H. (1995). The ERP and cognitive psychology: Conceptual issues. In M. D. Rugg & M. G. H. Coles (Eds.), *Electrophysiology of mind, event-related brain potentials and cognition* (pp. 27–39). Oxford: Oxford University Press.

Rugg, M. D., Fletcher, P. C., Allan, K., Frith, C. D., Frackowiak, R. S. J., & Dolan, R. J. (1998). Neural correlates of memory retrieval during recognition memory and cued recall. *NeuroImage, 8*(3), 262–273.

Rugg, M. D., & Henson, R. N. A. (in press). Episodic memory retrieval: An (event-related) functional neuroimaging perspective. In A. E. Parker, E. L. Wilding, & T. Bussey (Eds.), *The cognitive neuroscience of memory encoding and retrieval.* Hove, England: Psychology Press.

Rugg, M. D., Mark, R. E., Walla, P., Schloerscheidt, A. M., Birch, C. S., & Allan, K. (1998). Dissociation of the neural correlates of implicit and explicit memory. *Nature, 392,* 595–598.

Rugg, M. D., & Wilding, E. L. (2000). Retrieval processing and episodic memory. *Trends in Cognitive Sciences, 4,* 108–115.

Sanquist, T. F., Rohrbaugh, J. W., Syndulko, K., & Lindsley, D. B. (1980). Electrocortical signs of levels of processing: Perceptual analysis and recognition memory. *Psychophysiology, 17,* 568–76.

Schacter, D. L., Alpert, N. M., Savage, C. R., Rauch, S. L., & Albert, M. S. (1996). Conscious recollection and the human hippocampal formation: Evidence from positron emission tomography. *Proceedings of the National Academy of Sciences USA, 93,* 321–325.

Tulving, E. (1983). *Elements of episodic memory.* Oxford: Clarendon Press.

Tulving, E., & Thomson, D. M. (1973). Encoding specificity and retrieval processes in episodic memory. *Psychological Review, 80,* 353–373.

Wheeler, M. A., Stuss, D. T., & Tulving, E. (1997). Toward a theory of episodic memory: The frontal lobes and autonoetic consciousness. *Psychological Bulletin, 121,* 331–354.

Wilding, E. L. (1999). Separating retrieval strategies from retrieval success: An event-related potential study of source memory. *Neuropsychologia, 37,* 441–454.

Wilding, E. L., & Rugg, M. D. (1996). An event-related potential study of recognition memory with and without retrieval of source. *Brain, 119,* 889–905.

Yonelinas, A. P., Kroll, N. E., Dobbins, I., Lazzara, M., & Knight, R. T. (1998). Recollection and familiarity deficits in amnesia: Convergence of remember–know, process dissociation, and receiver operating characteristic data. *Neuropsychology, 12,* 323–339.

13

Functional Neuroimaging Studies of Memory Retrieval

KATHLEEN B. McDERMOTT
and RANDY L. BUCKNER

Functional neuroimaging techniques provide a window through which to view brain function in healthy, conscious humans. As such, these techniques offer an opportunity to gain insight into the neural underpinnings of human cognition. In the present chapter, we consider recent findings in basic research on episodic memory retrieval, or memory for episodes in one's past.

The principles underlying these functional neuroimaging techniques are roughly as follows. Positron emission tomography (PET) and functional magnetic resonance imaging (fMRI) both rely on the fortuitous physiological property that when a local region of the brain is actively used, blood flow to that region increases (e.g., regions within the occipital gyrus for vision; Posner & Raichle, 1994). PET allows blood flow increases to be observed through the administration of small amounts of radioactive isotope into the bloodstream. In this manner, the researcher can observe changes in radioactivity and infer from them the local changes in blood flow (Raichle, 1987). The most commonly employed fMRI techniques image derivatives of blood flow change associated with changes in oxygen content in the blood (the so-called "blood-oxygenation-level-dependent," or BOLD, contrast mechanism; Kwong et al., 1992; Ogawa et al., 1992). Because fMRI does not require radiation exposure, and because it offers better spatial and temporal resolution than does PET, fMRI is becoming the technique of choice for answering the types of questions outlined in the present chapter. In particular, utilization of the superior temporal resolution of fMRI has allowed increasingly sophisticated experimental designs, as will be described later.

We consider here some emerging findings with respect to retrieval of information from long-term episodic memory; discuss possible interpretations of these findings; and, in so doing, demonstrate an emerging understanding of the neural underpinnings of human memory retrieval.

REGIONS CORRELATED WITH RETRIEVAL SUCCESS

A fundamental question one might ask with respect to the neural underpinnings of memory retrieval is this: Which brain regions show preferential activity when people not only try to recollect the past, but are successful at doing so? Preferential activity in response to successfully retrieved items suggests neural correlates that may be used by subjects to remember the past. That is, although these linkages are based on correlation only, brain regions that show differential activity associated with retrieval success can be considered candidates for playing a direct role in the process of recollection.

Due to their theoretical importance, regions associated with retrieval success have been sought for a number of years (e.g., Buckner et al., 1998; Nyberg et al., 1995; Rugg, Fletcher, Frith, Frackowiak, & Dolan, 1996; Rugg et al., 1998; Schacter, Alpert, Savage, Rauch, & Albert, 1996; Tulving, Kapur, Craik, Moscovitch, & Houle, 1994). Recently developed methods for isolating a specific class of trials associated with retrieval success, based on event-related fMRI (Rosen, Buckner, & Dale, 1998), have allowed considerably more sophisticated explorations than were previously possible. The present review is focused on some of these most recent studies.

To anticipate, regions within the bilateral lateral inferior parietal cortex (within Brodmann's area [BA] 40, often left > right) have consistently shown preferential activation under conditions of retrieval success (Donaldson, Petersen, Ollinger, & Buckner, 2001; Henson, Rugg, Shallice, Josephs, & Dolan, 1999; Henson, Rugg, Shallice, & Dolan, 2000; Konishi, Wheeler, Donaldson, & Buckner, 2000; McDermott, Jones, Petersen, Lageman, & Roediger, 2000; see also Habib & Lepage, 2000; McDermott et al., 1999). These regions can be seen in the data from three independent studies shown in Plate 13.1 (see color plates, opposite page 238). To a lesser extent, a region within the left anterior prefrontal cortex (within or near BA 10, and sometimes a homologous region on the right) has shown this pattern (Donaldson et al., 2001; Henson et al., 2000; Konishi et al., 2000; McDermott et al., 2000; although see Henson et al., 1999). Other regions, such as those within the medial temporal lobes, have shown this pattern in some studies, although not as ubiquitously across studies as the parietal and frontal regions highlighted here (see also Schacter & Wagner, 1999).

How might researchers identify regions as related to retrieval success? One approach would be to use the "remember–know" technique (Tulving, 1985). People are presented with items (often words) on a recognition memory test and are asked for each word whether they recognize it as having occurred previously in the experiment; furthermore, for each word they recognize as previously encountered, people are asked to report whether they can vividly *remember* a particular aspect of having encountered the word, or whether they just *know* it appeared previously. Regions of the brain preferentially active for remembered words, relative to those just known to have been studied, should represent regions related to retrieval success; in addition, items remembered relative to new items correctly rejected should turn up regions associated with retrieval success.

Henson and colleagues (1999) recently used a variant of this procedure and found that regions within the left superior parietal cortex (BA 19), left inferior parietal cortex (BA 40), posterior cingulate, and left superior frontal gyrus showed greater activation for items remembered than for those just known to have occurred earlier. Eldridge, Knowlton, Furmanski, Bookheimer, and Engel (2000) applied a similar approach to examine regions of the hippocampus; specifically, they found hippocampal regions that were active during "remember" responses but not "know" responses (for a related finding, see Schacter et al., 1996). In addition, Eldridge and colleagues found greater activation for remembered than for known words in regions in the left inferior parietal cortex (BA 40), left middle frontal gyrus, and posterior cingulate, among other regions. One somewhat surprising aspect of these studies is that a region within the anterior prefrontal cortex (at or near BA 10), which is often active during memory retrieval (for reviews, see Buckner, 1996; Cabeza & Nyberg, 1997; Desgranges, Baron, & Eustache, 1998; Fletcher, Frith, & Rugg, 1997), did not show this particular pattern corresponding to retrieval success. However, before too much is made of this null effect, the following findings should be considered.

Another fruitful way of uncovering regions correlating with successful retrieval relative to failed retrieval attempts has been to compare "hits" (previously studied items correctly classified as such) to correct rejections (nonstudied items correctly classified as such) on recognition memory tests. Several recent studies have taken this approach (Donaldson et al., 2001; Henson et al., 2000; Konishi et al., 2000; McDermott et al., 2000; see also Stark & Squire, et al., 2000), and the results converge to suggest several regions that are consistently more active for hits than for correct rejections. These regions occur within the bilateral inferior parietal cortex (highlighted in Plate 13.1, opposite page 238), superior parietal and anterior prefrontal cortex (sometimes left-lateralized and sometimes bilateral), and medial parietal cortex (precuneus).

One potential concern in using a contrast between hit and correct-rejection trials to infer an association with retrieval success is that the comparison relies on items that have a different history (studied or not) and that receive different responses ("Yes, I studied it" or "No, I didn't study it"). McDermott and colleagues (2000) report a comparison that avoids these confounds by comparing two types of correct rejections: those that were mediated by retrieval success and those that were not. Specifically, after people study compound words such as "blackbird" and "airmail," "one potential way in which they are able to correctly classify the similar word "blackmail" as a nonstudied word is to remember the words that *were* studied (e.g., "The word seems familiar, but I remember 'blackbird' and 'airmail,' not 'blackmail'"; see Jones & Jacoby, 2001). Thus, under certain conditions, retrieval success can contribute to correct performance in this condition. By comparing correctly rejected words in this condition to correctly rejected unrelated words, McDermott and colleagues confirmed regions identified by the initial comparison discussed previously (hits vs. correct rejections). Sanders, Wheeler, and Buckner (2000) have also provided data that weigh in on this issue; they found that the parietal and frontal regions discussed above were more active for studied words correctly recognized (hits) than for those not correctly recognized (misses).

An important further caveat to this discussion is that the willful, directed attempt to retrieve the past does not appear necessary for these "retrieval success" signals to appear. Koutstaal and colleagues (2001; see also Donaldson, Petersen, & Buckner, in press) have found these regions in an object classification task in which studied and nonstudied words were embedded, but the words' old–new status was irrelevant to the task. This outcome is arguably attributable to what has been termed "involuntary conscious recollection" (Gardiner & Java, 1993; Schacter, 1987). That is, people can vividly recollect the past even when they are not attempting to do so; the fact that memories—even distant memories—can "pop to mind" is familiar to us all.

We consider now the implications and interpretation of these findings. What does it mean to have identified neural correlates of retrieval success? At this point, all that can be said is that these regions *correlate* with retrieval success. They may be contributing processes that tend to *lead to* retrieval success or that *accompany* retrieval success. Furthermore, it is unlikely that these multiple anatomically distinct regions contribute fully overlapping processes. Nonetheless, we believe that an important step has been made in identifying brain regions that are involved (somehow) in the successful retrieval of the past. Future investigations will be required to understand which, if any, of these regions directly supply neural signals that are used and/or are necessary for vivid recollection of one's past.

Another remaining, yet critical, question is whether (and, if so, how) these correlates of retrieval success depend on the medial temporal regions necessary for episodic remembering. That is, do these correlates of retrieval success (or a subset of them) appear in the brains of amnesic patients with damage to the medial temporal structures? The answer to this question will have theoretical consequences, in that their absence in amnesic patients would provide further evidence of an association to conscious remembering, and would also suggest a dependence on medial temporal structures. In addition, this finding could have practical consequences, in that the absence of these neural correlates of retrieval success in amnesics could suggest a marker of medial temporal dysfunction. That is, it may be possible to use the frontal and parietal correlates of retrieval success elucidated above to probe for signs of medial temporal dysfunction in, for example, early stages of dementia.

SENSORY-SPECIFIC RETRIEVAL SUCCESS

The previous section has been concerned with regions that are tentatively thought to be amodal correlates of retrieval success—perhaps signaling, in some manner, that studied information has been recovered. Evidence for their generality comes from their presence across stimulus forms and modalities (e.g., Habib & Lepage, 2000). We now turn to recent work suggesting that other regions can show sensory-specific patterns associated with retrieval success. It has long been held in the psychological literature that remembering is often accompanied by the reexperiencing of specific, vivid sensory details. This idea has been discussed at least since the time of William James (1890), who argued that such images arise from subsets of the same "nerve-tracks" that are concerned with sensation. Richard Semon wrote extensively on the topic; he described the process of "rousing into action of a disposition created by the original excitation" as the process of ecphory (Semon, 1921, p. 138; see also Schacter, 1982; Tulving, 1983). A conceptually similar idea is embedded in the more modern idea of "transfer-appropriate processing" (Morris, Bransford, & Franks, 1977), which holds that retrieval performance benefits to the extent that processes invoked during retrieval overlap with those performed during encoding. It has even been argued that one will not successfully retrieve an event unless one can reinstantiate the mental processes used during encoding (the "encoding specificity" principle; Tulving & Osler, 1968).

Given this rich literature concerned with the overlap in the processing requirements engaged by encoding and retrieval, it is perhaps not surprising that researchers have attempted to demonstrate such overlap via neuroimaging techniques. The groundwork for the studies we are about to review was laid by the literature showing that imagery tends to activate a subset of regions used in perception. For example, visual imagery leads to activation of a subset of those regions active during visual perception (see, e.g., D'Esposito et al., 1997; Kosslyn, Thompson, Kim, & Alpert, 1995), and auditory imagery leads to activation of a subset of regions active during auditory perception (see, e.g., Zatorre, Halpern, Perry, Meyer, & Evans, 1996). Thus higher-order processes can lead to activation of sensory-specific regions. O'Craven and Kanwisher (2000) recently extended this research by showing that within a perceptual domain (vision), stimulus-specific activation occurs for qualitatively different imagined events. Specifically, O'Craven and Kanwisher took advantage of the fact that perception of faces and places (locations) preferentially activates different regions within the extrastriate cortex. By contrasting the activation during imagery for recently seen faces and places, they demonstrated that this regional specificity within the extrastriate cortex holds for imagery much as for perception: The face- and place-specific regions were selectively activated through imagery.

There is sometimes a fine line between imagery and retrieval, which becomes apparent when one considers the similarities in design between the aforementioned study by O'Craven and Kanwisher (2000), which is framed in terms of imagery and perception, and the studies to be discussed next, which are framed in terms of memory retrieval. These differences are not terribly surprising, given the overlap between imagery and retrieval. Consider the similarities in processing that would be brought about by imagining the sound of an airplane flying overhead (imagery), recollecting the way an airplane tends to sound when flying overhead (semantic retrieval), and remembering the sound of the airplane that recently passed overhead (episodic retrieval).

Several recent papers have examined whether memory retrieval reactivates sensory-specific areas invoked during the encoding phase. For example, Nyberg, Habib, McIntosh, and Tulving (2000) paired some visual words (but not others) with sounds during an encoding phase. On a recognition task in which the words were again presented visually, those words previously paired with a sound showed greater activation in a region within the auditory cortex than those not previously paired with a sound. This reactivation effect was observed not only when the experimenters instructed subjects to attempt to remember the sounds (Experiment 1), but also when the task was a simple old–new judgment, and the auditory reactivation was incidental to the task (Experiment 2).

Wheeler, Petersen, and Buckner (2000) reported an effect similar to Nyberg and colleagues' (2000) first experiment: Words previously paired with sounds led to selective activation in auditory regions (the left superior temporal gyrus) when subjects were given words and asked to recollect the accompanying sound. In addition, Wheeler et al. extended these results by demonstrating the converse pattern: Words previously paired with pictures led to greater activation of visual regions (in the left extrastriate visual cortex, extending into the precuneus) than did words not previously paired with pictures. It is noteworthy that the sensory-specific regions reactivated during retrieval were a subset of those used during the initial encoding of the event. Specifically, visual and auditory areas putatively late in the processing hierarchy (e.g., visual areas probably beyond V4) showed modulation by memory retrieval, whereas areas earlier in the visual processing stream did not. The implication may be that during vivid remembering, sensory regions are recruited to the degree that they supply information relevant to the retrieval query. Future research will clearly be needed to investigate such a possibility.

In addition, it will be interesting to see whether more subtle aspects of prior experience are manifested during retrieval; for example, within the verbal domain, people can focus on phonological or semantic information during encoding. Presumably, these variations in encoding will be manifested during retrieval; thus, in theory, it may be possible to dissociate the effects of retrieving different types of information from within a broad domain of processing (e.g., verbal encoding of visually presented words).

SUMMARY

In the present chapter, we have reviewed some of the most recent neuroimaging evidence with respect to the neural underpinnings of episodic memory retrieval. We have argued that a network of regions is emerging as preferentially active when people successfully remember the past. Regions within the inferior parietal cortex and anterior prefrontal cortex seem to be the most ubiquitously observed of these regions at this point. In addition, activation of sensory-specific regions accompanies vivid recollection of prior sensory-specific experiences, much in the way mental imagery activates a subset of regions involved in perception.

ACKNOWLEDGMENTS

This work was supported by grants from the McDonnell–Pew Foundation, the National Science Foundation, and the National Institutes of Health.

REFERENCES

Buckner, R. L. (1996). Beyond HERA: Contributions of specific prefrontal brain areas to long-term memory retrieval. *Psychonomic Bulletin & Review, 3*, 149–158.

Buckner, R. L., Koutstaal, W., Schacter, D. L., Dale, A. M., Rotte, M., & Rosen, B. R. (1998). Functional–anatomic study of episodic retrieval: Selective averaging of event-related fMRI trials to test the retrieval success hypothesis. *NeuroImage, 7*, 163–175.

Cabeza, R., & Nyberg, L. (1997). Imaging cognition: An empirical review of PET studies with normal subjects. *Journal of Cognitive Neuroscience, 9*, 1–26.

D'Esposito, M., Detre, J. A., Aguirre, G. K., Stallcup, M., Alsop, D. C., Tippet, L. J., & Farah, M. J. (1997). A functional MRI study of mental image generation. *Neuropsychologia, 35*, 725–730.

Desgranges, B., Baron, J. C., & Eustache, F. (1998). The functional neuroanatomy of episodic memory: The role of frontal lobes, hippocampal formation, and other areas. *NeuroImage, 8*, 198–213.

Donaldson, D. I., Petersen, S. E., & Buckner, R. L. (in press). Dissociating implicit and explicit memory retrieval processes: fMRI evidence that conceptual priming does not support the contribution of familiarity to recognition. *Neuron.*

Donaldson, D. I., Petersen, S. E., Ollinger, J. M., & Buckner, R. L. (2001). Dissociating state- and item-related processes of recognition memory using fMRI. *NeuroImage, 13*, 129–142.

Eldridge, L. L., Knowlton, B. J., Furmanski, C. S., Bookheimer, S. Y., & Engel, S. A. (2000). Remembering episodes: A selective role for the hippocampus during retrieval. *Nature Neuroscience, 3*, 1149–1152.

Fletcher, P. C., Frith, C. D., & Rugg, M. D. (1997). The functional neuroanatomy of episodic memory. *Trends in Neurosciences, 20*, 213–218.

Gardiner, J. M., & Java, R. I. (1993). Recognising and remembering. In A. Collins, S. E. Gathercole, M. A. Conway, & P. E. Morris (Eds.), *Theories of memory* (pp. 163–188). Hillsdale, NJ: Erlbaum.

Habib, R., & Lepage, M. (2000). Novelty assessment in the brain. In E. Tulving (Ed.), *Memory, consciousness, and the brain* (pp. 265–277). Philadelphia: Psychology Press.

Henson, R. N. A., Rugg, M. D., Shallice, T., & Dolan, R. J. (2000). Confidence in recognition memory for words: Dissociating right prefrontal roles in episodic retrieval. *Journal of Cognitive Neuroscience, 12*, 913–923.

Henson, R. N. A., Rugg, M. D., Shallice, T., Josephs, O., & Dolan, R. J. (1999). Recollection and familiarity in recognition memory: An event-related functional magnetic resonance imaging study. *Journal of Neuroscience, 19*, 3962–3972.

James, W. J. (1890). *The principles of psychology.* New York: Dover.

Jones, T. C., & Jacoby, L. L. (2001). Feature and conjunction errors in recognition memory: Evidence for dual-process theory. *Journal of Memory and Language, 45*, 82–102.

Konishi, S., Wheeler, M. E., Donaldson, D. I., & Buckner, R. L. (2000). Neural correlates of episodic retrieval success. *NeuroImage, 12,* 276–286.

Kosslyn, S. M., Thompson, W. L., Kim, I. J., & Alpert, N. M. (1995). Topographical representations of mental images in primary visual cortex. *Nature, 378,* 496–498.

Koutstaal, W., Wagner, A. D., Rotte, M., Maril, A., Buckner, R. L., & Schacter, D. L. (2001). Perceptual specificity in visual object priming: Functional magnetic resonance imaging evidence for a laterality difference in fusiform cortex. *Neuropsychologia, 39,* 184–199.

Kwong, K. K., Belliveau, J. W., Chesler, D. A., Goldberg, I. E., Weisskoff, R. M., Poncelet, B. P., Kennedy, D. N., Hoppel, B. E., Cohen, M. S., & Turner, R. (1992). Dynamic magnetic resonance imaging of human brain activity during primary sensory stimulation. *Proceedings of the National Academy of Sciences USA, 89,* 5675–5679.

McDermott, K. B., Jones, T. C., Petersen, S. E., Lageman, S. K., & Roediger, H. L. (2000). Retrieval success is accompanied by enhanced activation in anterior prefrontal cortex during recognition memory: An event-related fMRI study. *Journal of Cognitive Neuroscience, 12,* 965–976.

McDermott, K. B., Ojemann, J. G., Petersen, S. E., Ollinger, J. M., Snyder, A. Z., Akbudak, E., Conturo, T. E., & Raichle, M. E. (1999). Direct comparison of episodic encoding and retrieval of words: An event-related fMRI study. *Memory, 7,* 661–678.

Morris, C. D., Bransford, J. D., & Franks, J. J. (1977). Levels of processing versus transfer appropriate processing. *Journal of Verbal Learning and Verbal Behavior, 16,* 519–533.

Nyberg, L., Habib, R., McIntosh, A. R., & Tulving, E. (2000). Reactivation of encoding-related brain activity during memory retrieval. *Proceedings of the National Academy of Sciences USA, 97,* 11120–11124.

Nyberg, L., Tulving, E., Habib, R., Nilsson, L.-G., Kapur, S., Houle, S., Cabeza, R., & McIntosh, A. R. (1995). Functional brain maps of retrieval mode and recovery of episodic information. *NeuroReport, 7,* 249–252.

O'Craven, K. M., & Kanwisher, N. (2000). Mental imagery of faces and places activates corresponding stimulus-specific brain regions. *Journal of Cognitive Neuroscience, 12,* 1013–1023.

Ogawa, S., Tank, D. W., Menon, R., Elerman, J. M., Kim, S. G., Merkle, H., & Ugurbil, K. (1992). Intrinsic signal changes accompanying sensory stimulation: Functional brain mapping with magnetic resonance imaging. *Proceedings of the National Academy of Sciences USA, 89,* 5951–5955.

Posner, M. I., & Raichle, M. E. (1994). *Images of mind.* New York: Scientific American Books.

Raichle, M. E. (1987). Circulatory and metabolic correlates of brain function in normal humans. In F. Plum & V. Mountcastle (Eds.), *Handbook of physiology: Section 1. The nervous system. Vol. 5. Higher functions of the brain. Part 1* (pp. 643–674). Bethesda, MD: American Physiological Association.

Rosen, B. R., Buckner, R. L., & Dale, A. M. (1998). Event related fMRI: Past, present, and future. *Proceedings of the National Academy of Sciences USA, 95,* 773–780.

Rugg, M. D., Fletcher, P. C., Allan, K., Frith, C. D., Frackowiak, R. S. J., & Dolan, R. J. (1998). Neural correlates of memory retrieval during recognition memory and cued recall. *NeuroImage, 8,* 262–273.

Rugg, M. D., Fletcher, P. C., Frith, C. D., Frackowiak, R. S. J., & Dolan, R. J. (1996). Differential activation of the prefrontal cortex in successful and unsuccessful memory retrieval. *Brain, 119,* 2073–2083.

Sanders, A. L., Wheeler, M. E., & Buckner, R. L. (2000). Episodic recognition modulates frontal and parietal cortex activity. *Journal of Cognitive Neuroscience, 12* (Suppl. 28).

Schacter, D. L. (1982). *Stranger behind the engram.* Hillsdale, NJ: Erlbaum.

Schacter, D. L. (1987). Implicit memory: History and current status. *Journal of Experimental Psychology: Learning, Memory, and Cognition, 13,* 501–518.

Schacter, D. L., Alpert, N. M., Savage, C. R., Rauch, S. L., & Albert, M. S. (1996). Conscious recollection and the human hippocampal formation: Evidence from positron emission tomography. *Proceedings of the National Academy of Sciences USA, 93,* 321–325.

Schacter, D. L., & Wagner, A. D. (1999). Medial temporal lobe activations in fMRI and PET studies of episodic encoding and retrieval. *Hippocampus*, *9*, 7–24.

Semon, R. (1921). *The mneme* (L. Simon, Trans.). New York: Macmillan.

Stark, C. E. L., & Squire, L. R. (2000). Functional magnetic resonance imaging (fMRI) activity in the hippocampal region during recognition memory. *Journal of Neuroscience*, *20*, 7776–7781.

Tulving, E. (1983). *Elements of episodic memory*. Oxford: Clarendon Press.

Tulving, E. (1985). Memory and consciousness. *Canadian Journal of Psychology*, *26*, 1–12.

Tulving, E., Kapur, S., Craik, F. I. M., Moscovitch, M., & Houle, S. (1994). Hemispheric encoding/retrieval asymmetry in episodic memory: Positron emission tomography findings. *Proceedings of the National Academy of Sciences USA*, *91*, 2016–2020.

Tulving, E., & Osler, S. (1968). Effectiveness of retrieval cues in memory for words. *Journal of Experimental Psychology*, *77*, 593–601.

Wheeler, M. E., Petersen, S. E., & Buckner, R. L. (2000). Memory's echo: Vivid remembering reactivates sensory-specific cortex. *Proceedings of the National Academy of Sciences USA*, *97*, 11125–11129.

Zatorre, R. J., Halpern, A. R., Perry, D. W., Meyer, E., & Evans, A. C. (1996). Hearing in the mind's ear: A PET investigation of musical imagery and perception. *Journal of Cognitive Neuroscience*, *8*, 29–46.

14

Cognitive Control and Episodic Memory

Contributions from Prefrontal Cortex

ANTHONY D. WAGNER

Cognitive and mnemonic control processes permit an individual to access and work with internal representations in a goal-directed manner. In so doing, these mechanisms are thought to guide stimulus processing and the online maintenance of internal representations through the sustained allocation of attention to specific stimulus features and long-term representations. Prefrontal cortex (PFC) is thought to be a component of the neural circuitry underlying cognitive control, including the control of memory (Fuster, 1997; Goldman-Rakic, 1987; Schacter, 1987; Shimamura, 1995; Stuss & Benson, 1984). Models of PFC function suggest that PFC represents the current task goal or context and supports top-down bias mechanisms that facilitate the processing and maintenance of goal-relevant representations in posterior cortices (Desimone & Duncan, 1995; Miller & Cohen, 2001; Shallice, 1988).

Importantly, the role of PFC control mechanisms does not appear restricted to stimulus processing and working memory functions. Rather, building on the human and nonhuman lesion and electrophysiological literatures, functional neuroimaging data suggest that PFC mechanisms—especially those supported by ventrolateral PFC regions (principally the inferior PFC)—play a fundamental role in episodic encoding, the process of transforming an experience into a durable memory trace such that it can be subsequently consciously remembered (Tulving, 1983). This chapter considers some of the most recent advances in our understanding of ventrolateral PFC contributions to cognitive and mnemonic control derived from functional imaging. The chapter first focuses on the nature of ventrolateral control mechanisms, including the role of anatomically separable ventrolateral PFC subregions in (1) controlled retrieval from semantic memory, (2) assembly and maintenance of phonological codes, and (3) attention to visuo-object and visuospatial representations (Figure 14.1). Subsequently, the contributions of these ventrolateral PFC mechanisms to episodic encoding are discussed, with attention also afforded recent data suggesting that explicit and implicit forms of memory interact during episodic encoding.

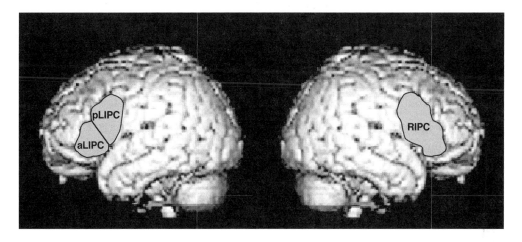

FIGURE 14.1. Lateral views of the left and right cerebral hemispheres. Three ventrolateral PFC regions are highlighted. The posterior LIPC region (pLIPC; ~BA 44/6) encompasses the posterior and dorsal extent of the left inferior frontal gyrus and portions of premotor cortex. The anterior LIPC region (aLIPC; ~BA 47/45) encompasses the anterior and ventral extent of the left inferior frontal gyrus. The RIPC region (~BA 44/6 and 47/45) encompasses both the posterior and anterior extents of the right inferior frontal gyrus and portions of premotor cortex. Subsequent research is likely to reveal further functional distinctions within these ventrolateral PFC regions.

THE CONTROL OF SEMANTIC MEMORY

One form of mnemonic control that is central to many types of cognition is the control of long-term semantic knowledge—that is, general knowledge about the world (Tulving, 1972, 1983), including facts, concepts, and vocabulary (Squire, 1987). Over the past decade, neuroimaging evidence has revealed that the left inferior prefrontal cortex (LIPC) is central to the control of semantic memory, including the recovery and evaluation of meaning (Fiez, 1997; Kapur et al., 1994; Martin, Haxby, Lalonde, Wiggs, & Ungerleider, 1995; Petersen, Fox, Posner, Mintun, & Raichle, 1988; Vandenberghe, Price, Wise, Josephs, & Frackowiak, 1996; Wagner, Desmond, Demb, Glover, & Gabrieli, 1997). For example, performance of semantic decision tasks (such as deciding whether a word represents an abstract or a concrete entity) and semantic generation tasks (such as generating a verb associated with a noun) consistently elicits robust activation in the anterior LIPC (~Brodmann's areas [BA] 47/45) and the posterior LIPC (~BA 44/6) (Buckner, 1996; Gabrieli et al., 1996; Poldrack et al., 1999; Wagner, 1999).

The nature of LIPC contributions to semantic control, though much investigated, remains controversial. Some theorists hypothesize that LIPC subserves semantic retrieval or semantic working memory processes (Demb et al., 1995; Fiez, 1997; Kapur et al., 1994; Petersen et al., 1988), and others hypothesize that LIPC mediates selection processes (Thompson-Schill, D'Esposito, Aguirre, & Farah, 1997; Thompson-Schill, D'Esposito, & Kan, 1999; Thompson-Schill et al., 1998). From the semantic retrieval perspective, LIPC is thought to guide recovery of goal-relevant semantic knowledge and to permit "working with" or evaluating the recovered knowledge (Buckner, 1996; Gabrieli, Poldrack, & Desmond, 1998; Kapur et al., 1994; Wagner, 1999). Alternatively, the selection hypothesis posits that LIPC does not mediate semantic retrieval per se. Rather, LIPC is thought to specifically guide the selection of task-relevant representations from among competing representations (Thompson-Schill et al., 1997, 1998, 1999). From this perspective, LIPC processes are engaged and are necessary only when a subset of knowledge must be recovered from amidst other, task-irrelevant knowledge.

Selection or Controlled Retrieval?

The selection and semantic retrieval hypotheses diverge on the role of LIPC in situations where selection demands are minimal during semantic retrieval. The selection hypothesis, but not the semantic retrieval hypothesis, posits that LIPC processes are unnecessary in the absence of competition and selection demands. Consistent with the selection perspective, fMRI data have revealed greater LIPC activation during high- compared to low-selection conditions (Thompson-Schill et al., 1997), and neuropsychological data have indicated that lesions of LIPC (~BA 44) result in impairment on high-selection—but not on low-selection—tasks (Thompson-Schill et al., 1998). Moreover, in contrast to the predictions of the semantic retrieval hypothesis, initial fMRI data have failed to reveal increased LIPC activation when semantic retrieval demands were putatively varied, but selection demands were held constant and kept to a minimum (Thompson-Schill et al., 1997). Although a null result, this latter finding was used to directly challenge the semantic retrieval hypothesis, which posits that LIPC control mechanisms mediate the recovery of semantic knowledge even in the absence of selection demands.

Recently it has been suggested that these results, which were argued to support selection, could also be accounted for by the hypothesis that LIPC specifically contributes to *controlled* semantic retrieval (Wagner, Paré-Blagoev, Clark, & Poldrack, 2001). That is, LIPC may guide the recovery of semantic knowledge in situations where preexperimental associations or prepotent responses do not support a more automatic recovery of semantic information. Considerable evidence suggests that PFC regions are particularly important for cognition and behavior under conditions where strong stimulus–stimulus or stimulus–response associations are absent (Cohen, Braver, & O'Reilly, 1996; Miller & Cohen, 2001; Norman & Shallice, 1986). Thus, from this perspective, LIPC may subserve controlled semantic retrieval when cue–target associations are weak, regardless of whether selection against competing knowledge is required. Importantly, the initial observation that LIPC activation did not vary as semantic retrieval demands putatively increased, but selection demands were held constant, does not address this hypothesis because the cue–target associative strength was quite strong in that study. This observation raises the possibility that performance was supported by more automatic retrieval processes not mediated by LIPC.

LIPC Contributions to Semantic Control

In a recent event-related fMRI study, the controlled semantic retrieval hypothesis was systematically assessed under conditions that held selection demands constant and to a minimum (Wagner, Paré-Blagoev, et al., 2001). In this study, subjects indicated which word from a set of possible targets (e.g., "flame," "bald," "design," "exist") was most globally related to a cue word (e.g., "candle"). Critically, controlled retrieval demands were manipulated by varying the preexperimental associative strength between the cue and target response in this global semantic comparison task, which selection proponents have suggested requires little to no selection (Thompson-Schill et al., 1997). The cue–target associative strength was either weak (e.g., "candle–halo") or strong (e.g., "candle–flame"), and semantic retrieval demands were further manipulated by varying the number of targets (either two or four) to be considered as possible responses (Thompson-Schill et al., 1997). The controlled retrieval account predicts that varying the cue–target associative strength and the number of targets should modulate LIPC activation, whereas the selection hypothesis predicts that these factors should not affect recruitment of LIPC control processes (Thompson-Schill et al., 1997).

The results from the study were clear: LIPC activation was modulated by both associative strength and number of targets. In contrast to the earlier-reported null result supporting the selection account (Thompson-Schill et al., 1997), in this experiment LIPC activation increased with the number of possible response targets, suggesting that LIPC recruitment increases as semantic and/or phonological processing demands rise, regardless of selection demands. This increase was observed in both the posterior and anterior LIPC. Moreover, LIPC activation also increased as cue–target associative strength decreased, providing striking evidence that LIPC subserves the controlled recovery of meaning even in the absence of competition. However, recent data also suggest that as competition increases, so too do demands on LIPC processes, as suggested by selection theorists (Thompson-Schill et al., 1999).

One possibility is that controlled retrieval and selection are emergent outcomes of a single LIPC control process. From this perspective, LIPC may represent goal or context information (Cohen et al., 1996) and may subserve a top-down bias signal that facilitates the recovery of goal-relevant knowledge (Figure 14.2A). This bias mechanism may be recruited under retrieval conditions that do not yield the target knowledge through more automatic processes, either because the cue–target associative strength is insufficient to result in automatic access or because task-irrelevant representations compete with task-relevant knowledge (Desimone & Duncan, 1995; Miller & Cohen, 2001). In this manner, controlled semantic retrieval may constitute the most basic functional outcome of this facilitative bias mechanism. However, controlled recruitment of the bias mechanism may further contribute to the recovery of meaning when relevant knowledge must be favored or selected from amidst competitive knowledge (Jonides, Smith, Marshuetz, & Koeppe, 1998; Thompson-Schill et al., 1997, 1998, 1999).

FUNCTIONALLY DISTINCT LIPC CONTROL MECHANISMS

Anatomically, the lateral PFC consists of multiple subregions that differ in cyctoarchitecture and connectivity (Petrides & Pandya, 1994), raising the possibility that PFC subregions may differentially guide goal-directed behavior and the control of memory through implementation of distinct mechanisms. Consistent with this possibility, imaging data suggest that anatomically separable subregions within LIPC subserve different control processes (Buckner, 1996; Fiez, 1997; Poldrack et al., 1999; Wagner, 1999). For example, although the controlled semantic retrieval and the selection hypotheses of LIPC function can be integrated at the mechanistic level (as just discussed), it is important to emphasize that extant data suggest that the neurobiology associated with each putative process may differ. Specifically, a posterior LIPC region (~BA 44) has been implicated in selection, with this region appearing to fall well posterior and dorsal to the anterior LIPC region (~BA 47/45) implicated in controlled semantic retrieval (Gabrieli et al., 1998; Poldrack et al., 1999; Wagner, Koutstaal, Maril, Schacter, & Buckner, 2000). Thus initial data suggest that distinct LIPC subregions may support controlled semantic retrieval and selection (see also Martin & Chao, 2001).

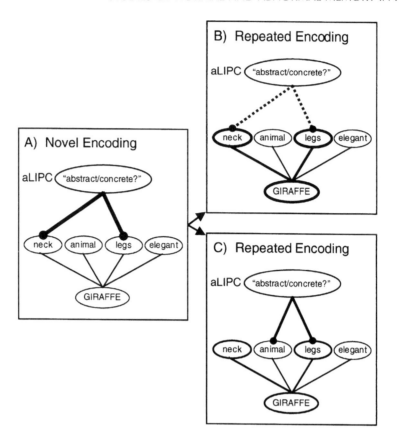

FIGURE 14.2. Illustrative example of the role of anterior LIPC (aLIPC) in semantic processing and episodic encoding, as well as an example of the effects of priming on LIPC processing demands and encoding variability. (A) During novel semantic processing of a stimulus (e.g., deciding whether the word "giraffe" refers to an abstract or a concrete entity), aLIPC represents the current task goal and biases long-term representations in semantic memory in favor of recovery of task-relevant knowledge. In so doing, aLIPC contributes to the episodic encoding of the recovered knowledge. (B) During repeated semantic processing of a stimulus, previously accessed task-relevant knowledge may be readily more accessible, giving rise to behavioral and neural priming effects (i.e., reduced demands on aLIPC control processes, as depicted by the dashed lines). When priming is robust, the previously accessed knowledge is likely to be reaccessed during the repeated processing of the stimulus, thus resulting in a stereotyped re-encoding of the item. (C) However, when priming is reduced (due to either decay or interference), the previously accessed knowledge is not as likely to be reaccessed, because it is not markedly more accessible than previously nonretrieved knowledge. Thus reprocessing of such items again places demands on aLIPC control processes and is likely to result in the encoding of features not encoded during novel stimulus processing. This encoding variability across the two processing events may ultimately benefit subsequent explicit remembering.

Segregation of Semantic and Phonological Control

More conclusive evidence for a functional segregation within LIPC has come from studies of semantic and phonological control (Table 14.1, Figure 14.1). Imaging data indicate that anterior LIPC may play a central role in the retrieval and evaluation of semantic knowledge, whereas posterior LIPC may mediate the assembly and maintenance of phonological codes (Awh et al., 1996; Fiez et al., 1996; Poldrack et al., 1999). For example, studies

TABLE 14.1. PFC Regions Mediating the Control of Memory and Hypothesized Functions

PFC subregion	~BA	Control functions	Role in episodic memory
Posterior left inferior (pLIPC)	44/6	Controlled phonological access, maintenance, and evaluation	Phonological encoding and retrieval
Anterior left inferior (aLIPC)	47/45	Controlled semantic access, maintenance, and evaluation	Semantic encoding and retrieval
Right inferior (RIPC)	44/6 and 47/45	Controlled visuospatial access, maintenance, and evaluation	Visuo-object and visuospatial encoding and retrieval
Left dorsolateral and Frontopolar	46/9 10	Material-independent monitoring and manipulation of representations in working memory	Retrieval and evaluation of episodic detail
Right dorsolateral and Frontopolar	46/9 10	Material-independent monitoring and manipulation of representations in working memory	Retrieval and evaluation of item strength

Note. ~BA, approximate Brodmann's area.

of phonological working memory have implicated posterior LIPC in phonological rehearsal (Paulesu, Frith, & Frackowiak, 1993; Smith, Jonides, Marshuetz, & Koeppe, 1998; Wagner, Maril, Bjork, & Schacter, 2001). Moreover, increased posterior LIPC activation has been observed during the processing of less familiar relative to familiar phonological forms, consistent with the hypothesis that posterior LIPC contributes to the construction of novel phonological representations (Poldrack et al., 1999; Wagner & Clark, 2001).

Importantly, functional dissociations between anterior LIPC and posterior LIPC have been observed in studies directly contrasting tasks that differentially depend on semantic and phonological control (Fiez, 1997; Poldrack et al., 1999; Price, Moore, Humphreys, & Wise, 1997). For example, Poldrack and colleagues (1999) directly compared semantic analysis of words (making an abstract–concrete decision) to phonological analysis of words (making a decision about the number of syllables). Results revealed that posterior LIPC activation occurred during performance of both tasks, but anterior LIPC activation occurred selectively during performance of the semantic control task. In a similar vein, activation of posterior LIPC—but not anterior LIPC—has been observed during performance of "nonsemantic" processing tasks that require or permit access to phonological codes (Poldrack et al., 1999; Wagner, Koutstaal, et al., 2000). Double dissociations that converge on a semantic–phonological distinction have also been observed between these two LIPC subregions (Otten & Rugg, in press; Price et al., 1997).

Evidence from Repetition Priming

Further evidence for distinct LIPC control processes has been derived from studies of repetition priming, with a recent fMRI study revealing that the pattern of repetition priming differs across anterior and posterior LIPC (Wagner, Koutstaal, et al., 2000). However, before discussing these dissociable priming patterns, we should consider more general characteristics of the neural correlates of repetition priming—that is, the influence of past experience on later neural responses in the absence of explicit or direct retrieval cues (Wiggs & Martin, 1998). Imaging studies of semantic repetition priming have consistently observed reduced anterior and posterior LIPC activation during repeated (primed) relative to initial (unprimed) semantic processing of stimuli (Gabrieli et al., 1996; Raichle et al., 1994; Schacter & Buckner, 1998; Wagner et al., 1997; Wagner & Koutstaal, in press). LIPC activation reductions have also been observed in patients with global amnesia, suggesting that such reductions reflect computational benefits deriving from implicit memory processes (Buckner & Koutstaal, 1998; Gabrieli et al., 1998). LIPC priming effects reflect long-term memory processes, because they occur even following delays of one to three days between the initial and the repeated episodes (van Turennout, Ellmore, & Martin, 2000; Wagner, Maril, & Schacter, 2000) (Figure 14.3A).

LIPC priming effects may mark decreased demands on LIPC control processes due to the "tuning" of posterior representational space by the initial experience (Fletcher, Shallice, & Dolan, 2000). More specifically, as mentioned above, during initial semantic processing of a stimulus, LIPC may represent the current task context or goal and may bias processing in posterior cortices toward task-relevant long-term knowledge (Figure 14.2A). In the course of facilitating controlled retrieval of relevant knowledge, this bias or attentional mechanism may render the recovered knowledge readily more available, such that computational demands on LIPC control processes are reduced during subsequent attempts to recover this knowledge (Figure 14.2B). These changes appear to occur independently of the medial temporal lobe memory system, and thus reflect a computational savings due to

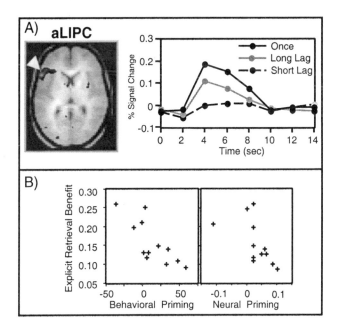

FIGURE 14.3. The effects of lag on anterior LIPC (aLIPC) priming and the relation between priming and subsequent explicit memory are depicted. (A) Relative to the processing of novel or once-presented items, repeated semantic processing of words is associated with reduced aLIPC activation. The magnitude of this neural priming effect is greater when there is a shorter lag between the two encounters with an item. (B) When the lag was held constant, negative correlations were observed between behavioral priming during the re-encoding or reprocessing of a word and the benefit in subsequent explicit memory derived from that second study episode. Similar negative correlations were observed between neural priming in aLIPC and subsequent memory. These data suggest that priming may hinder effective episodic encoding. From Wagner, Maril, and Schacter (2000). Copyright 2000 by the Massachusetts Institute of Technology. Reprinted by permission.

implicit memory. At present, it is unclear whether these savings constitute reduced selection demands because task-relevant knowledge is relatively more accessible than competing irrelevant knowledge (Thompson-Schill et al., 1999), or whether these savings also reflect the beginnings of a transition from controlled to automatic retrieval processes (Raichle et al., 1994).

Importantly, whereas priming in anterior LIPC may reflect a savings in recovering semantic knowledge, priming in posterior LIPC perhaps reflects a savings in accessing or assembling phonological codes. Initial tentative evidence for this possibility comes from the recent observation that the patterns of priming differ across anterior LIPC and posterior LIPC (Wagner, Koutstaal, et al., 2000). In this study, some words were initially processed in a semantic manner (e.g., making an abstract–concrete decision), whereas others were processed in a nonsemantic manner that permitted phonological access (e.g., making an uppercase–lowercase decision). Subsequently, all words were processed semantically, thus yielding within-task and across-task repetition conditions. Neural priming (i.e., activation reductions) was observed in anterior LIPC only in the within-task condition, thereby suggesting that such reductions specifically depend on having accessed task-relevant semantic knowledge during the initial experience. By contrast, priming in posterior LIPC was observed following both within-task and across-task repetition; priming tended to be greater in the within-task condition. This across-task priming effect is generally consistent with the hypothesis that posterior LIPC mediates phonological control, because access to phonological, but not semantic, knowledge was likely to have accompanied the initial nonsemantic processing.

Necessity of LIPC for Semantic and Phonological Control?

Although imaging studies have revealed correlations between LIPC activation and cognitive control, the necessity of these regions for phonological and semantic processing remains unclear. Posterior left PFC lesions impair lexical decision performance (Swick, 1998), whereas intraoperative stimulation directly to anterior left PFC appears to disrupt semantic processing but not word reading (Klein et al., 1997). Left PFC lesions can also yield phonological dyslexia (Fiez & Petersen, 1998)—an impairment in the ability to assemble phonological representations based upon orthographic information—and left ventrolateral PFC lesions can result in modest semantic processing deficits (Swick & Knight, 1996). Interpretation of these deficits is complicated, however, because the lesions often were not restricted to the posterior LIPC or anterior LIPC region observed with neuroimaging. Further complicating matters are paradoxical results (with respect to the imaging findings) suggesting that lesions of posterior LIPC (~BA 44) can result in selective semantic processing impairments (Thompson-Schill et al., 1998), whereas lesions of anterior LIPC may spare semantic processing (Price, Mummery, Moore, Frakowiak, & Friston, 1999; Thompson-Schill et al., 1998). Note that these latter results are ambiguous; the lesion site in one patient appeared to fall rostral to the anterior LIPC region typically associated with semantic processing (Thompson-Schill et al., 1998), and the behavioral results from the other patient suggested an impairment (Price et al., 1999). Nevertheless, these observations highlight the need for data from multiple subjects, perhaps with controlled "lesions" created through the focal application of transcranial magnetic stimulation.

THE CONTROL OF VISUO-OBJECT AND VISUOSPATIAL REPRESENTATIONS

The functional contributions of ventrolateral PFC to cognitive and mnemonic control differ not only within the left frontal lobe, but also between the frontal hemispheres (Milner, Corsi, & Leonard, 1991). For example, imaging investigations of working memory maintenance processes suggest that ventrolateral PFC activation tends to lateralize according to the nature of the material held in working memory. Whereas posterior LIPC is differentially active during phonological maintenance, right inferior prefrontal cortex (RIPC) is differentially active during attention to and maintenance of visuospatial and/or visuo-object representations (Awh & Jonides, 1998; D'Esposito et al., 1998; but see D'Esposito & Postle, Chapter 17, this volume; Nystrom et al., 2000). Similarly, goal-directed processing of words and of visual scenes yields dissociable patterns of activation across the left and right ventrolateral PFC (compare panel A of Figure 14.4 to panels D and F). RIPC has been posited to subserve visuo-object and/or visuospatial working memory processes (Table 14.1, Figure 14.1), which mediate access, maintenance, and/or evaluation of visual, icon-like representations of stimuli and of the position of stimuli in visual space (Haxby, Ungerleider, Horwitz, Rapoport, & Grady, 1995).

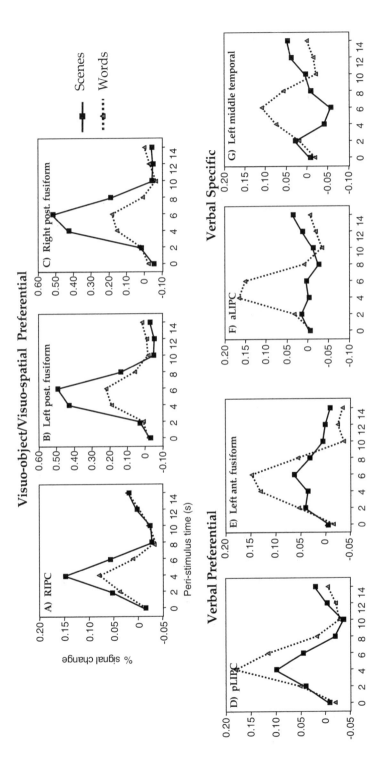

FIGURE 14.4. Three patterns of PFC–lateral temporal activation were observed during the processing and incidental encoding of words and visual scenes. (A–C) RIPC and bilateral posterior fusiform regions were differentially engaged during scene processing, consistent with their putative role in the control and representation of visuo-object/visuospatial knowledge. (D–E) In contrast, posterior LIPC (pLIPC) and left anterior fusiform regions were differentially engaged during word processing, but were also engaged during scene processing. These regions may subserve the control and representation of phonological or lexical knowledge. (F–G) Finally, anterior LIPC (aLIPC) and left middle temporal cortex were selectively engaged during word processing. These regions may guide the control and representation of long-term semantic knowledge. From Kirchhoff, Wagner, Maril, and Stern (2000). Copyright 2000 by the Society for Neuroscience. Reprinted by permission.

RIPC control mechanisms, like LIPC mechanisms, may constitute top-down facilitative signals that bias processing in posterior modules in favor of task-relevant stimulus codes. Consistent with this possibility, parallel patterns of content-sensitive activation were recently observed in PFC and lateral temporal structures (Kirchhoff, Wagner, Maril, & Stern, 2000). As in RIPC, bilateral posterior fusiform regions demonstrated greater activation during visual scene processing, suggesting that these frontal–temporal circuits subserve attention to and processing of visuo-object attributes (Figure 14.4). In contrast, as in LIPC, left anterior fusiform and middle temporal structures revealed greater activation during word processing, suggesting that these frontal–temporal circuits subserve attention to, and processing of, semantic and phonological or lexical attributes (Figure 14.4). Additional evidence from high-resolution temporal imaging methods may serve to further clarify the reliability and functional significance of these putative interactions between PFC control processes and more posterior cortical computations.

PFC CONTROL MECHANISMS AND EPISODIC MEMORY

Having considered ventrolateral PFC control processes, a central question is whether these mechanisms contribute to long-term memory. Among the striking features of the neuroimaging literatures on executive control and on episodic memory are the observed parallels in the patterns of ventrolateral PFC activation (Braver et al., 2001; Wagner, 1999). For example, like the content-sensitive effects observed in PFC during performance of working memory tasks, LIPC processes appear to be differentially recruited during episodic encoding and retrieval of verbal stimuli (e.g., words), whereas RIPC processes are differentially recruited during episodic memory for nonverbal stimuli (e.g., visual textures, novel faces, complex visual scenes) (Kelley et al., 1998; Kirchhoff et al., 2000; Klingberg & Roland, 1998; Wagner, Poldrack, et al., 1998). These parallels between PFC contributions to working memory and episodic memory suggest that the control processes that guide access to and maintenance of item representations may also play a fundamental role in episodic memory.

Subsequent Memory Effects

Recent fMRI studies of episodic encoding have focused on the relation between left and right PFC activation during an experience and subsequent explicit memory for that experience (Brewer, Zhao, Desmond, Glover, & Gabrieli, 1998; Henson, Rugg, Shallice, Josephs, & Dolan, 1999; Kirchhoff et al., 2000; Wagner, Schacter, et al., 1998). Taking advantage of developments in fMRI analysis procedures that permit measures of neural activation sorted at the event level (Dale & Buckner, 1997), and building on earlier electrophysiological studies (Paller, Kutas, & Mayes, 1987; Sandquist, Rohrbaugh, Syndulko, & Lindsley, 1980), these experiments sought to determine how neural activation during an experience that is later remembered differs from that during an experience that is later forgotten. This approach is powerful because it extends prior blocked-design studies of episodic encoding (Buckner, Kelley, & Petersen, 1999; Nyberg, Cabeza, & Tulving, 1996; Schacter & Wagner, 1999; Wagner, Koutstaal, & Schacter, 1999) by yielding a tighter correlation between fMRI measures of neural activation during episodic encoding and behavioral measures of effective episodic memory formation (i.e., whether the event is later remembered or forgotten).

In these studies of subsequent memory, fMRI scans were collected while subjects incidentally encoded words or visual scenes. Following encoding, memory for the stimuli was assessed via an explicit recognition test that required the participants to indicate whether they recognized each test stimulus as having been studied during scanning. Based on each participant's responses on this memory test, the fMRI data collected during encoding were sorted into events that were subsequently remembered or forgotten. Of central interest is whether encoding activation was predictive of later memory. Results revealed that, in addition to medial temporal lobe activation, the magnitude of LIPC activation consistently predicted subsequent memory for words, whereas RIPC activation predicted later memory for visual scenes (Brewer et al., 1998; Henson et al., 1999; Kirchhoff et al., 2000; Wagner, Schacter, et al., 1998). These correlations between activation in content-sensitive ventrolateral PFC regions and later episodic remembrance provides strong evidence implicating PFC control mechanisms in episodic learning (see also Otten, Henson, & Rugg, 2001; Paller & Wagner, 2001).

We have hypothesized that ventrolateral PFC control processes may act interdependently with medial temporal lobe mechanisms to promote the encoding of event attributes important for conscious remembrance (Kirchhoff et al., 2000; Wagner, Schacter, et al., 1998). For example, verbal experiences may be more memorable when semantic and phonological attributes of the experience are extensively processed via participation of LIPC regions. LIPC control processes, in the course of guiding goal-directed behavior, may serve to access and organize relevant stimulus attributes in working memory through the biasing of posterior cortical representations (Figure 14.2A), with the accessed information then serving as input to the medial temporal lobe memory system (Moscovitch, 1992). A specific experience may elicit the recruitment of these processes to a greater or lesser extent because of variable task demands, shifts in subjects' strategies, characteristics of target items, or attentional modulations. Regardless of the source of this variability, greater recruitment of PFC control processes will tend to produce more memorable experiences.

Interactions between Explicit and Implicit Memory

Consideration of the results from imaging studies of the subsequent-memory effect and of semantic repetition priming suggests that variability in the magnitude of priming may be one factor affecting the extent of recruitment of the PFC control processes that are important for effective episodic encoding (Wagner, Maril, & Schacter, 2000). Evidence that the magnitude of LIPC activation during encoding is predictive of later explicit memory, and that priming results in reduced LIPC activation during re-encoding of a stimulus, raises the possibility that priming for past experiences may hinder new episodic encoding.

To explore whether cross-talk exists between implicit and explicit forms of memory, we manipulated the magnitude of priming that accompanied the repeated encounter with a word by varying the temporal lag between the initial and repeated encoding or processing episodes with the word (2 minutes in a short-lag condition and 25 hours in a long-lag condition) (Wagner, Maril, & Schacter, 2000). Following these encoding episodes, subsequent recognition memory was assessed 2 days later, and the relation between priming during the second study episode and performance on the subsequent recognition test was considered. The results revealed that the behavioral and neural measures of priming were greater during the repeated encoding of an item in the short-lag relative to the long-lag condition (Figure 14.3A). Importantly, there was less of a benefit of the second study episode for later recognition in the short-lag condition, consistent with the well-known spacing effect (Ebbinghaus, 1885/1964). Thus greater priming was associated with worse explicit remembering. Moreover, similar negative correlations between behavioral priming and subsequent recognition memory, and between neural priming in LIPC and subsequent memory, were observed even when lag was held constant (Figure 14.3B). These negative correlations provide some of the first evidence pointing to a cost of priming: less effective episodic encoding.

Although the mechanism through which priming and explicit memory interact has yet to be specified, one possibility is that priming impairs new episodic encoding, and subsequent explicit memory, by reducing encoding variability. Behavioral studies suggest that encoding variability enhances subsequent explicit memory because it results in the encoding of multiple event features or attributes, thus providing multiple retrieval routes to a particular episodic memory (Martin, 1968). Priming may reduce encoding variability by increasing the probability that the same task-relevant stimulus features will be processed during a subsequent encoding event as were processed during an initial encoding event (Figure 14.2). In this manner, priming serves to bias re-encoding and to reduce encoding variability because the same task-relevant features would serve as input to the medial temporal memory system. From this perspective, priming tends to yield a stereotyped or sparse re-encoding experience (Wiggs & Martin, 1998). However, as priming declines, the probability of attending to other task-relevant or task-irrelevant features during re-encoding would increase (Figure 14.2C), thus increasing encoding variability and, ultimately, the efficacy of the encoding experience.

Multiple Forms of Cognitive and Mnemonic Control: Ventrolateral and Dorsolateral PFC

Although the focus of this chapter has been on cognitive and mnemonic control processes subserved by ventrolateral PFC, it is important to note before concluding that a number of theorists have suggested that functional distinctions between PFC subregions are not restricted to within ventrolateral PFC. Rather, fundamental functional differences may exist between ventrolateral and dorsolateral PFC, with one recent hypothesis focusing on the nature of the cognitive and mnemonic control processes supported by these PFC regions (Table 14.1). For example, based on lesion studies in nonhuman primates (Petrides, 1991), initial neuroimaging studies in humans (Petrides, Alivisatos, Evans, & Meyer, 1993; Petrides, Alivisatos, Meyer, & Evans, 1993), and structural/connectivity evidence (Petrides & Pandya, 1994), a two-stage model of PFC contributions to cognitive control has been proposed (Owen, Evans, & Petrides, 1996; Petrides, 1994a, 1994b, 1996). Within this framework, and broadly consistent with the hypotheses forwarded in this chapter, ventrolateral PFC is thought to subserve controlled retrieval of representations from posterior cortices, with some theorists also positing that ventrolateral PFC guides active online maintenance of the accessed representations (e.g., Christoff & Gabrieli, 2000; D'Esposito et al., 1998; D'Esposito & Postle, Chapter 17, this volume; Wagner, Maril, et al., 2001). In contrast, dorsolateral PFC is hypothesized to mediate the "monitoring" and "manipulation" of representations maintained by ventrolateral PFC. These monitoring operations may subserve the online coding and updating of the relative goal-specific status of items in working memory (Petrides, 2000) or the goal-directed selection between maintained representations

(Rowe, Toni, Josephs, Frackowiak, & Passingham, 2000). In this manner, ventrolateral and dorsolateral PFC processes are hypothesized to be hierarchically related, with dorsolateral processes operating on the products of ventrolateral PFC mechanisms.

It is also worth noting that whereas ventrolateral PFC has been consistently implicated in episodic encoding and retrieval, imaging studies of episodic memory have primarily observed dorsolateral PFC activation during the retrieval stage (Buckner et al., 1999; Rugg & Wilding, 2000; Schacter, Buckner, Koutstaal, Dale, & Rosen, 1997; Tulving, Kapur, Craik, Moscovitch, & Houle, 1994; Wagner, Desmond, Glover, & Gabrieli, 1998). Left dorsolateral and frontopolar regions appear to be engaged when retrieval requires recovery of specific episodic details, whereas right dorsolateral and frontopolar regions appear to be engaged when retrieval entails careful scrutiny of item strength or familiarity (Dobbins, Rice, Schacter, & Wagner, 2001; Henson et al., 1999; Nolde, Johnson, & D'Esposito, 1998; Ranganath, Johnson, & D'Esposito, 2000; Rugg, Fletcher, Chua, & Dolan, 1999). Undoubtedly, further functional segregation exists within these dorsolateral and anterior frontal regions (Christoff & Gabrieli, 2000; Henson, Rugg, Shallice, & Dolan, 2000).

The relative selectivity of episodic activation in dorsolateral and anterior PFC regions to retrieval should not be interpreted as indicating that these regions specifically mediate episodic retrieval processes. Rather, the "manipulation" and "monitoring" processes putatively subserved by these regions appear to be required in many retrieval contexts, perhaps in the service of postretrieval evaluation or monitoring of the products of retrieval (Rugg, Fletcher, Frith, Frackowiak, & Dolan, 1996). However, when encoding entails the monitoring or manipulation of the contents of working memory, dorsolateral processes also appear to be recruited and may contribute to learning (Davachi, Maril, & Wagner, in press).

CONCLUSIONS

As illustrated in this chapter, our approach to understanding the cognitive and functional neurobiology of memory focuses on exploring the relation between PFC control processes and long-term memory. These efforts to understand the "control of memory" place an emphasis on characterizing the basic units of control at the process and neuroanatomical levels. As discussed, it is likely that multiple forms and stages of memory depend on the recruitment of general control mechanisms—that is, mechanisms that are not specific to memory per se—with many of these control processes being subserved by distinct prefrontal subregions. It is anticipated that additional insights will derive from integration of this approach, which has principally relied on fMRI methods, with evidence regarding the relative timing of process engagement and with evidence regarding the necessity of the identified processes. Such efforts will undoubtedly facilitate continued development in our understanding of how PFC control processes give rise to learning and remembering.

ACKNOWLEDGMENTS

This work was supported in part by the National Institute on Deafness and Other Communication Disorders (DC04466), the National Institute of Mental Health (MH60941), the Ellison Medical Foundation, and P. Newton. I would like to thank members of the Learning and Memory Lab at MIT, the Schacter Lab at Harvard, and D. Schacter, J. Gabrieli, R. Poldrack, R. Buckner, W. Koutstaal, and L. Davachi for insightful comments and discussion.

REFERENCES

Awh, E., & Jonides, J. (1998). Spatial working memory and spatial selective attention. In R. Parasuraman (Ed.), *The attentive brain* (pp. 353–380). Cambridge, MA: MIT Press.

Awh, E., Jonides, J., Smith, E. E., Schumacher, E. H., Koeppe, R. A., & Katz, S. (1996). Dissociation of storage and rehearsal in verbal working memory: Evidence from PET. *Psychological Science, 7,* 25–31.

Braver, T. S., Barch, D. M., Kelley, W. M., Buckner, R. L., Cohen, N. J., Miezin, F. M., Snyder, A. Z., Ollinger, J. M., Akbudak, E., Conturs, T. E., & Petersen, S. E. (2001). Direct comparison of prefrontal cortex regions engaged by working memory and long-term memory tasks. *NeuroImage, 14,* 48–59.

Brewer, J. B., Zhao, Z., Desmond, J. E., Glover, G. H., & Gabrieli, J. D. (1998). Making memories: Brain activity that predicts how well visual experience will be remembered. *Science, 281,* 1185–1187.

Buckner, R. L. (1996). Beyond HERA: Contributions of specific prefrontal brain areas to long-term memory retrieval. *Psychonomic Bulletin and Review, 3,* 149–158.

Buckner, R. L., Kelley, W. M., & Petersen, S. E. (1999). Frontal cortex contributes to human memory formation. *Nature Neuroscience, 2,* 311–314.

Buckner, R. L., & Koutstaal, W. (1998). Functional neuroimaging studies of encoding, priming, and explicit memory retrieval. *Proceedings of the National Academy of Sciences USA, 95,* 891–898.

Christoff, K., & Gabrieli, J. D. E. (2000). The frontopolar cortex and human cognition: Evidence for a rostrocaudal hierarchical organization within the human prefrontal cortex. *Psychobiology, 28,* 168–186.

Cohen, J. D., Braver, T. S., & O'Reilly, R. C. (1996). A computational approach to prefrontal cortex, cognitive control and schizophrenia: Recent developments and current challenges. *Philosophical Transactions of the Royal Society of London, Series B, 351,* 1515–1527.

D'Esposito, M., Aguirre, G. K., Zarahn, E., Ballard, D., Shin, R. K., & Lease, J. (1998). Functional MRI studies of spatial and nonspatial working memory. *Cognitive Brain Research, 7,* 1–13.

Dale, A. M., & Buckner, R. L. (1997). Selective averaging of rapidly presented individual trials using fMRI. *Human Brain Mapping, 5,* 329–340.

Davachi, L., Maril, A., & Wagner, A. D. (in press). When keeping in mind supports later bringing to mind: Neural markers of phonological rehearsal predict subsequent remembering. *Journal of Cognitive Neuroscience, 13.*

Demb, J. B., Desmond, J. E., Wagner, A. D., Vaidya, C. J., Glover, G. H., & Gabrieli, J. D. E. (1995). Semantic encoding and retrieval in the left inferior prefrontal cortex: A functional MRI study of task difficulty and process specificity. *Journal of Neuroscience, 15,* 5870–5878.

Desimone, R., & Duncan, J. (1995). Neural mechanisms of selective visual attention. *Annual Review of Neuroscience, 18,* 193–222.

Dobbins, I. G., Rice, H. J., Schacter, D. L., & Wagner, A. D. (2001). *Cortical asymmetry during source and recency recognition: fMRI evidence for strategic reliance on recollection and familiarity.* Manuscript submitted for publication.

Ebbinghaus, H. (1964). *Memory: A contribution to experimental psychology.* New York: Dover. (Original work published 1885)

Fiez, J. A. (1997). Phonology, semantics, and the role of the left inferior prefrontal cortex. *Human Brain Mapping, 5,* 79–83.

Fiez, J. A., & Petersen, S. E. (1998). Neuroimaging studies of word reading. *Proceedings of the National Academy of Sciences USA, 95,* 914–921.

Fiez, J. A., Raife, E. A., Balota, D. A., Schwarz, J. P., Raichle, M. E., & Petersen, S. E. (1996). A positron emission tomography study of the short-term maintenance of verbal information. *Journal of Neuroscience, 16,* 808–822.

Fletcher, P. C., Shallice, T., & Dolan, R. J. (2000). "Sculpting the response space": An account of left prefrontal activation at encoding. *NeuroImage, 12,* 404–417.

Fuster, J. M. (1997). *The prefrontal cortex: Anatomy, physiology, and neuropsychology of the frontal lobe.* Philadelphia: Lippincott–Raven.

Gabrieli, J. D., Poldrack, R. A., & Desmond, J. E. (1998). The role of left prefrontal cortex in language and memory. *Proceedings of the National Academy of Sciences USA, 95,* 906–913.

Gabrieli, J. D. E., Desmond, J. E., Demb, J. B., Wagner, A. D., Stone, M. V., Vaidya, C. J., & Glover, G. H. (1996). Functional magnetic resonance imaging of semantic memory processes in the frontal lobes. *Psychological Science, 7,* 278–283.

Goldman-Rakic, P. S. (1987). Circuitry of primate prefrontal cortex and regulation of behavior by representational memory. In F. Plum & V. Mountcastle (Eds.), *Handbook of physiology: Section 1. The nervous system. Vol. 5. Higher functions of the brain. Part 1* (pp. 373–417). Bethesda, MD: American Physiological Society.

Haxby, J. V., Ungerleider, L. G., Horwitz, B., Rapoport, S. I., & Grady, C. L. (1995). Hemispheric differences in neural systems for face working memory: A PET-rCBF study. *Human Brain Mapping, 3,* 68–82.

Henson, R. N. A., Rugg, M. D., Shallice, T., & Dolan, R. J. (2000). Confidence in recognition memory for words: Dissociating right prefrontal roles in episodic retrieval. *Journal of Cognitive Neuroscience, 12,* 913–923.

Henson, R. N. A., Rugg, M. D., Shallice, T., Josephs, O., & Dolan, R. J. (1999). Recollection and familiarity in recognition memory: An event-related functional magnetic resonance imaging study. *Journal of Neuroscience, 19,* 3962–3972.

Jonides, J., Smith, E. E., Marshuetz, C., & Koeppe, R. A. (1998). Inhibition in verbal working memory revealed by brain activation. *Proceedings of the National Academy of Sciences USA, 95,* 8410–8413.

Kapur, S., Rose, R., Liddle, P. F., Zipursky, R. B., Brown, G. M., Stuss, D., Houle, S., & Tulving, E. (1994). The role of the left prefrontal cortex in verbal processing: Semantic processing or willed action? *NeuroReport, 5,* 2193–2196.

Kelley, W. M., Miezin, F. M., McDermott, K. B., Buckner, R. L., Raichle, M. E., Cohen, N. J., Ollinger, J. M., Akbudak, E., Conturo, T. E., Snyder, A. Z., & Petersen, S. E. (1998). Hemispheric specialization in human dorsal frontal cortex and medial temporal lobe for verbal and nonverbal memory encoding. *Neuron, 20,* 927–936.

Kirchhoff, B. A., Wagner, A. D., Maril, A., & Stern, C. E. (2000). Prefrontal–temporal circuitry for novelty encoding and subsequent memory. *Journal of Neuroscience, 20,* 6173–6180.

Klein, D., Olivier, A., Milner, B., Zatorre, R. J., Johnsrude, I., Meyer, E., & Evans, A. C. (1997). Obligatory role of the LIFG in synonym generation: Evidence from PET and cortical stimulation. *NeuroReport, 8,* 3275–3279.

Klingberg, T., & Roland, P. E. (1998). Right prefrontal activation during encoding, but not during retrieval, in a non-verbal paired-associates task. *Cerebral Cortex, 8,* 73–79.

Martin, A., & Chao, L. L. (2001). Semantic memory and the brain: Structure and processes. *Current Opinion in Neurobiology, 11,* 194–201.

Martin, A., Haxby, J. V., Lalonde, F. M., Wiggs, C. L., & Ungerleider, L. G. (1995). Discrete cortical regions associated with knowledge of color and knowledge of action. *Science, 270,* 102–105.

Martin, E. (1968). Stimulus meaningfulness and paired-associate transfer: An encoding variability hypothesis. *Psychological Review, 75,* 421–441.

Miller, E. K., & Cohen, J. D. (2001). An integrative theory of prefrontal cortex function. *Annual Review of Neuroscience, 24,* 167–202.

Milner, B., Corsi, P., & Leonard, G. (1991). Frontal-lobe contribution to recency judgements. *Neuropsychologia, 29,* 601–618.

Moscovitch, M. (1992). Memory and working-with-memory: A component process model based on modules and central systems. *Journal of Cognitive Neuroscience, 4,* 257–267.

Nolde, S. F., Johnson, M. K., & D'Esposito, M. (1998). Left prefrontal activation during episodic remembering: An event-related fMRI study. *NeuroReport, 9,* 3509–3514.

Norman, D. A., & Shallice, T. (1986). Attention to action: Willed and automatic control of behavior. In R. J. Davidson, G. E. Schwartz, & D. Shapiro (Eds.), *Consciousness and self-regulation* (pp. 1–18). New York: Plenum Press.

Nyberg, L., Cabeza, R., & Tulving, E. (1996). PET studies of encoding and retrieval: The HERA model. *Psychonomic Bulletin and Review, 3,* 135–148.

Nystrom, L. E., Braver, T. S., Sabb, F. W., Delgado, M. R., Noll, D. C., & Cohen, J. D. (2000). Working memory for letters, shapes, and locations: fMRI evidence against stimulus-based regional organization in human prefrontal cortex. *NeuroImage, 11,* 424–446.

Otten, L. J., Henson, R. N., & Rugg, M. D. (2001). Depth of processing effects on neural correlates of memory encoding: Relationship between findings from across- and within-task comparisons. *Brain, 124,* 399–412.

Otten, L. J., & Rugg, M. D. (in press). Task-dependency of the neural correlates of episodic encoding as measured by fMRI. *Cerebral Cortex.*

Owen, A. M., Evans, A. C., & Petrides, M. (1996). Evidence for a two-stage model of spatial working memory processing within the lateral frontal cortex: A positron emission tomography study. *Cerebral Cortex, 6,* 31–38.

Paller, K. A., Kutas, M., & Mayes, A. R. (1987). Neural correlates of encoding in an incidental learning paradigm. *Electroencephalography and Clinical Neurophysiology, 67,* 360–371.

Paller, K. A., & Wagner, A. D. (2001). Observing the transformation of experience into memory. *Trends in Cognitive Science.* Submitted for publication.

Paulesu, E., Frith, C. D., & Frackowiak, R. S. (1993). The neural correlates of the verbal component of working memory. *Nature, 362,* 342–345.

Petersen, S. E., Fox, P. T., Posner, M. I., Mintun, M., & Raichle, M. E. (1988). Positron emission tomographic studies of the cortical anatomy of single-word processing. *Nature, 331,* 585–589.

Petrides, M. (1991). Monitoring of selections of visual stimuli and the primate frontal cortex. *Proceedings of the Royal Society of London, Series B, 246,* 293–298.

Petrides, M. (1994a). Frontal lobes and behaviour. *Current Opinion in Neurobiology, 4,* 207–211.

Petrides, M. (1994b). Frontal lobes and working memory: Evidence from investigations of the effects of cortical excisions in nonhuman primates. In F. Boller & J. Grafman (Eds.), *Handbook of neuropsychology* (Vol. 9, pp. 59–82). Amsterdam: Elsevier.

Petrides, M. (1996). Specialized systems for the processing of mnemonic information within the primate frontal cortex. *Philosophical Transactions of the Royal Society of London, Series B, 351,* 1455–1462.

Petrides, M. (2000). Dissociable roles of mid-dorsolateral prefrontal and anterior inferotemporal cortex in visual working memory. *Journal of Neuroscience, 20,* 7496–7503.

Petrides, M., Alivisatos, B., Evans, A. C., & Meyer, E. (1993). Dissociation of human mid-dorsolateral from posterior dorsolateral frontal cortex in memory processing. *Proceedings of the National Academy of Sciences USA, 90,* 873–877.

Petrides, M., Alivisatos, B., Meyer, E., & Evans, A. C. (1993). Functional activation of the human frontal cortex during the performance of verbal working memory tasks. *Proceedings of the National Academy of Sciences USA, 90,* 878–882.

Petrides, M., & Pandya, D. N. (1994). Comparative architectonic analysis of the human and the macaque frontal cortex. In F. Boller & J. Grafman (Eds.), *Handbook of neuropsychology* (Vol. 9, pp. 17–58). Amsterdam: Elsevier.

Poldrack, R. A., Wagner, A. D., Prull, M. W., Desmond, J. E., Glover, G. H., & Gabrieli, J. D. E. (1999). Functional specialization for semantic and phonological processing in the left inferior frontal cortex. *NeuroImage, 10,* 15–35.

Price, C. J., Moore, C. J., Humphreys, G. W., & Wise, R. S. J. (1997). Segregating semantic from phonological processes during reading. *Journal of Cognitive Neuroscience, 9,* 727–733.

Price, C. J., Mummery, C. J., Moore, C. J., Frakowiak, R. S., & Friston, K. J. (1999). Delineating necessary and sufficient neural systems with functional imaging studies of neuropsychological patients. *Journal of Cognitive Neuroscience, 11,* 371–382.

Raichle, M. E., Fiez, J. A., Videen, T. O., Macleod, A. M. K., Pardo, J. V., Fox, P. T., & Petersen, S. E. (1994). Practice-related changes in human brain functional anatomy during nonmotor learning. *Cerebral Cortex, 4,* 8–26.

Ranganath, C., Johnson, M. K., & D'Esposito, M. (2000). Left anterior prefrontal activation increases with demands to recall specific perceptual information. *Journal of Neuroscience, 20,* RC108.

Rowe, J. B., Toni, I., Josephs, O., Frackowiak, R. S. J., & Passingham, R. E. (2000). The prefrontal cortex: Response selection or maintenance within working memory? *Science, 288,* 1656–1660.

Rugg, M. D., Fletcher, P. C., Chua, P. M., & Dolan, R. J. (1999). The role of the prefrontal cortex in recognition memory and memory for source: An fMRI study. *NeuroImage, 10,* 520–529.

Rugg, M. D., Fletcher, P. C., Frith, C. D., Frackowiak, R., S. J., & Dolan, R. J. (1996). Differential activation of the prefrontal cortex in successful and unsuccessful memory retrieval. *Brain, 119,* 2073–2083.

Rugg, M. D., & Wilding, E. L. (2000). Retrieval processing and episodic memory. *Trends in Cognitive Sciences, 4,* 108–115.

Sandquist, T. F., Rohrbaugh, J. W., Syndulko, K., & Lindsley, D. B. (1980). Electrophysiological signs of levels of processing: Perceptual analysis and recognition memory. *Psychophysiology, 17,* 568–576.

Schacter, D. L. (1987). Memory, amnesia, and frontal lobe dysfunction. *Psychobiology, 15,* 21–36.

Schacter, D. L., & Buckner, R. L. (1998). Priming and the brain. *Neuron, 20,* 185–195.

Schacter, D. L., Buckner, R. L., Koutstaal, W., Dale, A. M., & Rosen, B. R. (1997). Late onset of anterior prefrontal activity during true and false recognition: An event-related fMRI study. *NeuroImage, 6,* 259–269.

Schacter, D. L., & Wagner, A. D. (1999). Medial temporal lobe activations in fMRI and PET studies of episodic encoding and retrieval. *Hippocampus, 9,* 7–24.

Shallice, T. (1988). *From neuropsychology to mental structure.* New York: Cambridge University Press.

Shimamura, A. P. (1995). Memory and frontal lobe function. In M. S. Gazzaniga (Ed.), *The cognitive neurosciences* (pp. 803–813). Cambridge, MA: MIT Press.

Smith, E. E., Jonides, J., Marshuetz, C., & Koeppe, R. A. (1998). Components of verbal working memory: Evidence from neuroimaging. *Proceedings of the National Academy of Sciences USA, 95,* 876–882.

Squire, L. R. (1987). *Memory and brain.* New York: Oxford University Press.

Stuss, D. T., & Benson, D. F. (1984). Neuropsychological studies of the frontal lobes. *Psychological Bulletin, 95,* 3–28.

Swick, D. (1998). Effects of prefrontal lesions on lexical processing and repetition priming: An ERP study. *Cognitive Brain Research, 7,* 143–157.

Swick, D., & Knight, R. T. (1996). Is prefrontal cortex involved in cued recall?: A neuropsychological test of PET findings. *Neuropsychologia, 34,* 1019–1028.

Thompson-Schill, S. L., D'Esposito, M., Aguirre, G. K., & Farah, M. J. (1997). Role of left inferior prefrontal cortex in retrieval of semantic knowledge: A reevaluation. *Proceedings of the National Academy of Sciences USA, 94,* 14792–14797.

Thompson-Schill, S. L., D'Esposito, M., & Kan, I. P. (1999). Effects of repetition and competition on activity in left prefrontal cortex during word generation. *Neuron, 23,* 513–522.

Thompson-Schill, S. L., Swick, D., Farah, M. J., D'Esposito, M., Kan, I. P., & Knight, R. T. (1998). Verb generation in patients with focal frontal lesions: A neuropsychological test of neuroimaging findings. *Proceedings of the National Academy of Sciences USA, 95,* 15855–15860.

Tulving, E. (1972). Episodic and semantic memory. In E. Tulving & W. Donaldson (Eds.), *Organization of memory* (pp. 382–403). New York: Academic Press.

Tulving, E. (1983). *Elements of episodic memory.* Cambridge, England: Cambridge University Press.

Tulving, E., Kapur, S., Craik, F. I. M., Moscovitch, M., & Houle, S. (1994). Hemispheric encoding–retrieval asymmetry in episodic memory: Positron emission tomography findings. *Proceedings of the National Academy of Sciences USA, 91,* 2016–2020.

van Turennout, M., Ellmore, T., & Martin, A. (2000). Long-lasting cortical plasticity in the object naming system. *Nature Neuroscience, 3,* 1329–1334.

Vandenberghe, R., Price, C., Wise, R., Josephs, O., & Frackowiak, R. S. (1996). Functional anatomy of a common semantic system for words and pictures. *Nature, 383,* 254–256.

Wagner, A. D. (1999). Working memory contributions to human learning and remembering. *Neuron, 22,* 19–22.

Wagner, A. D., & Clark, D. (2001). *Prefrontal activation during phonological encoding predicts subsequent memory.* Manuscript submitted for publication.

Wagner, A. D., Desmond, J. E., Demb, J. B., Glover, G. H., & Gabrieli, J. D. E. (1997). Semantic repetition priming for verbal and pictorial knowledge: A functional MRI study of left inferior prefrontal cortex. *Journal of Cognitive Neuroscience, 9,* 714–726.

Wagner, A. D., Desmond, J. E., Glover, G. H., & Gabrieli, J. D. (1998). Prefrontal cortex and recognition memory: Functional-MRI evidence for context-dependent retrieval processes. *Brain, 121,* 1985–2002.

Wagner, A. D., & Koutstaal, W. (in press). Priming. In V. S. Ramachandran (Ed.), *Encyclopedia of the human brain.* San Diego, CA: Academic Press.

Wagner, A. D., Koutstaal, W., Maril, A., Schacter, D. L., & Buckner, R. L. (2000). Task-specific repetition priming in left inferior prefrontal cortex. *Cerebral Cortex, 10,* 1176–1184.

Wagner, A. D., Koutstaal, W., & Schacter, D. L. (1999). When encoding yields remembering: Insights from event-related neuroimaging. *Philosophical Transactions of the Royal Society of London, Series B, 354,* 1307–1324.

Wagner, A. D., Maril, A., Bjork, R. A., & Schacter, D. L. (2001). Prefrontal contributions to executive control: fMRI evidence for functional distinctions within lateral prefrontal cortex. *NeuroImage, 14,* 1337–1347.

Wagner, A. D., Maril, A., & Schacter, D. L. (2000). Interactions between forms of memory: When priming hinders new learning. *Journal of Cognitive Neuroscience, 12*(Suppl. 2), 52–60.

Wagner, A. D., Paré-Blagoev, E. J., Clark, J., & Poldrack, R. A. (2001). Recovering meaning: Left prefrontal cortex guides controlled semantic retrieval. *Neuron, 31,* 329–338.

Wagner, A. D., Poldrack, R. A., Eldridge, L. L., Desmond, J. E., Glover, G. H., & Gabrieli, J. D. (1998). Material-specific lateralization of prefrontal activation during episodic encoding and retrieval. *NeuroReport, 9,* 3711–3717.

Wagner, A. D., Schacter, D. L., Rotte, M., Koutstaal, W., Maril, A., Dale, A. M., Rosen, B. R., & Buckner, R. L. (1998). Building memories: Remembering and forgetting of verbal experiences as predicted by brain activity. *Science, 281,* 1188–1191.

Wiggs, C. L., & Martin, A. (1998). Properties and mechanisms of perceptual priming. *Current Opinion in Neurobiology, 8,* 227–233.

15

Where Encoding and Retrieval Meet in the Brain

LARS NYBERG

As noted by Frances Yates in *The Art of Memory*, Aristotle viewed memory as "a collection of mental pictures from sense impressions but with a time element added, for the mental images of memory are not from perception of things present but of things past" (Yates, 1966/1992, p. 47). Viewing memory[1] as "perception of things past" is consistent with modern theoretical views. For example, Craik (1983) has argued that retrieval is essentially an attempt to recapitulate processes involved in perception and comprehension of events, and encoding–retrieval interrelations are salient in the principles of "encoding specificity" (Tulving & Thomson, 1973) and "transfer-appropriate processing" (Morris, Bransford, & Franks, 1977; see also Roediger, Weldon, & Challis, 1989). In addition, encoding–retrieval interrelations are highlighted by findings of "state-dependent" (e.g., Ryan & Eich, 1999) and "context-dependent" (e.g., Godden & Baddeley, 1975) memory.

Encoding–retrieval interrelations have also been stressed in theories on the neural basis of memory. In one well-known proposal, Damasio (1989) argued that "Recalled experiences constitute an attempted reconstruction of perceptual experience based on activity in a set of pertinent sensory and motor cortices" (p. 44). Similarly, activation of overlapping brain regions during encoding and retrieval is a key aspect in neural network models of memory (Alvarez & Squire, 1994; McClelland, McNaughton, & O'Reilly, 1995).

In the present chapter, I review evidence from functional brain imaging studies that overlapping brain regions are involved during encoding and retrieval. Studies with positron emission tomography (PET) and functional magnetic resonance imaging (fMRI) are considered. The findings of these studies may also turn out to shed some light on the problem of where information is stored in the brain. Before the empirical studies are presented, some methodological issues are commented on.

---

[1]"Memory" refers here to "episodic memory."

METHODOLOGICAL ISSUES

A common factor in the PET and fMRI studies that are discussed in this chapter is that brain activity was measured *both* during initial perception/encoding and during subsequent retrieval. In that way, brain activity during encoding can be compared with brain activity during retrieval (for a discussion of how PET and fMRI measure brain activity, see Buckner & Logan, 2001). The comparison of brain activity during encoding and retrieval can be done in several ways. One way is to analyze the encoding and retrieval data separately, and then to compare the patterns in order to identify overlap. If the correspondence is high (close overlap between encoding and retrieval peaks), similarities in encoding- and retrieval-related activity can easily be detected. A somewhat more formal way of assessing overlap is to conduct a "conjunction analysis" (Price & Friston, 1997). This analysis identifies overlap in activity between multiple independent contrasts (e.g., encoding–baseline 1, retrieval–baseline 2). A related approach is to compute main effects involving both encoding and retrieval. Finally, those brain regions that show differential activity during encoding can be defined as a "mask" by which subsequent analyses of retrieval activity are constrained. In that way, regions that show differential activity in a retrieval contrast will only be identified if these regions were also engaged during encoding (i.e., regions that only show differential activity in the retrieval contrast will be ignored).

It should be stressed that in analyses of encoding–retrieval overlap, brain regions that are active during encoding or retrieval *only* may not be identified. Therefore, one should not be misled to believe that the regions found to be active in analyses of overlap constitute the full set of regions activated during encoding or retrieval. Instead, other strategies for data analysis are necessary for identifying regions that are specifically associated with encoding or retrieval. This approach can involve a direct contrast between encoding and retrieval conditions, or contrasts of encoding and retrieval conditions with baseline conditions. Such contrasts will reveal brain regions that are specifically active during encoding *or* retrieval.

A complicating factor in analyses of whether retrieval of information activates brain regions that were active when that information was originally encoded is that it can be difficult to determine whether a finding of overlap reflects *memory*-related processes or *sensory*-related processes. For example, suppose that a condition involving encoding of visual words is contrasted with a condition involving encoding of auditory words, and that a condition involving visual word recognition is contrasted with a condition involving auditory word recognition. Analyses of encoding–retrieval overlap, whether done in the form of testing for a main effect, conjunction analysis, or masked analysis, would most likely reveal overlapping activation in visual brain regions. However, it would be difficult if not impossible, based on such a design, to determine whether the overlap is attributable to reactivation of encoding regions during retrieval or to the fact that visual sensory regions were differentially stimulated during both encoding and retrieval. To rule out a sensory-related interpretation, it is important that there is some kind of modality shift between encoding and retrieval. This idea is exemplified in the next section.

Even if there is a shift in modality between encoding and retrieval, such that a finding of overlap should reflect memory-related rather than sensory-related processes, an additional complication has to do with selective attention. Several studies have shown that selectively attending to a certain modality (e.g., will a sound be heard?) or a certain stimulus dimension (e.g., will a stimulus move?) is associated with increased activity in brain regions that are involved if information in that modality or of that kind is actually presented (see Cabeza & Nyberg, 2000). This means that if a subject at test is asked to decide whether an auditory item was paired with a visual item during encoding, the process of attempting to retrieve visual information may lead to increased activity in visual brain regions—even if the subject does not remember the visual item. Therefore, in order to provide strong evidence that actual retrieval of information is what underlies an observation of encoding–retrieval overlap, potential confounding effects of selective attention need to be controlled for. This is also illustrated in the next section.

Still other factors may complicate analyses of overlap. For example, encoding processes can be operating during a retrieval task (see, e.g., Buckner, Wheeler, & Sheridan, 2001; Nyberg, Cabeza, & Tulving, 1996), and thereby cause "encoding–retrieval" overlap (or, rather, "encoding–encoding" overlap). Similarly, processes related to novelty detection have been found to play a major role during memory encoding (see, e.g., Dolan & Fletcher, 1997; Tulving, Markowitsch, Craik, Habib, & Houle, 1996). Activation related to novelty detection has been observed during retrieval tasks (see, e.g., Tulving, Markowitsch, Kapur, Habib, & Houle, 1994), which points to the possibility that encoding–retrieval overlap could also be related to common novelty detection processes. The focus here, however, is on overlap that appears to be related to actual recovery of information from memory during the retrieval phase.

BRAIN IMAGING STUDIES OF ENCODING–RETRIEVAL OVERLAP

Auditory Information

In a recent PET study, we provided evidence that auditory brain regions that are engaged during perception/encoding of sounds are reactivated during retrieval of sound information (Nyberg, Habib, McIntosh, & Tulving, 2000). Two experiments investigated what was termed "intentional reactivation." Briefly, the experimental design was as follows. Subjects were given two encoding conditions. In one condition, they were presented with pairs of visual words and unrelated sounds (e.g., the word "table" paired with the sound of a plane during takeoff). They were asked to try to memorize the pairs so that later on, when they were cued with one member of the pair, they would be able to retrieve the other member. In the other encoding condition, subjects were presented with visual words only and were asked to memorize the words for a later test. The encoding conditions were followed by two retrieval conditions (in a counterbalanced order). In both conditions, visual words were presented, and subjects were asked to (1) press one mouse button for words they recognized and thought had been presented alone at study, (2) press another mouse button when they recognized a word and remembered that it had been paired with a sound at study, and (3) press no button if they did not recognize a word. Thus, in both retrieval conditions, subjects intentionally had to remember whether visual words had been paired with sounds during encoding. Therefore, the conditions should not have differed with regard to selective attention to the auditory modality. The only difference between the retrieval conditions had to do with the type of words that was presented during the scan interval: In one retrieval condition, the words had been paired with sounds at study (paired condition); in the other condition, they had been presented alone at study (unpaired condition).

To examine whether brain regions activated during perception/encoding of auditory information were reactivated during retrieval of auditory information, the encoding condition involving words and sounds was contrasted with the encoding condition involving words only. As expected, in both experiments, the former relative to the latter condition was associated with increased activity in bilateral auditory regions in the temporal lobe. This is illustrated in Figure 15.1a. The activation map from the encoding contrast was then

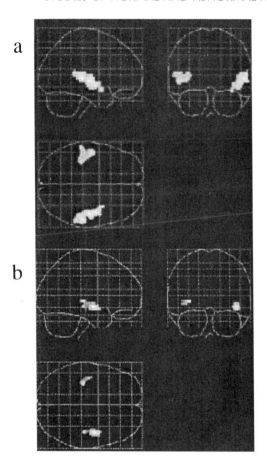

FIGURE 15.1. (a) Differential activation of the bilateral auditory cortex during encoding of visual words paired with sounds (relative to encoding of visual words only). (b) Activation of a subset of the encoding pattern during retrieval of sound information from visual word cues. In both a and b, activations are plotted on sagittal (upper left), coronal (upper right), and transverse (lower left) views of a glass brain. From Nyberg, Habib, McIntosh, and Tulving (2000, Exp. 2). Copyright 2000 by the National Academy of Sciences, USA. Reprinted by permission.

used as a mask for a subsequent contrast between the paired and unpaired retrieval conditions. As illustrated in Figure 15.1b, in both experiments, retrieval of sound information was associated with increased activity in auditory association areas in the temporal cortex. This finding provided support for the idea that some of the brain regions that are active during encoding of information are reactivated during subsequent retrieval of that information from memory. It should be noted that in addition to auditory activation, increased activity was observed in the left medial temporal lobe (MTL) during paired encoding relative to single-word encoding and during paired relative to unpaired retrieval. This observation is consistent with the suggestion that MTL regions are involved in binding together different kinds of event information (Cohen et al., 1999).

The second experiment also provided support for "incidental reactivation." The test of incidental reactivation was based on the proposal that when different components of an event have been consolidated, functional connections are established between the neuronal ensembles that represent the different components (with the support of MTL structures). As a result of these connections, reactivation of one component during retrieval will lead to reactivation of the other components, even if the situation does not demand retrieval of the other components (hence the term "incidental"). This proposal is formalized in the neural network models of memory referred to above (Alvarez & Squire, 1994; McClelland et al., 1995), and it was empirically supported by our observation of activation of auditory brain regions during simple "yes–no" recognition of visual words following word–sound pairings at encoding (for related observations in studies of conditioning, see Cahill, Ohl, & Scheich, 1996; McIntosh, Cabeza, & Lobaugh, 1998). It should be stressed that in the case of incidental reactivation, confounding effects of selective attention appear very unlikely, as there was no demand for retrieval of auditory information in the recognition task.

Visual Information

In independent but related work, Wheeler, Petersen, and Buckner (2000) also provided support for reactivation of auditory brain regions during retrieval of auditory information based on visual cues (verbal labels). This support was generated by event-related fMRI. In addition, Wheeler and colleagues showed that retrieval of pictorial information based on verbal labels led to reactivation of visual areas that were engaged during picture perception. The reactivation pattern included a medial occipital–parietal region, the precuneus. The precuneus was also found to be activated during encoding as well as during recall of visual geometrical patterns in a PET study by Roland and Gulyás (1995). Moreover, in a recent PET study (Nyberg, Persson, et al., 2000), we observed increasingly stronger activation in the left precuneus as more and more pictures were retrieved from memory (lowest in a recognition condition involving no targets, intermediate in a recognition condition involving 50% targets, and highest in a recognition condition involving 100% targets). It should be noted, though, that in the latter study the precuneus did not show differential activation during picture encoding (relative to encoding of visual sentences).

Spatial Information

The above-described studies provide support for reactivation of visual brain regions, notably the precuneus, during retrieval of pictorial information. A related set of studies provides evidence for reactivation of inferior parietal cortical regions during retrieval of the spatial location of visual objects. In an early study, Moscovitch, Kapur, Köhler, and Houle (1995) found that retrieval of object location in a two-item forced-choice recognition test, relative to retrieval of object identity in the same type of test, was associated with increased activity in the right inferior parietal cortex. The authors related their results to findings that regions in the dorsal visual pathway are engaged during perception of spatial location. In a subsequent study (Köhler, Moscovitch, Winocur, Houle, & McIntosh, 1998), it was found that the right inferior parietal cortex was activated during both a spatial matching task and during a spatial retrieval task (relative to object matching and object retrieval). Further evidence that the inferior parietal cortex is associated with encoding and retrieval of spatial location comes from a recent study (Persson & Nyberg, 2000) in which a condition involving encoding of the spatial location of visual words (left–right on a computer screen) was contrasted with encoding conditions that did not involve encoding of spatial location. In addition, a condition that involved retrieval of spatial location (deciding whether words presented in the center of a screen had been presented on the left or right side during encoding) was contrasted with retrieval conditions that did not involve spatial retrieval. A conjunction analysis revealed that increased activity in regions of the bilateral inferior parietal cortex was common to encoding and retrieval of spatial information. These results are consistent with the conclusion by Köhler and colleagues (1998) "that right inferior parietal cortex and bordering superior temporal sulcus are involved in spatial processing when conscious perceptual and memory judgements about the location of objects are required" (p. 137).

Motor Information

A final example of encoding–retrieval overlap in brain activity comes from a recent PET study on encoding and retrieval of motor information (Nyberg et al., 2001). At study, subjects encoded simple commands (e.g., "Make a fist") by using a verbal strategy (maintenance rehearsal) or by enacting the action described by each command (a third encoding condition involved motor imagery). At retrieval, subjects were verbally presented with the verb from each command and were asked to verbally recall the noun. When encoding by means of enactment was contrasted with encoding by means of maintenance rehearsal, increased activity associated with the enactment condition was observed in several motor areas in the left hemisphere (the actions were performed with the right arm/hand). This activation pattern was then used as a mask for a subsequent contrast between retrieval following encoding enactment and retrieval following maintenance rehearsal. This analysis revealed that increased activity in the left premotor cortex and left parietal cortex was common to encoding and retrieval of enacted events.

ENCODING AND RETRIEVAL: SIMILAR BUT ALSO DIFFERENT

The results discussed so far have highlighted similarities in brain activation patterns during initial perception/encoding and during subsequent retrieval. Importantly, though, this is not to say that differences do not exist. Rather, a number of studies have found that encoding and retrieval are associated with differential activity in several distinct brain regions, which has been taken as evidence for the existence of separate encoding and retrieval networks (Nyberg, McIntosh, et al., 1996; Nyberg, Persson, et al., 2000). Differences in regional activity between encoding and retrieval are perhaps especially striking in the prefrontal cortex. Encoding tends to be associated with differential activation in the left prefrontal cortex, whereas retrieval tends to be associated with differential activation in the right prefrontal cortex (Figure 15.2). This asymmetrical involvement of the prefrontal cortex during encoding and retrieval is captured by the HERA (hemispheric encoding–retrieval asymmetry) model (Tulving, Kapur, Craik, Moscovitch, & Houle, 1994; see also Nyberg, Cabeza, & Tulving, 1996). Independent support for the HERA model is provided by findings from transcranial magnetic stimulation that the left dorsolateral prefrontal cortex was involved in encoding of pictorial information whereas the right dorsolateral prefrontal cortex was crucial for retrieval of the same information (Rossi et al., 2001). More recent studies also show that the pattern of prefrontal activation during encoding and retrieval can be modulated by type of material—such that left prefrontal regions are preferentially activated by verbal material, whereas right prefrontal regions are preferentially activated by nonverbal material—but process-related differences in prefrontal activity nevertheless re-

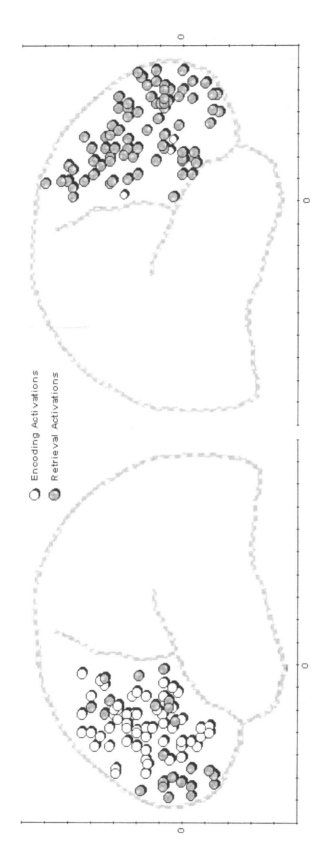

FIGURE 15.2. Differential activation of the left and right prefrontal cortex during encoding and retrieval. Published coordinates are plotted on left and right lateral brain outlines. Reprinted by permission of Roberto Cabeza.

main (e.g., McDermott, Buckner, Petersen, Kelley, & Sanders, 1999). Carefully designed PET and fMRI studies furthermore suggest that different component processes of encoding (e.g., Kapur et al., 1996; see also Nyberg, Cabeza, & Tulving, 1998) and retrieval (see Lepage, Ghaffar, Nyberg, & Tulving, 2000; Nolde, Johnson, & Raye, 1998; Nyberg, 1998; Rugg & Wilding, 2000) are associated with specific prefrontal regions.

Encoding–retrieval differences in brain activity have also been emphasized for other regions. For example, differences in parietal activation during encoding and retrieval were stressed in a recent fMRI study (McDermott, Ojemann, et al., 1999; see also Nyberg, Persson, et al., 2000). Also, it has been proposed that distinct regions in the MTL are engaged during encoding and retrieval (Gabrieli, Brewer, Desmond, & Glover, 1997; Lepage, Habib, & Tulving, 1998). Although it is clear that many PET and fMRI studies have observed increased MTL activity during encoding and retrieval, the existence and nature of encoding–retrieval differences in the MTL remain matters of debate (see Schacter & Wagner, 1999).

Regarding the existence of differences, a recent PET study presented a direct, within-subject comparison of MTL activation during encoding and retrieval (Schacter et al., 1999). It was found that encoding and retrieval activated overlapping posterior MTL regions. This observation can be related to the above-presented finding by Nyberg, Habib, and colleagues (2000) of increased activity in left MTL during paired encoding relative to single-word encoding and during paired relative to unpaired retrieval. Although both of these studies observed overlapping MTL activation during encoding and retrieval, the site of overlap was more anterior in the Nyberg, Habib, and colleagues study. As noted above, the Nyberg, Habib, and colleagues MTL activations were in keeping with a relational processing account (e.g., Cohen et al., 1999), and it has been suggested that anterior MTL activity will be observed under conditions that emphasize relational processing (Schacter et al., 1999; Schacter & Wagner, 1999). Nonetheless, despite the difference in the site for maximal overlap, the Schacter and colleagues and Nyberg, Habib, and colleagues studies point to similarities in MTL activity during encoding and retrieval. Regarding differences in encoding–retrieval MTL activity, Schacter and colleagues (1999) found in a direct contrast between encoding and retrieval that a posterior MTL region was more active during encoding than during retrieval. This finding is consistent with several previous PET and fMRI findings (see Schacter et al., 1999), but in opposition to the suggestion by Lepage and colleagues (1998) that encoding activations tend to fall in anterior parts of the MTL. Thus, although differences in MTL activity during encoding and retrieval have been demonstrated, the nature of these differences remains to be determined. Specifically, it needs to be explored whether basic differences between encoding and retrieval underlie such differences, or whether it simply is the case that encoding and retrieval tasks tend to put different emphasis on such factors as relational processing.

Taken together, some brain regions in the prefrontal and parietal cortices, and possibly also in the MTL, have been found to be differentially active during encoding and retrieval. A main challenge for the future is to explore how such encoding and retrieval regions interact with brain regions that are commonly engaged during encoding and retrieval. Analyses of functional and effective connectivity (Nyberg & McIntosh, 2001) are needed to shed light on this issue.

CONCLUSION

In conclusion, functional brain imaging techniques have made it possible to separately study brain regions involved in encoding and retrieval. Up to now, the focus has been on studying brain regions that are differentially involved during encoding and retrieval. However, as the present chapter has shown, several recent studies have also examined encoding–retrieval similarities in brain activity. The number of studies is still small, but collectively the results provide fairly strong support that specific areas are engaged during both encoding and retrieval of specific event information. Across studies, encoding–retrieval overlap tends to be observed in secondary rather than in primary areas. Thus only a subset of the encoding-related activity pattern is reactivated during retrieval (cf. Wheeler et al., 2000).

Findings that some brain regions are recruited during encoding as well as retrieval of information have implications for the issue of memory representation. Squire, Knowlton, and Musen (1993) noted that "permanent information storage is thought to occur in the same processing areas that are engaged during learning" (p. 484). According to this view, the areas of the brain where encoding and retrieval have been found to meet in PET and fMRI studies may be seen as storage sites. A challenge for future studies will be to examine additional stimulus dimensions, as well as to investigate the activation and reactivation patterns during encoding and retrieval of complex, multidimensional events.

ACKNOWLEDGMENTS

The coauthors of the papers that are discussed in this chapter are gratefully acknowledged. Special thanks to Endel Tulving for his comments on a previous version of the chapter, and to Roberto Cabeza and Reza Habib for help with figures. My work is supported by the Swedish Research Council.

REFERENCES

Alvarez, P., & Squire, L. R. (1994). Memory consolidation and the medial temporal lobe: A simple network model. *Proceedings of the National Academy of Sciences USA, 91,* 7041–7045.

Buckner, R. L., & Logan, J. M. (2001). PET and fMRI methods. In R. Cabeza & A. Kingstone (Eds.), *Handbook of functional neuroimaging of cognition* (pp. 27–48). Cambridge, MA: MIT Press.

Buckner, R. L., Wheeler, M. E., & Sheridan, M. (2001). Encoding processes during retrieval tasks. *Journal of Cognitive Neuroscience, 13,* 406–415.

Cabeza, R., & Nyberg, L. (2000). Imaging cognition: II. An empirical review of 275 PET and fMRI studies. *Journal of Cognitive Neuroscience, 12,* 1–47.

Cahill, L., Ohl, F., & Scheich, H. (1996). Alteration of auditory cortex activity with a visual stimulus through conditioning: A 2-deoxyglucose analysis. *Neurobiology of Learning and Memory, 65,* 213–222.

Craik, F. I. M. (1983). On the transfer of information from temporary to permanent memory. *Philosophical Transactions of the Royal Society of London, Series B, 302,* 341–359.

Cohen, N. J., Ryan, J., Hunt, C., Romine, L., Wszalek, T., & Nash, C. (1999). Hippocampal system and declarative (relational) memory: Summarizing the data from functional neuroimaging studies. *Hippocampus, 9,* 83–98.

Damasio, A. R. (1989). Time-locked multiregional retroactivation: A systems-level proposal for the neural substrates of recall and recognition. *Cognition, 33,* 25–62.

Dolan, R. J., & Fletcher, P. C. (1997). Dissociating prefrontal and hippocampal function in episodic memory encoding. *Nature, 388,* 582–585.

Gabrieli, J. D. E., Brewer, J. B., Desmond, J. E., & Glover, G. H. (1997). Separate neural bases of two fundamental memory processes in the human medial temporal lobe. *Science, 276,* 264–266.

Godden, D., & Baddeley, A. D. (1975). Context-dependent memory in two natural environments: On land and under water. *British Journal of Psychology, 66,* 325–331.

Kapur, S., Tulving, E., Cabeza, R., McIntosh, A. R., Houle, S., & Craik, F. I. M. (1996). The neural correlates of intentional learning of verbal materials: A PET study in humans. *Cognitive Brain Research, 4,* 243–249.

Köhler, S., Moscovitch, M., Winocur, G., Houle, S., & McIntosh, A. R. (1998). Networks of domain-specific and general regions involved in episodic memory for spatial location and object identity. *Neuropsychologia, 36,* 129–142.

Lepage, M., Ghaffar, O., Nyberg, L., & Tulving, E. (2000). Prefrontal cortex and episodic memory retrieval mode. *Proceedings of the National Academy of Sciences USA, 97,* 506–511.

Lepage, M., Habib, R., & Tulving, E. (1998). Hippocampal PET activations of memory encoding and retrieval: The HIPER model. *Hippocampus, 8,* 313–322.

McClelland, J. L., McNaughton, B. L., & O'Reilly, R. C. (1995). Why there are complementary learning systems in the hippocampus and neocortex: Insights from the successes and failures of connectionist models of learning and memory. *Psychological Review, 102,* 419–457.

McDermott, K. B., Buckner, R. L., Petersen, S. E., Kelley, W. M., & Sanders, A. L. (1999). Set- and code-specific activation in the frontal cortex: An fMRI study of encoding and retrieval of faces and words. *Journal of Cognitive Neuroscience, 11,* 631–640.

McDermott, K. B., Ojemann, J. G., Petersen, S. E., Ollinger, J. M., Snyder, A. Z., Akbudak, E., Conturo, T. E., & Raichle, M. E. (1999). Direct comparison of episodic encoding and retrieval of words: An event-related fMRI study. *Memory, 7,* 661–678.

McIntosh, A. R., Cabeza, R., & Lobaugh, N. J. (1998). Analysis of neural interactions explains the activation of occipital cortex by an auditory stimulus. *Journal of Neurophysiology, 80,* 2790–2796.

Morris, C. D., Bransford, J. D., & Franks, J. J. (1977). Levels of processing versus transfer appropriate processing. *Journal of Verbal Learning and Verbal Behavior, 16,* 519–533.

Moscovitch, M., Kapur, S., Köhler, S., & Houle, S. (1995). Distinct neural correlates of visual long-term memory for spatial location and object identity: A positron emission tomography study in humans. *Proceedings of the National Academy of Sciences USA, 92,* 3721–3725.

Nolde, S. F., Johnson, M. K., & Raye, C. L. (1998). The role of prefrontal cortex during tests of episodic memory. *Trends in Cognitive Sciences, 2,* 399–406.

Nyberg, L. (1998). Mapping episodic memory. *Behavioural Brain Research, 90,* 107–114.

Nyberg, L., Cabeza, R., & Tulving, E. (1996). PET studies of encoding and retrieval: The HERA model. *Psychonomic Bulletin and Review, 3,* 135–148.

Nyberg, L., Cabeza, R., & Tulving, E. (1998). Asymmetric frontal activation during episodic memory: What kind of specificity? *Trends in Cognitive Sciences, 2,* 419–420.

Nyberg, L., Habib, R., McIntosh, A. R., & Tulving, E. (2000). Reactivation of encoding-related brain activity during memory retrieval. *Proceedings of the National Academy of Sciences USA, 97,* 11120–11124.

Nyberg, L., & McIntosh, A. R. (2001). Functional neuroimaging: Network analyses. In R. Cabeza & A. Kingstone (Eds.), *Handbook of functional neuroimaging of cognition* (pp. 49–72). Cambridge, MA: MIT Press.

Nyberg, L., McIntosh, A. R., Cabeza, R., Habib, R., Houle, S., & Tulving, E. (1996). General and specific brain regions involved in encoding and retrieval of events: What, where, and when. *Proceedings of the National Academy of Sciences USA, 93,* 11280–11285.

Nyberg, L., Persson, J., Habib, R., Tulving, E., McIntosh, A. R., Cabeza, R., & Houle, S. (2000). Large scale neurocognitive networks underlying episodic memory. *Journal of Cognitive Neuroscience, 12,* 163–173.

Nyberg, L., Petersson, K.-M., Nilsson, L.-G., Sandblom, J., Åberg, C., & Ingvar, M. (2001). Reactivation of motor brain areas during explicit memory for actions. *NeuroImage, 14,* 521–528.

Persson, J., & Nyberg, L. (2000). Conjunction analysis of cortical activations common to encoding and retrieval. *Microscopy Research and Technique, 51,* 39–44.

Price, C. J., & Friston, K. J. (1997). Cognitive conjunction: A new approach to brain activation experiments. *NeuroImage, 5,* 261–270.

Roediger, H. L., III, Weldon, M. S., & Challis, B. H. (1989). Explaining dissociations between implicit and explicit measures of retention: A processing account. In H. L. Roediger III & F. I. M. Craik (Eds.), *Varieties of memory and consciousness: Essays in honour of Endel Tulving* (pp. 3–41). Hillsdale, NJ: Erlbaum.

Roland, P. E., & Gulyás, B. (1995). Visual memory, visual imagery, and visual recognition of large field patterns by the human brain: Functional anatomy by positron emission tomography. *Cerebral Cortex, 5,* 79–93.

Rossi, S., Cappa, S. F., Babiloni, C., Pasqualetti, P., Miniussi, C., Carducci, F., Babiloni, F., & Rossini, P. M. (2001). Prefrontal cortex in long-term memory: An "interference" approach using magnetic stimulation. *Nature Neuroscience, 4,* 948–952.

Rugg, M. D., & Wilding, E. L. (2000). Retrieval processing and episodic memory. *Trends in Cognitive Sciences, 4,* 108–115.

Ryan, L., & Eich, E. (1999). Mood dependence and implicit memory. In E. Tulving (Ed.), *Memory, consciousness and the brain: The Tallinn conference* (pp. 91–105). Philadelphia: Psychology Press.

Schacter, D. L., Curran, T., Reiman, E. M., Chen, K., Bandy, D. J., & Frost, J. T. (1999). Medial temporal lobe activation during episodic encoding and retrieval: A PET study. *Hippocampus, 9,* 575–581.

Schacter, D. L., & Wagner, A. D. (1999). Medial temporal lobe activations in fMRI and PET studies of episodic encoding and retrieval. *Hippocampus, 9,* 7–24.

Squire, L. R., Knowlton, B., & Musen, G. (1993). The structure and organization of memory. *Annual Review of Psychology, 44,* 453–495.

Tulving, E., Kapur, S., Craik, F. I. M., Moscovitch, M., & Houle, S. (1994). Hemispheric encoding/retrieval asymmetry in episodic memory: Positron emission tomography findings. *Proceedings of the National Academy of Sciences USA, 91,* 2016–2020.

Tulving, E., Markowitsch, H. J., Craik, F. I. M., Habib, R., & Houle, S. (1996). Novelty and familiarity activations in PET studies of memory encoding and retrieval. *Cerebral Cortex, 6,* 71–79.

Tulving, E., Markowitsch, H. J., Kapur, S., Habib, R., & Houle, S. (1994). Novelty encoding networks in the human brain: Positron emission tomography data. *NeuroReport, 5,* 2525–2528.

Tulving, E., & Thomson, D. M. (1973). Encoding specificity and retrieval processes in episodic memory. *Psychological Review, 80,* 352–373.

Wheeler, M. E., Petersen, S. E., & Buckner, R. L. (2000). Memory's echo: Vivid remembering reactivates sensory-specific cortex. *Proceedings of the National Academy of Sciences USA, 97,* 11125–11129.

Yates, F. A. (1992). *The art of memory.* London: Pimlico. (Original work published 1966)

16

Hippocampal Novelty Responses Studied with Functional Neuroimaging

R. J. DOLAN and B. A. STRANGE

Selection is the very keel on which our mental ship is built. And in the case of memory its utility is obvious. If we remembered everything, we should on most occasions be as ill off as if we remembered nothing.

—WILLIAM JAMES (1890, p. 680)

If one accepts James's (1890) proposal that not all sensory input can be committed to memory, it follows that novel information should have preferential access to memory systems. It is now widely accepted that mammalian brains require novelty-sensitive networks whose function includes indexing of information for long-term storage (Fabiani & Donchin, 1995; Metcalfe, 1993; von Restorff, 1933; Tulving & Kroll, 1995). A recent extension of this idea has been the novelty/encoding hypothesis developed by Tulving and Kroll (1995), who have proposed that novelty is a necessary, although not sufficient, condition for long-term information storage.

Most perspectives on novelty acknowledge that its investigation requires a dynamic perspective, in that biological systems show changing response profiles to repeated encounters with stimuli. Sokolov (1963) conjectured that the neocortex maintains a model of the environment, with novel stimuli producing a mismatch or error in this predictive signal. As a model of a stimulus is built up in the neocortex, this mismatch signal decreases, associated with habituation of the behavioral response to novelty. Sokolov attributed this mismatch detection to a neocortical–reticular formation interaction. This theme of mismatch was subsequently developed in a more anatomically specified manner by O'Keefe and Nadel (1978), who conceptualized novelty as a mismatch between expectation and experience. Thus these authors argued that exploratory behavior in response to novelty is driven by an occurrence of unpredicted events, and ceases when these events are incorporated within a hippocampal representation of the environment.

Hippocampal damage results in a dense anterograde amnesia (Scoville & Milner, 1957; Squire, 1992). This inability to acquire new episodic memories can be construed as consistent with a hippocampal role in selective processing of novel stimuli. In humans, intracranial electrophysiological recordings from epileptic patients have provided evidence for a hippocampal role in novelty processing. For example, single-unit recordings demonstrate differential neuronal activity in the human hippocampus to novel versus familiar stimuli (Fried, MacDonald, & Wilson, 1997), and hippocampal damage has been shown to attenuate medial temporal lobe evoked potentials to novel visually presented words without affecting responses to repetitive presentations (Grunwald, Lehnertz, Heinze, Helmstaedter, & Elger, 1998).

The emphasis in this chapter is on the study of novelty processing in the human brain as revealed by functional neuroimaging, either positron emission tomography (PET) or functional magnetic resonance imaging (fMRI). The specific biological questions addressed relate to the role of the hippocampus ("hippocampus" is used here to refer to the dentate gyrus, CA subfields, and subiculum) in indexing the occurrence of novelty. The outlined approach is predicated on an assumption that objects or items in the world are rarely completely novel. Indeed, we make two general assumptions about novelty. The first of these assumptions, which relates to the physical qualities of stimuli, is that novelty arises in most instances from a reconfiguration of familiar elements. An example of such a reconfiguration is the use of letter strings to create new items; the individual elements (the letters) are highly familiar, but a reconfiguration creates a novel item. The second assumption is that biological systems sensitive to novelty are likely to show changing response profiles to repeated encounters with stimuli. The proposal that novelty responses have a temporal component necessarily implies that the associated biological systems should show adaptation with repeated exposure to a stimulus. We illustrate our approach with experiments that first ask whether the hippocampus is sensitive to recency of prior occurrence. We then expand on this question by examining whether a novelty response in the hippocampus shows adaptation with repeated presentation of a stimulus. Finally, we describe an experimental approach testing the hypothesis that the critical variable for evoking novelty-dependent activity in the hippocampus is unpredictability.

HIPPOCAMPAL RESPONSES AND RECENCY
OF STIMULUS PRESENTATION

In an initial experiment, using auditory–verbal paired associates, we tested a hypothesis that hippocampal activation indexes relative stimulus novelty, defined on the basis of recency of prior occurrence (Dolan & Fletcher, 1997). As study material we used word paired associates, each pair consisting of a category (e.g., "dog") and an exemplar (e.g., "boxer") presented auditorily. We scanned subjects, using PET, while they performed an encoding task in relation to presentation of sets of 12 paired auditory–verbal paired associates. We used a design in which category and exemplar were independent factors, with two levels related to whether an item was novel (i.e., not previously presented) or old (i.e., presented on two occasions in the period immediately prior to scanning). The study thus involved four separate conditions representing two levels of novelty (new and old) with respect to either category or exemplar.

Activation of the left dorsolateral prefrontal cortex was sensitive to changing the association between a category and exemplar, or vice versa. An example of the former is a situation where a category ("dog") is changed to another category ("sportsman"), but the same exemplar (in two different senses) is used ("boxer"). By contrast, in the condition where both category and exemplar were novel, hippocampal activation was observed. This hippocampal response was evident when the condition involving presentation of a novel category and exemplar was compared to each of the other conditions. The profile of activation demonstrated a stepwise pattern, with highest values being expressed when category and exemplar were novel, intermediate levels where either a category or an exemplar was novel, and the lowest levels when neither were novel.

When a category and exemplar were presented for the first time, the critical processing emphasized was contextual novelty (relative recency of prior occurrence); as predicted, robust medial temporal activation was elicited for the most novel items. It is noteworthy that the magnitude of hippocampal activation reflected the overall degree of novelty of the material. One inference that can be made from these data is that the human hippocampus, and related medial temporal lobe structures, are sensitive to novelty that extends beyond mere item novelty to include contextual novelty.

THE TEMPORAL PROFILE OF NOVELTY RESPONSES IN THE HIPPOCAMPUS

One problem with using words to study novelty is that individual items are by necessity familiar to subjects, with recency and salience of the items varying across subjects. To overcome this difficulty, we subsequently used a finite-state "artificial grammar system" to generate entirely novel letter strings (see Figure 16.1a). An artificial grammar system embodies a set of arbitrary rules governing the concatenation of symbols. With such a system, it is possible to generate novel letter strings from previously familiar items (letters). In our experiments we used such a system to generate consonant strings, under the constraint that all strings must consist of four letters. Artificial grammar systems have been widely used to study implicit learning. In standard applications, subjects exposed to exemplars of such a grammar system learn to categorize as "grammatical" (i.e., conforming to the hidden rules) or "ungrammatical" subsequently presented symbol strings, with an accuracy greater than chance levels (Reber, 1967; Shanks, 1995). It is widely assumed that this type of learning reflects the application of an implicit learning system, although this idea is itself controversial (Shanks & St. John, 1994). Note, however, that in the experiments described here the emphasis was on explicit learning, in that subjects were provided with specific learning instructions and provided with performance details. Consequently, we used a modified approach to the standard use of the grammar system: Subjects were required to learn the grammatical status of consonant strings (the exemplars of the grammar system) that were presented repeatedly, with trial-by-trial feedback. Note that in standard applications, no feedback is provided.

Our previous experiment (Dolan & Fletcher, 1997) indicated a hippocampal response to novel items. In these studies, the question addressed was whether this hippocampal response reflects influences of perceptual novelty, pertaining to physical characteristics of stimuli (in this case, visual characteristics), or exemplar novelty, reflecting the semantic characteristics of stimuli (in this case, grammatical status within a rule system). By repeatedly presenting novel items, we were able to determine the temporal profile of hippocampal novelty responses.

Both our experiments using an artificial grammar system involved presenting subjects with a total of 30 strings, mixed with 30 arbitrarily chosen nongrammatical lures (Dolan & Fletcher, 1999; Strange, Fletcher, Henson, Friston, & Dolan, 1999). Each experiment comprised six blocks, and within each block, stimuli were visually presented up to a total of 10 consonant strings (50% grammatical, 50% lures). Subjects were required to respond to each item by indicating, via a keypad response, whether an item was grammatical or ungrammatical. Subjects received immediate visual feedback indicating whether a particular

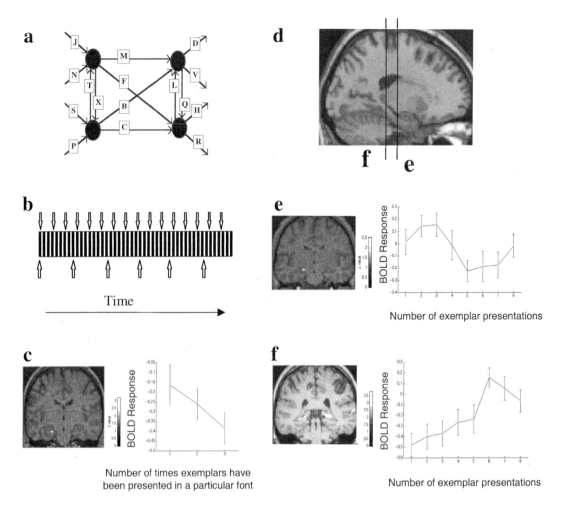

FIGURE 16.1. (a) The artificial grammar system. Grammatical four-consonant letter strings are formed by starting on the left and moving right in the direction of the arrows. (b) Experimental design. Every exemplar set presentation constitutes an activation epoch (black rectangle), each of which is followed by a control epoch (white rectangle). Upward arrows, introduction of exemplar novelty; downward arrows, introduction of perceptual novelty. (c) The left anterior hippocampal region, in which there is a significant time × condition interaction in response to perceptual novelty and adaptation with familiarity. The Statistical Parameter Map (SPM) (threshold at $p < .01$) indicating a left anterior hippocampal decreasing linear time × condition interaction following introduction of a novel font is superimposed on a coronal section of a T_1-weighted anatomical image (at $y = -16$). Activation at this voxel (x, y, z coordinates −22, −16, −24) is plotted relative to the baseline condition as a function of repeated presentation of fonts. The plotted time course shows the blood-oxygen-level-dependent (BOLD) response collapsed across the 16 font changes and averaged across 14 subjects. (d) Dissociation in the anterior–posterior hippocampal axis for exemplar novelty. T_1-weighted anatomical sagittal image, with vertical lines indicating the anterior–posterior positions of the coronal sections demonstrated in e and f. (e) SPM showing enhanced left anterior hippocampal activation after the introduction of exemplar novelty followed by adaptation (threshold at $p < .05$). Activation at this voxel (x, y, z coordinates −18, −16, −14), relative to the baseline condition, is plotted against number of presentations of an exemplar set. The plot shows the BOLD response collapsed across the six exemplar changes and averaged across all subjects. (f) SPM (threshold at $p < .01$) showing that increasing familiarity with exemplars activates the posterior hippocampus bilaterally. The coronal section demonstrates right posterior hippocampal activation (x, y, z coordinates 24, −34, −2) and also shows left posterior hippocampal activation (x, y, z coordinates −22, −38, −6). Activation of the right posterior hippocampal voxel is plotted relative to the baseline condition as for e. From Strange et al. (1999). Copyright 1999 by the National Academy of Sciences, USA. Adapted by permission.

response was correct or incorrect. In a single block the same 10 items were presented a total of either six times (Dolan & Fletcher, 1997) or eight times (Strange et al., 1999). Each presentation epoch was followed by a sensorimotor control condition, which consisted of serial visual presentation of either rows of the letter P or N, signaling a right or left keypad response, respectively. At the end of each block, a new block began, and 10 new items (5 grammatical, 5 ungrammatical) conforming to the same underlying rule system were presented. Thus, in the early stage of each experiment, subjects had no knowledge of the underlying grammatical rules and responded on the basis of guesses and explicit knowledge of outcomes of previous responses to individual items. Across blocks, subjects' responses were gradually modulated by an emerging knowledge of grammatical rules.

In our first experiment (Dolan & Fletcher, 1999), behavioral performance showed a significant linear improvement both within and across blocks. The effects seen with neuroimaging were then examined using two models. In the first model, we examined the effect of repeated presentation for the set of consonant strings presented in the first block (where there was little or no knowledge of underlying grammatical rules). In this analysis, a significant left anterior hippocampal effect was evident, with decreasing activation as a function of increasing item familiarity. In a subsequent analysis, which involved all six blocks, we examined how this anterior hippocampal response was modulated by increasing knowledge of the grammatical rules.

The observation of left anterior hippocampal response, within the first block, to initial presentation of exemplars emphasized encoding processes that were not contaminated by rule-based knowledge. The across-block time-dependent attenuation of this response mirrored a decreasing reliance on learning particular instances of the grammar (i.e., episodic encoding) and the emergence of rule-based task performance. In other words, the time × condition interaction for anterior hippocampal activation could reflect modulation of episodic encoding processes by the emergence of a rule-based system. Alternatively, it could reflect a "novelty of novelty" effect, insofar as there may have been a second-order adaptation to the occurrence of novel stimuli. The basic idea here is that repeated occurrences of novel items create a specific context where novel items are expected, and this leads to an attenuation of the associated response.

IS THE HIPPOCAMPUS SENSITIVE TO DISTINCT TYPES OF NOVELTY?

In our subsequent study, the question addressed was whether this hippocampal response reflects influences of perceptual novelty, pertaining to the physical characteristics of stimuli (in this case, visual characteristics), or exemplar novelty, reflecting the semantic characteristics of stimuli (in this case, grammatical status within a rule system) (Strange et al., 1999). To address these issues, we relied upon the same basic design as in the previous study, except that both exemplar and perceptual novelty were varied periodically. Exemplar novelty was introduced by periodically presenting novel consonant strings. Perceptual novelty was introduced by periodically changing the font in which individual exemplars were presented. Thus a given set of exemplars was presented eight times, and the font was changed after every three presentations of an exemplar set (see Figure 16.1b for the experimental time line). Critically, the manipulations of exemplar and perceptual novelty were orthogonal (i.e., uncorrelated), thus enabling characterization of hippocampal responses associated with each type of novelty.

The specific effect tested was a condition (exemplar or perceptual change) × time interaction, where "time" refers to the time elapsed following a change in either exemplar or font (i.e., the adaptation of hemodynamic responses following exemplar or perceptual changes). Figure 16.1c shows the hippocampal response to perceptual novelty and its modulation with time. A greater left anterior hippocampal response was seen for initial, relative to repeated, presentations of perceptually novel items, reflected in a significant linear time × condition interaction. This response showed adaptation with increasing font familiarity. A hippocampal response to exemplar novelty (again assessed as a condition × time interaction) was also evident, as shown in Figure 16.1e. Thus initial presentation of novel exemplars was associated with an activation in the left anterior hippocampus, 10 mm superior to the region indexed by perceptual novelty. With repeated exemplar presentations, activation in this region again showed significant adaptation. This pattern of response in the hippocampus was best modeled as an exponential decline. Thus a significant time × condition interaction was reflected in reducing activation, relative to the recurring baseline, in the anterior hippocampus.

Strikingly, a reverse effect, reflecting increasing familiarity with exemplars, was associated with augmented bilateral posterior hippocampal activation (Figure 16.1f). Hence familiarity with the meaningful characteristics of stimuli (i.e., grammatical status within a rule system) produced augmentation of posterior hippocampal responses bilaterally. By contrast, increasing font familiarity, which had no behavioral relevance, did not engage the posterior hippocampus. Thus, in the bilateral posterior hippocampus, we observed a time × condition interaction only for repeated exemplar presentations. Figure 16.1d demonstrates the location of these activations along the hippocampus with respect to the relative familiarity of study items. Neuronal responses in the anterior hippocampus would consequently seem to index generic novelty, whereas posterior hippocampal responses would seem to index familiarity to stimuli with behavioral relevance.

HIPPOCAMPAL ODDBALL RESPONSES

The previous experiments were predicated on a definition of novelty based upon recency of prior occurrence. Novelty can also be considered as a mismatch between expectation and experience. Indeed, the brain mechanisms for detecting such violations have been studied extensively in "oddball" paradigms. Intracranial (Halgren et al., 1980) and scalp (Knight, 1996) recordings of oddball-evoked event-related potentials have suggested a critical role for the hippocampus in oddball detection. Notably, functional neuroimaging experiments have singularly failed to find medial temporal lobe activation in response to visual (Downar, Crawley, Mikulis, Davis, & Davis, 2000; Linden et al., 1999; McCarthy, Luby, Gore, & Goldman-Rakic, 1997; Strange, Henson, Friston, & Dolan, 2000), auditory (Downar et al., 2000; Higashima et al., 1996; Linden et al., 1999; Opitz, Mecklinger, Friederici, & von Cramon, 1999), or tactile (Downar et al., 2000) oddball stimuli.

To address the issue of oddball-induced hippocampal activity, we used fMRI to measure hippocampal responses to three types of oddballs: perceptual, semantic, and emotional (Strange et al., 2000). During fMRI scanning, 11 subjects viewed sequential lists of 19 nouns, serially presented, where all nouns within a given list belonged to the same category except for one (the semantic oddball). In these lists, a further noun was presented either in a novel font (the perceptual oddball) or with an emotionally aversive content (the emotional oddball). The three oddball types were randomly positioned within the lists, with the constraints that the first 5 nouns were control nouns (i.e., nonoddballs). This arrangement allowed creation of a context for the oddballs, and also ensured that each oddball was followed by at least one control noun. Figure 16.2a gives examples of the stimuli for which subjects had to perform a shallow or deep encoding task. The experiment consisted of four sequential scanning sessions, with half of the subjects following one encoding task order (deep, shallow, shallow, deep) and the other half another order (shallow, deep, deep, and shallow). As the first oddball was completely unexpected, we hypothesized that the response indexing mismatch, or surprise, would be greatest to the first oddballs encountered (e.g., the presentation of "group" in a novel font; see Figure 16.2a). Consequently, we hypothesized that this decreasing mismatch between expectation and outcome would be reflected in an adaptation in anterior hippocampal responses expressed across successive presentations of oddballs.

For each oddball type, we compared the habituating neural response evoked by an oddball with that evoked by a randomly chosen control noun in the same list, yielding an independent control for each oddball. To determine common activation profiles evoked by all oddball types, we conducted a conjunction analysis of the three oddball types versus their respective controls. A conjunction analysis requires an independent baseline for each effect tested; hence three nonoddball words were randomly assigned as the controls for the three oddball types. Figure 16.2b shows that, as predicted, adaptive activation was expressed in the left anterior hippocampus for all oddball types. The parameter estimates for the response to each oddball type versus control for session 1 versus session 2 are plotted for both encoding tasks. The plot demonstrates that the adaptive hippocampal response, common to all oddball types, was not modulated by encoding task.

In contrast to previous functional imaging studies of oddball detection (Downar et al., 2000; Higashima et al., 1996; Linden et al., 1999; McCarthy et al., 1997; Opitz et al., 1999; Strange et al., 2000), we demonstrated hippocampal activation in response to oddball stimuli. Specifically, the left anterior hippocampus was differentially engaged by stimuli that violated, across a number of different dimensions, the prevailing context in which they were presented. The fact that the hippocampal oddball response was not modulated by depth of processing suggests a high degree of automaticity in the underlying process. Furthermore, we demonstrated that this anterior hippocampal response adapted following presentation of multiple oddballs. The adaptive response profile we observed in the anterior hippocampus is consistent with this region being engaged by mismatches between expectancy and experience (Ploghaus et al., 2000; Strange et al., 1999). The initial presentations of oddballs were unexpected, but this breach of expectancy diminished as subjects were exposed to more and more oddballs, reflected in a habituating anterior hippocampal response. The adaptive nature of the hippocampal response to oddballs may explain why previous neuroimaging studies of oddball detection have failed to find hippocampal activation. Given that the oddball-evoked hippocampal signal rapidly attenuates, averaging oddball-evoked hemodynamic responses across the entire experiment is unlikely to detect hippocampal responses (Strange et al., 2000).

The majority of functional imaging studies of novelty have demonstrated activation of the anterior hippocampus (Constable et al., 2000; Dolan & Fletcher, 1997; Fischer, Furmark, Wik, & Fredrikson, 2000; Haxby et al., 1996; Martin, Wiggs, & Weisberg, 1997; Saykin et al., 1999; Tulving, Markowitsch, Craik, Habib, & Houle, 1996). Although some studies report posterior hippocampal responses to novelty (Rombouts, 1997; Stern et al., 1996), the majority of novelty-evoked activations in the posterior medial temporal lobe have been observed in the parahippocampal gyrus (see Schacter & Wagner, 1999, for a review). The fact that novelty activations are in the anterior hippocampus supports previ-

a

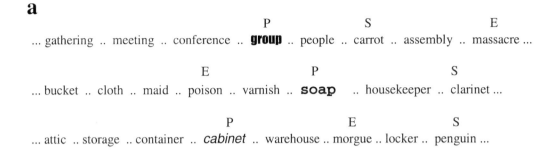

P   S   E

... gathering .. meeting .. conference .. **group** .. people .. carrot .. assembly .. massacre ...

E   P   S

... bucket .. cloth .. maid .. poison .. varnish .. **soap** .. housekeeper .. clarinet ...

P   E   S

... attic .. storage .. container .. *cabinet* .. warehouse .. morgue .. locker .. penguin ...

b i

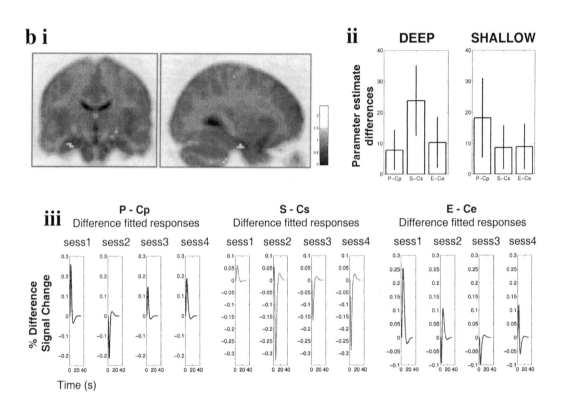

FIGURE 16.2. (a) Examples of presented nouns. Abbreviations: P, perceptual oddball; S, semantic oddball; E, emotional oddball. (b) The left anterior hippocampus is activated by all oddball types, and this response adapts across the experiment. (i) The SPM (threshold at $p < .001$) is superimposed on a coronal section of the mean functional image at $y = -12$ and on a sagittal section at $x = -30$ to demonstrate left anterior hippocampal activation (-30, -12, -27). (ii) The parameter estimates pertain to the canonical hemodynamic response for the three oddballs minus their respective control nouns for the first minus the second session, and are plotted for both deep and shallow encoding. (iii) The fitted responses for each oddball type minus its control, averaged across all subjects and collapsed across deep and shallow encoding, are plotted for the four sessions. Error bars represent ± 1 standard error; the bar indicates the t statistic of the activation. Abbreviations: P, perceptual oddball; S, semantic oddball; E, emotional oddball; Cp, control noun for perceptual oddball; Cs, control noun for semantic oddball; Ce, control noun for emotional oddball. From Strange and Dolan (2001). Copyright 2001 by Wiley. Adapted by permission.

ous claims for functional segregation within the human hippocampus, which propose that the anterior hippocampus mediates episodic memory encoding and novelty detection (Lepage, Habib, & Tulving, 1998; Saykin et al., 1999; Strange et al., 1999), but see Schacter & Wagner, 1999). Support for segregated functional properties of the anterior and posterior hippocampus is also provided by anatomical and biochemical studies, which demonstrate that both connectivity profiles and neuroreceptor densities are segregated along the hippocampal longitudinal axis (Moser & Moser, 1998).

Animal cellular recordings demonstrate novelty-sensitive cells in the medial temporal cortex (Brown & Xiang, 1998) as well as the hippocampus (Vinogradova, 1975). Medial temporal cortical (specifically, perirhinal) responses are typically stimulus-specific, responding differentially to the relative familiarity of certain stimuli and not others (Young, Otto, Fox, & Eichenbaum, 1997), and are thought to possess the firing properties that enable recognition memory for simple visual stimuli (Brown & Xiang, 1998). By contrast, novelty responses in the hippocampus do not show this stimulus selectivity (Otto & Eichenbaum, 1992; Rolls, Cahusac, Feigenbaum, & Miyashita, 1993; Vinogradova, 1975; Wiebe & Staubli, 1999), suggesting that the hippocampus mediates abstracted, stimulus-general mismatch detection. In agreement with this proposal is the observation that hippocampal responses to oddballs show adaptation expressed across successive presentations of *different* oddballs that deviate from context along the same dimension.

SUMMARY

In summary, we have extended the general finding that the hippocampus is sensitive to recency of prior occurrence by proposing that a critical process underlying hippocampal responses to novelty is the detection of mismatch between expectation and experience. Functional neuroimaging data would seem to provide evidence for what has been termed a "comparator theory" of hippocampal function (Gray, 1982; Vinogradova, 1975). Our data suggest that this function is a specialization of the anterior hippocampus. The engagement of mismatch detection in response to an unpredictable stimulus may be the physiological basis for awarding a stimulus preferential access to storage in long-term memory. A breakdown in this process, consequent upon hippocampal damage, may explain phenomena seen in patients with anterograde amnesia.

REFERENCES

Brown, M. W., & Xiang, J. Z. (1998). Recognition memory: Neuronal substrates of the judgement of prior occurrence. *Progress in Neurobiology, 55*, 149–189.

Constable, R. T., Carpentier, A., Pugh, K., Westerveld, M., Oszunar, Y., & Spencer, D. D. (2000). Investigation of the human hippocampal formation using a randomized event-related paradigm and Z-shimmed functional MRI. *NeuroImage, 12*, 55–62.

Dolan, R. J., & Fletcher, P. C. (1997). Dissociating prefrontal and hippocampal function in episodic memory encoding. *Nature, 388*, 582–585.

Dolan, R. J., & Fletcher, P. F. (1999). Encoding and retrieval in human medial temporal lobes: An empirical investigation using functional magnetic resonance imaging (fMRI). *Hippocampus, 9*, 25–34.

Downar, J., Crawley, A. P., Mikulis, D., Davis, J., & Davis, K. D. (2000). A multimodal cortical network for detecting changes in the sensory environment. *Nature Neuroscience, 3*, 277–283.

Fabiani, M., & Donchin, E. (1995). Encoding processes and memory organization: A model of the von Restorff effect. *Journal of Experimental Psychology: Learning, Memory, and Cognition*, *21*, 224–240.

Fischer, H., Furmark, T., Wik, G., & Fredrikson, M. (2000). Brain representation of habituation to repeated complex visual stimulation studied with PET. *NeuroReport*, *11*, 123–126.

Fried, I., MacDonald, K. A., & Wilson, C. L. (1997). Single neuron activity in human hippocampus and amygdala during recognition of faces and objects. *Neuron*, *18*, 753–765.

Gray, J. A. (1982). *The neuropsychology of anxiety*. Oxford: Oxford University Press.

Grunwald, T., Lehnertz, K., Heinze, H. J., Helmstaedter, C., & Elger, C. E. (1998). Verbal novelty detection within the human hippocampus proper. *Proceedings of the National Academy of Sciences USA*, *95*, 3193–3197.

Halgren, E., Squires, N. K., Wilson, C. L., Rohrbaugh, J. W., Babb, T. L., & Crandall, P. H. (1980). Endogenous potentials generated in the human hippocampal formation and amygdala by infrequent events. *Science*, *210*, 803–805.

Haxby, J. V., Ungerleider, L. G., Horwitz, B., Maisog, J. M., Rapoport, S. I., & Grady, C. L. (1996). Face encoding and recognition in the human brain. *Proceedings of the National Academy of Sciences USA*, *93*, 922–927.

Higashima, M., Kawasaki, Y., Urata, K., Maeda, Y., Sakai, N., Mizukoshi, C., Nagasawa, T., Kamiya, T., Yamaguchi, N., Koshino, Y., Matsuda, H., Tsuji, S., Sumiya, H., & Hisada, K., (1996). Simultaneous observation of regional cerebral blood flow and event-related potential during performance of an auditory task. *Brain Research and Cognitive Brain Science*, *4*, 289–296.

James, W. (1890). *The principles of psychology*. New York: Holt.

Knight, R. T. (1996). Contribution of human hippocampal region to novelty detection. *Nature*, *383*, 256–259.

Lepage, M., Habib, R., & Tulving, E. (1998). Hippocampal PET activations of memory encoding and retrieval: The HIPER model. *Hippocampus*, *8*, 313–322.

Linden, D., Prvulovic, D., Formisano, E., Vollinger, M., Zanella, F. E., Goebel, R., & Dierks, T. (1999). The functional neuroanatomy of target detection: an fMRI study of visual and auditory oddball tasks. *Cerebral Cortex*, *9*, 815–823.

Martin, A., Wiggs, C. L., & Weisberg, J. (1997). Modulation of human medial temporal lobe activity by form, meaning, and experience. *Hippocampus*, *7*, 587–93.

McCarthy, G., Luby, M., Gore, J., & Goldman-Rakic, P. (1997). Infrequent events transiently activate human prefrontal and parietal cortex as measured by functional MRI. *Journal of Neurophysiology*, *77*, 1630–1634.

Metcalfe, J. (1993). Novelty monitoring, metacognition, and control in a composite holographic associative recall model: Implications for Korsakoff amnesia. *Psychological Review*, *100*, 3–22.

Moser, M.B., & Moser, E. (1998). Functional differentiation in the hippocampus. *Hippocampus*, *8*, 608–619.

O'Keefe, J., & Nadel, L. (1978). *The hippocampus as a cognitive map*. Oxford: Clarendon Press.

Opitz, B., Mecklinger, A., Friederici, A. D., & von Cramon D. Y. (1999). The functional neuroanatomy of novelty processing: Integrating ERP and fMRI results. *Cerebral Cortex*, *9*, 379–391.

Otto, T., & Eichenbaum, H. (1992), Neuronal activity in the hippocampus during delayed nonmatch to sample performance in rats: Evidence for hippocampal processing in recognition memory, *Hippocampus*, *2*, 323–334.

Ploghaus, A., Tracey, I., Clare, S., Gati, J. S., Rawlins J. N., & Matthews, P. M. (2000). Learning about pain: The neural substrate of the prediction error for aversive events. *Proceedings of the National Academy of Sciences USA*, *97*, 9281–9286.

Reber, A. S. (1967). Implicit learning of artificial grammars. *Journal of Verbal Learning and Verbal behavior*, *6*, 855–863.

Rolls, E. T., Cahusac, P. M., Feigenbaum, J. D., & Miyashita, Y. (1993). Responses of single neurons in the hippocampus of the macaque related to recognition memory. *Experimental Brain Research*, *93*, 299–306.

Rombouts, S. A., Machielsen, W. C., Witter, M. P., Barkhof, F., Lindeboom, J., & Scheltens, P. (1997). Visual association encoding activates the medial temporal lobe: A functional magnetic resonance imaging study. *Hippocampus, 7,* 594–601.

Saykin, A. J., Johnson, S. C., Flashman, L. A., McAllister, T. W., Sparling, M., Darcey, T. M., Moritz, C. H., Guerin, S. J., Weaver, J., & Mamourian, A. (1999). Functional differentiation of medial temporal and frontal regions involved in processing novel and familiar words: An fMRI study. *Brain, 122,* 1963–1971.

Schacter, D. L., & Wagner, A. D. (1999). Medial temporal lobe activations in fMRI and PET studies of episodic encoding and retrieval. *Hippocampus, 9,* 7–24.

Scoville, W. B., & Milner, B. (1957). Loss of recent memory after bilateral hippocampal lesions. *Journal of Neurology, Neurosurgery and Psychiatry, 20,* 11–21.

Shanks, D. (1995). *The psychology of associative learning.* Cambridge, England: Cambridge University Press.

Shanks, D. R., & St John, M. F. (1994). Characterisitcs of dissociable human learning systems. *Behavioral and Brain Sciences, 17,* 367–447.

Sokolov, E. N. (1963). Higher nervous functions: The orienting reflex. *Annual Review of Physiology, 25,* 545–580.

Squire, L. R. (1992). Memory and the hippocampus: A synthesis from findings in rats, monkeys, and humans. *Psychological Review, 99,* 195–231.

Stern, C. E., Corkin, S., González, R. G., Guimaraes, A. R., Baker, J. R., Jennings, P. J., Carr, C. A., Sugiura, R. M., Vedantham, V., & Rosen, B. R. (1996). The hippocampal formation participates in novel picture encoding: Evidence from functional magnetic resonance imaging. *Proceedings of the National Academy of Sciences USA, 93,* 8660–8665.

Strange, B. A., & Dolan, R. J. (2001). Adaptive anterior hippocampal responses to oddball stimuli. *Hippocampus, 11,* 690–698.

Strange, B. A., Fletcher, P. C., Henson, R. N., Friston, K. J., & Dolan, R. J. (1999). Segregating the functions of human hippocampus. *Proceedings of the National Academy of Sciences USA, 96,* 4034–4039.

Strange, B. A., Henson, R. N. A., Friston, K. J., & Dolan, R. J. (2000). Brain mechanisms for detecting perceptual, semantic and emotional deviance. *NeuroImage, 12,* 425–433.

Tulving, E., & Kroll, N. (1995). Novelty assessment in the brain and long-term memory encoding. *Psychonomic Bulletin and Review, 2,* 387–390.

Tulving, E., Markowitsch, H. J., Craik, F. E., Habib, R., & Houle, S. (1996). Novelty and familiarity activations in PET studies of memory encoding and retrieval. *Cerebral Cortex, 6,* 71–79.

Vinogradova, O. (1975). Functional organization of the limbic system in the process of registration of information: Facts and hypotheses. In R. L. Isaacson & K. H. Pribram (Eds.) *The hippocampus* (pp. 3–69). New York: Plenum Press.

von Restorff, H. (1933). Uber die wirkung von bereichsbildungen im spurenfeld [On the effect of spheres formation in the trace field]. *Psycholische Forschung, 18,* 299–342.

Wiebe, S. P., & Staubli, U. V. (1999). Dynamic filtering of recognition memory codes in the hippocampus. *Journal of Neuroscience, 19,* 10562–10574.

Young, B. J., Otto, T., Fox, G. D., & Eichenbaum, H. (1997). Memory representation within the parahippocampal region. *Journal of Neuroscience, 17,* 5183–5195.

17

The Neural Basis of Working Memory Storage, Rehearsal, and Control Processes

Evidence from Patient and Functional Magnetic Resonance Imaging Studies

MARK D'ESPOSITO and BRADLEY R. POSTLE

"Working memory" is an evolving concept that refers to the temporary online maintenance and manipulation of information that can be used to guide behavior, even though that information is no longer present in the environment. It has been implicated as a critical contributor to such complex cognitive tasks as language comprehension, learning, planning, and reasoning (Baddeley, 1992; Jonides, 1995; Miller, Galanter, & Pribram, 1960). Elucidation of the cognitive and neural architectures underlying human working memory has been an important focus of cognitive neuroscience for much of the past decade (D'Esposito, Aguirre, Zarahn, & Ballard, 1998; Smith & Jonides, 1999; Ungerleider, 1995). Two conclusions that arise from this research are that working memory can be viewed as neither a unitary nor a dedicated system. For example, behavioral and functional neuroanatomical dissociations of working memory for different kinds of stimulus information attest to its componential nature (D'Esposito et al., 1998; Halbig, Mecklinger, Schriefers, & Friederici, 1998; Postle, Jonides, Smith, Corkin, & Growdon, 1997), and working memory performance recruits neuroanatomical systems that are also responsible for online analysis of sensory information (Courtney, Ungerleider, Keil, & Haxby, 1997; Zarahn, Aguirre, & D'Esposito, 1999).

To maintain and manipulate information when that information is not accessible in the environment, the brain needs (1) "storage" processes; (2) "rehearsal" processes, which can prevent the contents of the storage system from decaying; and (3) "executive control" processes, to perform transformations upon these mnemonic representations and to govern their accessibility to goal-appropriate processes. The first two of these can be considered mnemonic processes, because their function is decidedly memory-related. The latter of these can be classified as extramnemonic in nature, because many such executive control processes can also contribute to behaviors that do not involve working memory. For example, such processes include shifting attention within a task (Garavan, 1998; Postle &

D'Esposito, 1998) or between tasks (Rogers & Monsell, 1995); resolving interference be-
tween stimuli (D'Esposito, Postle, Jonides, & Smith, 1999; May, Hasher, & Kane, 1999);
inhibiting inappropriate responses to prepotent stimuli (Diamond, 1988, 1990; Hasher &
Zacks, 1979; Roberts, Hager, & Heron, 1994); gating behaviorally irrelevant stimuli (Chao
& Knight, 1995); selecting among competing responses (Thompson-Schill, D'Esposito,
Aguirre, & Farah, 1997); and maintaining/refreshing information in a noisy environment
(Johnson, 1992). It is the complex interaction among storage, rehearsal, and extramnemonic
executive control processes that gives rise to the behavioral phenomenon of working
memory.

In this chapter, we review evidence from studies of patients with focal lesions and from
functional MRI (fMRI) studies of healthy human subjects that converge to suggest a model
of the neuroanatomical organization of working memory. This evidence supports the notion that posterior brain regions subserve storage processes contributing to working memory
capacity, and that prefrontal regions subserve rehearsal and executive control processes.

ANALYSIS OF STUDIES OF PATIENTS
WITH FOCAL FRONTAL LESIONS

Beginning with the classic studies of Jacobsen (1935, 1936) on delayed response in monkeys with large bilateral lesions of the prefrontal cortex (PFC), this region has been viewed
as critical for working memory performance, although the precise functions supported by
the PFC were difficult to specify (Warren & Akert, 1964). An important breakthrough
occurred when single-unit electrophysiological recording techniques were applied to the
PFC. Studies of delayed response revealed PFC neurons whose activity bridged the delay
period between target stimulus and go signal (Fuster & Alexander, 1971), and thus appeared to be a neural manifestation of the reverberatory activity that had been proposed
decades earlier as a mechanism of the short-term storage of information (Hebb, 1949).
Subsequent electrophysiological studies indicated that the delay-period activity of PFC
neurons could be restricted to specific types of stimuli, representing, for example, "memory
fields" of retinotopic space (Funahashi, Bruce, & Goldman-Rakic, 1990), by analogy to
receptive fields of cells in the visual system.

As we have indicated in our introduction, however, working memory is supported by
many theoretically dissociable mechanisms. To determine the contribution of the PFC to
the mnemonic components of working memory (i.e., to storage and rehearsal processes)
in humans, we analyzed reports of the performance of patients with lateral PFC lesions on
tests of working memory. We focused on published reports of group studies with simple
span and delayed-response tasks (D'Esposito & Postle, 1999). We selected these measures
because we believe that they offer reasonably direct measures of working memory storage
and rehearsal, respectively. Storage is measured in terms of capacity, and can be indexed
by span tasks: digit span for verbal working memory (Wechsler, 1945), and block span for
visuospatial working memory (Milner, 1971). Although we consider span tasks an index
of storage processes, it is important to note that these span tasks are not "pure" tests of
storage, because these tests also recruit rehearsal processes. This feature is manifested in
the "articulatory suppression effect" (Levy, 1971; Murray, 1968) and the "word length
effect" (Baddeley, Thomson, & Buchanan, 1975). These effects exemplify experimental
manipulations believed to tie up articulatory rehearsal resources, and the effect of each is
to decrease memory span. Such results provide reasonable evidence that rehearsal processes
contribute to performance on a span test. Nevertheless, patients with intact articulatory

abilities (and thus intact rehearsal) can have severely circumscribed spans (Vallar & Baddeley, 1984), suggesting that storage processes make a critical contribution to span performance. Digit span—a widely used clinical and experimental measure—is likely to minimize rehearsal processes, because subjects repeat the remembered information immediately following presentation.

As noted above, "rehearsal" refers to the processes necessary to refresh and maintain information held in working memory. Tests of delayed recognition are often used to measure rehearsal processes (Awh et al., 1996; Paulesu, Frith, & Frackowiak, 1993), because such tests tax a subject's ability to maintain information over a period of time. The typical delayed-recognition task presents one or a few stimulus items to be remembered at the beginning of a trial, conceals the stimuli during a delay period, and then probes memory for the stimulus (or stimuli) at the end of the trial by requiring the classification of a newly presented stimulus as an identity match or nonmatch with the memorandum. In contrast to span tests, delayed-recognition tests rarely require memory for a large number of items, and thus do not provide a measure of working memory storage capacity. Conversely, because delayed-recognition tests *always* require maintenance of information across intervals that exceed the passive decay properties of working memory storage, these tests necessarily index rehearsal.

Span and delayed-recognition tasks have the additional feature that they are relatively uncontaminated by the extramnemonic executive control processes that can contribute to performance on more complex tests of working memory. That is, neither simple span nor simple delayed-recognition tests place appreciable demands on such functions as shifting attention among items held in working memory, reordering or otherwise manipulating these items, or inhibiting responses to the most prepotent among them. More complex working memory tasks, such as *n*-back (Gevins & Cutillo, 1993; see Jonides et al., 1997b, and Postle, Stern, Rosen, & Corkin, 2000, for task analyses), self-ordered pointing (Petrides & Milner, 1982), reading span (Daneman & Carpenter, 1980), and operation span (Turner & Engle, 1989), by contrast, require the involvement of such extramnemonic control functions for their successful performance. And because these tasks can require the simultaneous function of mnemonic and extramnemonic processes, performance on them typically reflects important contributions from both these types of processes. Therefore, these complex working memory tasks can be ill suited for the purpose of isolating the mnemonic role of the PFC. For all these reasons, in this chapter span measures serve as an acceptable operationalization of working memory storage processes, and delayed-recognition measures serve as an acceptable operationalization of working memory rehearsal processes.

Our literature review, spanning the years from 1960 to 1997, uncovered eight group studies reporting digit span results that used the standardized procedures of the Wechsler Adult Intelligence Scale—Revised (Wechsler, 1981). None of the reports of digit span found a statistically significant deficit in patients with frontal lobe lesions (total number of patients from the eight studies = 115), as compared to groups of normal control subjects. It can be seen from Figure 17.1 that the locations of the lesions in these studies do not appear to spare any portion of the PFC. Therefore, the consistently spared performance on span tasks cannot be linked reliably to any one spared region of the PFC. Importantly, one of the eight studies reporting the span performance of patients with PFC lesions also reported data from patients with posterior cortical lesions that spared the PFC (Ghent, Mishkin, & Teuber, 1962). The patients with posterior lesions, in contrast to patients with PFC lesions, were impaired on the test of digit span, with the left-hemisphere group demonstrating the largest impairment. This result is consistent with reports linking impaired span performance with lesions of the left inferior parietal lobe (Vallar & Papagno, 1995).

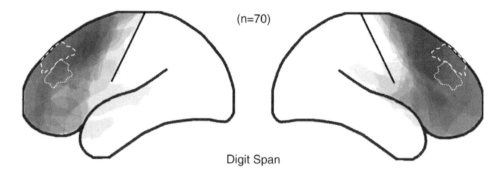

FIGURE 17.1. Composite diagrams illustrating extent of PFC lesions in patients showing no deficit in digit span performance, from four of the eight studies reviewed that published imaging data amenable to our lesion overlap technique (D'Esposito & Postle, 1999). Areas with overlapping lesions appear darker. Dashed line denotes Brodmann's area 9; dotted line denotes area 46. From D'Esposito and Postle (1999). Copyright 1999 by Elsevier Science. Adapted by permission.

Our review of studies of performance on delayed-recognition tasks in patients with PFC lesions encompassed seven reports, many featuring multiple experiments that varied stimulus materials. Also, in some studies the delay interval was filled with a distraction. Patients in only three of the nine experiments that employed delay periods without distraction were significantly impaired relative to normal control subjects, as contrasted with significant impairment of patient performance in four of the six experiments that featured distraction during the delay period. Three studies of delayed recognition that included patients with posterior lesions found no evidence of delayed-recognition impairment in these patients (Chao & Knight, 1995; Ghent et al., 1962; Verin et al., 1993). These results, paired with the report of impaired digit span in posterior-lesioned patients (Ghent et al., 1962), form a functional neuroanatomical double dissociation: They strengthen our claim that span tests (and thus working memory storage processes) exhibit greater dependence on posterior cortex, whereas delayed-recognition performance (and thus working memory rehearsal processes) exhibits a greater dependence on the PFC. Moreover, our review of the literature is consistent with the idea that the working memory function is not a unitary process, but comprises dissociable processes that are subserved by distinct neural circuitry.

Our literature review also suggests that the dependence of delayed-recognition performance on the PFC may increase with the presence of distraction during delay periods. This finding may be understood as a reflection of the effects of this manipulation on information processing demands: the rehearsal processes that suffice to support delayed-recognition function without distraction may require the mediation of other PFC-supported processes (such as executive control processes) when distraction during the delay interval presents a source of interference or attentional salience. The executive control processes that may be necessary to protect the contents of working memory against distraction, and rehearsal processes, may depend on the same or distinct regions of the lateral PFC. Patient studies performed to date have not been able to answer this question, either because the patients studied had lesions too large for this level of segregation of function to be assessed, or because the studies have not addressed this question. A review of decades of neuropsychological research reveals that it is difficult for any single group of investigators to accumulate sufficient numbers of patients with lesions limited to discrete subregions of the lateral PFC to determine adequately whether these types of functional subdivisions exist. In contrast, the spatial resolution afforded by functional neuroimaging studies of healthy subjects allows one to probe whether functional subdivisions within the lateral PFC exist.

FMRI STUDIES OF WORKING MEMORY

Using fMRI, we tested the hypothesis that the processes supporting the strictly mnemonic demands of a letter working memory task can be dissociated anatomically from the processes supporting the extramnemonic control demands of the same task. As previously stated, we predicted that posterior perisylvian regions would be engaged by storage processes; that the PFC would be engaged by rehearsal and executive control processes; and, moreover, that different regions of the lateral PFC may be engaged by rehearsal and executive control processes. The preponderance of neuroimaging studies investigating the neural basis of working memory thus far have featured blocked experimental designs, and thus have not permitted direct assessment of the relative contributions of mnemonic and extramnemonic processes to cortical activation (Aguirre & D'Esposito, 1999; D'Esposito, Zarahn, & Aguirre, 1999). In the studies to be reviewed in the remainder of this chapter, we used an event-related fMRI approach for experimental design and analysis that permitted temporal isolation of the neural correlates of processes contributing to different components of the working memory task (i.e., target presentation/encoding, delay, probe/response; Postle, Zarahn, & D'Esposito, 2000; Zarahn, Aguirre, & D'Esposito, 1997).

In the first study (D'Esposito, Postle, Ballard, & Lease, 1999), the behavioral paradigm was a delayed-recognition task in which a set of five letters was presented simultaneously, in a randomly determined order, followed immediately by an instruction cue ("Forward" or "Alphabetize"). After the cue, there was an 8-second delay during which only a fixation cross appeared on the screen, followed by a probe that subjects evaluated against the memory set, indicating "match" or "nonmatch" with a button press. Thus subjects were presented with two types of trials (in random order) in which they were required either to (1) *maintain* a randomly ordered sequence of five letters across a delay period, or (2) *manipulate* a comparable sequence of letters by arranging them into alphabetical order during the delay period. In both conditions, the probe consisted of a letter and number. In the maintenance condition, subjects were instructed to determine whether the letter had been in the ordinal position represented by the number. This condition, therefore, simply required retention of the letters in the same format as presented at the beginning of the trial. In the manipulation condition, subjects were instructed to determine whether the probe letter would be in the ordinal position represented by the probe number if the items in the memory set had been rearranged into alphabetical order. This condition, therefore, required subjects to transpose the order of the five items presented at the beginning of the trial during the delay period.

In each subject, activity during the delay period was found throughout the lateral PFC in both types of trials. However, in every subject only activity within the dorsolateral PFC (and not the ventrolateral PFC) was significantly greater in trials during which information held in working memory was manipulated (see Figure 17.2). Thus our results were broadly consistent with a two-stage processing model of the organization of working memory function in the PFC, in that they revealed a consistently greater contribution of the dorsolateral than the ventrolateral PFC to the alphabetization process—one type of extramnemonic control process.

The second event-related fMRI study of maintenance versus manipulation of letters replicated the results of the first such study, providing corroborative evidence for dorso-

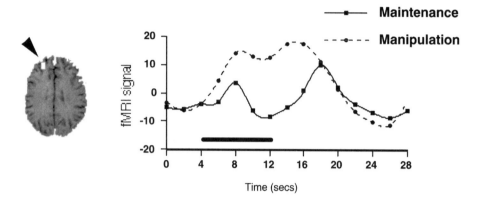

FIGURE 17.2. Trial-averaged time series from voxels that were significant in the direct contrast between manipulation and maintenance in a representative subject. Note the two peaks in the maintenance condition, corresponding to the stimulus presentation and the probe periods of the trial. In the manipulation condition, by contrast, the voxel displayed maintained a high level of activity throughout the delay period. The solid bar represents the duration of the delay period. From D'Esposito, Postle, Ballard, and Lease (1999). Copyright 1999 by Academic Press. Adapted by permission.

and ventrolateral PFC activity during the delay period of working memory maintenance trials, and consistently greater activity during manipulation trials only in the dorsolateral PFC (Postle, Berger, & D'Esposito, 1999). This second study also extended our earlier results in two important ways. First, it established that the maintenance–manipulation organization of the dorsolateral PFC is not confounded by differences in difficulty, because performance on "Forward" and "Alphabetize" trials (each presenting five letters) was equivalent. Second, the inclusion of a condition requiring maintenance ("Forward") of two letters permitted investigation of working memory load effects. We did not find consistent delay-specific load effects in the dorsolateral PFC, and, importantly, there was no evidence of delay-specific load effects in any voxels that showed greater manipulation than maintenance activity. Delay-specific load effects were observed, however, in the left posterior perisylvian cortex of each of the five subjects in this study.

These results, therefore, provided the first evidence that the manipulation-related processes ascribed to the dorsolateral PFC are fundamentally extramnemonic in nature. That is, whereas they play an important role in the exercise of executive control of working memory, they do not govern the storage per se of the information held in working memory. Indeed, the alphabetization-related processes required by our manipulation working memory trials are probably the same as those required when one alphabetizes a string of letters that are present on a piece of paper throughout the trial (i.e., in a task that does not require working memory). This result has implications not only for hierarchical processing models of the organization of working memory function in the PFC (Petrides, 1994), but also for the interpretation of "load effects" observed in the PFC in experiments that manipulate parametrically the number of items maintained in an *n*-back task (Braver et al., 1997; Cohen et al., 1997; Jonides et al., 1997a). Such effects may be attributable to extramnemonic processes contributing to performance of these tasks (e.g., attention shifting and/or inhibiting prepotent responses), rather than to information storage or maintenance processes. They may also reflect variation of memory-encoding and memory-scanning demands with load (Rypma & D'Esposito, 1999). This interpretation is broadly consistent with the conclusions we have drawn from the neuropsychology literature, reviewed earlier in this chapter.

The results from this study also indicated that truly mnemonic load effects were only observed reliably in the left posterior perisylvian cortex—a finding replicated in our laboratory (Rypma & D'Esposito, 1999). This result is also consistent with what the neuropsychology literature has told us about working memory storage of verbal material: that it is independent of the PFC and likely to be dependent on posterior perisylvian regions associated with the representation of abstract numerical and linguistic codes.

CONCLUSION

Our review of studies of patients with focal cortical lesions is consistent with the broad view that posterior brain regions subserve storage functions contributing to working memory capacity, and that prefrontal regions subserve rehearsal and executive control processes. The fMRI data extend and refine this notion by providing evidence for a functional neuroanatomical double dissociation of storage and extramnemonic executive control processes that contribute to the storage and manipulation, respectively, of information in memory. Moreover, they provide evidence that rehearsal and executive control processes are supported by distinct regions of the lateral PFC. These findings are thus consistent with our view that working memory function arises from the coordinated recruitment of several independent cognitive processes, which are differentially engaged depending on the demands of the particular task. Finally, it is important to note that PFC-supported extramnemonic executive control processes, in particular, probably influence other cognitive systems such as long-term memory (see the fMRI studies presented by Wagner in Chapter 14 of this volume, and the description of memory deficits in patients with frontal lobe pathology by Schacter, 1987). This notion highlights the interactive relationship between memory systems (Fuster, 1995).

The empirical results presented here can be used to constrain information-processing models and neurophysiological models of working memory. The fMRI studies alone, however, cannot be taken as conclusive evidence about the necessary neural substrates of storage, rehearsal, and control processes. The inference of the necessity of a brain area to a particular function cannot be made without a demonstration that the inactivation of a brain system disrupts the function in question (Sarter, Berntson, & Cacioppo, 1996). Such evidence comes from the neuropsychological studies of patients with focal lesions that we have reviewed in this chapter. Thus converging evidence supports the notions that the left posterior perisylvian cortex represents a critical neural substrate for short-term storage of verbal information; that rehearsal of this information is associated with activation in the left ventral PFC (Awh et al., 1996; Jonides et al., 1998; Paulesu et al., 1993); and that manipulation of this information can be carried out by executive control processes that are dependent on dorsolateral PFC (D'Esposito & Postle, 2000; Postle et al., 1999). Moreover, within the ventral PFC, there may be further functional subdivisions depending on the type of information being maintained (e.g., semantic vs. phonological or verbal vs. spatial; see Wagner, Chapter 14, this volume, and Postle & D'Esposito, 2000). Also, components of working memory such as rehearsal and executive control processes may be differentially influenced by subcortical modulatory systems, such as the dopaminergic system (D'Esposito & Postle, 2000). The combined application of methods of disruption (e.g., lesion and transcranial magnetic stimulation; Walsh & Rushworth, 1999) and physiological measurement (e.g., fMRI, event-related potentials, and magnetoencephalography) represents a powerful means of testing and refining cognitive neuroscientific models of complex behavioral phenomena such as working memory.

ACKNOWLEDGMENTS

This research was supported by National Institutes of Health Grants No. NS01762, No. AG13483, No. AG15793, and No. AG09253, and by the American Federation for Aging Research.

REFERENCES

Aguirre, G. K., & D'Esposito, M. (1999). Experimental design for brain fMRI. In C. T. W. Moonen & P. A. Bandettini (Eds.), *Functional MRI* (pp. 369–380). Berlin: Springer-Verlag.

Awh, E., Jonides, J., Smith, E. E., Schumacher, E. H., Koeppe, R. A., & Katz, S. (1996). Dissociation of storage and rehearsal in verbal working memory: Evidence from PET. *Psychological Science, 7,* 25–31.

Baddeley, A. (1992). Working memory. *Science, 255,* 556–559.

Baddeley, A. D., Thomson, N., & Buchanan, M. (1975). Word length and the structure of short-term memory. *Journal of Verbal Learning and Verbal Behavior, 14,* 575–589.

Braver, T. S., Cohen, J. D., Nystrom, L. E., Jonides, J., Smith, E. E., & Noll, D. C. (1997). A parametric study of prefrontal cortex involvement in human working memory. *NeuroImage, 5,* 49–62.

Chao, L. L., & Knight, R. T. (1995). Human prefrontal lesions increase distractibility to irrelevant sensory inputs. *NeuroReport, 6,* 1605–1610.

Cohen, J. D., Perlstein, W. M., Braver, T. S., Nystrom, L. E., Noll, D. C., Jonides, J., & Smith, E. E. (1997). Temporal dynamics of brain activation during a working memory task. *Nature, 386,* 604–607.

Courtney, S. M., Ungerleider, L. G., Keil, K., & Haxby, J. V. (1997). Transient and sustained activity in a distributed neural system for human working memory. *Nature, 386,* 608–611.

D'Esposito, Aguirre, G. K., Zarahn, E., & Ballard, D. (1998). Functional MRI studies of spatial and non-spatial working memory. *Cognitive Brain Research, 7,* 1–13.

D'Esposito, M., & Postle, B. R. (1999). The dependence of span and delayed-response performance on prefrontal cortex. *Neuropsychologia, 37,* 89–101.

D'Esposito, M., & Postle, B. R. (2000). Neural correlates of component processes of working memory: Evidence from neuropsychological and pharmacological studies. In S. Monsell & J. Driver (Eds.), *Attention and performance XVIII: Control of cognitive processes* (pp. 579–602). Cambridge, MA: MIT Press.

D'Esposito, M., Postle, B. R., Ballard, D., & Lease, J. (1999). Maintenance versus manipulation of information held in working memory: An event-related fMRI study. *Brain and Cognition, 41,* 66–86.

D'Esposito, M., Postle, B. R., Jonides, J., & Smith, E. E. (1999). The neural substrate and temporal dynamics of interference effects in working memory as revealed by event-related functional MRI. *Proceedings of the National Academy of Sciences USA, 96,* 7514–7519.

D'Esposito, M., Zarahn, E., & Aguirre, G. K. (1999). Event-related functional MRI: Implications for cognitive psychology. *Psychological Bulletin, 125,* 155–164.

Daneman, M., & Carpenter, P. A. (1980). Individual differences in working memory and reading. *Journal of Verbal Learning and Verbal Behavior, 19,* 450–466.

Diamond, A. (1988). Differences between adult and infant cognition: Is the crucial variable presence or absence of language? In L. Weiskrantz (Ed.), *Thought without language* (pp. 337–370). Oxford: Oxford University Press.

Diamond, A. (1990). The development and neural bases of memory functions as indexed by the A-not-B and delayed response tasks in human infants and infant monkeys. *Annals of the New York Academy of Sciences, 68,* 267–317.

Funahashi, S., Bruce, C. J., & Goldman-Rakic, P. S. (1990). Visuospatial coding in primate prefrontal neurons revealed by oculomotor paradigms. *Journal of Neurophysiology, 63,* 814–831.

Fuster, J. M. (1995). *Memory in the cerebral cortex.* Cambridge, MA: MIT Press.

Fuster, J. M., & Alexander, G. E. (1971). Neuron activity related to short-term memory. *Science*, *173*, 652–654.

Garavan, H. (1998). Serial attention within working memory. *Memory and Cognition*, *26*, 263–276.

Gevins, A. S., & Cutillo, B. S. (1993). Neuroelectric evidence for distributed processing in human working memory. *Electroencephalography and Clinical Neurophysiology*, *87*, 128–143.

Ghent, L., Mishkin, M., & Teuber, H.-L. (1962). Short-term memory after frontal-lobe injury in man. *Journal of Comparative and Physiological Psychology*, *5*, 705–709.

Halbig, T., Mecklinger, A., Schriefers, H., & Friederici, A. (1998). Double dissociation of processing temporal and spatial information in working memory. *Neuropsychologia*, *36*, 305–311.

Hasher, L., & Zacks, R. T. (1979). Automatic and effortful processes in memory. *Journal of Experimental Psychology*, *108*, 356–388.

Hebb, D. O. (1949). *Organization of behavior*. New York: Wiley.

Jacobsen, C. F. (1935). Functions of frontal association areas in primates. *Archives of Neurology and Psychiatry*, *33*, 558–560.

Jacobsen, C. F. (1936). The functions of the frontal association areas in monkeys. *Comparative Psychology Monographs*, *13*, 1–60.

Johnson, M. K. (1992). MEM: Mechanisms of recollection. *Journal of Cognitive Neuroscience*, *4*, 268–280.

Jonides, J. (1995). Working memory and thinking. In E. E. Smith & D. N. Osherson (Eds.), *An invitation to cognitive science* (pp. 215–265). Cambridge, MA: MIT Press.

Jonides, J., Schumacher, E. H., Smith, E. E., Koeppe, R. A., Awh, E., Reuter-Lorenz, P. A., Marshuetz, C., & Willis, C. R. (1998). The role of parietal cortex in verbal working memory. *Journal of Neuroscience*, *18*, 5026–5034.

Jonides, J., Schumacher, E. H., Smith, E. E., Lauber, E., Awh, E., Minoshima, S., & Koeppe, R. A. (1997a). Verbal working memory load affects regional brain activation as measured by PET. *Journal of Cognitive Neuroscience*, *9*, 462–475.

Jonides, J., Schumacher, E. H., Smith, E. E., Lauber, E. J., Awh, E., Minoshima, S., & Koeppe, R. A. (1997b). Verbal working memory load affects regional brain activation as measured by PET. *Journal of Cognitive Neuroscience*, *9*, 462–475.

Levy, B. A. (1971). The role of articulation in articulatory and visual short-term memory. *Journal of Verbal Learning and Verbal Behavior*, *10*, 123–132.

May, C. P., Hasher, L., & Kane, M. J. (1999). The role of interference in memory span. *Memory and Cognition*, *27*, 759–767.

Miller, G. A., Galanter, E., & Pribram, K. H. (1960). *Plans and the structure of behavior*. New York: Holt.

Milner, B. (1971). Interhemispheric differences in the localization of psychological processes in man. *British Medical Bulletin*, *27*, 272–277.

Murray, D. J. (1968). Articulation and acoustic confusability in short-term memory. *Journal of Experimental Psychology*, *78*, 679–684.

Paulesu, E., Frith, C. D., & Frackowiak, R. S. (1993). The neural correlates of the verbal component of working memory. *Nature*, *362*, 342–345.

Petrides, M. (1994). Frontal lobes and working memory: Evidence from investigations of the effects of cortical excisions in nonhuman primates. In F. Boller & J. Grafman (Eds.), *Handbook of neuropsychology* (Vol. 9, pp. 59–82). Amsterdam: Elsevier.

Petrides, M., & Milner, B. (1982). Deficits on subject-oriented tasks after frontal- and temporal-lobe lesions in man. *Neuropsychologia*, *20*, 249–262.

Postle, B. R., Berger, J. S., & D'Esposito, M. (1999). Functional neuroanatomical double dissociation of mnemonic and executive control processes contributing to working memory performance. *Proceedings of the National Academy of Sciences USA*, *96*, 12959–12964.

Postle, B. R., & D'Esposito, M. (1998). Homologous cognitive mechanisms and neural substrates underlie dissociable components of set-shifting and task-switching phenomena. *Society for Neuroscience Abstracts*, *24*, 507.

Postle, B. R., & D'Esposito, M. (2000). Evaluating models of the topographical organization of working memory function in frontal cortex with event-related fMRI. *Psychobiology, 28,* 132–145.

Postle, B. R., Jonides, J., Smith, E., Corkin, S., & Growdon, J. H. (1997). Spatial, but not object, delayed response is impaired in early Parkinson's disease. *Neuropsychology, 11,* 1–9.

Postle, B. R., Stern, C. E., Rosen, B. R., & Corkin, S. (2000). An fMRI investigation of cortical contributions to spatial and nonspatial visual working memory. *NeuroImage, 11,* 409–423.

Postle, B. R., Zarahn, E., & D'Esposito, M. (2000). Using event-related fMRI to assess delay-period activity during performance of spatial and nonspatial working memory tasks. *Brain Research Protocols, 5,* 57–66.

Roberts, R. J., Hager, L. D., & Heron, C. (1994). Prefrontal cognitive processes: Working memory and inhibition in the antisaccade task. *Journal of Experimental Psychology: General, 123,* 374–393.

Rogers, R. D., & Monsell, S. (1995). Costs of a predictable switch between simple cognitive tasks. *Journal of Experimental Psychology: General, 124,* 207–231.

Rypma, B., & D'Esposito, M. (1999). The roles of prefrontal brain regions in components of working memory: Effects of memory load and individual differences. *Proceedings of the National Academy of Sciences USA, 96,* 6558–6563.

Sarter, M., Berntson, G. G., & Cacioppo, J. T. (1996). Brain imaging and cognitive neuroscience: Toward strong inference in attributing function to structure. *American Psychologist, 51,* 13–21.

Schacter, D. L. (1987). Memory, amnesia, and frontal lobe dysfunction. *Psychobiology, 15,* 21–36.

Smith, E. E., & Jonides, J. (1999). Storage and executive processes of the frontal lobes. *Science, 283,* 1657–1661.

Thompson-Schill, S. L., D'Esposito, M., Aguirre, G. K., & Farah, M. J. (1997). Role of left inferior prefrontal cortex in retrieval of semantic knowledge: A reevaluation. *Proceedings of the National Academy of Sciences USA, 94,* 14792–14797.

Turner, M. L., & Engle, R. W. (1989). Is working memory capacity task dependent? *Journal of Memory and Language, 28,* 127–154.

Ungerleider, L. G. (1995). Functional brain imaging studies of cortical mechanisms for memory. *Science, 270,* 769–775.

Valler, G., & Baddeley, A. D. (1984). Fractionation of working memory: Neuropsychological evidence for a phonological short-term store. *Journal of Verbal Learning and Verbal Behavior, 23,* 151–161.

Vallar, G., & Papagno, C. (1995). Neuropsychological impairments of short-term memory. In A. D. Baddeley, B. A. Wilson, & F. N. Watts (Eds.), *Handbook of memory disorders* (pp. 135–165). Chichester, England: Wiley.

Verin, M., Partiot, A., Pillon, B., Malapani, C., Agid, Y., & Dubois, B. (1993). Delayed response tasks and prefrontal lesions in man: Evidence for self generated patterns of behavior with poor environmental modulation. *Neuropsychologia, 31,* 1379–1396.

Walsh, V., & Rushworth, M. (1999). A primer of magnetic stimulation as a tool for neuropsychology. *Neuropsychologia, 37,* 125–135.

Warren, J. M., & Akert, K. (Eds.). (1964). *The frontal granular cortex and behavior.* New York: McGraw-Hill.

Wechsler, D. (1945). A standardized memory scale for clinical use. *Journal of Psychology, 19,* 87–95.

Wechsler, D. (1981). *Wechsler Adult Intelligence Scale—Revised: Manual.* New York: Psychological Corporation.

Zarahn, E., Aguirre, G. K., & D'Esposito, M. (1997). A trial-based experimental design for functional MRI. *NeuroImage, 6,* 122–138.

Zarahn, E., Aguirre, G. K., & D'Esposito, M. (1999). Temporal isolation of the neural correlates of spatial mnemonic processing with fMRI. *Cognitive Brain Research, 7,* 255–268.

18

Functional Anatomy of Motor Skill Learning

JULIEN DOYON and LESLIE G. UNGERLEIDER

In everyday life, we use a variety of motor skills that have been acquired gradually through practice and interactions with our environment. These skills include, for example, the use of smooth coarticulation of finger movements into a specific sequence (e.g., playing a musical instrument like the piano), regular multijoint movement synergies (e.g., reaching for and grasping small objects), and smoothly executed eye–body coordinated actions (e.g., playing sports such as golf). In order to study in the laboratory the cognitive processes and the neural substrates mediating the ability to learn such skilled behaviors, investigators have used experimental paradigms that fall into two categories. The first measures the incremental acquisition of movements into a well-executed behavior ("motor sequence learning"), whereas the second tests the capacity to compensate for environmental changes ("motor adaptation") (e.g., Doyon, Owen, Petrides, Sziklas, & Evans, 1996; Flament, Ellermann, Kim, Ugurbil, & Ebner, 1996; Grafton, Hazeltine, & Ivry, 1995; Grafton, Woods, & Mike, 1994; Karni et al., 1995, 1998; Shadmehr & Brashers-Krug, 1994; Shadmehr & Holcomb, 1997). Operationally defined, these two forms of motor skill learning refer to the process by which movements, produced either alone or in a sequence, come to be performed effortlessly through repeated practice (Willingham, 1998).

In both animals and humans, motor skill learning is usually measured by a reduction in reaction time and errors, and/or by a change in movement synergy and kinematics (e.g., Doyon et al., 1997, 1998; Hikosaka, Rand, Miyachi, & Miyashita, 1995; Shadmehr & Brashers-Krug, 1997; for reviews, see Doyon, 1997; Karni, 1996; Squire, 1992). For some skills, such as learning to play a new melody on a musical instrument, early learning can be facilitated by using explicit knowledge (i.e., employing thought). For most motor skills, however, performance is ultimately overlearned to a point where it can be performed implicitly (i.e., without thought). As opposed to other forms of memory (e.g., episodic memory), these changes in performance are known to evolve slowly, requiring many repetitions over several training sessions (Karni, 1996; Squire, 1992). Indeed, psychophysical studies have demonstrated that the incremental acquisition of motor skills follows two distinct stages: (1) an early, fast learning stage in which considerable improvement in performance occurs within a single training session; and (2) a later, slow stage in which further gains occur across several sessions (and even weeks) of practice (Brashers-Krug, Shadmehr, & Bizzi,

1996; Karni et al., 1998; Nudo, Milliken, Jenkins, & Merzenich, 1996). In addition to these two stages, an intermediate, consolidation phase of motor skill acquisition has recently been proposed, as gains in performance have been reported following a latent period of more than 6 hours after the first training session without additional practice on the task (e.g., Jackson et al., 1997; Karni & Sagi, 1993). In addition, there is little or no interference from a competing task, provided that it is administered beyond a critical time window of about 4–6 hours (Brashers-Krug et al., 1996; Rey-Hipolito, Adams, Ungerleider, & Karni, 1997; Shadmehr & Brashers-Krug, 1997). Finally, with extended practice, the skilled behavior is thought to become resistant both to interference and to the simple passage of time. Once overlearned, a motor skill can thus be readily retrieved despite long periods without practice.

Based on animal and human work, several brain structures, including the striatum, cerebellum, and motor cortical regions of the frontal lobe, are thought to be critical for the acquisition and/or retention of skilled motor behaviors (for reviews, see, e.g., Bloedel, 1992a, 1992b; Doyon, 1997; Georgopoulos, 2000; Graybiel, 1995; Karni, 1996; Sanes & Donoghue, 2000; Thach, 1997; van Mier, 2000; Ungerleider, 1995). Anatomical studies have demonstrated that these cortical and subcortical structures form two distinct circuits: a cortico-striato-thalamo-cortical loop and a cortico-cerebello-thalamo-cortical loop (Middleton & Strick, 1997; Picard & Strick, 1996; Tanji, 1996) (see Figure 18.1). Evidence supporting the role of these cortical and subcortical systems in motor skill learning has come from impairments found in patients with striatal dysfunction (e.g., in Parkinson's or Huntington's disease), with damage to the cerebellum, or with a circumscribed lesion involving the frontal motor areas (e.g., Ackermann, Daum, Schugens, & Grodd, 1996; Doyon et al., 1997, 1998; Gabrieli, Stebbins, Singh, Willingham, & Goetz, 1997; Harrington, Haaland, Yeo, & Marder, 1990; Pascual-Leone et al., 1993; Sanes, Dimitrov, & Hallett, 1990; Willingham & Koroshetz, 1993). Further support has come from neurophysiological studies (e.g., Graybiel, Aosaki, Flaherty, & Kimura, 1994; Nudo, Milliken, et al., 1996; Tanji, 1996), as well as from lesion experiments in rodents (e.g., MacDonald & White, 1993; see White, 1997, for a review) and nonhuman primates (e.g., Lu, Hikosaka, & Miyachi, 1998; Milak, Shimansky, Bracha, & Bloedel, 1997). More recently, modern brain imaging techniques have confirmed the functional contribution of both corticostriatal and corticocerebellar systems in motor skill learning, and also identified *in vivo* the neural substrates mediating this type of memory and the functional dynamic changes that occur over the entire course of the acquisition process (for reviews, see, e.g., Doyon, 1997; Karni, 1996; van Mier, 2000; Ungerleider, 1995).

In the following sections, we discuss the results of a large body of studies in healthy human subjects that have examined the functional anatomy and the cerebral plasticity associated with motor skill learning using brain imaging technology, including positron emission tomography (PET) and functional magnetic resonance imaging (fMRI). Special emphasis is given to the results of studies that have used either motor sequence or motor adaptation paradigms, and to the role that both the corticostriatal and corticocerebellar systems play in these types of motor learning.

IMAGING MOTOR SKILL LEARNING

Reviews of studies investigating the neuroanatomy of motor skill learning have often pointed out the heterogeneity in the results obtained (Doyon, 1997; Grafton et al., 1995; van Mier, 2000). Several reasons may explain this variability in previous findings. First, many differ-

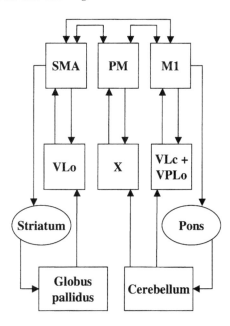

FIGURE 18.1. Diagram illustrating the major cortical and subcortical structures involved in motor skill learning, and their interconnections. These structures are organized into two main circuits: a cortico-striato-thalamo-cortical loop and a cortico-cerebello-thalamo-cortical loop. Dynamic changes within these loops occur during motor sequence learning and motor adaptation (see text for more details). Cortical regions: SMA, supplementary motor area; PM, premotor cortex; M1, primary motor cortex. Thalamic nuclei: Vlo, ventrolateral nucleus, oral division; X, area X; VLc, ventrolateral nucleus, caudal division; VPLo, ventroposterior nucleus, oral division.

ent training paradigms have been employed, which may require the acquisition of very different motor routines. Such diverse paradigms include learning to (1) repeat a sequence of finger or limb movements (Doyon et al., 1996; Grafton et al., 1995; Hazeltine, Grafton, & Ivry, 1997; Jenkins, Brooks, Nixon, Frackowiak, & Passingham, 1994; Jueptner, Frith, Brooks, Frackowiak, & Passingham, 1997; Rauch et al., 1995; Toni, Krams, Turner, & Passingham, 1998); (2) maintain contact between a metal stylus and a small target located on a disk that may rotate at different velocities (Grafton et al., 1992, 1994); (3) move a pen through a cutout maze by trial and error (van Mier, Tempel, Perlmutter, Raichle, & Petersen, 1998; Petersen, van Mier, Fiez, & Raichle, 1998); and (4) adapt to changes in the relationship between the movements of a joystick and those of a cursor on a screen (Flament et al., 1996; Imamizu et al., 2000), or to the force field applied to a robotic arm when pointing to visual targets (Krebs et al., 1998; Shadmehr & Holcomb, 1997, 1999).

A second source of variability in previous findings is that even when the same task is used, activations have been measured during conditions that elicit different cognitive processes. For example, in studies of motor sequence learning, some investigators have used an implicit form of learning during which subjects must acquire a sequence of movements through practice without knowledge of the sequence, whereas others have employed an explicit form of learning during which they are practicing a motor sequence for which they have complete declarative knowledge (e.g., Doyon et al., 1996; Grafton et al., 1995; Rauch et al., 1995). A third source of variability comes from the different baseline conditions that have been employed to control for nonspecific factors during learning, such as the sensory and purely motoric components of the task. To identify the neural network mediating the learning of motor sequences, for instance, some researchers have used simple rest as a baseline condition, whereas others either have used a random motor condition or have compared activity obtained in two separate phases (e.g., early vs. late) of the acquisition process (e.g., Doyon et al., 1996; Seitz, Roland, Bohm, Greitz, & Stone-Elander, 1990; Toni et al., 1998).

A fourth source of variability is that different experimental designs and data-analytic approaches have been employed. For example, when measuring the dynamic changes occurring during the fast phase of learning, some studies have used the standard subtraction design, in which the pattern of activity in the experimental condition is compared with that in a control condition—either rest or the same experimental condition at a different phase of learning (Doyon et al., 1996; Jenkins et al., 1994; Rauch et al., 1995, 1997). By contrast, others have exploited the use of a parametric design, in which cerebral structures are identified by their correlated activity with improved performance on the task over time (e.g., Friston, Frith, Passingham, Liddle, & Frackowiak, 1992; Grafton et al., 1995; Grafton, Hazeltine, & Ivry, 1998; Sakai et al., 1998; Toni et al., 1998).

Yet another source of variability is that across studies, subjects have been scanned at different phases of the learning process. Even in studies examining within-session (fast) learning, there is little consistency in the amount of practice subjects have received and the degree to which the motor skill has been acquired (e.g., Jenkins et al., 1994; Jueptner, Stephan, et al., 1997; Jueptner, Frith, et al., 1997). Finally, individual differences among subjects in their cognitive, perceptual, motoric, and learning abilities have typically been ignored both in the designs of imaging experiments and in analyses of the data. Such individual differences may interact with task demands, and thus produce variability in both behavioral and functional data as well as individual differences in the temporal course of learning (see Frutiger et al., 2000, for a more detailed discussion of this factor inherent in studies of motor skill learning).

Despite the many differences in methodological approaches used in imaging experiments of motor learning, much of the variability in the pattern of results across studies can be accounted for if one considers the type of motor task and the learning phase at which subjects are scanned. Here we propose that the corticocerebellar and corticostriatal systems contribute differentially to motor adaptation and motor sequence learning, respectively, and that this difference is most apparent at the end of the training period (i.e., during slow learning), when subjects achieve asymptotic performance.

FUNCTIONAL ANATOMY OF MOTOR ADAPTATION

Several studies have examined the neural systems that are involved in motor adaptation. Tasks have included target reaching with the upper limb, in which the relationship between movements of a manipulandum and movements of a cursor on a monitor is reversed (Flament et al., 1996; Imamizu et al., 2000), and pointing to a target with a robotic arm to which different force fields are applied (Krebs et al., 1998; Shadmehr & Holcomb, 1997, 1999). In these studies, subjects have been tested both early in the fast learning process and later, when they have achieved asymptotic performance on the task. In addition, in some studies, the relative changes in activation between sessions after variable time intervals have been considered in order to identify the cerebral structures mediating the memory consolidation (Shadmehr & Holcomb, 1997) or the long-term retention

(Nezafat, Shadmehr, & Holcomb, 2001) of skilled motor behaviors. Finally, a similar between-session paradigm has also been used to investigate subjects' abilities to inhibit competing motor memories during learning of a novel motor task (Shadmehr & Holcomb, 1999).

In a series of PET studies, Shadmehr and Holcomb (1997, 1999) found that at the beginning of the acquisition process, the capacity of subjects to adapt to a perturbing force field when reaching to randomly presented targets with a robotic arm was associated with increased activity in the left putamen and dorsolateral prefrontal cortex (DLPFC) bilaterally. Later in the fast learning phase of the first training session, when subjects failed to show further gains in performance, decreased activity in the putamen was seen. This pattern of findings in the striatum has been corroborated by Krebs and colleagues (1998), who have used a similar force field task with PET. In the latter study, early (fast) learning was associated with activations in the ventral striatum, as well as in the contralateral primary sensory cortex and bilateral parietal association areas. By contrast, when the skill was well learned and the subjects produced smooth reaching movements, there was a shift of activity from the striatum and parietal areas to the left motor and premotor regions and to the right cerebellar cortex. This shift suggests that the corticostriatal circuit contributes more importantly during early motor adaptation learning, whereas the corticocerebellar circuit plays a more critical role during late adaptation learning.

The distinct contribution of the cerebellum to motor adaptation has also been studied by Imamizu and colleagues (2000) and by Flament and colleagues (1996) with fMRI technology, using tasks in which subjects are required to adjust to a change in their sensorimotor coordinate system. Both groups of researchers found an inverse relationship between the subjects' level of performance and the extent of cerebellar activation: Better performance on the task was associated with decreased activity in the cerebellum, supporting the notion that this structure participates in the detection and correction of errors. In addition, however, these studies showed a sustained increase in activity in specific areas of the cerebellum with continued practice—that is, in an area near the posterior superior fissure in Imamizu and colleagues (2000) (see Figure 18.2), and possibly in the dentate nucleus in Flament and colleagues (1996). This increase suggests that these cerebellar regions may be part of the neuronal system engaged in the creation of a long-term representation of the skilled movements necessary to execute these motor adaptation tasks proficiently.

FUNCTIONAL ANATOMY OF MOTOR SEQUENCE LEARNING

In brain imaging investigations designed to clarify the neuroanatomy of motor skill learning, subjects are typically required to produce a sequence of movements that they know explicitly before scanning (Doyon et al., 1999; Karni et al., 1995, 1998; Schlaug, Knorr, & Seitz, 1994; Seitz et al., 1990), to discover a particular sequence by trial and error (Jenkins et al., 1994; Jueptner, Frith, et al., 1997; Jueptner, Stephan, et al., 1997; Sakai et al., 1998; Toni et al., 1998), or to follow the display of visual stimuli appearing sequentially on a screen (Doyon et al., 1997, 1999; Grafton et al., 1995; Hazeltine et al., 1997; Rauch et al., 1995, 1997). The motor responses in those tasks involve finger-to-thumb opposition movements (e.g., Karni et al., 1995, 1998; Seitz et al., 1990), finger presses on response boxes (e.g., Grafton et al., 1995; Rauch et al., 1995, 1997), or movements of the whole arm (e.g., Doyon et al., 1996; Grafton et al., 1998). However, other sequence tasks, including rotor pursuit (Grafton et al., 1992, 1994), the tracing of cutout mazes (van Mier et al., 1998), and the practice of

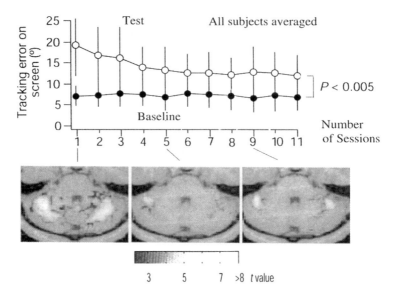

FIGURE 18.2. Behavioral and neural changes associated with learning a motor adaptation task, during which subjects moved a cursor with a computer mouse to reach a randomly moving target on a screen. During the test period, the cursor appeared in a position rotated 120 degrees around the center of the screen, whereas in the baseline period, the cursor was not rotated. *Top:* Mean tracking errors over the training sessions. *Bottom: t*-statistic maps showing two types of changes in learning-dependent activity within the cerebellum. One is spread over wide areas of the cerebellum, but decreases proportionally with the reduction in error signal that guides the acquisition of this skill; the second is located in an area near the posterior superior fissure and remains stable even after subjects have reached asymptotic performance (see session 9). Adapted from Imamizu et al. (2000). Copyright 2000 by Nature Publishing Group. Adapted by permission.

repeating two-dimensional trajectory movements (Seitz et al., 1994), have also been employed in previous brain imaging studies to examine this form of motor learning.

In studies using such paradigms, changes in activity in both the corticostriatal and corticocerebellar circuits have been reported. For example, activity in the striatum and the cerebellum has been associated with both the encoding of motor sequence programs (e.g., Doyon et al., 1996; Grafton et al., 1995; Jenkins et al., 1994; Jueptner, Frith, et al., 1997; Rauch et al., 1995; Schlaug et al., 1994; Seitz et al., 1990; Toni et al., 1998) and the retrieval of learned sequences of movements (Boecker et al., 1998; Jenkins et al., 1994; Jueptner, Frith, et al., 1997). On the few occasions in which learning-related activation in the cerebellum has not been observed (Grafton et al., 1992, 1995; Rauch et al., 1995), it has been hypothesized that the negative findings result from the limited field of view of the PET camera, thereby precluding full visualization of the inferior portions of this structure (Doyon, 1997; van Mier, 2000). Either the striatum or the cerebellum or both, in concert with motor cortical regions, have also been activated during implicit learning (Doyon et al., 1996; Grafton et al., 1995; Rauch et al., 1995, 1997), when subjects are practicing a motor sequence for which they have complete explicit knowledge (Doyon et al., 1999; Grafton et al., 1995; Schlaug et al., 1994; Seitz et al., 1990; Toni et al., 1998). These regions have also been activated during tasks in which subjects need to utilize problem-solving strategies to find a repeating sequence of finger movements (Jenkins et al., 1994; Jueptner, Frith, et al., 1997; Toni et al., 1998).

Changes in activity in both the striatum and cerebellum have also been observed at different stages of the acquisition process of motor sequence learning. Studies have demonstrated that the cerebellum is active during the fast learning phase (e.g., Doyon et al., 1996; Jenkins et al., 1994). However, this activity decreases with practice and may become undetectable when the sequential movements are well learned (Doyon et al., 1999; Friston et al., 1992; Grafton et al., 1994; Jueptner, Frith, et al., 1997; Seitz et al., 1994; Toni et al., 1998). Some investigators have reported striatal activations as well in the early acquisition phase of motor sequence learning, when subjects have to rely more strongly on the use of cognitive strategies and working memory (Jenkins et al., 1994; Jueptner, Frith, et al., 1997; Toni et al., 1998). However, the results of other studies have shown that the striatum is significantly more activated when subjects have reached asymptotic performance on the task than at the beginning of the acquisition process (e.g., Doyon et al., 1996; Grafton et al., 1994; Jueptner, Frith, et al., 1997). Furthermore, unlike the pattern of activity changes in the cerebellum, no decrease in striatal activity is observed with extended practice. Together, the latter findings suggest that the striatum (and motor cortical areas discussed below) may be critical for the long-term storage of well-learned sequences of movements.

Evidence to support the role of the corticostriatal system in memory storage comes from a PET study by Grafton and colleagues (1994), who scanned subjects on two separate occasions: (1) on day 1, while they were learning to keep a stylus on a rotating disk (rotary pursuit task); and (2) on day 2, after they had completed an extensive practice session on the task. On day 1, learning-dependent changes were observed in the ipsilateral anterior cerebellum and parasagittal vermal area. Additional activations were seen in the primary motor cortex (M1) contralaterally, in the supplementary motor area (SMA) bilaterally, and in the cingulate and inferior parietal regions. By contrast, on day 2, after the subjects had received additional practice and achieved an asymptotic level of performance, activations were observed in the putamen bilaterally, as well as in the parietal cortex bilaterally and the left inferior premotor area, but not in the cerebellum.

Other evidence supporting the role of the corticostriatal system in storing well-learned behaviors come from our recent fMRI study (Doyon et al., 1999). Subjects were scanned during motor sequence learning using a version of the serial reaction time task, in which they were required to press as quickly as possible one of four buttons corresponding to the location of a red circle that appeared on a screen. The stimuli either were presented in an unpredictable order (random condition) or followed a repeating 10-item sequence of movements that was taught to each subject prior to scanning (explicit learning condition). Subjects were scanned over three separate sessions, with intervening periods of practice of the 10-item sequence administered just prior to the second and third scan sessions. As a group, the subjects showed consistent improvement in executing the sequence of finger movements across scanning sessions (see Figure 18.3) and attained the slow learning phase, as their level of performance became stable in session 3. Analysis of the functional imaging data in the early phase of learning revealed activations in the cerebellum, as well as in the right anterior cingulate, dorsal premotor, and inferior parietal regions. At the end of session 3, however, these cerebellar and cortical regions showed significant reductions in activity, whereas right-hemispheric activations were now observed in the striatum (see Figure 18.3), as well as in the SMA, ventrolateral prefrontal cortex, precuneus, and inferior parietal area. The latter findings suggest that when a sequence of movements is well learned and its execution has become "automatic," a distributed neural system composed of the striatum and related motor cortical regions, but not the cerebellum, may be sufficient to express and retain the learned behavior.

Changes in Striatum During Motor Sequence Learning

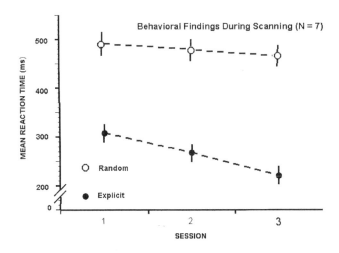

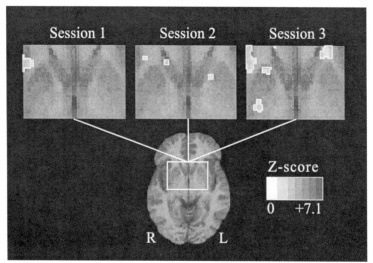

FIGURE 18.3. Behavioral and neural changes associated with performance of a task requiring motor sequence learning, during which subjects pressed as quickly as possible one of four buttons corresponding to the location of a visual stimulus that appeared either randomly, or in a repeating sequence that they knew explicitly prior to scanning (see text for more details). The subjects were scanned over three separate sessions, with intervening periods of practice administered just before the second and third scan sessions. *Top:* A repeated analysis of variance revealed that subjects improved their ability to execute the finger sequence in both the explicit and random conditions ($p < .01$), but that their level of improvement in reaction time across sessions was greater in the explicit than in the random condition ($p < .05$). *Bottom:* Z-score maps showing the dynamic changes in activity in the striatum over the three sessions of scanning. Significant activity in the striatum was observed in session 3 only, when subjects attained high levels of performance on this task.

CHANGES IN MOTOR REPRESENTATIONS
OVER THE COURSE OF LEARNING

A very limited number of imaging studies have investigated the changes in motor representation that occur in the brain over the entire course of motor learning (Grafton et al., 1994; Karni et al., 1995, 1998; Toni et al., 1998). Consequently, little is known about the neural circuitry mediating the acquisition of new motor skills that become fully mastered (i.e., completely automatic). Furthermore, the relative contribution of the corticostriatal and corticocerebellar systems during the consolidation and long-term retention of motor skills remains largely unknown. Nevertheless, one indisputable finding emerging from the studies reviewed above is that practice of a motor task elicits plastic neuronal changes in both cortical and subcortical structures within these two circuits.

A few investigators have proposed that modifications in the representation of motor skills with learning occur within the same cerebral structures used to execute the task. Evidence supporting such a model of plasticity comes from a PET study by Grafton and colleagues (1992), who showed that learning-dependent changes associated with performance of a rotorary pursuit task were located in areas that were part of a more distributed network active during motor execution. Additional evidence stems from Karni and colleagues (1995, 1998), who have reported the emergence of a specific, more extensive representation of a trained motor sequence in the contralateral M1 after 4 weeks of practice on a sequence of finger movements. Finally, the results from Nudo and colleagues (Nudo, Milliken, et al., 1996; Nudo, Wise, SiFuentes, & Milliken, 1996) using conventional intracortical microstimulation techniques in squirrel monkeys are also in accord with this view, inasmuch as the distal forelimb zone of M1 was found to undergo significant changes in cortical representation following extended practice on a reach-and-grasp task requiring skilled finger manipulations.

There is also evidence supporting an alternative view—namely, that the acquisition of motor skills produces representational changes in different cerebral structures over the course of learning (e.g., Doyon, 1997). This model of cerebral plasticity suggests that representational changes depend not only on the stage of learning, but also on whether subjects are required to learn a new sequence of movements or learn to adapt to environmental perturbations. We propose that early in learning, during the fast learning phase, both motor sequence and motor adaptation tasks recruit similar cerebral structures: the striatum, cerebellum, and motor cortical regions (e.g., the premotor cortex, SMA, pre-SMA, and anterior cingulate), as well as prefrontal and parietal areas. Dynamic interactions between these structures are likely to be critical for establishing the motor routines necessary to learn the skilled motor behavior. As learning progresses, however, representational changes can be observed. For example, Krebs and colleagues (1998) have demonstrated that learning to adapt to a force field first elicits activation in the striatum, which is followed by a change of activity in the cerebellum; others (e.g., Doyon et al., 1999; Grafton et al., 1994) have shown that during motor sequence learning, the cerebellar contribution to the task precedes that of the striatum. Finally, when a task is well learned and asymptotic performance is achieved, the representation of the motor skill may be distributed in a network of structures that involves either the corticocerebellar or the corticostriatal circuit, depending on the type of learning acquired.

We suggest that at this final stage of motor adaptation, the striatum is no longer necessary for the retention and execution of the acquired skill; regions representing the skill will now involve the cerebellum and related cortical regions. By contrast, a reverse pattern of plasticity is proposed to occur in motor sequence learning, such that with extended practice the cerebellum is no longer essential, and the long-lasting retention of the skill will now involve representational changes in the striatum and its associated motor cortical regions.

At the level of the cortex, the evidence thus far indicates that significant experience-related functional reorganization develops within specific motor and associative areas (e.g., Classen, Liepert, Wise, Hallett, & Cohen, 1998; Doyon et al., 1999; Jueptner, Frith, et al., 1997; Karni et al., 1995, 1998; Tanji & Shima, 1996). In most imaging studies, decreases in activity have been observed in the DLPFC as subjects acquire both motor adaptation and motor sequence skills (e.g., Doyon et al., 1999; Seitz et al., 1990; Shadmehr & Holcomb, 1997, 1999). Although scarce, the imaging data on motor adaptation suggest that a consolidated representation of this ability may include the dorsal premotor cortex and posterior parietal regions (Shadmehr & Holcomb, 1997). On the other hand, findings from motor sequence learning studies indicate that the creation of a long-term representation of this skill necessitates, at the very least, the contribution of both the SMA and M1 (Classen et al., 1998; Gordon, Lee, Flament, Ugurbil, & Ebner, 1998; Karni et al., 1995, 1998; Hund-Georgiadis & von Cramon, 1999).

The model of cerebral plasticity during motor learning that we have proposed generates predictions that can be tested experimentally. For example, based on the results from Shadmehr and Holcomb (1997), who have shown that the cerebellum is critical for consolidating adaptation learning, and those from Imamizu and colleagues (2000), who have demonstrated that this structure constitutes a storage site for this form of motor memory, one would expect that the striatum would play an equally important role in the consolidation of movement sequences, because this structure is known to contribute to the development and maintenance of the final representation of this skill. At present, however, this remains a working hypothesis, awaiting experimental investigation.

ACKNOWLEDGMENTS

We wish to thank Miriam Beauchamp, Eva Gutierrez, and Kimberly Montgomery for their technical assistance in preparing the manuscript. This work was supported in part by grants from the Natural Sciences and Engineering Research Council of Canada and the Medical Research Council of Canada to Julien Doyon, and through funding from the National Institute of Mental Health— to Leslie G. Ungerleider.

REFERENCES

Ackermann, H., Daum, I., Schugens, M. M., & Grodd, W. (1996). Impaired procedural learning after damage to the left supplementary motor area (SMA). *Journal of Neurology, Neurosurgery and Psychiatry*, 60(1), 94–97.

Bloedel, J. R. (1992a). Functional heterogeneity with structural homogeneity: How does the cerebellum operate? *Behavioral and Brain Sciences*, 15, 666–678.

Bloedel, J. R. (1992b). Concepts of cerebellar integration: Still more questions than answers. *Behavioral and Brain Sciences*, 15(4), 833–838.

Boecker, H., Dagher, A., Ceballos-Baumann, A. O., Passingham, R. E., Samuel, M., Friston, K. J., Poline, J., Dettmers, C., Conrad, B., & Brooks, D. J. (1998). Role of the human rostral supplementary motor area and the basal ganglia in motor sequence control: Investigations with H2 15O PET. *Journal of Neurophysiology*, 79(2), 1070–1080.

Brashers-Krug, T., Shadmehr, R., & Bizzi, E. (1996). Consolidation in human motor memory. *Nature*, 382(6588), 252–255.

Classen, J., Liepert, J., Wise, S. P., Hallett, M., & Cohen, L. G. (1998). Rapid plasticity of human cortical movement representation induced by practice. *Journal of Neurophysiology, 79*(2), 1117–1123.

Doyon, J. (1997). Skill learning. In J. D. Schmahmann (Ed.), *The cerebellum and cognition* (pp. 273–294). San Diego, CA: Academic Press.

Doyon, J., Gaudreau, D., Laforce, R. J., Castonguay, M., Bedard, P. J., Bedard, F., & Bouchard, J. P. (1997). Role of the striatum, cerebellum, and frontal lobes in the learning of a visuomotor sequence. *Brain and Cognition, 34*(2), 218–245.

Doyon, J., Laforce, R. J., Bouchard, J. P., Gaudreau, D., Roy, J., Poirier, M., Bédard, P. J., Bédard, F., & Bouchard, J.-P. (1998). Role of the striatum, cerebellum and frontal lobes in the automatization of a repeated visuomotor sequence of movements. *Neuropsychologia, 36*(7), 625–641.

Doyon, J., Owen, A. M., Petrides, M., Sziklas, V., & Evans, A. C. (1996). Functional anatomy of visuomotor skill learning in human subjects examined with positron emission tomography. *Europrean Journal of Neuroscience, 8*(4), 637–648.

Doyon, J., Song, A. W., Lalonde, F., Karni, A., Adams, M. M., & Ungerleider, L. G. (1999). Plastic changes within the cerebellum associated with motor sequence learning: A fMRI study. *NeuroImage, 9*(6), S506.

Flament, D., Ellermann, J. M., Kim, S. G., Ugurbil, K., & Ebner, T. J. (1996). Functional magnetic resonance imaging of cerebellar activation during the learning of a visuomotor dissociation task. *Human Brain Mapping, 4*, 210–226.

Friston, K. J., Frith, C. D., Passingham, R. E., Liddle, P. F., & Frackowiak, R. S. (1992). Motor practice and neurophysiological adaptation in the cerebellum: A positron tomography study. *Proceedings of the Royal Society of London, Series B, 248*(1323), 223–228.

Frutiger, S. A., Strother, S. C., Anderson, J. R., Sidtis, J. J., Arnold, J. B., & Rottenberg, D. A. (2000). Multivariate predictive relationship between kinematic and functional activation patterns in a PET study of visuomotor learning. *NeuroImage, 12*(5), 515–527.

Gabrieli, J. D., Stebbins, G. T., Singh, J., Willingham, D. B., & Goetz, C. G. (1997). Intact mirror-tracing and impaired rotary-pursuit skill learning in patients with Huntington's disease: Evidence for dissociable memory systems in skill learning. *Neuropsychology, 11*(2), 272–281.

Georgopoulos, A. P. (2000). Neural aspects of cognitive motor control. *Current Opinion in Neurobiology, 10*(2), 238–241.

Gordon, A. M., Lee, J. H., Flament, D., Ugurbil, K., & Ebner, T. J. (1998). Functional magnetic resonance imaging of motor, sensory, and posterior parietal cortical areas during performance of sequential typing movements. *Experimental Brain Research, 121*(2), 153–166.

Grafton, S. T., Hazeltine, E., & Ivry, R. (1995). Functional mapping of sequence learning in normal humans. *Journal of Cognitive Neuroscience, 7*(4), 497–510.

Grafton, S. T., Hazeltine, E., & Ivry, R. B. (1998). Abstract and effector-specific representations of motor sequences identified with PET. *Journal of Neuroscience, 18*(22), 9420–9428.

Grafton, S. T., Mazziotta, J. C., Presty, S., Friston, K. J., Frackowiak, R. S., & Phelps, M. E. (1992). Functional anatomy of human procedural learning determined with regional cerebral blood flow and PET. *Journal of Neuroscience, 12*(7), 2542–2548.

Grafton, S. T., Woods, R. P., & Mike, T. (1994). Functional imaging of procedural motor learning: Relating cerebral blood flow with individual subject performance. *Human Brain Mapping, 1*, 221–234.

Graybiel, A. M. (1995). Building action repertoires: Memory and learning functions of the basal ganglia. *Current Opinion in Neurobiology, 5*(6), 733–741.

Graybiel, A. M., Aosaki, T., Flaherty, A. W., & Kimura, M. (1994). The basal ganglia and adaptive motor control. *Science, 265*(5180), 1826–1831.

Harrington, D. L., Haaland, K. Y., Yeo, R. A., & Marder, E. (1990). Procedural memory in Parkinson's disease: Impaired motor but not visuoperceptual learning. *Journal of Clinical and Experimental Neuropsychology, 12*(2), 323–339.

Hazeltine, E., Grafton, S. T., & Ivry, R. (1997). Attention and stimulus characteristics determine the locus of motor-sequence encoding. A PET study. *Brain, 120*(1), 123–140.

Hikosaka, O., Rand, M. K., Miyachi, S., & Miyashita, K. (1995). Learning of sequential movements in the monkey: Process of learning and retention of memory. *Journal of Neurophysiology*, 74(4), 1652–1661.

Hund-Georgiadis, M., & von Cramon, D. Y. (1999). Motor-learning-related changes in piano players and non musicians revealed by functional magnetic-resonance signals. *Experimental Brain Research*, 25(4), 417–425.

Imamizu, H., Miyauchi, S., Tamada, T., Sasaki, Y., Takino, R., Putz, B., Yoshioka, T., & Kawato, M. (2000). Human cerebellar activity reflecting an acquired internal model of a new tool. *Nature*, 403(6766), 192–195.

Jackson, P. L., Forget, J., Soucy, M.-C., Leblanc, M., Cantin, J.-F., & Doyon, J. (1997). Consolidation of visuomotor skills in humans: A psychophysical study. *Society for Neuroscience Abstracts*, 23, 1052.

Jenkins, I. H., Brooks, D. J., Nixon, P. D., Frackowiak, R. S., & Passingham, R. E. (1994). Motor sequence learning: A study with positron emission tomography. *Journal of Neuroscience*, 14(6), 3775–3790.

Jueptner, M., Frith, C. D., Brooks, D. J., Frackowiak, R. S., & Passingham, R. E. (1997). Anatomy of motor learning: II. Subcortical structures and learning by trial and error. *Journal of Neurophysiology*, 77(3), 1325–1337.

Jueptner, M., Stephan, K. M., Frith, C. D., Brooks, D. J., Frackowiak, R. S., & Passingham, R. E. (1997). Anatomy of motor learning: I. Frontal cortex and attention to action. *Journal of Neurophysiology*, 77(3), 1313–1324.

Karni, A. (1996). The acquisition of perceptual and motor skills: A memory system in the adult human cortex. *Cognitive Brain Research*, 5(1–2), 39–48.

Karni, A., Meyer, G., Jezzard, P., Adams, M. M., Turner, R., & Ungerleider, L. G. (1995). Functional MRI evidence for adult motor cortex plasticity during motor skill learning. *Nature*, 377(6545), 155–158.

Karni, A., Meyer, G., Rey-Hipolito, C., Jezzard, P., Adams, M. M., Turner, R., & Ungerleider, L. G. (1998). The acquisition of skilled motor performance: Fast and slow experience-driven changes in primary motor cortex. *Proceedings of the National Academy of Sciences USA*, 95(3), 861–868.

Karni, A., & Sagi, D. (1993). The time course of learning a visual skill. *Nature*, 365(6443), 250–252.

Krebs, H. I., Brashers-Krug, T., Rauch, S. L., Savage, C. R., Hogan, N., Rubin, R. H., Fischman, A. J., & Alpert, N. M. (1998). Robot-aided functional imaging: Application to a motor learning study. *Human Brain Mapping*, 6(1), 59–72.

Lu, X., Hikosaka, O., & Miyachi, S. (1998). Role of monkey cerebellar nuclei in skill for sequential movement. *Journal of Neurophysiology*, 79(5), 2245–2254.

MacDonald, R., & White, N. M. (1993). A triple dissociation of memory systems: Hippocampus, amygdala, and dorsal striatum. *Behavioral Neuroscience*, 107, 3–22.

Middleton, F. A., & Strick, P. L. (1997). Cerebellar output channels. *International Review of Neurobiology*, 41, 61–82.

Milak, M. S., Shimansky, Y., Bracha, V., & Bloedel, J. R. (1997). Effects of inactivating individual cerebellar nuclei on the performance and retention of an operantly conditioned forelimb movement. *Journal of Neurophysiology*, 78(2), 939–959.

Nezafat, R., Shadmehr, R., & Holcomb, H. H. (2001). Long-term adaptation to dynamics of reaching movements: A PET study. *Experimental Brain Research*, 140, 66–76.

Nudo, R. J., Milliken, G. W., Jenkins, W. M., & Merzenich, M. M. (1996). Use-dependent alterations of movement representations in primary motor cortex of adult squirrel monkeys. *Journal of Neuroscience*, 16(2), 785–807.

Nudo, R. J., Wise, B. M., SiFuentes, F., & Milliken, G. W. (1996). Neural substrates for the effects of rehabilitative training on motor recovery after ischemic infarct. *Science*, 272(5269), 1791–1794.

Pascual-Leone, A., Grafman, J., Clark, K., Stewart, M., Massaquoi, S., Lou, J. S., & Hallett, M.

(1993). Procedural learning in Parkinson's disease and cerebellar degeneration. *Annals of Neurology, 34*(4), 594–602.

Petersen, S. E., van Mier, H., Fiez, J. A., & Raichle, M. E. (1998). The effects of practice on the functional anatomy of task performance. *Proceedings of the National Academy of Sciences USA, 95*(3), 853–860.

Picard, N., & Strick, P. L. (1996). Motor areas of the medial wall: A review of their location and functional activation. *Cerebral Cortex, 6*(3), 342–353.

Rauch, S. L., Savage, C. R., Alpert, N. M., Brown, H. D., Curran, T., Kendrick, A., Fischman, A. J., & Kosslyn, S. (1995). Functional neuroanatomy of implicit sequence learning studied with PET. *Human Brain Mapping, 3*, 409.

Rauch, S. L., Whalen, P. J., Savage, C. R., Curran, T., Kendrick, A., Brown, H. D., Bush, G., Breiter, H. C., & Rosen, B. R. (1997). Striatal recruitment during an implicit sequence learning task as measured by functional magnetic resonance imaging. *Human Brain Mapping, 5*(2), 124–132.

Rey-Hipolito, C., Adams, M. M., Ungerleider, L. G., & Karni, A. (1997). When practice makes perfect: Time dependent evolution of skilled motor performance. *Society for Neuroscience Abstracts, 23*, 1052.

Sakai, K., Hikosaka, O., Miyauchi, S., Takino, R., Sasaki, Y., & Putz, B. (1998). Transition of brain activation from frontal to parietal areas in visuomotor sequence learning. *Journal of Neuroscience, 18*(5), 1827–1840.

Sanes, J. N., Dimitrov, B., & Hallett, M. (1990). Motor learning in patients with cerebellar dysfunction. *Brain, 113*(1), 103–120.

Sanes, J. N., & Donoghue, J. P. (2000). Plasticity and primary motor cortex. *Annual Review of Neuroscience, 23*, 393–415.

Schlaug, G., Knorr, U., & Seitz, R. (1994). Inter-subject variability of cerebral activations in acquiring a motor skill: A study with positron emission tomography. *Experimental Brain Research, 98*(3), 523–534.

Seitz, R. J., Canavan, A. G., Yaguez, L., Herzog, H., Tellmann, L., Knorr, U., Huang, Y., & Homberg, V. (1994). Successive roles of the cerebellum and premotor cortices in trajectorial learning. *NeuroReport, 5*(18), 2541–2544.

Seitz, R. J., Roland, E., Bohm, C., Greitz, T., & Stone-Elander, S. (1990). Motor learning in man: A positron emission tomographic study. *NeuroReport, 1*(1), 57–60.

Shadmehr, R., & Brashers-Krug, T. (1997). Functional stages in the formation of human long-term motor memory. *Journal of Neuroscience, 17*(1), 409–419.

Shadmehr, R., & Holcomb, H. H. (1997). Neural correlates of motor memory consolidation. *Science, 277*(5327), 821–825.

Shadmehr, R., & Holcomb, H. H. (1999). Inhibitory control of competing motor memories. *Experimental Brain Research, 126*(2), 235–251.

Squire, L. R. (1992). Declarative and nondeclarative memory: Multiple brain systems supporting learning and memory. *Journal of Cognitive Neuroscience, 4*, 232–243.

Tanji, J. (1996). New concepts of the supplementary motor area. *Current Opinion in Neurobiology, 6*(6), 782–787.

Tanji, J., & Shima, K. (1996). Contrast of neuronal activity between the supplemental motor area and other cortical motor areas. *Advances in Neurology, 70*, 95–103.

Thach, W. T. (1997). Context–response linkage. *International Review of Neurobiology, 41*, 599–611.

Toni, I., Krams, M., Turner, R., & Passingham, R. E. (1998). The time course of changes during motor sequence learning: A whole-brain fMRI study. *NeuroImage, 8*(1), 50–61.

Ungerleider, L. G. (1995). Functional brain imaging studies of cortical mechanisms for memory. *Science, 270*(5237), 769–775.

van Mier, H. (2000). Human learning. In A. W. Toga & J. C. Mazziotta (Eds.), *Brain mapping: The systems* (pp. 605–620). San Diego, CA: Academic Press.

van Mier, H., Tempel, L. W., Perlmutter, J. S., Raichle, M. E., & Petersen, S. E. (1998). Changes in brain activity during motor learning measured with PET: Effects of hand of performance and practice. *Journal of Neurophysiology, 80*(4), 2177–2199.

White, N. M. (1997). Mnemonic functions of the basal ganglia. *Current Opinion in Neurobiology, 7*(2), 164–169.

Willingham, D. B. (1998). A neuropsychological theory of motor skill learning. *Psychological Review, 105*(3), 558–584.

Willingham, D. B., & Koroshetz, W. J. (1993). Evidence for dissociable motor skills in Huntington's disease patients. *Psychobiology, 21*, 173–182.

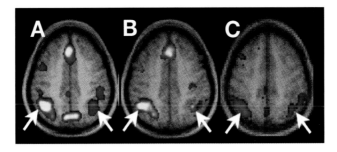

PLATE 13.1. Commonalities in regions identified as related to retrieval success. Data in the three panels from (A) Konishi, Wheeler, Donaldson, and Buckner (2000); (B) McDermott, Jones, Petersen, Lageman, and Roediger (2000); and (C) Donaldson, Petersen, Ollinger, and Buckner (2001). Bilateral inferior parietal regions (within BA 40) are indicated by arrows. All slices shown are 40 mm superior to the anterior commissure–posterior commissure plane.

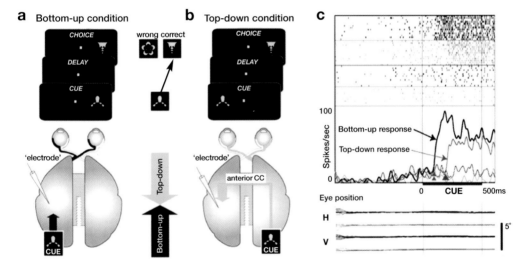

PLATE 24.1. Top-down signal from the prefrontal cortex to the temporal cortex in posterior-split-brain monkeys. (a–b) Experimental design in the posterior-split-brain monkey. (a) Bottom-up condition. Visual stimuli (cue and choice pictures) were presented in the hemifield contralateral to the recording site ("electrode") in the IT cortex. The monkey had to make the correct choice specified by the cue. Fixation was required throughout a trial. Bottom-up sensory signals (black arrow) would be detected in this condition. (b) Top-down condition; as in a, but the cue was presented in the hemifield ipsilateral to the recording site, whereas the choice was presented contralaterally. In this condition, the bottom-up sensory signal from the retina did not reach the recording site, and only the top-down signal (blue arrow) could activate IT neurons in the recording site through feedback connections from the prefrontal cortex. (c) Neuronal activity of a single IT cell in the bottom-up and top-down conditions (top-down, blue; bottom-up, black). Raster displays, spike density functions (SDFs), and eye position traces were aligned at the cue onset. In the SDFs, thick lines show responses to the optimal cue, whereas thin lines show responses to a null cue. Onset of the top-down response (arrowhead) was later than that of the bottom-up response (double arrowhead). Horizontal (H) and vertical (V) eye positions in all the trials for the optimal cue are shown.

Therefore, in the absence of bottom-up visual inputs, single IT neurons were robustly activated by the effect of the top-down signal from the prefrontal cortex in the retrieval of long-term memory stored in the IT cortex. From Tomita et al. (1999). Copyright 1999 by Nature Publishing Group. Adapted by permission.

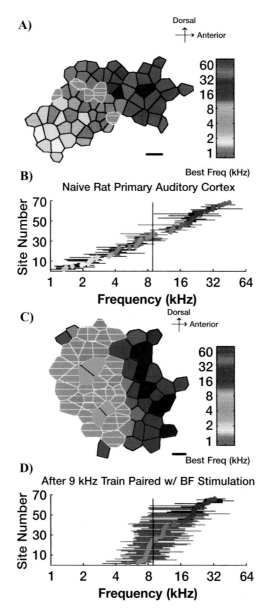

PLATE 32.1. Topographic organization of tone frequency preference in rat primary auditory cortex. (A and B) Example of normal organization in naïve animals. (C and D) Example of the map reorganization following 4 weeks of NB stimulation paired with 9-kHz tone trains. Each polygon represents one microelectrode penetration. The color indicates the best frequency for each site. The region of the map that responded selectively to 9 kHz is indicated by white hatching. Calibration bar: 0.25 mm. (B and D) Every A1 receptive field is shown to illustrate the increased receptive field size and shift toward 9 kHz in the experimental group. Each line indicates the width of each receptive field 10 dB above threshold. The color dots represent the best frequency at each site. Receptive fields that include 9 kHz are colored in red. Adapted from Kilgard and Merzenich (1998a). Copyright 1998 by the American Association for the Advancement of Science. Adapted by permission.

19

Searching for the Neural Correlates of Object Priming

ALEX MARTIN and MIRANDA VAN TURENNOUT

"Object priming" is characterized by increased efficiency in identifying an object as a result of prior exposure to that object. A particularly striking example of this form of implicit learning comes from object-naming studies: Previously named object pictures are named faster than novel object pictures. This facilitation of naming speed is extremely long-lasting (up to 48 weeks, the longest interval tested; Cave, 1997). Amnesic patients show normal levels of object name priming with up to a week intervening between repetitions (Cave & Squire, 1992). These findings suggest that naming an object produces a more or less permanent change in processing efficiency, and that the development of this change is not dependent on the medial temporal lobe memory system.

Functional brain imaging has revealed that this seemingly simple act of naming an object is mediated by a hierarchically organized, interactive network of discrete cortical regions (Bouchart et al., 2000; Martin, Wiggs, Ungerleider, & Haxby, 1996). This network typically includes bilateral regions of occipital, temporal, left inferior frontal cortices and the left insula. Activity in these regions reflects different component processes necessary for object naming, including visual processing of the physical stimulus, and retrieval of semantic, lexical, and phonological representations (for reviews, see Martin, 2001; Martin & Chao, 2001; and Price, Indefrey, & van Turennout, 1999). In this chapter, we highlight our recent experiments that have explored the association between object priming and changes in neural activity in different regions of the object-naming system.

DECREASED ACTIVITY IN POSTERIOR CORTEX: CREATION OF SPARSER YET MORE OBJECT-SPECIFIC REPRESENTATIONS

In 1992, Squire and colleagues (1992) used positron emission tomography (PET) to record regional cerebral activity while subjects generated words to three-letter word stems. Completing the stems with previously studied words resulted in less neural activity in occipital cortex (right lingual gyrus), compared with generating words to stems that could not be completed with previously studied words (Squire et al., 1992). Following this report, decreased neural activity with repetition of words, as well as objects, was found in studies using PET (Buckner et al., 1995; Schacter, Alpert, Savage, Rauch, & Albert, 1996) and functional magnetic resonance imaging (fMRI) (Buckner et al., 1998; Buckner, Koutstaal, Schacter, & Rosen, 2000; Martin et al., 1995; Wagner, Maril, & Schacter, 2000). Moreover, decreases, though commonly including occipital cortex, were not limited to this region, but rather tended to include most of the cortical regions engaged by the task (for reviews, see Schacter & Buckner, 1998; Wiggs & Martin, 1998).

An early demonstration of this phenomenon using fMRI can be seen in Figure 19.1. Subjects were scanned while silently naming pictures of objects. The first block of trials consisted of pictures that the subjects had not previously seen. This block was followed approximately 30 seconds later by a repetition of these pictures in a different order, followed by another set of novel object pictures. Interspersed between these object blocks were series of visual noise stimuli that subjects were told to stare at, and that served as a baseline condition (Martin et al., 1995). As illustrated by Figure 19.1, relative to the visual noise baseline, silent object naming produced a robust response that was significantly decreased when the same objects were again named, and then returned to its initial level of

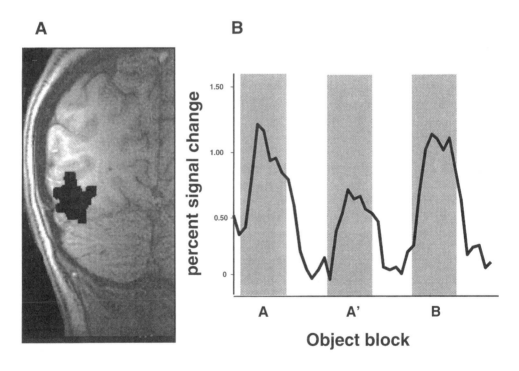

FIGURE 19.1. (A) Coronal section of the left hemisphere of a single subject. Shown is a region in the posterior temporal cortex (black) that was more active during silent object naming relative to viewing noise patterns. Recording was made with a surface coil place along the left side of the subject's head. (B) fMRI time series showing how activity in this region was modulated by silent naming of a series of novel objects (A), repeated presentation of these novel objects (A'), and a new set of objects (B). Data were averaged across all active voxels in the region and across six runs of the A-A'-B series. Different objects were presented in each run. Alternating blocks of object (gray bars) and visual noise (white bars) lasted 21 seconds. Data from Martin et al. (1995).

activity when new objects were presented. These and similar findings (Buckner et al., 1998) suggested that fMRI could be used to investigate modulation of neural activity across different regions of the cortex within a relatively short time frame.

As Squire and colleagues (1992) noted in their original report, two types of explanations could account for priming-related reductions in neural activity. One possibility is that they reflect changes in the processing demands of the task. For example, in the Squire and colleagues report, subjects may have recognized that the stems were beginnings of words they had recently studied, thereby requiring less attention than the novel word stems presented during the baseline condition. Indeed, when subjects were explicitly instructed to complete stems with recently studied words, reduced activity was again noted, albeit to a lesser extent than in the priming condition (Squire et al., 1992). A similar explanation could be offered for the fMRI time series illustrated in Figure 19.1. In this study, novel and repeated objects were presented in sequential blocks. As a result, it could be argued that subjects quickly became aware of this sequence, resulting in less attention devoted to the repeated objects, and a corresponding reduction in neural activity. Thus, within this framework, priming-related reductions in neural activity reflect changes in attention as a consequence of explicit memory of the recent past.

Modulation of the fMRI signal by attentional task demands is certainly of interest. Indeed, many studies have shown that selective attention can either suppress or enhance neural activity (see Kastner & Ungerleider, 2000, for a review). However, if reduced neural activity with object repetition reflects reduced attention as a result of explicit memory processes, then it cannot be the mechanism for object priming. Object priming is intact in patients with severely limited episodic memory (see, e.g., Cave & Squire, 1992) and relatively impervious to manipulations of attention and awareness in normal individuals (for a review, see Roediger & McDermott, 1993).

An alternative view is that reduced activity reflects a change in the neural representation of a previously encountered stimulus, resulting in more efficient processing when that stimulus is encountered again. Single-unit recordings from cortical neurons in alert, behaving monkeys provide evidence for a mechanism that could lead to enhanced processing efficiency as a result of stimulus repetition. Beginning with reports by Brown, Wilson, and Riches (1987) and Baylis and Rolls (1987), many investigators have observed reduced firing rates in subsets of neurons with repeated presentation of stimuli. As reviewed elsewhere, the properties of repetition-related reductions in neural firing rates mirror many of the properties of behavioral priming in humans (Wiggs & Martin, 1998). For example, repetition-related reductions in neural activity are stimulus-specific, graded, unaffected by manipulations of object size and location, automatic, and long-lasting.

A critical point about these single-cell recording studies is that repetition-induced reductions in firing rate are observed in only a subset of neurons that initially respond to an object. For example, Miller, Li, and Desimone (1991) observed repetition-related reductions in approximately one-third of neurons recorded from inferior temporal cortex. Importantly, other neurons that initially responded strongly to a particular object maintained their firing rate with subsequent object repetitions. As suggested by Desimone (1996), this stimulus-specific pattern of maintained response in some neurons, coupled with reduced response in others, might provide a mechanism for repetition priming. Specifically, as object-specific features are learned through experience, neurons strongly tuned to these features maintain their firing rates, whereas neurons less strongly tuned gradually drop out of the responsive pool. As a result, repeated exposure to an object leads to a sparser and yet more object-specific representation, which in turn results in enhanced object identification. Thus, within this view, facilitation of performance in priming tasks does not result specifically from reduced attentional demands, but rather from the formation of sparser yet more stimulus-specific representations, leading to more efficient stimulus processing.

In a recent experiment (van Turennout, Ellmore, & Martin, 2000), we sought to tighten the link between the reduced neural activity and the sparse representation view by using a design that should greatly reduce, if not eliminate, changes in attentional demands for processing novel versus repeated objects. In addition, we sought to determine whether repetition-related reductions as measured by fMRI would extend to two characteristics of behavioral priming. First, reductions should occur regardless of whether the object has a preexisting representation in memory (see, e.g., Gabrieli, Milberg, Keane, & Corkin, 1990; Schacter, Cooper, & Delaney, 1990). Second, they should be long-lasting. As mentioned previously, behavioral studies report object priming using a naming task with lags of nearly a year (Cave, 1997), suggesting a permanent change in processing efficiency that can be established after a single experience.

In our study, we took advantage of a relatively new development in fMRI methodology: event-related designs (Buckner et al., 1998; D'Esposito, Zarahn, & Aguirre, 1999). In contrast to presenting stimuli blocked by condition, event-related designs allow different types of stimuli or conditions to occur in a randomly intermixed order. As a result, subjects are unable to anticipate the next stimulus event, and thus are discouraged from developing strategies that could confound the interpretation of the results.

Several days prior to the scanning session, subjects engaged in an object-naming task. Each object was presented for 200 milliseconds (msec) at a rate of one item every 2 seconds. Interspersed between the pictures of real objects that the subjects named aloud were pictures of nonsense objects. Subjects were instructed to attend carefully to each object, even if they could not name it. Three days later, subjects participated in the scanning session. Again, objects were presented as in the prior training session. Subjects were told to name each object silently, and to look carefully at the nonsense objects. During scanning, subjects saw real objects and nonsense objects that had been presented previously, objects and nonsense objects that they had not previously seen, and repetitions of these novel objects after a delay of approximately 30 seconds. In addition, visual noise stimuli were included to provide a low-level baseline (van Turennout et al., 2000). Presentation of these seven stimulus types in a random, intermixed order, with items appearing for only 200 msec, made it highly unlikely that a reduced neural response associated with object repetition would result from reduced attentional demands for processing repeated versus novel objects.

Relative to naming new objects, neural activity in posterior cortex was markedly reduced when objects were repeated after a 30-second delay. Moreover, reduced activity was present, although to a weaker extent, after a 3-day lag (see Figure 19.2; see also Wagner et al., 2000, for reduced neural activity in a word-priming task after a 1-day lag). These findings mirrored the behavioral data collected outside the scanner with a different group of subjects. Object-naming speed was strongly facilitated at the short delay, and to a lesser extent at the longer delay.

The same pattern of results was found for viewing nonsense objects. Repetition of nonsense objects was associated with a robust reduction in neural activity after a 30-second delay. Relative to viewing nonsense objects for the first time, activity was also reduced for nonsense objects presented 3 days earlier. These reductions tended to be confined to occipital cortex, whereas the reductions extended into the posterior region of ventral temporal cortex for real objects (see van Turennout et al., 2000, for details). Thus a single, brief (200-msec) presentation of an object can lead to long-term changes in neural activity, even when that object has no prior representation in memory.

A. Real objects

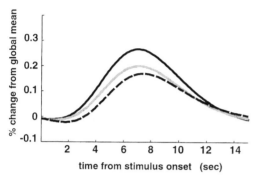

B. Nonsense objects

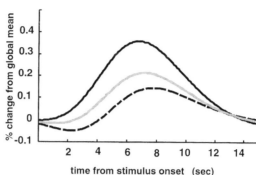

FIGURE 19.2. (A) Fitted responses for novel real objects (black), repeated objects at a 30-second delay (dashed line), and repeated objects at a 3-day delay (gray). Shown are group-averaged event-related hemodynamic responses computed from all voxels within the left occipitotemporal cortex active during object naming, showing an effect of object repetition. (B) Same as in A, but showing an effect in occipital cortex for viewing nonsense objects (see the original paper for details). Data from van Turennout, Ellmore, and Martin (2000).

These findings are consistent with the idea that behavioral priming is attributable to changes in object representations stored in posterior cortex. In addition, they cast doubt on the usefulness of explanations of priming-related neural reductions that appeal solely to changes in attention or other processing strategies. However, additional findings from this study indicate that no single mechanism is likely to account fully for neural changes associated with object priming in naming tasks.

INCREASED ACTIVITY IN THE INSULAR CORTEX: A FORM OF PROCEDURAL LEARNING?

In the van Turennout and colleagues (2000) study, silently naming objects produced increased activity in left inferior frontal cortex (Broca's area) and the anterior region of the left insula, as is typically seen during object naming and other language tasks (Martin et al., 1996; Price, Moore, Humphreys, Frackowiak, & Friston, 1996). However, repetition-related changes in these anterior sites were in stark contrast to those seen in posterior cortical regions. Whereas decreases were stronger at the short (30-second) than at the long (3-day) delay in posterior cortex, activity in Broca's area showed a minimal decrease after 30 seconds and a large decrease when 3 days intervened between the first and second object presentations. Moreover, whereas activity in Broca's area declined as a function of delay, the left anterior insula showed the opposite pattern: Activity was minimal when objects were first named, increased in response to objects repeated after 30 seconds, and increased further when naming objects that were first seen 3 days prior to the scan session (Figure 19.3). (Neither the insula nor Broca's area was active for viewing nonsense objects.)

These findings have been replicated and extended in a more recent event-related study that investigated the time course of these changes in greater detail (van Turennout, Biela-mowicz, Ellmore, & Martin, 2001). Again, activity in Broca's area decreased and activity

A. Left inferior frontal

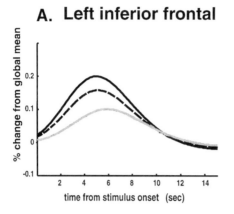

B. Left insula

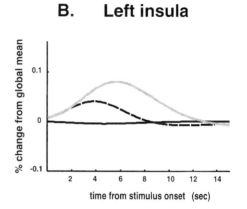

FIGURE 19.3. (A) Fitted responses for novel real objects (black), repeated objects at a 30-second delay (dashed line), and repeated objects at a 3-day delay (gray). Shown are group-averaged event-related hemodynamic responses computed from all voxels within the left inferior frontal cortex active during object naming, showing an effect of object repetition. (B) Same as in A, but for the left insular cortex (see the original paper for details). Data from van Turennout, Ellmore, and Martin (2000).

in the insula increased, with repetition lags that now included 1 hour, 6 hours, and 3 days. An added feature of this study was that a set of novel objects were repeated multiple times during scanning (three repetitions at approximately 30-second intervals). For these objects, the same contrasting patterns of activity in Broca's area and the insula were observed: Activity decreased in Broca's region and increased in the left insula as objects were named repeatedly. In addition, increased activity with repeated practice was found in the left basal ganglia.

To what can we attribute these complex patterns of response? Clearly, the increased activity in the insular cortex is at odds with both the attention and sparse encoding hypotheses. Both of these ideas would predict the greatest amount of activity to novel objects, which would then decrease with repetition. An alternative possibility is that this increased activity reflects explicit remembering. Activity may be increasing with repetition because subjects are becoming more and more aware of having seen the object previously. This explanation, however, is not supported by the data for objects repeated only once at different time lags. Subjects should be more aware, and thus insular activity should be greater, for objects repeated after short delays than after long delays. Yet the opposite pattern of activation was found.

Another alternative is that the increased activation in the anterior insula, coupled with decreased activity in Broca's area, reflects a form of procedural learning whereby performance becomes more automatic with practice. This idea was first proposed by Raichle and colleagues (1994) to account for the practice-related changes in verb generation. As subjects continued to generate the same verb in response to the same noun, activity increased in insular cortex bilaterally (and in left medial occipital cortex), and decreased in left inferior frontal cortex (and in left posterior temporal cortex, left anterior cingulate, and right cerebellum). These changes were reversed when new nouns were presented, suggesting a change in neural circuitry as task performance became more automatic (see Petersen, van Mier, Fiez, & Raichle, 1998, and Raichle, 1998, for additional findings and extended discussion).

Studies of patients with focal lesions of left inferior frontal cortex (see Caplan, 1992, for a review) or left anterior insular cortex (Dronkers, 1996) indicate that these regions play central roles in lexical and phonological processes. Our data may reflect a learning-related reorganization of neural circuitry, whereby the link between a preexisting lexical–phonological representation (the object name) and a novel picture of that object becomes stronger with practice and time. Specifically, we propose that whereas lexical–phonological retrieval is initially subserved by Broca's area, it is at least partially taken over by the left anterior insula, perhaps in concert with the basal ganglia, as naming a specific object becomes more automatic. In addition, it appears that this switch can develop even after a single exposure to an object, as long as some minimal amount of time, perhaps on the order of hours, has elapsed (for reviews of the functions of the insula and its connections to other structures, including the basal ganglia, see Augustine, 1996; Flynn, Benson, & Ardila, 1999).

CONCLUSIONS AND FUTURE DIRECTIONS

These findings have a number of implications for understanding the functional neuro-anatomy of memory systems in the brain. First, changes in neural activity occur automatically with object repetition. These changes reflect the object's presentation history and the brain's response to it, not reduced attentional demands resulting from remembering that history. Second, the data suggest that object name priming is mediated by two distinct mechanisms. The first mechanism is the formation of a sparser yet more object-specific representation, yielding enhanced object identification. This view is consistent with models viewing priming as a change in presemantic, perceptual representational systems that results in improved recognition (Tulving & Schacter, 1990). Single-unit recordings from monkey cortex suggest that the neural correlates of this process are a progressive decline in the firing rate of a subset of neurons that initially responded to the object, coupled with the continued firing of neurons that code the critical features necessary to identify that object (Desimone, 1996; Wiggs & Martin, 1998; see also Rolls & Tovee, 1995, for a discussion of the role of sparse encoding in object recognition). Because the fMRI signal reveals the aggregate activity of large populations of neurons, this process is reflected as a signal reduction (but see James, Humphrey, Gati, Menon, & Goodale, 2000, for a different interpretation of repetition-related reductions measured by fMRI).

The second mechanism may be a form of procedural learning characterized by increased efficiency in name retrieval in response to a specific object picture. This view is consistent with the idea that object name priming results from facilitation in the linking of an object's features and its associated phonological representation (Wheeldon & Monsell, 1992). The neural correlates of this process appear to be a progressive decline in activity in Broca's area, coupled with a progressive increase in activity in the left insula and basal ganglia. It remains to be determined whether patients with lesions of the left insula or basal ganglia show impaired object name priming, especially with long delays between presentations. The present data suggest that this pattern of results should be observed.

Clearly, many questions remain concerning the neural correlates of object priming. The most common feature reported across studies is a repetition-related decrease in posterior cortical activity. However, there is no universal agreement on the interpretation of this effect (see, e.g., James et al., 2000). Moreover, contrary to our findings with nonsense objects, object repetition-related *increases* in posterior cortex have been reported in studies using novel stimuli (Henson, Shallice, & Dolan, 2000; Schacter et al., 1995). Much work is needed to characterize the effects that different stimulus characteristics (e.g., familiarity) and priming paradigms have on repetition-related changes in neural activity. Finally, we have argued throughout this chapter that these neural changes reflect implicit memory phenomena (priming and procedural learning). Nevertheless, subjects are perfectly capable of explicitly recognizing objects they have previously named. In fact, object recognition memory can remain above chance levels even after nearly a year has elapsed between presentations (Cave, 1997). How the changes described here interact with explicit memory processes (Wagner et al., 2000) remains to be determined.

REFERENCES

Augustine, J. R. (1996). Circuitry and functional aspects of the insular lobe in primates including humans. *Brain Research Reviews, 22*, 229–244.

Baylis, G. C., & Rolls, E. T. (1987). Responses of neurons in inferotemporal cortex in short term and serial recognition memory tasks. *Experimental Brain Research, 65*, 614–622.

Bouchart, M., Meyer, M. E., Pins, D., Humphreys, G. W., Scheiber, C., Gounod, D., & Foucher, J. (2000). Automatic object identification: An fMRI study. *NeuroReport, 11*, 2379–2383.

Brown, M. W., Wilson, F. A. W., & Riches, I. P. (1987). Neuronal evidence that inferomedial temporal cortex is more important than hippocampus in certain processes underlying recognition memory. *Brain Research, 409*, 158–162.

Buckner, R. L., Goodman, J., Burock, M., Rotte, M., Koutstaal, W., Schacter, D., Rosen, B., & Dale, A. M. (1998). Functional–anatomic correlates of object priming in humans revealed by rapid presentation event-related fMRI. *Neuron, 20*, 285–296.

Buckner, R. L., Koutstaal, W., Schacter, D. L., & Rosen, B. (2000). Functional MRI evidence for a role of frontal and inferior temporal cortex in amodal components of priming. *Brain, 123*, 620–640.

Buckner, R. L., Petersen, S. E., Ojemann, J. G., Miezen, F. M., Squire, L. S., & Raichle, M. E. (1995). Functional anatomical studies of explicit and implicit memory retrieval processes. *Journal of Neuroscience, 15*, 12–29.

Caplan, D. (1992). *Language: Structure, processing, and disorders.* Cambridge, MA: MIT Press.

Cave, B. C. (1997). Very long-lasting priming in picture naming. *Psychological Science, 8*, 322–325.

Cave, B. C., & Squire, L. R. (1992). Intact and long-lasting repetition priming in amnesia. *Journal of Experimental Psychology: Learning, Memory, and Cognition, 18*, 509–520.

D'Esposito, M., Zarahn, E., & Aguirre, G. K. (1999). Event-related functional MRI: Implications for cognitive psychology. *Psychological Bulletin, 125*, 155–164.

Desimone, R. (1996). Neural mechanisms for visual memory and their role in attention. *Proceedings of the National Academy of Sciences USA, 93*, 13494–13499.

Dronkers, N. F. (1996). A new brain region for coordinating speech articulation. *Nature, 384*, 159–161.

Flynn, F. G., Benson, D. F., & Ardila, A. (1999). Anatomy of the insula: Functional and clinical correlates. *Aphasiology, 13*, 55–78.

Gabrieli, J. D. E., Milberg, W. P., Keane, M. M., & Corkin, S. (1990). Intact priming of patterns despite impaired memory. *Neuropsychologia, 28*, 417–427.

Henson, R., Shallice, T., & Dolan, R. (2000). Neuroimaging evidence for dissociable forms of repetition priming. *Science, 287*, 1269–1272.

James, T. W., Humphrey, G. K., Gati, J. S., Menon, R. S., & Goodale, M. A. (2000). The effects of visual object priming on brain activation before and after recognition. *Current Biology, 10*, 1017–1024.

Kastner, S., & Ungerleider, L. G. (2000). Mechanisms of visual attention in the human cortex. *Annual Review of Neuroscience, 23*, 315–341.

Martin, A. (2001). Functional neuroimaging of semantic memory. In R. Cabeza & A. Kingstone (Eds.), *Handbook of functional neuroimaging of cognition* (pp. 153–186). Cambridge, MA: MIT Press.

Martin, A., & Chao, L. L. (2001). Semantic memory and the brain: Structure and processes. *Current Opinion in Neurobiology, 11,* 194–201.

Martin, A., Lalonde, F. M., Wiggs, C. L., Weisberg, J., Ungerleider, L. G., & Haxby, J. V. (1995). Repeated presentation of objects reduces activity in ventral occipitotemporal cortex: A fMRI study of repetition priming. *Society for Neuroscience Abstracts, 21,* 1497.

Martin, A., Wiggs, C. L., Ungerleider, L. G., & Haxby, J. V. (1996). Neural correlates of category-specific knowledge. *Nature, 379,* 649–652.

Miller, E. K., Li, L., & Desimone, R. (1991). A neural mechanism for working memory and recognition memory in inferior temporal cortex. *Science, 254,* 1377–1379.

Petersen, S. E., van Mier, H., Fiez, J. A., & Raichle, M. E. (1998). The effects of practice on the functional neuroanatomy of task performance. *Proceedings of the National Academy of Sciences USA, 95,* 853–860.

Price, C. J., Indefrey, P., & van Turennout, M. (1999). The neural architecture underlying the processing of written and spoken word forms. In C. M. Brown & P. Hagoort (Eds.), *Neurocognition of language processing* (pp. 211–240). New York: Oxford University Press.

Price, C. J., Moore, C. J., Humphreys, G. W., Frackowiak, R. S. J., & Friston, K. J. 1996). The neural regions sustaining object recognition and naming. *Proceedings of the Royal Society of London, Series B, 263,* 1501–1507.

Raichle, M. E. (1998). The neural correlates of consciousness: An analysis of cognitive skill learning. *Philosophical Transactions of the Royal Society of London, Series B, 353,* 1889–1901.

Raichle, M. E., Fiez, J. A., Videen, T. O., MacLeod, A. M. K., Pardo, J. V., Fox, P. T., & Petersen, S. E. (1994). Practice-related changes in human brain functional anatomy during nonmotor learning. *Cerebral Cortex, 4,* 8–26.

Roediger, H. L., & McDermott, K. B. (1993). Implicit memory in normal human subjects. In H. Spinnler & F. Boller (Eds.), *Handbook of neuropsychology* (Vol. 8, pp. 63–131). Amsterdam: Elsevier.

Rolls, E. T., & Tovee, M. J. (1995). Sparseness of neuronal representation of stimuli in the primate temporal visual cortex. *Journal of Neurophysiology, 73,* 713–726.

Schacter, D. L., Alpert, N. M., Savage, C. R., Rauch, S. L., & Albert, M. S. (1996). Conscious recollection and the human hippocampal formation: Evidence from positron emission tomography. *Proceedings of the National Academy of Sciences USA, 93,* 321–325.

Schacter, D. L., & Buckner, R. (1998). Priming and the brain. *Neuron, 20,* 185–195.

Schacter, D. L., Cooper, L. A., & Delaney, S. M. (1990). Implicit memory for unfamiliar objects depends on access to structural descriptions. *Journal of Experimental Psychology: General, 119,* 5–24.

Schacter, D. L., Reiman, E., Uecker, A., Polster, M. R., Yun, L. S., & Cooper, L. A. (1995). Brain regions associated with retrieval of structurally coherent visual information. *Nature, 376,* 587–590.

Squire, L. S., Ojemann, J. G., Miezen, F. M., Petersen, S. E., Videen, T. O., & Raichle, M. E. (1992). Activation of the hippocampus in normal humans: A functional anatomical study of memory. *Proceedings of the National Academy of Sciences USA, 89,* 1837–1841.

Tulving, E., & Schacter, D. L. (1990). Priming and human memory systems. *Science, 247,* 301–306.

van Turennout, M., Bielamowicz, L., Ellmore, T., & Martin, A. (2001). *Modulation of neural activity during object naming: The effects of time and practice.* Manuscript submitted for publication.

van Turennout, M., Ellmore, T., & Martin, A. (2000). Long-lasting cortical plasticity in the object naming system. *Nature Neuroscience, 3,* 1329–1334.

Wagner, A. D., Maril, A., & Schacter, D. L. (2000). Interactions between forms of memory: When priming hinders new episodic learning. *Journal of Cognitive Neuroscience, 12*(Suppl. 2), 52–60.

Wheeldon, L. R., & Monsell, S. (1992). The locus of repetition priming of spoken word production. *Quarterly Journal of Experimental Psychology, 44,* 723–761.

Wiggs, C. L., & Martin, A. (1998). Properties and mechanisms of perceptual priming. *Current Opinion in Neurobiology, 8,* 227–233.

20

Neuropsychological Approaches to Preclinical Identification of Alzheimer's Disease

MARILYN S. ALBERT and MARK B. MOSS

Alzheimer's disease (AD) is the most common cause of dementia among older persons, and is estimated to affect 4.9 million individuals in the United States alone (Evans et al., 1989). It is particularly appropriate to discuss AD in a book about the neuropsychology of memory, because the earliest symptom in the vast majority of patients is a gradually progressive memory disorder. The underlying nature of this memory disorder has been extensively studied in recent years, along with efforts to understand its neurobiological substrate. The present chapter focuses on preclinical identification of persons with AD, but it is helpful first to briefly review the initial identification of AD as a disorder, as well as recent research efforts that have led to a better understanding of its neurobiological and neuropsychological characteristics.

The first patient with AD was described in 1907 by Alois Alzheimer. He had followed a patient who demonstrated a progressive loss of cognition, and who eventually died. Taking advantage of the development of a new silver stain, he was able to describe a set of pathological changes in the patient's brain on autopsy, which he hypothesized had caused her progressive brain disease (Alzheimer, 1907). For the following 60 years, this disorder was thought to be rare and to affect only individuals under the age of 65. However, by the late 1970s it had become clear that the pathology seen in patients with AD under the age of 65 was essentially identical to that seen in the majority of patients with dementia aged 65 and over, and that most individuals with so-called "senility" or "hardening of the arteries" actually had AD (Katzman, 1976). This recognition, and the subsequent publication of clinical (McKhann et al., 1984) and pathological (National Institute on Aging [NIA]–Reagan Working Group, 1997) research criteria for AD, led to an explosion of studies in this area. Thus, in the last 20 years, much has been learned about the neuropsychological, pathological, and genetic manifestations of AD.

Neuropsychologically, the memory disorder that characterizes the onset of disease in the majority of patients is most evident on tests of delayed recall. Experimental studies comparing patients with AD to controls, and to patients with other forms of amnesia and dementia, have shown that patients with mild AD recall less information over brief delay intervals (of approximately 10 minutes' duration) than other patient groups studied to date (Hart, Kwentus, Harkins, & Taylor, 1988; Kopelman, 1985; Milberg & Albert, 1989; Moss, Albert, Butters, & Payne, 1986; Welsh, Butters, Hughes, Mohs, & Heyman, 1991). Early in the course of disease, the majority of patients with AD also have difficulty with executive function, particularly on tests that require sequencing and set shifting (Grady et al., 1988; Lafleche & Albert, 1995). As the disease spreads, other cognitive domains (such as language and spatial skill) become impaired (Rosen & Mohs, 1982), and patients ultimately become dependent in all activities of daily living (Cummings & Benson, 1983).

Neuropathologically, the progression of disease is marked by the development of neuritic plaques and neurofibrillary tangles (the pathological changes first described by Alois Alzheimer). As these pathological changes accumulate, synapses are lost and neurons die (for a review, see Kemper, 1994). Initially, these pathological alterations are seen in the entorhinal cortex, which loses up to 30% of its neurons in the earliest stages of disease (Gomez-Isla et al., 1996). This neuronal loss then spreads throughout the perforant pathway, affecting the hippocampus and adjacent structures (Hyman, Van Hoesen, Kromer, & Damasio, 1984). Ultimately, these changes are evident throughout the association cortices; however, several regions, including the primary motor cortex, the sensory cortex, and the occipital cortex, are relatively spared. Thus the pathological changes of the disease initially appear in a fairly focal manner and, even in end-stage disease, do not affect all parts of the brain equally.

Studies at the molecular level have demonstrated that the neuritic plaques seen in autopsy tissue are primarily composed of a form of β-amyloid protein with a particular molecular weight, known as $A\beta_{1-42}$ (Glenner & Wong, 1984). The neurofibrillary tangles are composed of tau, a substance involved in the cytoskeleton of the nerve cells (Lee, Balin, Otvos, & Tojanowski, 1991). For many years, researchers have debated which of these two abnormalities represents the initial step in the biological cascade that leads to AD.

The genetic mutations now known to be associated with the development of AD have led to the current consensus that the accumulation of the β-amyloid protein is the initiating molecular event in AD. Three dominant mutations have been found that inevitably lead to AD among all individuals who possess the mutation. These mutations are seen on chromosomes 21, 14, and 1 (Goate et al., 1991; Levy-Lahad et al., 1995; Schellenberg et al., 1992). Each of these mutations leads to the accumulation of $A\beta_{1-42}$, and thus a consensus has been reached that its accumulation represents the first step in the development of AD (for a review, see Selkoe, 2000). In addition, a variant of at least one other gene has been shown to increase the risk for AD. This gene, known as the apolipoprotein E (APOE) gene, has three forms; it is the APOE-4 form that alters risk for AD (Saunders et al., 1993). It is hypothesized that APOE-4 alters the clearance of $A\beta_{1-42}$, but this conclusion is still under study (Bales et al., 1997). The increasing consensus about this "amyloid hypothesis" has led to new approaches to the development of drugs for AD, and to increasing optimism that effective therapies will soon be available.

Therefore, the current focus within the field of AD research is on the development of medications that retard or stop progression of disease, and on the identification of patients in the preclinical phase of disease. The rationale for the latter emphasis is based on the assumption, mentioned above, that the development of AD pathology (and neuronal loss) precedes the appearance of full-blown symptoms by many years. If preclinical identification is possible, then medicines may be used to slow or halt progression of the disease before substantial neuronal loss has taken place. Thus the discrimination of those destined to develop AD from the larger pool of individuals with mild memory loss would be crucial to the development of strategies for the prevention or delay of AD. This goal is the underlying motivation for the studies described here.

METHODOLOGY FOR PREDICTING WHO WILL DEVELOP AD

Our studies have focused on the identification of specific factors that predict who, among a group of individuals with memory problems, will ultimately be diagnosed as having AD. Toward that end, as part of a multidisciplinary program on cognition and aging, we recruited from a population of several thousand screened individuals a study sample of over 300 individuals who met specific exclusion and inclusion cognitive and health criteria. Approximately one-quarter of these individuals met criteria for normal cognition when they were first evaluated, and approximately three-quarters had evidence of memory problems but did not meet clinical criteria for AD. These latter individuals met criteria for "questionable AD" when they were first evaluated.

After recruitment, each participant received a detailed neuropsychological assessment, a variety of neuroimaging studies, and a series of genetic analyses. The participants were then followed prospectively to determine those who progressed to meeting clinical criteria for AD, those who remained normal, and those who continued to be categorized as "questionable" (i.e., to have mild memory problems but without evidence of dementia).

This methodology has made it possible to examine the data obtained at baseline to determine which measures predict subsequent development of AD. Since the data obtained at baseline included measures of brain structure and function, as well as genetic status, it has also been possible to determine the interrelationships among domains that suggest the underlying brain–behavior relationships involved in the preclinical phase of AD. Implicit in this study design is the assumption that AD starts many years prior to the point where symptoms are fully expressed, and that the techniques of neuropsychology, imaging, and genetics can measure these changes in a meaningful way and shed light on the progression of symptoms over time. This approach also assumes that an interdisciplinary integration of information, which combines measurements of the brain with those of cognition and genetics, will yield a more comprehensive understanding of the prodromal phase of AD than will any one technique alone.

RECRUITMENT AND FOLLOW-UP OF SUBJECTS

Two cohorts of individuals have been recruited for these studies of preclinical prediction of AD. The data to be described here pertain to the first cohort of individuals, who have been followed for 5–7 years. The second cohort of individuals was only recruited in the last few years, and thus there is insufficient follow-up for their data to be integrated and analyzed in a meaningful manner.

Characteristics of Subjects at Baseline

The first cohort of subjects consisted of 165 individuals, who were evaluated in detail. Functional status was determined by a highly reliable semistructured interview (Daly et al., 2000) that was conducted by skilled interviewers. The interview was used to generate a

Clinical Dementia Rating (CDR) score for each individual (Hughes, Berg, Danziger, Cohen, & Martin, 1982). The CDR scale is designed to stage individuals according to their functional ability, from 0 (representing normal function) and 1 (representing mild dementia) through 5 (representing the terminal phase of dementia). The subjects who were judged neither to be normal nor to have clear-cut dementia were considered "questionable" and received an overall CDR rating of 0.5. Their general characteristics can be summarized by the fact that they (1) had memory complaints, but (2) had normal activities of daily living, (3) had normal general cognitive function, and (4) were not demented.

At baseline, the 165 subjects were divided into two groups, based on their CDR rating. One group consisted of 42 subjects with normal cognition (CDR = 0.0), and the other group consisted of 123 individuals who met criteria for "questionable AD" (CDR = 0.5). The groups' mean ages were 71.4 years and 72.2 years, respectively. The educational levels of the two groups were equivalent (14.4 years and 14.9 years, respectively). Similarly, performance on a brief mental status test, the Mini-Mental State Exam (Folstein, Folstein, & McHugh, 1975), was equivalent across the two groups at baseline (29.4 ± 0.7 and 29.1 ± 1.2, respectively). The gender distribution within both groups was also similar (approximately 60% female and 40% male).

Characteristics of Subjects after 3 Years of Follow-Up

The semistructured interview was administered annually to assess changes in functional status. After 3 years of follow-up, nine subjects were deceased. One of these individuals died prior to the first follow-up assessment and is not included in this report. For those who remained alive, the annual follow-up rate was 99%.

Based on their 3-year trajectory of functional change, the subjects could be categorized into six groups:

1. *Group 1—Normals.* These subjects had normal cognition at baseline (CDR = 0) and continued to be categorized as normal at follow-up (*n* = 32). This group represented 76% of the normal subjects. Of 42 subjects with a CDR rating of 0 at baseline, 10 were categorized as questionable after 3 years of follow-up, but *none* converted to AD.

2. *Group 2—Questionables.* These subjects who met criteria for "questionable AD" at baseline (CDR = 0.5) and were still categorized as CDR = 0.5 after 3 years of follow-up (*n* = 91). This group represented 73% of the subjects with "questionable AD" at baseline.

3. *Group 3—Converters.* These subjects met CDR criteria for "questionable AD" at baseline, but progressed to the point where they were coded CDR = 1 within 3 years of follow-up and met clinical research criteria for probable AD (McKhann et al., 1984) (*n* = 23). Three Converters are now deceased, and an autopsy was obtained on two of them, which confirmed a diagnosis of definite AD in both cases (NIA–Reagan Working Group, 1997). This group of Converters represented 19% of the subjects who had been categorized as having "questionable AD" at baseline; thus the annual conversion rate among the Questionables was about 6% per year (as compared with 0% per year for the Controls).

Groups 4, 5, and 6 consisted of three smaller sets of individuals. Group 4 consisted of subjects who had "questionable AD" at baseline and were coded CDR = 1 on follow-up, but did not meet clinical research criteria for probable AD (*n* = 3). These three individuals had developed strokes, and therefore vascular disease was the cause of their cognitive impairment. Group 5 consisted of subjects with "questionable AD" at baseline who improved and were categorized as normal at follow-up ($n = 6$). Group 6 consisted of normal subjects who declined and were categorized as having "questionable AD" at follow-up ($n = 10$). Groups 4–6 have not yet been examined in detail. Data from groups 1–3 are the focus of the present report.

COLLECTION OF DATA FROM MULTIPLE DOMAINS

Data from multiple domains were collected from each of the subjects at baseline. These data included neuropsychological, neuroimaging, and genetic information. The findings from each of these assessments have been published previously (see Albert, Moss, Tanzi, & Jones, 2001; Johnson et al., 1998; Killiany et al., 2000) and are summarized below.

Neuropsychological Procedures

The neuropsychological battery that was administered to the participants at baseline consisted of 20 test scores based on 17 tests.

1. Five memory tests: the California Verbal Learning Test (CVLT), the Cued Selective Reminding Test, the Rey–Osterrieth Complex Figure Test, the Delayed Word Recall Test, and the Visual Reproduction subtest of the Wechsler Memory Scale (WMS) (Delis, Kramer, Kaplan, & Ober, 1987; Grober & Buschke, 1987; Knopman & Ryberg, 1989; Rey, 1941; Wechsler, 1945).
2. Six tests of executive function: the Trail Making Test (TMT), Part B; the Stroop Interference Test; the Self-Ordering Test (SOT); the Porteus Mazes; the Alpha Span Test; and the Digit Span (backward) subtest of the Wechsler Adult Intelligence Scale—Revised (WAIS-R) (Craik, 1986; Petrides & Milner, 1982; Porteus, 1959; Reitan, 1958; Stroop, 1935; Wechsler, 1988).
3. Three language tests: the Controlled Word Association Test for letters and for categories, and 15 items from the Boston Naming Test (Benton & Hamsher, 1976; Kaplan, Goodglass, & Weintraub, 1982).
4. Two tests of spatial ability: copying the Rey–Osterrieth Complex Figure, and copying the figures from the WMS (Rey, 1941; Wechsler, 1945).
5. Three tests of sustained attention: the Digit Span (forward) subtest of the WAIS-R; the TMT, Part A; and Cued Reaction Time (Baker, Letz, & Fidler, 1985; Reitan, 1958; Wechsler, 1988).
6. An assessment of general intelligence (estimated IQ based on a reduced version of the WAIS-R; Satz & Mogel, 1962).

These tests were not administered by the same individuals who conducted the semistructured interview that was used to generate the CDR ratings, and the test scores were not used in the assignment of the CDR ratings.

MRI Procedures

The MRI data consisted of regions of interest (ROIs) derived from three-dimensional T_1-weighted gradient echo scans of the brain (TR = 35 milliseconds [msec], TE = 5 msec, FOV = 220, flip angle = 45 degrees, slice thickness = 1.5 mm, matrix size = 256 × 256).

Each ROI was adjusted by the total intracranial volume on the scan, calculated by a semi-automated computer program (Sandor et al., 1992).

Two types of MRI measures were employed: a set that was manually drawn, and a set that was defined by an automated algorithm. Both types of measures used images that were normalized so that they could be resliced in standard planes.

The first set of ROIs consisted of five manually drawn ROIs for each subject that were obtained from the MRI images, with the operator unaware of the group status of the subject. They included the volume of the entorhinal cortex; the volume of the banks of the superior temporal sulcus (both of which were calculated on three consecutive coronal slices); and the volume of the cingulate gyrus, which was subdivided into three sections as follows: the rostral portion of the anterior cingulate, the caudal portion of the anterior cingulate, and the posterior cingulate. The methods for identifying these ROIs have been previously described (Killiany et al., 2000). The semiautomated procedures used to calculate the volume of the ROIs are described elsewhere (Sandor et al., 1990).

The second set of ROIs consisted of six automated measures of cerebrospinal fluid spaces that either provided a reflection of the integrity of the medial temporal lobe (e.g., the temporal horn) or assessed the generalized atrophy that is evident in the middle and late stages of disease (e.g., the third ventricle). These latter ROIs, which have been previously used in other studies (Sandor et al., 1992), were as follows: the temporal horns, the suprasellar cisterns, the third ventricle, the lateral ventricles, the sylvian fissures, and the interhemispheric fissure.

SPECT Procedures

The SPECT data were obtained from a brain imaging system (CERESPECT, Digital Scintigraphics, Inc., Waltham, MA) consisting of a stationary annular NAI crystal and rotating collimator system (Genna & Smith, 1988). Subjects were scanned 20 minutes after injection of 20.0 mCi (± 1.0 mCi) of 99mTc-HMPAO (Ceretec, Amersham, England) with the subjects supine at rest, with eyes open, in a darkened room with ambient white noise. Datasets were displayed as a set of 64 slices (slice thickness = 1.67 mm), using a 128×128 matrix (pixels = $1.67 \times 1.67 \times 2$ mm). Anatomical orientation, surface contouring, and scaling procedures for the SPECT data were performed as detailed previously (Johnson et al., 1993). The measured resolution was 7.3 mm at 9 mm from center for 99mTc (Holman et al., 1990).

The statistical method of singular value decomposition (SVD) was used to examine the SPECT data (Jones et al., 1998). For each subject, 20 weighted scores were calculated, based on 20 vectors derived from a normative sample ($n = 152$). The normative group was used to compute the weighting coefficients for the 20 vectors, which together represented the covariance pattern of brain activity. The 20 vector scores for each subject were then used in the analysis of the subjects in the longitudinal study (Johnson et al., 1998).

Genetic Assessment

The APOE gene was also examined in the participants, because the APOE-4 allele of this gene is overrepresented in patients with AD compared to the general population (Saunders et al., 1993), and is now widely recognized as a risk factor for AD. We therefore sought to determine whether APOE status, either alone or in combination with the neuropsychological or neuroimaging measures, was useful as a predictor of which individuals would "convert" to having AD over time.

PARALLEL METHODS OF DATA ANALYSIS

Each of the data sets related to neuropsychological and imaging status were analyzed separately, and the results have been published (Albert et al., 2001; Johnson et al., 1998; Killiany et al., 2000). As the data were analyzed in a parallel manner, it is possible to compare the findings directly with one another, as discussed below.

For the neuropsychological and MRI data, a series of parallel discriminant-function analyses were performed (Press, 1972). These analyses were as follows:

1. The first discriminant analysis was conducted to determine whether the primary scores in each of the three domains, when taken together, would significantly differentiate the three groups from one another (Controls vs. Questionables vs. Converters). This discriminant function also included a measure of age and gender (number of years of education was also included in the neuropsychological analyses, because of the potential impact of education on test performance). It should be noted that these covariates (age, gender, and years of education) were not significant, but were included in all of the discriminant-function analyses. This procedure was used to assure that any subtle, though nonsignificant, effect of these variables was reduced as much as possible.

2. The second discriminant function (which was only performed if the first analysis was statistically significant) was a stepwise discriminant-function analysis. The goal of this analysis was to select the variables within each domain that best differentiated the Controls, Questionables, and Converters from one another. The term "best" refers here to the process by which each variable was selected by the algorithm, and the fact that specific variables were selected in sequence, in order to improve the significance of the overall function. In the stepwise analysis, the covariates were entered at the first step, and then the algorithm of the discriminant function selected the variables that, when combined, "best" differentiated the groups from one another.

3. Separate post hoc discriminant function analyses were then performed within each domain in which the groups were compared pairwise (i.e., Controls vs. Converters, Controls vs. Questionables, Questionables vs. Converters). These pairwise comparisons included only the covariates mentioned above, and the variables that had been deemed "best" by the stepwise analysis.

The analysis of the SPECT data departed slightly from this procedure, due to the use of the SVD method. For the SPECT data, the overall discriminant-function analysis was performed (adjusted for age and gender) in the same manner described above, using 20 SPECT vector scores for each subject. The vectors that contributed to the discrimination were then "back-projected" in order to identify the brain regions that were involved in differentiating the groups (see Jones et al., 1998, and Johnson et al., 1998, for additional details).

It should be emphasized that all of the data were obtained at baseline, but that group membership was based on a subject's status following three annual follow-up visits. It should also be noted that the sample sizes varied depending upon the domain of analysis, as some subjects were missing relevant data or had data that contained artifacts and thus could not be used.

NEUROPSYCHOLOGICAL AND NEUROIMAGING RESULTS

Neuropsychological Test Results

Four of the 20 neuropsychological measures obtained at baseline were useful in discriminating the groups on the basis of their status 3 years after the tests were given. The four discriminating tests pertained to assessments of memory and executive function. They were (1) the total learning score on the CVLT, (2) the immediate recall of the figures from the WMS (F-WMS), (3) the time to completion on Part B of the TMT, and (4) the total score on the SOT.

In the CVLT, the subject is presented with a 16-word list of words that is read five times in succession (each time in a different order). The subject is asked to recall the words after each reading of the list, and then again after both long and short delays (during which a list with a different set of words is read). The total learning score is the total number of words the subject recalls over the first five learning trials, and thus reflects the number of words the subject can learn with repeated exposure. For the F-WMS, the subject is presented with four moderately complex drawings and is asked to draw each one approximately 10 seconds after having seen it. This measure pertains to the ability to recall drawings rather than words, and assesses immediate recall after a single exposure, rather than cumulative learning over multiple exposures. It should be noted that the F-WMS was not significantly different among the groups in the pairwise comparisons, but when all of the measures were combined with one another, it improved the accuracy of discrimination significantly. Both of these memory tasks evaluate the ability to learn new information; one assesses total learning over multiple trials, and one assesses the amount of information learned over a single trial.

In Part B of the TMT, the subject is asked to draw a line between numbers and letters in order, alternating between each number and letter (i.e., A-1-2-B-3-C, etc.). The numbers and letters are scattered across the page; thus the subject must search for the next number or letter in the series, and keep track of where he or she is in the series. In order to maintain the alternating principle of the task, the subject must alternate between these overlearned series and inhibit the impulse to go to the next number or letter in the series. In the SOT, the subject sees sheets of paper on which are lists of words of varying lengths (e.g., a six-word list, an eight-word list, etc). Each sheet contains the entire list, but there is more than one sheet for each list; the number of sheets per trial corresponds to the number of words on the list (e.g., six sheets for a six-word trial). The subject is presented with the sheets for each word list one at a time, and is asked to point to a different word on each sheet. Thus the subject decides the order in which the words will be pointed to, but must keep track of that order in order to perform well. Both of these executive function tasks require sequencing, self-monitoring, and set shifting.

The accuracy with which these four tasks could differentiate the groups was related to the clinical similarity between them. When the Controls were compared to the individuals with memory impairments who ultimately developed AD (the Converters), the accuracy of discrimination was 89%, based on the neuropsychological measures at baseline. The discrimination of the Controls from the individuals with mild memory problems who did not progress to the point where they met clinical criteria for probable AD over the 3 years of follow-up (the Questionables) was 74%, and the discrimination of the Questionables from the Converters was 80%. (See Albert et al., 2001, for further details.)

MRI Results

Three of the 11 MRI measures obtained at baseline were useful in discriminating the groups on the basis of their status 3 years after the scans were obtained. These measures were the entorhinal cortex, the banks of the superior temporal sulcus, and the caudal portion of the anterior cingulate. As with the neuropsychological results, the accuracy of discrimination was related to the clinical similarity between groups. When the Controls were compared to the Converters, the accuracy of discrimination was 93%. The discrimination of the Controls from the Questionables was 85%, and the discrimination of the Questionables from the Converters was 75%. (See Killiany et al., 2000, for further details.)

SPECT Results

SPECT perfusion abnormalities in four brain regions at baseline were found to differentiate the groups on the basis of their status 3 years after the scans were obtained. These regions were as follows: the hippocampal–amygdaloid complex, the posterior cingulate, the anterior thalamus, and the caudal portion of the anterior cingulate. When the Controls were compared to the Converters, the accuracy of discrimination was 83%. The discrimination of the Controls from the Questionables was 72.6%, and the discrimination of the Questionables from the Converters was 84%. (See Johnson et al., 1998, for further details.)

Genetic Results

When APOE status alone was used to differentiate the three groups, the discriminant function was not statistically significant. APOE status was then added to each of the discriminant-function analyses for each domain. Addition of APOE status did not significantly improve the discrimination of the three groups above that of the neuropsychological or neuroimaging data alone (Albert et al., 2001; Johnson et al., 1998; Killiany et al., 2000).

BRAIN NETWORKS IMPLICATED IN PRECLINICAL AD

These findings indicate that individuals in the preclinical phase of AD have measurable difficulties with memory and executive function. The memory measure obtained at baseline that best predicted a subsequent diagnosis of AD was the total learning score from the CVLT. As this is a measure of the total number of words recalled over the course of five learning trials, it is primarily a reflection of consistency of learning over time. A measure of delayed recall was also useful in discriminating the groups (data not shown), but the total learning score of the CVLT was a better indicator of subsequent progression of memory difficulty than the measure of delayed recall was. This was an unexpected finding, as numerous studies have shown that recall after a delay is best at discriminating patients with mild AD from controls and from patients with other dementias or amnesias (Kopelman, 1985; Milberg & Albert, 1989; Moss et al., 1986). We hypothesize that the CVLT total learning score was the best discriminator in this setting because it is a more stable measure of memory function than delayed recall, particularly among individuals with very mild impairments.

The two executive function tasks that were predictors of subsequent decline both involved sequencing and set shifting. This finding is entirely consistent with previous studies in patients with mild AD showing that tasks of sequencing and set shifting are impaired at an early stage of disease, particularly as compared to tests that evaluate conceptualization (Grady et al., 1988; Lafleche & Albert, 1995; Morris & Baddeley, 1988; Sahakian et al., 1990).

These findings with respect to memory performance are consistent with previous reports conducted among those destined to develop dementia (e.g., Bondi et al., 1994; Howieson, Camicioli, Sexton, Payami, & Kane, 1997; Jacobs et al., 1995; Petersen, Smith, Ivnik, Kokmen, & Tangalos, 1994; Rubin et al., 1998; Small, Herlitz, Fratiglioni, Almkvist, & Cakman, 1997; Small, LaRue, Komo, Kaplan, & Mandelkern, 1995; Tierney et al., 1996; Tuokko, Vernon-Wilkinson, Weir, & Beattie, 1991). At least one previous study reported that a test involving the reversal of a well-known sequence (i.e., the Mental Control subtest of the WMS) was useful in predicting subsequent development of AD (Tierney et al., 1996).

Atrophy in the entorhinal cortex and the adjacent hippocampus has likewise been reported among individuals with preclinical AD by a few research groups (Bobinski et al., 1999; Convit et al., 1993; Fox et al., 1996; Kaye et al., 1997; Xu et al., 2000). Moreover, a single MRI measure of the entorhinal cortex is more accurate at discriminating individuals with preclinical or mild AD from controls than is a comparable measure of the hippocampus. This suggests that the entorhinal cortex is affected earlier in AD, leading to its more accurate discrimination when individuals with incipient or mild disease are compared with normal controls (Killiany et al., 2001).

Decreases in perfusion in the hippocampal region and the anterior and posterior cingulate are consistent with several reports. This change has recently been seen among individuals who have a genetic mutation that causes AD but who remain asymptomatic (Johnson et al., 2001). In addition, alterations in the posterior cingulate have been seen among individuals who are homozygous for the APOE-4 allele, both with and without memory problems (Reiman et al., 1996; Small, Mazziotta, et al., 1995). Decreases in temporoparietal perfusion among prodromal cases of AD have also been reported (Kennedy et al., 1995).

Taken together, the overall importance of these findings primarily pertains to the parallels that are evident between the neuropsychological and neuroimaging results. They suggest that a selected group of brain regions develop neuropathology during preclinical AD, and that this pathology in turn influences the cognitive deficits of the individuals.

The memory deficit seen in preclinical AD appears to be related to the brain regions that influence memory function and that show pathological change early in the course of AD. The initial neuronal lesions of AD (e.g., the neurofibrillary tangles and neuritic plaques) develop in the entorhinal cortex (Braak & Braak, 1991), with some layers of the entorhinal cortex undergoing 40–60% neuronal loss even in the earliest phase of disease (Gomez-Isla et al., 1996). The entorhinal cortex is part of a memory-related neural system in the brain (Squire & Zola, 1997). The superior temporal sulcus is a multimodal association area that appears to be necessary for holding information during a delay, and that has been hypothesized to play a role in memory or the attentional capacities necessary for normal memory (Eskander, Richmond, & Optican, 1992; Salzman, 1995).

Similarly, it has been hypothesized that the caudal portion of the anterior cingulate plays a major role in executive function abilities, primarily through reciprocal connections with the prefrontal cortex (Arikuni, Sako, & Murata, 1994). This region also has reciprocal connections with memory-related structures, including the entorhinal cortex (Van

Hoesen, Morecraft, & Vogt, 1993). The anterior cingulate is known to develop severe neuronal loss in AD (Vogt, Crino, & Volicer, 1991), but the stage at which this occurs is not yet known. The present findings suggest that neuronal loss in the anterior cingulate may begin early in the disease, and may be responsible in part for the executive function deficits seen in the early stage of disease.

The negative findings regarding APOE status as a predictor of "conversion" to AD are consistent with several recent studies, including a large multicenter study that examined the use of the APOE genotype as a diagnostic test for AD (Mayeux et al., 1998). Although there is consensus that APOE-4 status confers increased lifetime risk for AD, the present findings suggest that this genotype cannot be used to predict conversion to AD within 3 years.

In summary, these findings suggest that an interdisciplinary approach involving neuropsychological testing (with an emphasis on the characterization of memory function), neuroimaging, and genetics can yield important insights into the development of AD. Identification of individuals in a preclinical or prodromal phase will be critical in testing existing therapies for their ability to alter the course of the illness and for developing novel strategies to prevent or delay dementia.

ACKNOWLEDGMENTS

This work was supported by Grant No. P01-AG04953 from the National Institute on Aging. We would like to thank Dr. Kenneth Jones for assistance with statistical analysis, and Dr. Mary Hyde for assistance with data management.

REFERENCES

Albert, M. S., Moss, M. B., Tanzi, R., & Jones, K. (2001). Preclinical prediction of AD using neuropsychological tests. *Journal of the International Neuropsychological Society, 7,* 631–639.

Alzheimer, A. (1907). Uber eine eigenatrige Erkraukung der Hirwrinde. *Allegmeine Zeitschrift für Psychiatrie, 64,* 146–148.

Arikuni, T., Sako, H., & Murata, A. (1994). Ipsilateral connections of the anterior cingulate with the frontal and medial temporal cortices in the macaque monkey. *Neuroscience Research, 21,* 19–39.

Baker, E. L., Letz, R., & Fidler, A. T. (1985). A computer administered neurobehavioral evaluation system for occupational and environmental epidemiology. *Journal of Occupational Medicine, 27,* 206–212.

Bales, K. R., Verina, T., Dodel, R. C., Du, Y., Altstiel, L., Bender, M., Hyslop, P., Johnstone, E.M., Little, S. P., Cummins, D. J., Piccardo, P., Ghetti, B., & Paul, S. M. (1997). Lack of apolipoprotein E dramatically reduces amyloid beta-peptide deposition. *Nature Genetics, 3,* 263–264.

Benton, A. L., & Hamsher, K. (1976). *Multilingual Aphasia Examination.* Iowa City: University of Iowa Press.

Bobinski, M., deLeon, M., Convit, A., DeSanti, S., Weigiel, J., Tarshish, C., Saint Louis, L., & Wisniewski, H. (1999). MRI of entorhinal cortex in mild Alzheimer's disease. *Lancet, 353,* 38–40.

Bondi, M., Monsch, A., Galasko, D., Butters, N., Salmon, D., & Delis, D. (1994). Preclinical cognitive markers of dementia of the Alzheimer type. *Neuropsychology, 4,* 374–384.

Braak, H., & Braak, E. (1991). Neuropathological staging of Alzheimer-related changes. *Acta Neuropathologica, 82,* 239–259.

Convit, A., de Leon, M., Golomb, J., Goerge, A., Tarshish, C., Bobinski, M., Tsui, W., De Santi, S., Wegiel, J., & Wisniewski, H. (1993). Hippocampal atrophy in early Alzheimer's disease: Anatomic specificity and validation. *Psychiatric Quarterly, 64,* 371–387.

Craik, F. I. M. (1986). A functional account of age differences in memory. In F. Klix & H. Hagendorf (Eds.), *Human memory and cognitive capabilities* (pp. 409–422). Amsterdam: Elsevier.

Cummings, J., & Benson, D. (1983). *Dementia: A clinical approach.* Boston: Butterworth.

Daly, E., Zaitchik, D., Copeland, M., Schmahmann, J., Gunther, J., & Albert, M. (2000). Predicting "conversion" to AD using standardized clinical information. *Archives of Neurology, 57,* 675–680.

Delis, D., Kramer, J., Kaplan, E., & Ober, B. (1987). *The California Verbal Learning Test.* New York: Psychological Corporation.

Eskander, E., Richmond, B., & Optican, L. (1992). Role of inferior temporal neurons in visual memory: I. Temporal encoding of information about visual images, recalled images, and behavioral context. *Journal of Neurophysiology, 68,* 1277–1295.

Evans, D., Funkenstein, H., Albert, M., Scherr, P., Cook, N., Chown, M., Hebert, L., Hennekens, C., & Taylor, J. (1989). Prevalence of Alzheimer's disease in a community dwelling population of older persons: Higher than previously reported. *Journal of the American Medical Association, 262,* 2551–2556.

Folstein, M., Folstein, S., & McHugh, P. (1975). "Mini-Mental State": A practical method for grading the cognitive state of patients for the clinician. *Journal of Psychiatric Research, 2,* 189–198.

Fox, N., Warrington, E., Freeborough, P., Hartikainene, P., Kennedy, A., Stevens, M., & Rossor, M. (1996). Presymptomatic hippocampal atrophy in Alzheimer's disease: A longitudinal study. *Brain, 119,* 2001–2007.

Genna, S., & Smith, A. (1988). The development of ASPECT, an annular single crystal brain camera for high efficiency SPECT. *IEEE Transactions in Nuclear Science, 35,* 654–658.

Glenner, G., & Wong, C. (1984). Alzheimer's disease: Initial report of purification and characterization of a novel cerebrovascular amyloid protein. *Biochemical and Biophysics Research Communications, 120,* 885–890.

Goate, A., Chartier-Harlin, M., Mullan, M., Brown, J., Crawford, F., Fidani, L., Giuffra, L., Haynes, A., Irving, N., James, L., Mant, R., Newton, P., Rooke, K., Roques, P., Talbot, C., Pericak-Vance, M., Roses, A., Williamson, R., Rossor, M., Owen, M., & Hardy, J. (1991). Segregation of a missense mutation in the amyloid precursor protein gene with familial Alzheimer's disease. *Nature, 349,* 704–706.

Gomez-Isla, T., Price, J., McKeel, D., Morris, J., Growdon, J., & Hyman, B. (1996). Profound loss of layer II entorhinal cortex neurons occurs in very mild Alzheimer's disease. *Journal of Neuroscience, 16,* 4491–4500.

Grady, C., Haxby, J., Horwitz, B., Sundaram, M., Berg, G., Schapiro, M., Friedland, R., & Rapoport, S. (1988). Longitudinal study of the early neuropsychological and cerebral metabolic changes in dementia of the Alzheimer type. *Journal of Clinical and Experimental Neuropsychology, 10,* 576–596.

Grober, E., & Buschke, H. (1987). Genuine memory deficits in dementia. *Developmental Neuropsychology, 3,* 13–36.

Hart, R., Kwentus, J., Harkins, S., & Taylor, J. (1988). Rate of forgetting in mild Alzheimer's-type dementia. *Brain and Cognition, 7,* 31–38.

Holman, B., Carvalho, P., Zimmerman, R., Johnson, K., Tumeh, S., Smith, A., & Genna., S. (1990). Brain perfusion SPECT using an annular single crystal camera: Initial clinical experience. *Journal of Nuclear Medicine, 31,* 1456–1561.

Howieson, D., Camicioli, R., Sexton, G., Payami, H., & Kaye, J. (1997). Cognitive markers preceding Alzheimer's dementia in the healthy oldest old. *Journal of the American Geriatrics Society, 44,* 584–589.

Hughes, C. P., Berg, L., Danziger, W. L., Coben, L. A., & Martin, R. L. (1982). A new clinical scale for the staging of dementia. *British Journal of Psychiatry, 140,* 566–572.

Hyman, B. T., Van Hoesen, G. W., Kromer, C., & Damasio, A. R. (1984). Alzheimer's disease: Cell specific pathology isolates the hippocampal formation. *Science, 225,* 1168–1170.

Jacobs, D., Sano, M., Doonerief, G., Marder, K., Bell, K., & Stern, Y. (1995). Neuropsychological detection and characterization of preclinical Alzheimer's disease. *Neurology, 45,* 957–962.

Johnson, K. A., Jones, K., Holman, B. L., Becker, J. A., Spiers, P., Satlin, A., & Albert, M. S. (1998). Preclinical prediction of Alzheimer's disease using SPECT. *Neurology, 50,* 1563–1571.

Johnson, K. A., Kijewski, M., Becker, J., Garada, B., Satlin, A., & Holman, B. L. (1993). Quantitative brain SPECT in Alzheimer's disease and normal aging. *Journal of Nuclear Medicine, 34,* 2044–2048.

Johnson, K. A., Lopera, F., Jones, K., Becker, A., Sperling, R., Hilson, J., Londono, J., Siegert, I., Arcos, M., Moreno, S., Madrigal, L., Ossa, J., Pineda, N., Ardila, A., Roselli, M., Albert, M., Kosik, K., & Rios, A. (2001). Presenilin-1-associated abnormalities in regional cerebral perfusion. *Neurology, 56,* 1545–1551.

Jones, K., Johnson, K. A., Becker, A., Spiers, P., Albert, M. S., & Holman, L. B. (1998). Use of singular value decomposition to characterize age and gender differences in SPECT cerebral perfusion. *Journal of Nuclear Medicine, 39,* 965–973.

Kaplan, E., Goodglass, H., & Weintraub, S. (1982). *Boston Naming Test.* Philadelphia: Lea & Febiger.

Katzman, R. (1976). The prevalence and malignancy of Alzheimer disease. *Archives of Neurology, 33,* 217–218.

Kaye, J., Swihart, T., Howieson, D., Dame, A., Moore, M., Karnos, B., Camicioli, R., Ball, M., Oken, B., & Sexton, G. (1997). Volume loss of the hippocampus and temporal lobe in healthy elderly persons destined to develop dementia. *Neurology, 48,* 1297–1304.

Kemper, T. (1994). Neuroanatomical and neuropathological changes during aging. In M. L. Albert and J. Knoefel (Eds.), *Clinical neurology of aging* (2nd ed., pp. 3–67). New York: Oxford University Press.

Kennedy, A. M., Frackowiak, R. S., Newman, S. K., Bloomfield, P. M., Seaward, J., Roques, P., Lewington, G., Cunningham, V. J., & Rossor, M. N. (1995). Deficits in cerebral glucose metabolism demonstrated by positron emission tomography in individuals at risk of familial Alzheimer's disease. *Neuroscience Letters, 186,* 17–20.

Killiany, R., Gomez-Isla, T., Moss, M., Kikinis, R., Sandor, T., Jolesz, F., Tanzi, R., Jones, K., Hyman, B., & Albert, M. (2000). Use of structural magnetic resonance imaging to predict who will get alzheimer's disease. *Annals of Neurology, 47,* 430–439.

Killiany, R., Hyman, B., Gomez-Isla, T., Moss, M., Kikinis, R., Jolesz, F., Tanzi, R., Jones, K., & Albert, M. (2001). *The entorhinal cortex is selectively atrophied in preclinical AD: Comparison of MRI measures of the entorhinal cortex and hippocampus.* Manuscript submitted for publication.

Knopman, D. S., & Ryberg, S. (1989). A verbal memory test with high predictive accuracy for dementia of the Alzheimer type. *Archives of Neurology, 46,* 141–145.

Kopelman, M. (1985). Rates of forgetting in Alzheimer-type dementia and Korsakoff's syndrome. *Neuropsychologia, 23,* 623–638.

Lafleche, G., & Albert, M. S. (1995). Executive function deficits in mild Alzheimer's disease. *Neuropsychology, 9,* 313–320.

Lee, V.-Y., Balin, B., Otvos, L., & Tojanowski, J. (1991). A68: A major subunit of paired helical filaments and derivatized forms of normal tau. *Science, 251,* 675–678.

Levy-Lahad, E., Wasco, W., Poorkaj, P., Romano, D. M., Oshima, J., Pettingell, W., Yu, C., Jondro, P., Schmidt, S., Wang, K., Crowley, A., Fu, Y.-H., Guenette, S., Galas, D., Nemens, E., Wijsman, E., Bird, T., Schellenberg, G., & Tanzi, R. (1995). Candidate gene for the chromosome 1 familial Alzheimer's disease locus. *Science, 269,* 973–977.

Mayeux, R., Saunders, A. M., Shea, S., Mirra, S., Evans, D., Roses, A., Hyman, B. T., Crain, B., Tang, M. X., & Phelps, C. H. (1998). Utility of the apolipoprotein E genotype in the diagnosis of Alzheimer's disease. *New England Journal of Medicine, 338,* 506–511.

McKhann, G., Drachman, D., Folstein, M. F., Katzman, R., Price, D., & Stadlan, E. (1984). Clinical diagnosis of Alzheimer's disease: Report of the NINCDS–ADRDA Workgroup under the auspices of Department of Health and Human Services Task Force. *Neurology, 34*, 939–944.

Milberg, M., & Albert, M. S. (1989). Cognitive differences between patients with progressive supranuclear palsy and Alzheimer's disease. *Journal of Clinical and Experimental Neuropsychology 11*, 605–614.

Morris, R., & Baddeley, A. (1988). Primary and working memory functioning in Alzheimer-type dementia. *Journal of Clinical and Experimental Neuropsychology, 10*, 279–276.

Moss, M. B., Albert, M. S., Butters, N., & Payne, M. (1986). Differential patterns of memory loss among patients with Alzheimer's disease, Huntington's disease and Alcoholic Korsakoff's Syndrome. *Archives of Neurology, 43*, 239–246.

National Institute on Aging (NIA)–Reagan Working Group. (1997). Consensus recommendations for the postmortem diagnosis of Alzheimer's disease. *Neurobiology of Aging, 18*, S1–S27.

Petersen, R., Smith, G., Ivnik, R., Kokmen, E., & Tangalos, E. (1994). Memory function in very early Alzheimer's disease. *Neurology, 44*, 867–872.

Petrides, M., & Milner, B. (1982). Deficits in subject-ordered tasks after frontal and temporal lobe lesions in man. *Neuropsychologia, 20*, 249–262.

Porteus, S. (1959). *The Maze Test and clinical psychology*. Palo Alto, CA: Pacific Books.

Press, E. J. (1972). *Applied multivariate analysis*. New York: Holt, Rinehart & Winston.

Reiman, E. M., Caselli, R. J., Yun, L. S., Chen, K., Bandy, D., Minoshima, S., Thibodeau, S. N., & Osborne, D. (1996). Preclinical evidence of Alzheimer's disease in persons homozygous for the epsilon 4 allele for apolipoprotein E. *New England Journal of Medicine, 334*, 752–758.

Reitan, R. M. (1958). Validity of the Trail Making Test as an indicator of organic brain damage. *Perceptual and Motor Skills, 8*, 271–276.

Rey, A. (1941). L'examen psychologique dans les cas d'encephalopathie traumatique. *Archives de Psychologie, 28*, 286–340.

Rosen, W., & Mohs, R. (1982). Evolution of cognitive decline in dementia. In S. Corkin, K. L. Davis, J. H. Growdon, E. Usdin, & R. J. Wurtman (Eds.), *Aging: Vol. 19. Alzheimer's disease: A report of progress* (pp. 183–188). New York: Raven Press.

Rubin, E. H., Storandt, M., Miller, J. P., Kinscherf, D. A., Grant, E. E., Morris, J. C., & Berg, L. (1998). A prospective study of cognitive function and onset of dementia in cognitively healthy elders. *Archives of Neurology, 55*, 395–401.

Sahakian, B., Downes, J., Eagger, S., Evenden, J., Levy, R., Philpot, M., Roberts, A., & Robbins, T. (1990). Sparing of attentional relative to mnemonic function in a subgroup of patients with dementia of the Alzheimer type. *Neuropsychologia, 28*, 1197–1213.

Salzman, E. (1995). Attention and memory trials during neuronal recording from the primate pulvinar and posterior parietal cortex (area PG). *Behavioral Brain Research, 67*, 241–253.

Sandor, T., Jolesz, F., Tieman, J., Kikinis, R., Jones, K., & Albert, M. S. (1992). Comparative analysis of computed tomographic and magnetic resonance imaging scans in Alzheimer patients and controls. *Archives of Neurology, 49*, 381–384.

Sandor, T., Jolesz, F., Tieman, J., Kikinis, R., LeMay, M., & Albert, M. S. (1990). Extraction of morphometric information from dual echo magnetic resonance images. *Proceedings of the Society for Photo Optical Instruments and Engineering, 1360*, 665–675.

Satz, P., & Mogel, S. (1962). An abbreviation of the WAIS for clinical use. *Journal of Clinical Psychology, 18*, 77–79.

Saunders, A. M., Strittmatter, W. J., Schmechel, D., St. George-Hyslop, P., Pericak-Vance, M., Joo, S., Rosi, B., Gusella, J., Crapper-MacLachlan, D., Alberts, M., Hulette, C., Crain, B., Goldgaber, D., & Roses, A. (1993). Association of apolipoprotein E allele 4 with late-onset familial and sporadic Alzheimer's disease. *Neurology, 43*, 1467–1472.

Schellenberg, G., Bird, T., Wijsman, E., Orr, H., Anderson, L., Nemens, E., White, J., Bonnycastle, L., Weber, J., Alonso, M., Potter, H., Heston, L., & Martin, J. (1992). Genetic linkage evidence for a familial Alzheimer's disease locus on chromosome 14. *Science, 258*, 668–671.

Selkoe, D. (2000). The genetics and molecular pathology of Alzheimer's disease: Roles of amyloid and the presenilins. *Neurologic Clinics, 18*, 903–922.

Small, B., Herlitz, A., Fratiglioni, L., Almkvist, O., & Cakman, L. (1997). Cognitive predictors of incident Alzheimer's disease: A prospective longitudinal study. *Neuropsychology, 11*, 1–8.

Small, G. W., LaRue, A., Komo, S., Kaplan, A., & Mandelkern, M. (1995). Predictors of cognitive change in middle-aged and older adults with memory loss. *American Journal of Psychiatry, 152*, 1757–1764.

Small, G. W., Mazziotta, J. C., Collins, M. T., Baxter, L. R., Phelps, M. E., Mandelkern, M. A., Kaplan, A., LaRue, A., Adamson, C. F., Chang, L., et al. (1995). Apolipoprotein E type 4 allele and cerebral glucose metabolism in relatives at risk for familial Alzheimer disease. *Journal of the American Medical Association, 273*, 942–947.

Squire, L., & Zola, S. (1997). Amnesia, memory and brain systems. *Philosophical Transactions of the Royal Society of London, Series B, 29*, 1663–1673.

Stroop, J. R. (1935). Studies of interference in serial verbal reactions. *Journal of Experimental Psychology, 18*, 643–662.

Tierney, M., Szalai, J., Snow, W., Fisher, R., Nores, A., Nadon, G., Dunn, E., & St. George-Hyslop, P. (1996). Prediction of probable Alzheimer's disease in memory-impaired patients: A prospective longitudinal study. *Neurology, 46*, 661–665.

Tuokko, H., Vernon-Wilkinson, J., Weir, J., & Beattie, W. (1991). Cued recall and early identification of dementia. *Journal of Clinical and Experimental Neuropsychology, 13*, 871–879.

Van Hoesen, G., Morecraft, R., & Vogt, B. (1993). Connections of the monkey cingulate cortex. In B. Vogt & M. Gabriel (Eds.), *The neurobiology of the cingulate cortex and limbic thalamus* (pp. 249–284). Boston: Birchauser.

Vogt, B., Crino, P., & Volicer, L. (1991). Laminar alterations in γ-aminobutyric acid$_a$, muscarinic and β adrenoceptors and neuron degeneration in cingulate cortex in Alzheimer's disease. *Journal of Neurochemistry, 57*, 282–290.

Wechsler, D. (1945). A standardized memory scale for clinical use. *Journal of Psychology, 19*, 87–95.

Wechsler, D. (1988). *The Wechsler Adult Intelligence Scale—Revised.* New York: Psychological Corporation.

Welsh, K., Butters, N., Hughes, J., Mohs, R., & Heyman, A. (1991). Detection of abnormal memory decline in mild cases of Alzheimer's disease using CERAD neuropsychological measures. *Archives of Neurology, 48*, 278–281.

Xu, Y., Jack, C., O'Brien, P., Kokmen, E., Smith, G., Ivnik, R., Boeve, B., Tangalos, R., & Petersen, R. (2000). Usefulness of MRI measures of entorhinal cortex versus hippocampus in AD. *Neurology, 54*, 1760–1767.

21

Memory Rehabilitation

BARBARA A. WILSON

Rehabilitation is not synonymous with recovery or restitution of lost functioning. For most people with organic memory deficits, recovery or restitution of lost memory skills is unobtainable. Although rehabilitation may include attempts to restore lost functioning, it goes far beyond this approach. It is concerned with helping people to understand, come to terms with, and compensate for their difficulties. "Cognitive rehabilitation" may be defined as "a process whereby people with brain injury work together with health service professionals to remediate or alleviate cognitive deficits arising from a neurological insult" (Wilson, 1997, p. 488). Memory difficulties are among the commonest cognitive problems arising from injury to the brain; consequently, much cognitive rehabilitation is devoted to helping people with memory deficits reduce or avoid everyday problems. This chapter describes some of the ways people with memory deficits can be helped to live as independent and stress-free lives as possible.

ASSESSMENT FOR REHABILITATION

Before memory rehabilitation begins, it is customary to carry out an assessment of clients' general intellectual ability, together with a more detailed assessment of their memory functioning. In addition, most neuropsychologists assess language, perceptual, attentional, and executive functioning to build up a picture of each person's cognitive strengths and weaknesses. Assessment of memory and other cognitive functioning will enable an evaluator to determine such things as the person's present level of intellectual functioning, the estimated premorbid level of functioning, whether there are widespread cognitive deficits or whether the person has a pure amnesic syndrome, whether the memory problems are global or restricted to certain kinds of material, and so forth. Useful as this information is, it is insufficient to determine how memory problems are affecting the individual in his or her everyday life. For example, poor scores on standardized tests do not show how the memory deficits identified are manifested in everyday life. These scores also cannot indicate how family members cope, what the memory-impaired person and relatives want particular help with, what kind of treatment should be offered, and so forth. To identify these problems, neuropsychologists need to use other types of measures, such as direct observations, self-report measures (from family members, therapists, and others), and interviews. Information from both standardized and more functional measures should be combined in the planning of a treatment program. (See Wilson, 1999, for examples of this approach in clinical practice.)

SELECTING GOALS FOR TREATMENT

Treatment in many rehabilitation centers is focused around a goal-planning approach, whereby the goals for treatment are negotiated among the memory-impaired person, family members or carers, and the rehabilitation staff. Goal planning in rehabilitation is not new and has been used for a number of years with people who have spinal injuries, learning difficulties, or cerebral palsy, as well as those with brain injury (McMillan & Sparkes, 1999).

Houts and Scott (1975) have stated five principles of goal planning: (1) Involve the patient, (2) set reasonable goals, (3) describe the patient's behavior when the goal is reached, (4) set a deadline, and (5) spell out the method so that anyone reading it will know what to do. McMillan and Sparkes (1999) expand on these principles by suggesting that there should be long-term and short-term goals. Long-term goals are concerned with the reduction of disabilities and handicaps, and should be achievable by the time of discharge from the center. Short-term goals are steps required to achieve long-term goals. McMillan and Sparks elaborate further on the principles of Houts and Scott by stating that goals should be (1) client-centered, (2) realistic and potentially attainable during admission, (3) clear and specific, (4) presented with a definite time deadline, and (5) measurable.

Given the principles described above, a goal-planning approach for a man with memory problems might include the following:

Goal 1: Develop an understanding of his cognitive strengths and weaknesses.
Goal 2: Help him develop a system for remembering and scheduling his everyday activities.
Goal 3: Have him learn how to use a computer program for managing his own finances.
Goal 4: Assist him in developing a range of leisure pursuits.
Goal 5: Identify the tasks required for his return to work.

Each of these long-term goals will be broken down and attempted through a series of short-term goals. (See Wilson, Evans, & Keohane, 2001, for an example of this approach with a man who sustained both a head injury and a stroke.)

COMPENSATING FOR MEMORY DEFICITS

The ultimate goal of rehabilitation is to enable people with disabilities to function as adequately as possible in their own most appropriate environment (McLellan, 1991). Compensating for an inadequate memory is one of the major ways people with organic memory impairment can achieve independence or partial independence in their own environments. Elsewhere (Wilson & Watson, 1996), a colleague and I describe a framework for understanding compensatory behavior. The framework, based on one by Bäckman and Dixon (1992), suggests that compensation involves four processes: origins (a mismatch between environmental demands and cognitive capacity), mechanisms (the means by which the mismatch is reduced), forms (the manner and extent to which compensatory behavior differs from the behavior of a normal person in a given situation), and consequences (the successful or unsuccessful results of the compensatory behavior). We (Wilson & Watson, 1996) have provided evidence to show that it is easier for people with a relatively pure amnesic syndrome to compensate adequately for their difficulties than it is for those with more widespread cognitive deficits. (See Wilson, 2000, for a more detailed discussion of compensation.)

A recent study (Evans, Wilson, Needham, & Brentnall, 2001) found that in a group of 96 memory-impaired people living in the community, all but 2 were using some kind of compensatory strategy, and that a total of 44 different strategies were employed. The most commonly used aids were calendars, lists, notebooks, and diaries. These results are similar to those of an earlier study (Wilson, 1991b). Very few people in either study were using electronic aids. This lack of use may be because such aids are too complex to learn to use following the onset of memory impairment. However, it *is* possible to teach people the use of such aids (Wright et al., 2001).

One of the most successful compensatory aids evaluated by our team over the past few years is NeuroPage, a small pager worn on a belt. NeuroPage was developed in California by Larry Treadgold, the engineer father of a head-injured son, working together with Neil Hersh, a neuropsychologist (Hersh & Treadgold, 1994). NeuroPage uses an arrangement of microcomputers linked to a conventional computer memory and, by telephone, to a paging company. The scheduling of reminders or prompts for each individual is entered into a computer, and from then on, no further human interaction is necessary. At the appropriate time and date, the reminder is transmitted to the individual, who simply has to press a button to receive and clear (and, if necessary, re-receive) the message.

In all our NeuroPage studies, the memory-impaired subjects and their families decide on the reminders they want. Thus we always target real-life problems. Following a successful pilot study (Wilson, Evans, Emslie, & Malinek, 1997) and two single-case studies (Evans, Emslie, & Wilson, 1998; Wilson, Emslie, Quirk, & Evans, 1999), we carried out a randomized, controlled, crossover study (whereby patients were allocated to pager or no pager for 7 weeks and then switched over) with 143 people referred from throughout the United Kingdom (Wilson, Emslie, Quirk, & Evans, 2001). The results are shown in Figure 21.1.

As can be seen from Figure 21.1, there were no differences in the target behaviors achieved between group A (pager first) and group B (waiting list first) during the baseline. There was a significant difference at the end of the first treatment phase, when group A had the pager and group B did not. At the end of the final phase, when group B had the pager and group A did not, group B achieved significantly more targets than group A. People in group A had declined a little but were still significantly better than during baseline.

Teaching the use of compensatory strategies is not always easy because their use involves memory, but it is nonetheless possible. Our research (Kime, Lamb, & Wilson, 1996; Wilson, 1999; and the NeuroPage studies) shows that when compensatory strategies are used effectively, independent living is possible even for people with severe memory problems.

IMPROVING LEARNING IN PEOPLE
WITH ORGANIC MEMORY DEFICITS

Despite the fact that compensatory strategies are the most effective for helping memory-impaired people achieve a measure of independence, there are times when it is necessary

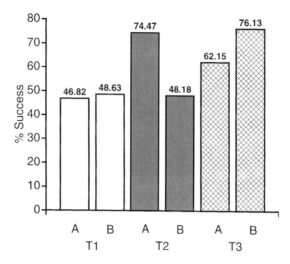

FIGURE 21.1. Percentage success rate for participants in group A (pager first) and group B (pager later) at time 1 (baseline), time 2 (weeks 8 and 9), and time 3 (weeks 15 and 16). From Wilson, Emslie, Quirk, and Evans (2001). Copyright 2001 by BMJ Publishing Group. Reprinted by permission.

for them to learn new information. Consider people's names, for example. Although it is possible to write names in a book and even to pair each name with a photograph, when people meet other persons in the street or at the hospital, they need to greet these others by name. For memory-impaired people to look up the names in their system would be very disruptive to normal human interaction.

Learning new information is one of the major handicaps faced by people with organic memory deficits. However, there are ways to enhance or improve learning for them. Employing mnemonics, for example, leads to faster learning than rote rehearsal (Wilson, 1987); so too does "spaced retrieval," also known as "expanding rehearsal" (Landauer & Bjork, 1978; Schacter, Rich, & Stampp, 1985). Other strategies to improve learning have come from the fields of study techniques (e.g., Glasgow, Zeiss, Barrera, & Lewinsohn, 1977; Robinson, 1970; Wilson, 1991a) and of learning disability (Yule & Carr, 1987). Perhaps one of the most important techniques is that of "errorless learning," which has recently become one of the most important components of memory rehabilitation.

Errorless learning is a teaching technique whereby people are prevented, as far as possible, from making mistakes while they are learning a new skill or acquiring new information. Instead of teaching by demonstration, which may involve the learner in trial and error, the experimenter, therapist, or teacher presents the correct information or procedure in ways that minimize the possibility of erroneous responses.

There are two theoretical backgrounds to investigations of errorless learning in people with organic memory impairment. The first is the work on errorless discrimination learning in the field of behavioral psychology, first described by Terrace (1963, 1966). Sidman and Stoddard (1967) soon applied errorless learning principles to children with developmental learning difficulties. They were able to teach these children to discriminate ellipses from circles. Others soon took up the idea (e.g., Cullen, 1976; Jones & Eayrs, 1992; Walsh & Lamberts, 1979).

The second theoretical impetus comes from studies of implicit memory and implicit learning in the fields of cognitive psychology and cognitive neuropsychology (e.g., Brooks & Baddeley, 1976; Graf & Schacter, 1985; Tulving & Schacter, 1990; and many others). Although it has been known for decades that memory-impaired people can learn some skills and information normally, through their intact (or relatively intact) implicit learning abilities, it has been difficult to apply this knowledge to reduce the real-life problems such people encounter. The main studies attempting to accomplish this task were done by Glisky and colleagues (Glisky & Schacter, 1987; Glisky, Schacter, & Tulving, 1986). They used a method known as "vanishing cues," where prompts were progressively reduced.

A colleague and I (Baddeley & Wilson, 1994) posed this question: Do amnesic patients learn better if prevented from making mistakes during the learning process? In a study with 16 young and 16 elderly control participants, and 16 densely amnesic people, employing a stem completion procedure, we found that every one of the amnesic people learned better if prevented from making mistakes during learning. Following this study, errorless learning principles were quickly adopted in the rehabilitation of memory-impaired people (Clare, Wilson, Breen, & Hodges, 1999; Clare et al., 2000; Evans et al., 2000; Squires, Aldrich, Parkin, & Hunkin, 1998; Squires, Hunkin, & Parkin, 1996, 1997; Wilson, Baddeley, Evans, & Shiel, 1994; Wilson & Evans, 1996).

We (Baddeley & Wilson, 1994) contended that errorless learning is superior to trial and error because it depends on implicit memory. As the amnesic people in our study could not use explicit memory effectively, they were forced to rely on implicit memory. Without adequate episodic memory that enables one to remember mistakes, it seems better to prevent the injection of errors in the first place. In the absence of an efficient episodic memory, the very fact of making an incorrect response may strengthen or reinforce an error. Hunkin, Squires, Parkin, and Tidy (1998) believed that the success of errorless learning is due to the effects of error prevention on the residual explicit memory capacities of people with amnesia. A third explanation is that it may be attributable to both implicit and explicit forms of memory.

In an attempt to clarify the situation, we (Wilson, Carter, Norris, & Page, 2001) gave memory-impaired people stem completion tasks presented in either an errorful or errorless way, using both implicit and explicit recall instructions to try to determine how errorless learning works. We tested 24 people with stable organic memory impairment (all at more than 1 year postinsult). Of these people, 16 were males and 8 were females. The age range was 26–69 years (mean = 46.16 years, SD = 12.17 years). Ten people had sustained a traumatic head injury, four a stroke, four encephalitis, two hypoxic brain damage, one Korsakoff's syndrome, one idiopathic epilepsy, one surgery for a cyst, and one chronic hydrocephalus. We divided the main group into two subgroups, depending on the severity of memory impairment. There were 11 participants with a severe memory impairment, operationally defined as scoring 0 on delayed recall of the stories from the Wechsler Memory Scale—Revised (WMS-R), along with a screening score of 3 or less on the Rivermead Behavioural Memory Test (RBMT). There were 13 participants with a moderate memory impairment, operationally defined as having a delayed story recall score of less than 50% on the WMS-R and a screening score of 4, 5, or 6 on the RBMT.

Twenty-four words were divided into two sets, roughly matched for frequency. Half of these words were presented in an errorful manner, and half in an errorless way. In addition, we requested explicit recall for half the words and implicit recall for the remaining words. Errorless and errorful conditions were counterbalanced across participants, and testing of each condition was separated by approximately 1 week. We made the following predictions:

1. If errorless learning depends on implicit memory, then both groups should benefit from the implicit/errorless learning condition, because both groups are able to use implicit memory.

2. If errorless learning works by capitalizing on residual explicit memory, then those people with some episodic memory functioning (i.e., the moderately impaired people) should benefit from the explicit errorless condition more than those with no or very little episodic memory functioning (i.e., the severely impaired group).

3. If both explanations are partly correct, then we would expect the severely impaired group to benefit from the implicit/errorless learning condition, whereas those with some episodic functioning should benefit from both errorless learning conditions.

The results (see Table 21.1) demonstrated that there was a significant difference between errorful and errorless learning in the implicit condition for both the severely impaired group ($p < .05$) and the moderately impaired group ($p < .01$). Similar results were found in the explicit condition, where again the difference between errorful and errorless was at the 5% level for the severe group and the 1% level for the moderate group. There were no significant differences between the two groups in the *implicit* condition for errorless or errorful conditions, nor for explicit errorful learning. There was, however, a difference between the two groups for *explicit* errorless learning. Here the moderately impaired group benefited more from the errorless procedure than did the severely impaired group.

Both groups therefore benefited from implicit errorless learning compared with implicit errorful learning. The moderately impaired group showed greater benefit. In the explicit condition, once again, both groups performed at a higher level with errorless than errorful learning, but the moderately impaired group benefited more. Thus the first two predictions were borne out. We also noted that if both explanations were correct, the severely impaired group would only benefit under the implicit errorless condition, and the moderately impaired group would benefit under both errorless conditions. This outcome was less clear-cut, but the nature of responses suggested that the severely impaired group used implicit memory even when requested to use explicit recall. It is difficult to see how we could have prevented this process.

We suggest that these results indicate errorless learning can work both by capitalizing on implicit memory and, for those with some episodic memory functioning, by also strengthening explicit memory. Further work is underway both to replicate these findings and to clarify further the effects of errorless learning on explicit and implicit memory.

TABLE 21.1. Mean Number of Correct Responses (Maximum = 6)

	Errorful		Errorless		$p <$
	Implicit task				
Severe group	0.80	(0.91)	2.30	(1.41)	.05
Moderate group	1.07	(1.26)	2.87	(1.61)	.01
	Explicit task				
Severe group	0.60	(0.69)	2.0	(1.15)	.05
Moderate group	1.21	(1.36)	3.28	(1.48)	.01
Severe vs. moderate	n.s.	(0.2)			.05

Note. Data from Wilson, Carter, Norris, and Page (2001).

ENVIRONMENTAL ADAPTATIONS

For memory-impaired people with severe and widespread cognitive deficits, the most that we may be able to do is change or adapt the environment in some way in order to reduce or avoid the need for memory. In Norman's (1988) words, from his book *The Psychology of Everyday Things*, "knowledge is in the world rather than in the head" (p. 54). An example of this idea is given by Harris (1980) when he describes a geriatric unit in the United States with a high rate of incontinence until somebody painted all the lavatory doors a distinctive color. The rate of incontinence decreased, presumably because more people could remember that the lavatories were behind the distinctively colored doors.

Similar approaches can be used in a variety of settings. Signposts, for example, can be placed strategically around the hospital or home. Doors can be labeled so that patients know which is the dining room, which is the bedroom, and so forth. A patient's bed itself can be labeled. As well as providing signposts and labels, therapists should make sure that (1) the printing is large enough to be legible to those with failing eyesight, (2) the labels/ signs are placed in prominent positions, (3) the labels are discriminable against their backgrounds, and (4) the terminology used is familiar to each patient. (Further examples of environmental adaptation can be found in Wilson, 1995, and Wilson & Evans, 2000.)

The origins of environmental modification or restructuring can be found in the field of behavior modification, particularly in the area of severe learning disability (Murphy & Oliver, 1987). Severely disruptive behaviors, for example, can sometimes be prevented through environmental changes. For example, a child who is easily distracted in the classroom may be able to work at a task if a screen is placed around the work table so that no other children can be seen and, apart from the task in hand, there are no other stimuli present to act as distractors. For some people with severe intellectual impairment and memory problems, environmental restructuring is the best chance of attaining some degree of independence. People with encephalitis, severe head injury, or Korsakoff's syndrome have been known to live happily in structured, organized environments that greatly decrease the need for them to remember.

REDUCING EMOTIONAL PROBLEMS ASSOCIATED WITH MEMORY IMPAIRMENTS

"Memory is a very important part of who we are. . . . It is no surprise that memory problems often have major emotional consequences, including feelings of loss and anger and increased levels of anxiety" (Clare & Wilson, 1997, p. 41). People with severe memory difficulties sometimes think they are going crazy, or are stupid or worthless. They may become socially isolated and withdrawn, or terrified of making a mistake. Their anxiety levels are high (Evans & Wilson, 1992), and depression is common (Kopelman & Crawford, 1996). Reducing distress, anxiety, and depression, together with increasing awareness, understanding, and self-esteem, should be part of every memory rehabilitation program. Enabling clients to talk, ask questions, and express their feelings may reduce their distress and enable them to accept more readily the strategies we neuropsychologists have to offer.

Providing information is one of the cheapest, simplest, and most easily implemented strategies for reducing anxiety. A question frequently asked by family members and people with memory problems is why something that happened several years ago is remembered, but something that happened a short while ago is forgotten. Sometimes a simple explanation will suffice, such as "Old memories are stored differently in the brain than new memories are." Other people may need more detailed and sophisticated references. Simple reassurance that the pattern of difficulties seen is typical of people with memory problems may help to reduce anxiety. Written explanations should supplement oral explanations; this is true even for family members with good memories, as well as for those with poor memories. It is easy to forget or distort spoken information, especially when one is tired or distressed.

Other strategies worth considering are relaxation therapy, cognitive-behavioral therapy, and psychological support (see Prigatano, 1999, and Wilson et al., 2000, for further discussion of these issues). Reminiscence therapy and other memory therapy in groups can also result in the reduction of depression and anxiety (see Moffat, 1992; Wilson & Moffat, 1992). Finally, psychologists and other therapists involved in memory rehabilitation can act as a resource for putting families in touch with local services, self-help groups, and written material to help reduce the stress, isolation, and helplessness they often feel.

REFERENCES

Bäckman, L., & Dixon, R. A. (1992). Psychological compensation: A theoretical framework. *Psychological Bulletin, 112*, 259–283.

Baddeley, A. D., & Wilson, B. A. (1994). When implicit learning fails: Amnesia and the problem of error elimination. *Neuropsychologia, 32*, 53–68.

Brooks, D. N., & Baddeley, A. D. (1976). What can amnesic patients learn? *Neuropsychologia, 14*, 111–122.

Clare, L., & Wilson, B. A. (1997). *Coping with memory problems: A practical guide for people with memory impairments, relatives, friends and carers.* Bury St. Edmunds, England: Thames Valley Test Company.

Clare, L., Wilson, B. A., Breen, E. K., & Hodges, J. R. (1999). Errorless learning of face–name associations in early Alzheimer's disease. *NeuroCase, 5*, 37–46.

Clare, L., Wilson, B. A., Carter, G., Breen, E. K., Gosses, A., & Hodges, J. R. (2000). Intervening with everyday memory problems in dementia of Alzheimer type: An errorless learning approach. *Journal of Clinical and Experimental Neuropsychology, 22*, 132–146.

Cullen, C. N. (1976, March 25). Errorless learning with the retarded. *Nursing Times*, pp. 43–47.

Evans, J. J., Emslie, H., & Wilson, B. A. (1998). External cueing systems in the rehabilitation of executive impairments of action. *Journal of the International Neuropsychological Society, 4*, 399–408.

Evans, J. J., & Wilson, B. A. (1992). A memory group for individuals with brain injury. *Clinical Rehabilitation, 6*, 75–81.

Evans, J. J., Wilson, B. A., Schuri, U., Andrade, J., Baddeley, A., Bruna, O., Canavan, T., Della Sala, S., Green, R., Laaksonen, R., Lorenzi, L., & Taussik, I. (2000). A comparison of "errorless" and "trial-and-error" learning methods for teaching individuals with acquired memory deficits. *Neuropsychological Rehabilitation, 10*, 67–101.

Evans, J. J., Wilson, B. A., Needham, P., & Brentnall, S. (2001). *Who makes good use of memory-aids: Results of a survey of 100 people with acquired brain injury.* Manuscript submitted for publication.

Glasgow, R. E., Zeiss, R. A., Barrera, M. J., & Lewinsohn, P. M. (1977). Case studies on remediating memory deficits in brain-damaged individuals. *Journal of Clinical Psychology, 33*, 1049–1054.

Glisky, E. L., & Schacter, D. L. (1987). Acquisition of domain-specific knowledge in organic amnesia: Training for computer-related work. *Neuropsychologia, 25*, 893–906.

Glisky, E. L., Schacter, D. L., & Tulving, E. (1986). Computer learning by memory impaired patients: Acquisition and retention of complex knowledge. *Neuropsychologia, 24*, 313–328.

Graf, P., & Schacter, D. L. (1985). Implicit and explicit memory for new associations in normal and amnesic subjects. *Journal of Experimental Psychology: Learning, Memory, and Cognition, 11*, 501–518.

Harris, J. E. (1980). We have ways of helping you remember. *Concord: The Journal of the British Association of Service to the Elderly*, *17*, 21–27.

Hersh, N., & Treadgold, L. (1994). NeuroPage: The rehabilitation of memory dysfunction by prosthetic memory and cueing. *NeuroRehabilitation*, *4*, 187–197.

Houts, P. S., & Scott, R. A. (1975). *Goal planning with developmentally disabled persons: Procedures for developing an individualized client plan*. Hershey: Department of Behavioral Science, Pennsylvania State University College of Medicine.

Hunkin, M. M., Squires, E. J., Parkin, A. J., & Tidy, J. A. (1998). Are the benefits of errorless learning dependent on implicit memory? *Neuropsychologia*, *36*, 25–36.

Jones, R. S. P., & Eayrs, C. B. (1992). The use of errorless learning procedures in teaching people with a learning disability. *Mental Handicap Research*, *5*, 304–312.

Kime, S. K., Lamb, D. G., & Wilson, B. A. (1996). Use of a comprehensive program of external cuing to enhance procedural memory in a patient with dense amnesia. *Brain Injury*, *10*, 17–25.

Kopelman, M., & Crawford, S. (1996). Not all memory clinics are dementia clinics. *Neuropsychological Rehabilitation*, *6*, 187–202.

Landauer, T. K., & Bjork, R. A. (1978). Optimum rehearsal patterns and name learning. In M. M. Gruneberg, P. E. Morris, & R. N. Sykes (Eds.), *Practical aspects of memory* (pp. 625–632). London: Academic Press.

McLellan, D. L. (1991). Functional recovery and the principles of disability medicine. In M. Swash & J. Oxbury (Eds.), *Clinical neurology* (pp. 768–790). Edinburgh: Churchill Livingstone.

McMillan, T., & Sparkes, C. (1999). Goal planning and neurorehabilitation: The Wolfson Neurorehabilitation Centre approach. *Neuropsychological Rehabilitation*, *9*, 241–251.

Moffat, N. (1992). Strategies of memory therapy. In B. A. Wilson & N. Moffat (Eds.), *Clinical management of memory problems* (2nd ed., pp. 86–119). London: Chapman & Hall.

Murphy, G., & Oliver, C. (1987). Decreasing undesirable behaviour. In W. Yule & J. Carr (Eds.), *Behaviour modification for people with mental handicaps* (pp. 102–142). London: Croom Helm.

Norman, D. A. (1988). *The psychology of everyday things*. New York: Basic Books.

Prigatano, G. (1999). Commentary: Beyond statistics and research design. *Journal of Head Trauma Rehabilitation*, *14*, 308–311.

Robinson, F. P. (1970). *Effective study*. New York: Harper & Row.

Schacter, D. L., Rich, S. A., & Stampp, M. S. (1985). Remediation of memory disorders: Experimental evaluation of the spaced-retrieval technique. *Journal of Clinical and Experimental Neuropsychology*, *7*, 79–96.

Sidman, M., & Stoddard, L. T. (1967). The effectiveness of fading in programming simultaneous form discrimination for retarded children. *Journal of the Experimental Analysis of Behavior*, *10*, 3–15.

Squires, E. J., Aldrich, F. K., Parkin, A. J., & Hunkin, N. M. (1998). Errorless learning and the acquisition of word processing skills. *Neuropsychological Rehabilitation*, *8*, 433–449.

Squires, E. J., Hunkin, N. M., & Parkin, A. J. (1996). Memory notebook training in a case of severe amnesia: Generalising from paired associate learning to real life. *Neuropsychological Rehabilitation*, *6*, 55–65.

Squires, E. J., Hunkin, N. M., & Parkin, A. J. (1997). Errorless learning of novel associations in amnesia. *Neuropsychologia*, *35*, 1103–1111.

Terrace, H. S. (1963). Discrimination learning with and without "errors". *Journal of the Experimental Analysis of Behavior*, *6*, 1–27.

Terrace, H. S. (1966). Stimulus control. In W. K. Honig (Ed.), *Operant behavior: Areas of research and application* (pp. 271–344). New York: Appleton-Century-Crofts.

Tulving, E., & Schacter, D. L. (1990). Priming and human memory systems. *Science*, *247*, 301–306.

Walsh, B. F., & Lamberts, F. (1979). Errorless discrimination and fading as techniques for teaching sight words to TMR students. *American Journal of Mental Deficiency*, *83*, 473–479.

Wilson, B. A. (1987). *Rehabilitation of memory*. New York: Guilford Press.

Wilson, B. A. (1991a). Behavior therapy in the treatment of neurologically impaired adults. In P. R. Martin (Ed.), *Handbook of behavior therapy and psychological science: An integrative approach* (pp. 227–252). New York: Pergamon Press.

Wilson, B. A. (1991b). Long term prognosis of patients with severe memory disorders. *Neuropsychological Rehabilitation, 1*, 117–134.

Wilson, B. A. (1995). Memory rehabilitation: Compensating for memory problems. In R. A. Dixon & L. Bäckman (Eds.), *Compensating for psychological deficits and declines: Managing losses and promoting gains* (pp. 171–190). Hillsdale, NJ: Erlbaum.

Wilson, B. A. (1997). Cognitive rehabilitation: How it is and how it might be. *Journal of the International Neuropsychological Society, 3*, 487–496.

Wilson, B. A. (1999). *Case studies in neuropsychological rehabilitation*. New York: Oxford University Press.

Wilson, B. A. (2000). Compensating for cognitive deficits following brain injury. *Neuropsychology Review, 10*, 233–243.

Wilson, B. A., Baddeley, A. D., Evans, J. J., & Shiel, A. (1994). Errorless learning in the rehabilitation of memory impaired people. *Neuropsychological Rehabilitation, 4*, 307–326.

Wilson, B. A., Carter, G., Norris, D., & Page, M. (2001). Does errorless learning work through implicit or explicit memory? *Journal of the International Neuropsychological Society, 7*, 250.

Wilson, B. A., Emslie, H., Quirk, K., & Evans, J. (1999). George: Learning to live independently with NeuroPage®. *Rehabilitation Psychology, 44*, 284–296.

Wilson, B. A., Emslie, H. C., Quirk, K., & Evans, J. J. (2001). Reducing everyday memory and planning problems by means of a paging system: A randomised control crossover study. *Journal of Neurology, Neurosurgery and Psychiatry, 70*, 477–482.

Wilson, B. A., & Evans, J. J. (1996). Error free learning in the rehabilitation of individuals with memory impairments. *Journal of Head Trauma Rehabilitation, 11*, 54–64.

Wilson, B. A., & Evans, J. J. (2000). Practical management of memory problems. In G. E. Berrios & J. R. Hodges (Eds.), *Memory disorders in psychiatric practice* (pp. 291–310). Cambridge, England: Cambridge University Press.

Wilson, B. A., Evans, J. J., Brentnall, S., Bremner, S., Keohane, C., & Williams, H. (2000). The Oliver Zangwill Centre for Neuropsychological Rehabilitation: A partnership between health care and rehabilitation research. In A.-L. Christensen & B. P. Uzzell (Eds.), *International handbook of neuropsychological rehabilitation* (pp. 231–246). New York: Kluwer Academic/ Plenum Press.

Wilson, B. A., Evans, J. J., Emslie, H., & Malinek, V. (1997). Evaluation of NeuroPage: A new memory aid. *Journal of Neurology, Neurosurgery and Psychiatry, 63*, 113–115.

Wilson, B. A., Evans, J. J., & Keohane, C. (2001). *Cognitive rehabilitation: A goal-planning approach with a man who sustained a head injury and cerebro-vascular complications*. Manuscript submitted for publication.

Wilson, B. A., & Moffat, N. (1992). The development of group memory therapy. In B. A. Wilson & N. Moffat (Eds.), *Clinical management of memory problems* (2nd ed., pp. 243–273). London: Chapman & Hall.

Wilson, B. A., & Watson, P. C. (1996). A practical framework for understanding compensatory behaviour in people with organic memory impairment. *Memory, 4*, 465–486.

Wright, P., Rogers, N., Bartram, C., Wilson, B. A., Evans, J. J., Emslie, H., & Hall, C. (2001). Comparison of pocket-computer aids for people with brain injury. *Brain Injury, 15*(9), 787–800.

Yule, W., & Carr, J. (Eds.). (1987). *Behaviour modification for people with mental handicaps*. London: Croom Helm.

22

Circadian Rhythms and Memory in Aged Humans and Animals

GORDON WINOCUR and LYNN HASHER

People have strong preferences for the times at which they engage in everyday activities, such as shopping, reading newspapers, and listening to music (Yoon, 1998). These preference patterns are quite different across the adult lifespan, with college-age young adults preferring to perform many activities in the afternoon and evening, and older adults preferring the morning (Hasher, Zacks, & May, 1999; May, Hasher, & Stoltzfus, 1993). One explanation for these patterns is that by the afternoon, older adults are tired and lack motivation, whereas young people are more likely to be alert and functioning at near-optimal levels. In fact, the scenario may be more complicated than this; it may relate to diurnal biological rhythms that are different for older and younger adults, and that in addition are disrupted in old age. The altered behavioral patterns are consistent with a substantial shift toward peak arousal and activity in the morning that has been found for both older humans and lower animals (see, e.g., Hoch et al., 1992; Ingram, London, & Reynolds, 1982; Peng & Kang, 1984). This age-related shift has been linked to changes in a wide range of circadian rhythms that affect, for example, sleep–wake cycles, eating and drinking patterns, glucose uptake, and heart rate, as well as circulating hormones (e.g., melatonin, adrenocorticotropic hormone) and neurotransmitter function (e.g., acetylcholine, norepinephrine; Brock, 1991; Burwell, Whealin, & Gallagher, 1994; Edgar, 1994; Horne & Ostberg, 1977; Hrushesky, 1994; Ingram et al., 1982; Stone, 1989).

Recent work in several laboratories suggests that variations in circadian arousal rhythms may also influence human cognitive function, with optimal performance associated with testing that occurs near peak times of arousal as opposed to off-peak times. This pattern is termed the "synchrony effect" (May & Hasher, 1998). Given considerable evidence that older and younger adults experience peak arousal times at different times of day (e.g., Adan & Almirall, 1990; May & Hasher, 1998; Mecacci & Zani, 1983; Yoon, 1998), the suggestion is that age-related patterns of performance could well differ across the day, from morning (a peak time for as many as 75% of older adults) to late afternoon (near a peak time for at least 35% of college students).

Indeed, a growing literature suggests that levels of cognitive performance for some tasks do change across the day. With respect to age comparisons, however, they change in different directions: Older adults show better performance in the morning than in the afternoon, and younger adults show the reverse pattern (see Hasher et al., 1999; Intons-Peterson, Rocchi, West, McLellan, & Hackney, 1998; May & Hasher, 1998; Yoon, May, & Hasher, 1998). In humans, the synchrony effect has been demonstrated in a variety of paradigms, most reliably on tasks that incorporate a substantial inhibitory component—that is, tasks that require ignoring concurrent distraction, ignoring no longer relevant information, or suppressing inappropriate response tendencies.

For example, one task involved presenting a verbal puzzle (three unrelated words that could be related by a missing fourth word) in either the presence or absence of verbal distraction. All participants were instructed to ignore the distraction while solving the word problem. Although young adults were able to ignore the distraction in an afternoon testing period, they were unable to do so in a morning testing period. Older adults (consistent with views that inhibitory control declines with age) were unable to ignore the distraction at either time of testing, but distraction was far more disruptive (in terms of reductions in the numbers of problems solved) in the afternoon than in the morning (May, 1999).

Another study in this series used a version of a stop-signal paradigm, in which on most trials, people must respond as quickly as possible to make a simple category decision (e.g., is a couch an instance of the category "furniture"?). On a small proportion of trials in this study, a signal indicated that a classification response should be withheld. Although there were no differences as a function of time of testing on the standard classification trials, there were substantial differences on the stop-signal trials. In particular, both younger and older adults were more likely to fail at withholding when tested at a nonoptimal time than when tested at an optimal time (May & Hasher, 1998).

From a neuropsychological perspective, an interesting feature of the various inhibitory tasks is that they are associated with frontal lobe function. For example, the stop-signal test is reminiscent of other tasks (e.g., alternation, go/no-go) that require suppression of a prepotent response following a discrete signal, and that are sensitive to impairments in attentional processes and response control in animals and humans with frontal lobe damage (see, e.g., Freedman & Oscar-Berman, 1986; Winocur, 1991). Indeed, it has been suggested that the synchrony effect in aged humans is the direct result of circadian disruption of frontal lobe function (Intons-Peterson et al., 1999; May & Hasher, 1998).

The question arises as to whether a synchrony-like effect can be demonstrated in an animal model. Although research in this area is in its infancy, this effect does appear to occur. Work in our laboratory and others (e.g., Gallagher & Burwell, 1989; Stone, 1989; Winocur & Hasher, 1999) has shown that age differences on tests of learning and memory in rats are greater late in the animals' activity cycle, when arousal levels are lowest, than at the beginning of the cycle. Of particular interest, this pattern of performance coincides with significant alterations in measures of circadian rhythmicity in the older rats.

In this chapter, we review recent and current work that demonstrates a link between altered circadian patterns in old age and cognitive performance, with a particular emphasis on memory function. Two research programs, involving aged humans and animals, are described; although the respective paradigms and strategies necessarily differ, there is a remarkable convergence in the findings. The results of this research highlight the potential importance of disrupted circadian rhythms for cognitive aging, as well as providing some insights into their neuropsychological correlates.

HUMAN STUDIES

In a study highlighting the impact of the synchrony effect on even very simple memory performance in aged humans, a simple word span task was administered to groups of young and old adults. Participants were asked to recall an increasingly long series of words (from two to six items) immediately after each list was presented, with span measured as the longest series correct (Yoon et al., 1998). Testing took place in the morning (at 8:00 or 9:00 A.M.) or in the afternoon (at 4:00 or 5:00 P.M.). Performance on the immediate memory test revealed a synchrony effect (see Figure 22.1): Older and younger adults were virtually equivalent in the morning. However, they differed substantially in the afternoon, with the pattern for older adults showing a decline in performance from morning to afternoon testing, whereas performance for young adults showed an improvement. Thus the performance on a simple span task measure of immediate memory changes across the day, and does so differently for younger and older adults. And it does so in a manner consistent with each group's general circadian arousal pattern, since the older adults were strong "morning-type" individuals and the younger adults were strong "evening-type" people (see Yoon et al., 1998, for norms).[1]

A similar synchrony pattern was observed in a series of studies on recognition of prose information (Intons-Peterson, Rocchi, West, McLellan, & Hackney, 1999; May et al., 1993; Yoon, 1998). In the May and colleagues (1993) and Yoon (1998) studies, participants read a prose passage and were tested after a brief delay with an "old–new" decision procedure. This procedure included, as foils (or never-presented items), statements that were either related or unrelated to information in the original passage. The Yoon study varied the similarity of foils to target items as well. Both studies showed a substantial increase in false

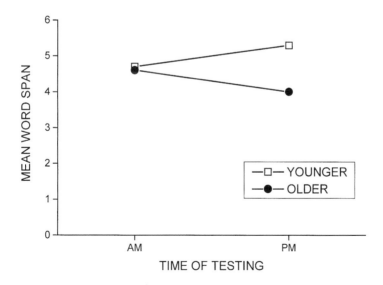

FIGURE 22.1. Mean word span for older and younger adults tested in the morning or the afternoon. Data from May and Hasher (2001).

[1]All participants in the Hasher, May, and Yoon studies were administered the Horne and Ostberg (1977) Morningness–Eveningness Questionnaire, a paper-and-pencil inventory that has been shown to correlate highly with physiological markers of circadian arousal (see, e.g., May et al., 1993).

alarms to related items (i.e., calling a new, related item "old") at nonoptimal as compared to optimal times. When the corrected recognition data (hits – false alarms) were arrayed as a function of time of day (see Figure 22.2), the pattern of recognition performance mirrored that of the span task: Younger and older adults looked quite similar in the morning and quite different in the afternoon, with accuracy declining for older adults in the afternoon and increasing for younger adults. Again, this pattern is consistent with what is known about each group's general circadian arousal pattern.

In a recently completed study (May & Hasher, 2001), recall of two short passages was tested both immediately after reading each passage and following a 20-minute filled interval. Figure 22.3 shows a forgetting score, indicating the difference between the number of ideas recalled on the immediate test and the number recalled on the delayed test. Once again, there were small differences between older and younger adults when they were tested in the morning, and substantial differences when tested in the afternoon. Here, the young adults showed a small decline in the rate of forgetting (actually, an improvement in retention) in the afternoon compared with the morning. Older adults, however, showed a dramatic increase in forgetting from the morning to the afternoon. The data from the span and the prose recognition studies show once again that performance changes across the day in a manner consistent with each group's circadian arousal patterns.

It is important to note that the memory findings for both younger and older adults cannot simply be attributed to tiredness. In the case of each of the studies mentioned, there was additional evidence that time of testing did not influence performance on other measures. For example, in the stop-signal study, the speed of responding on unsignaled or go trials did not change across the day for either younger or older adults (May & Hasher, 1998). In the memory studies, verbal ability was tested using a difficult vocabulary test. Once again, verbal ability, which was not at ceiling level for any group tested at any time, did not show changes across the day. Thus neither tiredness nor lack of motivation is a

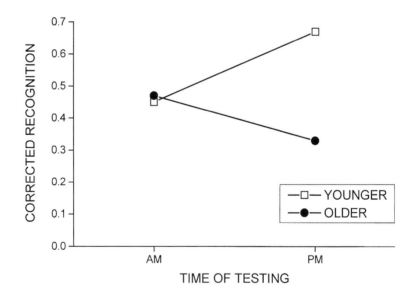

FIGURE 22.2. Corrected recognition (hits – false alarms) for older and younger adults tested in the morning or the afternoon. From May, C. P., Hasher, L., & Stoltzfus, E. R. (1993). Optimal time of day and the magnitude of age differences in memory. *Psychological Science*, *4*, 326–330. Copyright 1993 by Blackwell Publishers. Reprinted by permission.

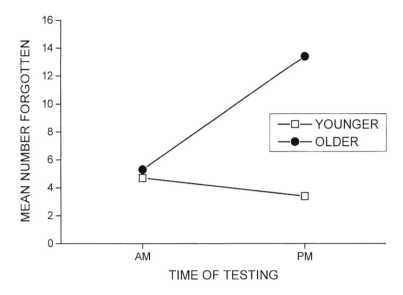

FIGURE 22.3. Mean number of words forgotten (test 1 – test 2) for older and younger adults tested in the morning or the afternoon. Data from May and Hasher (2001).

likely explanation for these findings. Instead, these data are all consistent in showing reduced memory performance at nonoptimal times of day.

The studies with human subjects were not designed specifically to assess underlying brain mechanisms, but there is evidence that frontal functions are implicated in the synchrony effect, at least in some tasks (e.g., the span effect; false recognition with related foils). At the same time, medial temporal lobe impairment may have contributed to the false recognition (Melo, Winocur, & Moscovitch, 1999; Schacter, Verfaellie, & Pradere, 1996), as well as to poor recall in the delayed test. The issue of neural correlates of the synchrony effect is taken up again in the next section.

It has also been suggested that memory failures associated with the synchrony effect are related to a basic disruption in inhibitory control over working memory functioning. Such control allows irrelevant information from various sources (perceptual and conceptual; the immediate present and the recent past) to disrupt the acquisition and retrieval of information (Hasher et al., 1999). Other work in this series suggests that (in adult humans at least) working memory functions, which of course are linked to frontal lobe function, also vary in efficiency across the day (see Hasher et al., 1999; Yoon et al., 1998).

ANIMAL STUDIES

In its initial stages, our animal research had several objectives. The first was to determine whether the synchrony effect (or some approximation of it) could be demonstrated in a rat model, and whether the effect could be related to independent measures of circadian rhythmicity. Second, tasks with neuropsychological validity were selected in an attempt to relate any such effects to dysfunction in specific brain regions. Third, employing multidimensional tests that measure different aspects of learning and memory made it possible to determine whether time-of-testing effects are general, or whether they act selectively on specific processes. An important implication of this research is that although aged rats reliably perform worse than young rats on various behavioral tests, time of testing is rarely taken into account. Because light–dark periods and testing schedules vary considerably between labs, uncontrolled time of testing, combined with age-related circadian disruption, may have contributed to some of the observed differences in performance.

In the first study (see Winocur & Hasher, 1999), old and young rats were administered a variable-interval, delayed-alternation (VIDA) test and a runway test of inhibitory avoidance conditioning (IAC). These tests were selected because they (1) measure a variety of learning and memory processes; (2) are sensitive to dysfunction in specific brain regions (e.g., frontal lobes, hippocampus; see Winocur, 1985, 1991); and (3) require a rat to inhibit competing responses to obtain reward—an important component that emerged from Hasher and colleagues' work with humans.

Before behavioral training, rats were housed in individual cages and maintained on a 12-hour light–dark schedule with lights on between 8:00 P.M. and 8:00 A.M. Rhythmic entrainment to this schedule was confirmed by measuring water intake patterns at the end of the light and dark periods. After about 3 weeks, when the rats had adjusted to the schedule, there were no age differences in daily water intake. There was, however, an important difference in the groups' drinking patterns: Old rats drank significantly less water than young rats during the dark periods, and more during the light periods.

For the IAC task, rats were water-deprived and trained to run down an alley and drink from a water spout. When this response had stabilized, shock was administered on one of the training trials, followed by shock avoidance testing 24 hours and 6 weeks later. Each test session consisted of a single trial in which rats were allowed up to 5 minutes to contact the spout and drink for 10 seconds (sec). No shock was administered on these trials.

After the 24-hour IAC test, water was made available on an *ad libitum* basis, but food was restricted in anticipation of VIDA testing. This test, conducted in a Skinner box with a single retractable lever, is a go/no-go alternation task with a variable interval (0–80 sec) between the go and no-go trials. The lever was present during the trials, but retracted during the intertrial intervals (ITIs). During go trials, each lever press produced a food pellet, whereas lever presses during no-go trials were not reinforced. Each ITI occurred twice after go trials and twice after no-go trials, with the ITI sequence varied in each test session. Rats received 15 daily sessions on the VIDA task, before being placed on *ad lib.* food and water. A few weeks later, the water deprivation schedule was reinstated prior to the 6-week IAC test. (See Winocur, 1991, for a detailed description of the procedure.)

All rats received the same behavioral testing, except that approximately half the subjects in each age group were tested within 1 hour of the beginning of the dark cycle (AM), and the other half were tested within 1 hour of the end of the dark cycle (PM).

VIDA test results, averaged over the final block of three sessions, are presented in Figure 22.4 in the form of go/no-go latency ratios. At each ITI, ratios were calculated by dividing the mean latency to the first response in the go trials by the mean latency to the first response in the no-go trials. A low ratio would result from shorter latencies in the go trials than in the no-go trials. Thus a low ratio signifies good performance.

The block 5 data confirm a significant effect of age on performance at all ITIs, including ITI-0, where there was virtually no delay between trials. Of particular interest is the clear evidence of a time-of-day (TOD) effect in old rats. Old rats tested early in the dark cycle (group O-AM) performed significantly better than the old rats tested late in the dark cycle (group O-PM), but only at ITIs 40 and 80. Notably, at the longer ITIs, the performance of the O-AM group approached (but did not equal) that of the younger groups. Importantly, time of testing did not affect performance in the younger rats, indicating a

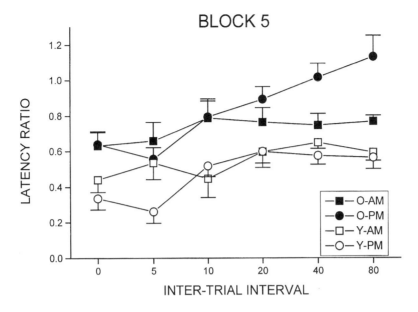

FIGURE 22.4. Latency ratios for old (O) and young (Y) rats on block 5 of the VIDA test. AM, testing in the morning (early in the dark cycle); PM, testing in the afternoon (late in the dark cycle). From Winocur and Hasher (1999). Copyright 1999 by American Psychological Association. Reprinted by permission.

failure to demonstrate the full synchrony effect that has been reported in young and old human adults.

It is also important that the TOD effect was selective for longer ITIs, in that previous research has shown that successful VIDA performance at these delays is controlled by hippocampal function (Winocur, 1985). By comparison, acquisition of the VIDA rule, as reflected in ITI-0 performance and where no TOD effect was observed, has been linked to frontal cortex and thalamic function (Winocur, 1991).

With respect to performance on the IAC task, there were no age differences in acquiring the approach response, but there was a clear age effect on postshock avoidance behavior at both test sessions (see Figure 22.5). There was a significant TOD effect as well, in that the O-AM group performed better than the O-PM group at the 6-week test. Once gain, this effect was not seen in the younger rats.

Th IAC results are also important from a neuropsychological perspective, in that previous work has shown that performance at long delays (beyond 2 weeks), but not short delays (24 hours), is selectively affected by damage to the hippocampus (Winocur, 1985). Thus, although there are numerous differences between the VIDA and IAC tasks, it is noteworthy that in both cases the TOD effect was limited to measures that appear to be under hippocampal control.

In a recently completed study (reported here for the first time), the generality of the TOD effect in rats was further assessed. As before, old and young rats were entrained to a 12-hour light–dark schedule and tested early or late in the dark cycle, but this time in a nonspatial nonmatching-to-sample (NMS) test, conducted in a Morris water maze. This test involved a series of paired study and test trials. In each study trial, the location of a hidden platform was cued by a conspicuous black or white dowel that was suspended directly above the platform. On the subsequent test trial, both dowels were present, but the

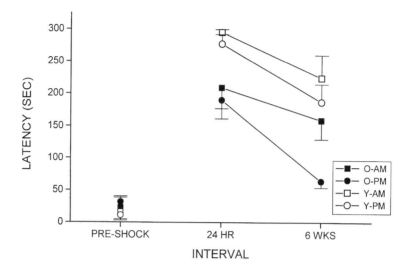

FIGURE 22.5. Response latencies for old (O) and young (Y) rats at short and long delays in the IAC task. AM, testing in the morning (early in the dark cycle); PM, testing in the afternoon (late in the dark cycle). From Winocur and Hasher (1999). Copyright 1999 by American Psychological Association. Reprinted by permission.

platform was in a different location (beneath the dowel that was not present in the preceding study trial). Initially, rats were trained with minimal delay (approximately 5 sec) between study and test trials. After 10 daily sessions of training (four trials/session), rats were administered 5 additional four–trial test sessions, with ITIs of 0, 20, 40, or 80 sec. Finally, after the completion of delayed testing, rats received an additional five sessions of delayed testing, but this time with test times reversed. That is, those rats that were previously tested early in the dark cycle were now tested at the end of the cycle, and vice versa. This reversal was conducted in an attempt to provide a powerful within-subjects demonstration of the TOD effect.

The most reliable measure of performance on the NMS task was the animal's latency to find the hidden platform on the test trials. On this measure, there was no main effect of age on NMS rule acquisition (see Figure 22.6). As well, there was no TOD effect in the old rats, but, interestingly, the data indicate that the Y-PM subgroup learned the rule at a faster rate than the Y-AM subgroup. This outcome is the opposite of that typically observed in old rats, but is reminiscent of reports that young human adults sometimes show a similar pattern (e.g., May & Hasher, 1998; Yoon et al., 1998).

Age differences in performance persisted into the acquisition–delay condition (see Figure 22.7, left), but here the main result was the disproportionately poor performance of the O-PM group at ITIs 40 and 80. At this ITI, the O-PM group performed worse than the other three groups, which, interestingly, did not differ from each other. It is also noteworthy that indications of a possible TOD effect in young rats in the acquisition condition did not extend to the acquisition–delay condition.

In the reversal–delay condition, a highly significant age × delay interaction reflected the continued poor performance of old rats at longer ITIs (see Figure 22.7, right). This

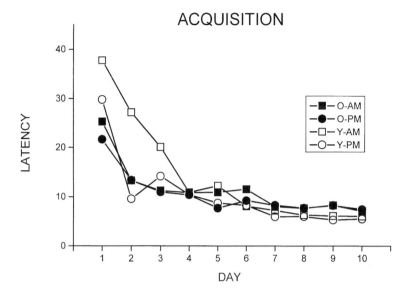

FIGURE 22.6. Response latencies of old (O) and young (Y) rats on test trials during NMS acquisition training. AM, testing in the morning (early in the dark cycle); PM, testing in the afternoon (late in the dark cycle).

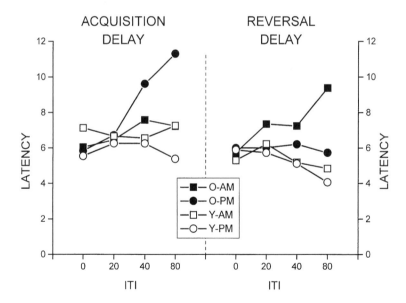

FIGURE 22.7. Response latencies of old (O) and young (Y) rats on test trials of NMS acquisition–delay and reversal–delay conditions. AM, testing in the morning (early in the dark cycle); PM, testing in the afternoon (late in the dark cycle); ITI, intertrial interval.

pattern was especially apparent in the O-PM subgroup, providing further evidence of the adverse effects of testing aged rats during suboptimal periods. In this case, the demonstration is particularly dramatic because, in the reversal–delay condition, when the same rats were tested early in the dark cycle, they performed much better than they did when tested late in the cycle. Once again, there was no evidence of a TOD effect in the young rats.

Overall, the NMS data are consistent with the results of VIDA and IAC testing. Age differences in performance were qualified by significant effects of time of testing and length of ITI in the acquisition–delay and reversal–delay conditions. These results show that cognitive performance in aged rats is strongly influenced by the stage of the activity cycle in which testing occurs, although the influence may be limited to memory processes under hippocampal control.

As in the human studies (see above), a concern about data such as these is that TOD effects are related to performance factors such as general fatigue or lack of motivation. Several points argue against this interpretation. For example, in all three tasks, TOD effects were limited to long-delay conditions that challenged hippocampus-controlled memory function, and were not linked to other cognitive processes, as would be expected if they were the result of performance-related variables. Similarly, it is significant that in the VIDA and IAC tasks, old rats advanced through all stages of shaping and training as quickly as the younger rats did. Moreover, there were no age differences in learning the NMS rule. Finally, in the IAC task, the TOD effect was reflected in shorter latencies in the O-PM subgroup—a finding that is clearly inconsistent with excessive fatigue or diminished motivation. Taken together, the evidence favours the view that old rats, tested late in their activity cycle, exhibited cognitive dysfunction that was related to changes in biological rhythmicity.

The consistent finding that the TOD effect in aged rats was manifested selectively on measures of memory function under hippocampal control and not on tests of frontal lobe function is somewhat at odds with the human data, which suggest a more general effect. Because only a limited number of behavioral tests have been utilized in TOD research, it is premature to draw firm conclusions about the generality of such effects. The frontal lobe is a complex structure with numerous subregions that control a diverse range of attentional, mnemonic, and executive functions (Moscovitch & Winocur, 1995; Stuss & Benson, 1986), and it is entirely possible that future research with brain-damaged and aged animals will reveal meaningful relationships between some of these functions and circadian patterns.

One of the aims of the animal research was to assess the importance of task-related inhibitory demands on the TOD effect. As indicated above, Hasher and colleagues (1999) have suggested that disruption of circadian rhythms may be directly related to an exaggerated loss of inhibitory control that occurs in normal aging and contributes to impairment on many cognitive tasks. Our tasks all had inhibitory components to varying degrees, but in general, TOD effects were independent of any difficulties with response control. The one important exception occurred in the VIDA study, where the O-PM subgroup exhibited exaggerated lever pressing after long ITIs in the no-go trials. However, it could not be determined whether that tendency contributed to the overall deficit or was a symptom that resulted from the memory failure during the long delays. This issue may relate to the nature of the tests employed and the underlying processes that support successful performance. For example, the frontal lobe (Mishkin, 1964) and the hippocampus (Kimble, 1968) both participate in inhibitory control, but in different ways, and it may be important to consider these differences in assessing the time-of-testing impact on inhibitory mechanisms.

Finally, an important objective of this research program was to determine whether variations in cognitive performance among aged rats are related directly to changes in their rhythmically controlled drinking patterns. Despite clear evidence that water intake by aged rats in the dark cycle was accompanied by relatively poor cognitive performance, the two measures did not correlate with each other in any of the tasks. This result does not rule out a link between circadian rhythmicity and cognitive function, but it is more likely to reflect the sensitivity of this particular measure of rhythmicity. Age-related disruptions in drinking patterns are undoubtedly related to other circadian changes in old age that more directly affect brain function. This complex issue requires systematic investigation of relationships between specific circadian changes and various aspects of cognitive function.

SUMMARY AND CONCLUSIONS

Cognitive aging in humans is influenced by a wide range of biological, environmental, and psychosocial factors (Craik & Trehub, 1982; Zacks, Hasher, & Li, 2000). Many of the same influences are known to contribute to age differences in learning and memory in lower animals (Winocur, 1988, 1998). There is now convincing evidence that time of testing must be added to the list of variables that can affect cognitive performance generally and memory in particular, in both animals and humans. Indeed, with respect to humans, it is interesting to speculate that if all cognitive studies were run early in the morning, our views of age-related changes in memory might be quite different from the view of dominant, inevitable decline that is prevalent in the cognitive gerontology literature. In fact, there is reason to believe that the majority of participants, both young and old, are actually tested in the afternoon (May et al., 1993). To that extent, it is necessary to consider the possibility that conclusions regarding human age differences in memory may be at least slightly exaggerated.

Although considerable work is needed in this area, there is promising evidence that synchrony and TOD effects on memory performance are related to a mismatch between circadian arousal levels and the time of testing. At this point, we know that memory function in aged animals and humans are closely linked to circadian rhythms that are reflected in variable patterns of wakefulness, activity, and water consumption. The challenge is to specify those circadian rhythms that have a direct impact on cognitive processes, as well as those processes and neural mechanisms that are particularly vulnerable to age-related circadian disruption.

ACKNOWLEDGMENTS

The work reported here and the preparation of this chapter were supported by grants from the Natural Sciences and Engineering Research Council of Canada (No. OGP-8181) and the Canadian Institutes of Health Research (No. MRC-6694) to Gordon Winocur, and by grants (No. R37 4306 and No. RO1 2753) from the U.S. National Institute on Aging to Lynn Hasher.

REFERENCES

Adan, A., & Almirall, H. (1990). Adaptation and standardization of a Spanish version of the Morningness–Eveningness Questionnaire: Individual differences. *Personality and Individual Differences, 11*, 1123–1130.

Brock, M. A. (1991). Chronobiology and aging. *Journal of the American Geriatrics Society, 39*, 74–91.

Burwell, R. D., Whealin, J., & Gallagher, M. (1992). Effects of aging on the diurnal pattern of water intake in rats. *Behavioral and Neural Biology, 58*, 196–203.

Craik, F. I. M., & Trehub, S. (1982). *Aging and cognitive processes: Advances in the study of communication and affect*. New York: Plenum Press.

Edgar, D. M. (1994). Sleep–wake circadian rhythms and aging: Potential etiologies and relevance to age-related changes in integrated physiological systems. *Neurobiology of Aging, 15*, 499–501.

Freedman, M., & Oscar-Berman, M. (1986). Bilateral frontal lobe disease and selective delayed response deficits in humans. *Behavioral Neuroscience, 100*, 332–342.

Gallagher, M., & Burwell, R. D. (1989). Relationship of age-related decline across several behavioral domains. *Neurobiology of Aging, 10*, 691–708.

Hasher, L., Zacks, R. T., & May, C. P. (1999). Inhibitory control, circadian arousal, and age. In D. Gopher & A. Koriat (Eds.), *Attention and performance XVII: Cognitive regulation of performance. Interaction of theory and application* (pp. 653–675). Cambridge, MA: MIT Press.

Hoch, C. C., Reynolds, C. F., Jennings, J. R., Monk, T. H., Buysse, D. J., Machen, M. A., & Kupler, D. J. (1992). Daytime sleepiness and performance among healthy 80 and 20 year olds. *Neurobiology of Aging, 13*, 353–356.

Horne, J., & Ostberg, O. (1977). Individual differences in human circadian rhythms. *Biological Psychology, 5*, 179–190.

Hrushesky, W. (1994). Timing is everything. *The Sciences, 4*, 32–37.

Ingram, D. K., London, E. D., & Reynolds, M. A. (1982). Circadian rhythmicity and sleep: Effects of aging in laboratory animals. *Neurobiology of Aging, 3*, 287–297.

Intons-Peterson, M. J., Rocchi, P., West, T., McLellan, K., & Hackney, A. (1998). Aging, optimal testing times and negative priming. *Journal of Experimental Psychology: Learning, Memory, and Cognition, 24*, 362–376.

Intons-Peterson, M. J., Rocchi, P., West, T., McLellan, K., & Hackney, A. (1999). Age, testing at preferred times (testing optimality), and false memory. *Journal of Experimental Psychology: Learning, Memory, and Cognition, 25*, 23–40.

Kimble, D. P. (1968). Hippocampus and internal inhibition. *Psychological Bulletin, 70*, 185–195.

May, C. P. (1999). Synchrony effects in cognition: The costs and a benefit. *Psychonomic Bulletin and Review, 6*, 142–147.

May, C. P., & Hasher, L. (1998). Synchrony effects in inhibitory control over thought and action. *Journal of Experimental Psychology: Human Perception and Performance, 24*, 363–379.

May, C. P., & Hasher, L. (2001). *Story recall: Circadian synchrony effects*. Manuscript in preparation.

May, C. P., Hasher, L., & Stoltzfus, E. R. (1993). Optimal time of day and the magnitude of age differences in memory. *Psychological Science, 4*, 326–330.

Mecacci, L., & Zani, A. (1983). Morningness–eveningness preferences and sleep–waking diary data of morning and evening types in student and worker samples. *Ergonomics, 26*, 1147–1153.

Melo, B., Winocur, G., & Moscovitch, M. (1999). False recall and false recognition: An examination of the effects of selective and combined lesions to the medial temporal lobe/diencephalon and frontal lobe structures. *Cognitive Neuropsychology, 16*, 343–359.

Mishkin, M. (1964). Perseveration of central sets after frontal lesions in monkeys. In J. M. Warren & K. Akert (Eds.), *The Frontal granular cortex and behavior* (pp. 219–241). New York: McGraw-Hill.

Moscovitch, M., & Winocur, G. (1995). Frontal lobes, memory, and aging. *Annals of the New York Academy of Sciences, 769*, 119–150.

Peng, M. T., & Kang, M. (1984). Circadian rhythms and patterns of running-wheel activity, feeding and drinking behaviors of old male rats. *Physiology and Behavior, 33*, 615–620.

Schacter, D. L., Verfaellie, M., & Pradere, D. (1996). The neuropsychology of memory illusions: False recall and recognition in amnesic patients. *Journal of Memory and Language, 35*, 319–334.

Stone, W. S. (1989). Sleep and aging in animals: Relationships with circadian rhythms and memory. *Clinical Geriatric Medicine, 5*, 363–379.

Stuss, D. T., & Benson, D. F. (1986). *The frontal lobes*. New York: Raven Press.

Winocur, G. (1985). The hippocampus and thalamus: Their roles in short- and long-term memory and the effects of interference. *Behavioural Brain Research*, *16*, 135–152.

Winocur, G. (1988). A neuropsychological analysis of memory loss with age. *Neurobiology of Aging*, *9*, 487–494.

Winocur, G. (1991). Functional dissociation of the hippocampus and prefrontal cortex in learning and memory. *Psychobiology*, *19*, 11–20.

Winocur, G. (1998). Environmental influences on cognitive decline in aged rats. *Neurobiology of Aging*, *19*(6), 589–597.

Winocur, G., & Hasher, L. (1999). Aging and time-of-day effects on cognition in rats. *Behavioral Neuroscience*, *113*(5), 991–997.

Yoon, C. (1998). Age differences in consumers' processing strategies: An investigation of moderating influences. *Journal of Consumer Research*, *24*, 329–342.

Yoon, C., May, C. P., & Hasher, L. (1998). When does synchrony matter?: Evidence from studies of cognitive aging and inhibition. In N. Schwarz, D. Park, B. Knauper, & S. Sudman (Eds.), *Aging, cognition and self reports* (pp. 117–143). Washington, DC: Psychological Press.

Zacks, R. T., Hasher, L., & Li, K. Z. H. L. (2000). Aging and memory. In T. A. Salthouse & F. I. M. Craik (Eds.), *Handbook of aging and cognition* (pp. 293–357). Mahwah, NJ: Erlbaum.

PART II

STUDIES OF MEMORY IN NONHUMAN PRIMATES

Beginning with the classical studies by Carlyle Jacobsen in the 1930s, research with monkeys has provided enormously useful information about the neuropsychology of memory. In the late 1960s, it became possible to obtain single-neuron recordings from awake, behaving monkeys that had been trained to perform sensory or motor tasks. Since that time, single-neuron recordings have been obtained from monkeys while they learn and remember. Work with monkeys has also benefited from improved neuroanatomical information and from continuing studies of how selective brain lesions affect memory.

This section consists of five chapters describing progress in the neuropsychology of memory based on studies of monkeys. Chapter 23 presents findings from anatomical and single-unit neurophysiological studies of the medial temporal lobe, which illuminate how the structures within the medial temporal lobe contribute differently to memory function. Chapter 24 summarizes studies combining single-cell recording and surgical disconnection procedures, which have illuminated how the temporal lobe stores and retrieves long-term visual memories under the top-down control of frontal cortex. Chapter 25 describes several ways that neuronal activity in the anterior temporal cortex can be modulated during the formation or expression of memory. Chapter 26 summarizes studies, using the lesion technique, that suggest how the anatomical structures of the medial temporal lobe memory system contribute to the capacity to recognize recently encountered objects as familiar. Chapter 27 discusses the neural basis of rapid sensorimotor mapping in monkeys and places this memory ability in an ethological perspective.

23

Cortical Memory Systems in the Nonhuman Primate

An Anatomical and Physiological Perspective

WENDY A. SUZUKI

Which areas of the brain are important for memory? We have known since the description of the well-known amnesic patient H. M. (Scoville & Milner, 1957), and early work on preserved functions in amnesia (Cohen & Squire, 1980), that bilateral damage to the medial temporal lobes produces a profound and permanent impairment in declarative memory—the ability to form and retain new information about facts and events. Since that time, the study of the brain basis of memory has benefited not only from the study of human amnesic patients, but also from the development of animal models of human amnesia in monkeys, rats, and mice. Experimental lesion studies in these animal model systems, taken together with findings from neuroanatomical studies, have led to the understanding that the medial temporal lobe structures important for declarative memory include the hippocampus and the surrounding and strongly interconnected entorhinal, perirhinal, and parahippocampal cortices (Figure 23.1).

Although there is now a strong consensus about the identity of the medial temporal lobe structures important for declarative memory, substantial controversy still remains concerning exactly how these structures contribute to memory. Do all medial temporal lobe areas support similar types of mnemonic information, or do certain areas specialize in particular forms of memory? This chapter describes findings from two complementary approaches that my colleagues and I have used to address these questions. First, to identify the patterns of sensory inputs to the medial temporal lobe, we have used anterograde and retrograde tract-tracing techniques. Findings from these anatomical studies have not only provided a detailed "wiring diagram" of this region, they have also generated specific predictions concerning the contributions of individual medial temporal lobe structures to memory. To test some of these predictions, we have used single-unit neurophysiological techniques to examine the patterns of neural activity observed in the medial temporal lobe as animals perform various memory-demanding tasks. Together, these studies have begun to reveal general principles of organization that underlie the anatomy and the physiology of memory in the medial temporal lobe.

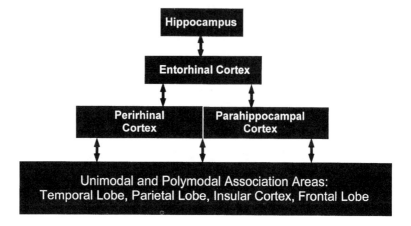

FIGURE 23.1. Schematic representation of medial temporal lobe connections, based on early findings from anterograde degeneration studies (Jones & Powell, 1970; Van Hoesen et al., 1975; Van Hoesen & Pandya, 1975a, 1975b). These studies showed that the medial temporal lobe structures—including the perirhinal cortex, parahippocampal cortex, entorhinal cortex, and hippocampus—are the recipient of a strong convergence of sensory inputs from the visual, somatosensory, and auditory modalities. The relative strengths of the inputs from these sensory areas, however, could not be determined from the anterograde degeneration studies alone.

ANATOMICAL EXPLORATIONS OF THE MEDIAL TEMPORAL LOBE

Medial Temporal Lobe Areas Involved in Memory

Ever since the dramatic description of patient H. M., findings from neuroanatomical investigations have provided important clues toward understanding the mnemonic functions of the medial temporal lobe. The seminal studies by Jones, Powell, Van Hoesen, and Pandya in the 1970s were some of the first to examine the patterns of interconnections between the hippocampal formation (including the hippocampus, subicular complex, and entorhinal cortex) and the rest of the neocortical mantle (Jones & Powell, 1970; Van Hoesen & Pandya, 1975a, 1975b; Van Hoesen, Pandya, & Butters, 1972, 1975). Using anterograde degeneration techniques, these studies showed that the medial temporal lobe in general, and the perirhinal and parahippocampal cortices in particular, are the recipients of a convergence of sensory inputs from the visual, auditory, and somatosensory modalities. The perirhinal and parahippocampal cortices then project to the entorhinal cortex, which provides the major input and output of the hippocampus—an area considered to be the pinnacle of this anatomical hierarchy (Figure 23.1).

Despite these early studies highlighting the interconnections of the hippocampus with the surrounding entorhinal, perirhinal, and parahippocampal cortices, studies of the brain basis of memory in the 1970s and 1980s focused on the hippocampus and the amygdala (Mishkin, 1978). Convergent studies in monkeys, rats, and humans have confirmed the important role of the hippocampus in declarative memory (Vargha-Khadem et al., 1997; Zola et al., 2000). However, it is now clear that the amygdala does not play a central role in this function (Zola-Morgan, Squire, & Amaral, 1989). Instead, findings from a series of influential studies reexamining the anatomical organization of the monkey entorhinal cortex (Amaral, Insausti, & Cowan, 1987; Insausti, Amaral, & Cowan, 1987a, 1987b) focused attention on the possible role of the perirhinal and parahippocampal cortices in memory.

Specifically, these studies showed that the entorhinal cortex receives nearly two-thirds of its cortical input from the adjacent perirhinal and parahippocampal cortices. This findings raised the possibility that these adjacent cortical areas may also be participating in normal memory function. Selective lesion studies in monkeys confirmed these anatomical predictions by showing that animals with damage limited to the perirhinal and parahippocampal cortices exhibited a profound memory impairment. This impairment not only was long-lasting, but extended to both the visual and tactual modalities (Suzuki, Zola-Morgan, Squire, & Amaral, 1993; Zola-Morgan, Squire, Amaral, & Suzuki, 1989). These findings, taken together with other studies (Gaffan & Murray, 1992; Leonard, Amaral, Squire, & Zola-Morgan, 1995; Meunier, Bachevalier, Mishkin, & Murray, 1993), suggested that the medial temporal lobe areas important for memory include not only the hippocampus and entorhinal cortex, but also the adjacent and anatomically related perirhinal and parahippocampal cortices.

Contributions of Specific Medial Temporal Lobe Areas to Memory

Although the combination of findings from lesion studies and anatomical studies was essential in identifying the specific medial temporal lobe areas important for memory, it was still unclear exactly how each of these areas contributes to memory. Early anatomical studies stressed the idea that the entorhinal, perirhinal, and parahippocampal cortices are zones of convergence for multiple sensory modalities (Jones & Powell, 1970; Van Hoesen et al., 1975; Van Hoesen & Pandya, 1975a, 1975b). However, because these studies were based solely on anterograde tracing studies, it was not clear whether all the cortical inputs to these areas had been identified. To address this question, my colleagues and I subsequently used retrograde tract-tracing techniques to reexamine the organization of cortical inputs to two of these medial temporal lobe structures, the perirhinal and parahippocampal cortices. By identifying the full complement and relative strength of cortical inputs to these areas, we hoped to gain a better understanding of the kinds of mnemonic functions in which these areas are involved (Suzuki & Amaral, 1994a). Our findings showed that, consistent with earlier reports, the perirhinal and parahippocampal cortices receive a prominent convergence of sensory inputs from the visual, somatosensory, and auditory modalities. However, these studies also revealed striking differences in the patterns of sensory inputs to these two areas, particularly with respect to information in the visual modality.

The perirhinal cortex is characterized by its strong inputs from visual association areas TE and TEO, which make up approximately 63% of its total cortical input (Figure 23.2). Areas TE and TEO are part of the ventral visual processing pathway important for object identification (Ungerleider & Mishkin, 1982). In contrast, the parahippocampal cortex receives a disproportionately larger input from regions associated with the dorsal visual processing pathway, which are important for conveying information about the spatial location of objects (Ungerleider & Mishkin, 1982). Together, inputs from dorsal stream areas—including the parietal cortex, the retrosplenial cortex, and the dorsal bank of the superior temporal sulcus—make up approximately 55% of the total inputs to the parahippocampal cortex (Figure 23.2). Another noteworthy observation concerned the organization of reciprocal projections between the perirhinal and parahippocampal cortices. Whereas the perirhinal cortex receives strong projections from the parahippocampal cortex, comprising approximately 24% of its total cortical input, the reciprocal projection is substantially weaker, comprising approximately 4% of total cortical input to the parahippocampal cortex.

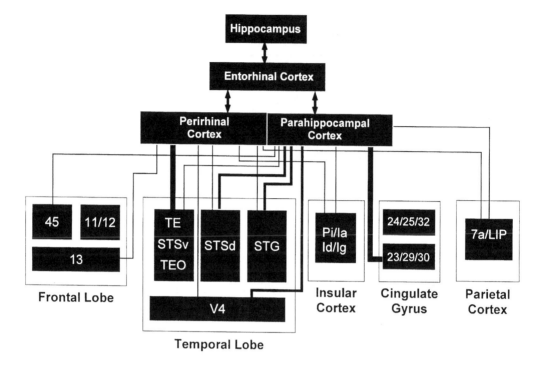

FIGURE 23.2. Simplified view of our current understanding of cortical inputs to the macaque monkey medial temporal lobe. The projections to the perirhinal and parahippocampal cortices are emphasized here. The thickness of the lines represents the relative strength of projections to the perirhinal or parahippocampal cortices. The thickest lines represent inputs that make up more than 30% of the total cortical input to either of these areas. Medium lines represent inputs that make up between 10% and 30% of the total cortical inputs, while the thin lines represent inputs that make up less than 10% of the total input to these areas. All quantitative data are from Suzuki and Amaral (1994a). Areas 45, 11, 12, 13, 24, 25, 32, 23, 29, 30, and 7a after the nomenclature of Brodmann (1919); Areas TE and TEO after the nomenclature of Bonin and Bailey (1947); Ia, agranular insula; Id, dysgranular insula; Ig, granular insula; LIP, lateral interparietal area; Pi, parainsular cortex; STG, superior temporal gyrus; STSd, dorsal bank of the superior temporal sulcus; STSv, ventral bank of the superior temporal sulcus.

These striking and differential patterns of cortical inputs suggested equally striking and differential functions. Specifically, these findings suggested that the parahippocampal cortex is involved in processing spatial memory but not object memory. The connections of the perirhinal cortex, in contrast, suggested that this area may be involved in processing object memory as well as certain forms of spatial memory. Recent evidence from selective lesion studies as well as from functional imaging studies supports these predictions. For example, a recent PET study showed activation of the human parahippocampal gyrus, but not the perirhinal cortex, during the performance of a virtual reality computer game requiring memory for spatial/topographic information (Maguire et al., 1998). Lesions including the parahippocampal cortex produce impairments on spatial tasks (Murray & Wise, 1996), but not on a task of object recognition memory (Ramus, Zola-Morgan, & Squire, 1994). In contrast, selective damage of the perirhinal cortex produces a severe impairment on a task of visual object recognition (Buffalo et al., 1999; Gaffan, 1995; Meunier et al., 1993). Some studies report no spatial memory impairment following perirhinal lesions

(Gaffan, 1995), but others have reported evidence for a mild spatial deficit following peri-rhinal lesions (Wiig & Burwell, 1998).

Although the studies described above have started to examine the role of the perirhi-nal and parahippocampal cortices in object and spatial memory, many more predictions generated by the anatomical studies described above have yet to be tested. For example, preferential inputs from the parietal cortex and auditory association areas to the lateral and medial portions of the parahippocampal cortex, respectively, suggest that lateral regions may be more involved in spatial memory, whereas medial regions may be more involved in auditory memory. Projections from somatosensory association areas to both the perirhinal and parahippocampal cortices suggest that both these areas are involved in processing tactile information in memory. The lack of prominent olfactory projections to these areas suggests that olfactory memory may not be supported by these areas in the macaque monkey.

Summary of Anatomical Findings

Our progress in understanding the neuroanatomical organization of the medial temporal lobe can be appreciated by comparing a wiring diagram based on early anatomical descriptions of this region (Figure 23.1) to a wiring diagram based on the most recent anatomical data (Figure 23.2). The findings illustrated in Figure 23.2 provide detailed new information on both the similarities and differences in cortical inputs to the structures of the medial temporal lobe. This information, together with findings from selective lesion studies and functional imaging techniques, has allowed us to formulate and test specific new hypotheses concerning how individual medial temporal lobe areas contribute to memory. Thus, whereas early views did not even consider the perirhinal and parahippo-campal cortices as important for memory, a convergence of findings including convincing data from anatomical studies showed that these areas not only are important for memory, but appear to contribute differentially to object and spatial memory. Importantly, neuro-anatomical considerations are also being incorporated into the newest theories of medial temporal lobe memory function (Eichenbaum, Dudchenko, Wood, Shapiro, & Tanila, 1999; Mishkin, Suzuki, Gadian, & Vargha-Khadem, 1997; Squire & Zola, 1998). Although the details of these recent theories may differ significantly, these anatomical findings are starting to provide increasingly detailed constraints on the various mnemonic computations proposed for the medial temporal lobe.

THE NEUROPHYSIOLOGY OF MEMORY IN THE MEDIAL TEMPORAL LOBE

Findings from anatomical studies have provided useful insights into the specific functions of individual medial temporal lobe areas. However, these studies alone cannot provide information concerning the patterns of neural activity that underlie normal memory function. Perhaps one of the most powerful techniques available to address this issue is single-unit neurophysiology correlated with behavior. My colleagues and I were particularly interested in understanding how object and spatial memories may be signaled by neurons in the medial temporal lobe. To address this question, we examined the patterns of neural activity as two monkeys performed an object recognition memory task and a third monkey performed a spatial recognition memory task (Suzuki, Miller, & Desimone, 1997). We focused our studies on neural activity in the entorhinal cortex because of its role as a major zone of convergence, both for object information arriving from the perirhinal cortex and for spatial information arriving from the parahippocampal cortex (Insausti et al., 1987a; Suzuki & Amaral, 1994b). We found that entorhinal neurons signal memory for object and spatial information in similar ways. Entorhinal neurons respond selectively to particular objects or cued spatial locations (i.e., stimulus-selective response), and memory is signaled by enhancing or suppressing these stimulus-selective responses. Moreover, comparisons of the mnemonic signals in the entorhinal cortex with findings from other areas have revealed an extensive network of structures throughout the medial temporal lobe and prefrontal cortex that signal either similar or complementary patterns of mnemonic signals. Taken together, these studies suggest that memory for objects and spatial locations is signaled by a complex network of structures in both the medial temporal lobe and prefrontal cortex.

Delayed-Matching-to-Sample and Delayed-Matching-to-Place Tasks

To study the neural correlates of memory in the entorhinal cortex, we used two tasks of recognition memory: the delayed matching-to-sample (DMS) task and the delayed matching-to-place (DMP) task (Figure 23.3). In these tasks, animals are asked to distinguish between a recently seen stimulus (either an object or a cued spatial location) and distractor or "test" stimuli. The DMS task begins with the presentation of a sample picture followed by a

A. Delayed Match to Sample Task

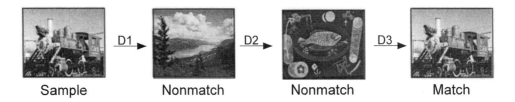

| | | | |
| Sample | Nonmatch | Nonmatch | Match |

B. Delayed Match to Place Task

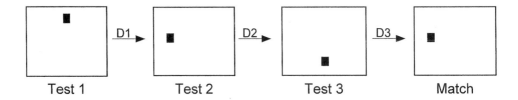

| | | | |
| Test 1 | Test 2 | Test 3 | Match |

FIGURE 23.3. Schematic diagram of the delayed-matching-to-sample (DMS; A) and delayed-matching-to-place (DMP; B) tasks. For both tasks, the visual stimuli (i.e., pictures or spatial cues) were shown for 500 milliseconds (msec), and the delay intervals (D1, D2, and D3) were 700 msec long. For the DMS task, the trial always ended with the repetition of the sample stimulus shown at the beginning of the trial (i.e., the match). Unlike the DMS task, in which a response was required for the repetition of the sample stimulus, any one of the previously shown test locations could be repeated for the DMP task. For this task, the animal learned to release the bar after any repeated cued location. See Suzuki, Miller, and Desimone (1997) for a full description of both these tasks.

variable sequence of nonmatching test pictures. The trial always ends with the repetition of the sample picture, or match. For the DMP task, a cue is presented at a variable sequence of places on a computer screen, always ending with a repetition of one of the previously shown places (i.e., a match). For the DMP task, any one of the previously shown places can be shown as a match. For both tasks, the monkeys are rewarded with a drop of fruit juice for responding to the matching stimulus. There are three main requirements for solving these tasks. First, the animals must discriminate between the different stimuli presented; second, the animals must maintain a memory of the sample stimulus during the delay periods (i.e., a working memory signal); and third, they must evaluate whether a test stimulus matches any of the previously presented stimuli. We found evidence that entorhinal neurons participate in all three of these task requirements for both the object and spatial memory tasks (Suzuki et al., 1997). In the following sections, I consider each of these three requirements in turn. I also compare our findings in the entorhinal cortex with findings in other brain areas.

Stimulus Discrimination

A prominent characteristic of neurons in the entorhinal cortex is their selective response to particular visual stimuli. During the object memory task, for example, entorhinal neurons responded in a highly selective way to particular visual stimuli (Figure 23.4A). Similarly, during the performance of the place memory task, entorhinal neurons responded selectively to the location of the cue on the computer screen. Not only do these patterns of neural activity signal selective information about particular sensory stimuli; as we shall see below, modulation (either up or down) of these sensory-selective responses provides a powerful recognition memory signal.

Working Memory Signals during the Delay Interval

We next asked whether entorhinal neurons signaled information about the to-be-remembered sample stimulus during the delay intervals of the object memory task. We found that the response of some entorhinal neurons during the delay intervals of the DMS task was dependent on which sample stimulus was being held in mind. Thus, if a preferred sample stimulus was shown at the beginning of the trial, a high level of activity was observed during each of the subsequent delay intervals (Figure 23.4B, dark bars). If a nonpreferred stimulus was shown, little or no delay activity was observed (Figure 23.4B, white bars). Similarly, during the place memory task, entorhinal neurons signaled selective information about a particular cue location during the delay interval that immediately proceeded that cue presentation.

These working memory signals in the entorhinal cortex were particularly surprising, because similar studies using the same object memory task in the monkey perirhinal cortex reported no such working memory signal (Miller, Erickson, & Desimone, 1996). In contrast, robust working memory signals for both object and spatial information have been reported throughout the prefrontal cortex (Funahashi, Bruce, & Goldman-Rakic, 1989; Miller et al., 1996). Although early studies did not emphasize the working memory signals in the monkey medial temporal lobe, there is growing evidence that medial temporal lobe structures participate in a wider range of working memory processes than previously appreciated. For example, studies of olfactory recognition memory in rats reported stimulus-

A. Stimulus-Selective Response

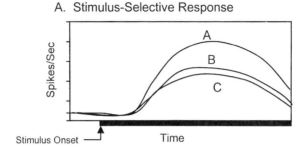

B. Selective Delay Activity

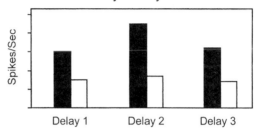

C. Match-Nonmatch Response

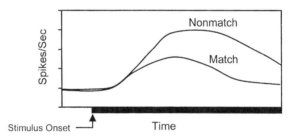

FIGURE 23.4. Schematic representation of the three major patterns of neural activity observed in the entorhinal cortex during performance of either the object or spatial recognition memory task. (A) Some entorhinal neurons responded selectively to particular sensory stimuli. In this illustration, a prototypical cell responded with its highest firing rate to stimulus A, and less to stimuli B and C. (B) Some neurons in the entorhinal cortex responded selectively during the delay intervals of the task (i.e., D1, D2, D3 of Figure 23.3), depending on which sample stimulus was shown. The dark bars represent the activity in response to the sample stimulus that elicited the highest level of activity during the delay, while the white bars represent the level of delay activity observed after a nonpreferred sample stimulus was shown as a sample. (C) Illustration of a selective match suppression response. Compared to the response of this neuron's preferred stimulus when it was shown as a nonmatch, the response to the same stimulus was suppressed when it was shown as a match. Other entorhinal neurons signaled the repetition of any stimulus that was shown as a match with a significantly suppressed response (abstracted match–nonmatch signal). These patterns of responses have been observed not only in the entorhinal cortex, but also in the perirhinal cortex, hippocampus, and prefrontal cortex (see text).

selective delay activity in both the perirhinal and entorhinal cortices (Young, Otto, Fox, & Eichenbaum, 1997). Moreover, recent functional imaging studies reported prominent working memory signals in both the entorhinal cortex (Fernandez, Brewer, Zhao, Glover, & Gabrieli, 1999) and the hippocampus (Ranganath & D'Esposito, 2000). Taken together, these findings suggest that working memory signals are observed not only in prefrontal cortex but also throughout the medial temporal lobe.

Recognition Memory Signals

We next asked whether entorhinal neurons signaled information about whether an object or spatial cue matched or did not match stimuli being held in memory. To address this question, we focused on neurons that exhibited selective responses to particular objects or spatial locations. Specifically, we compared the response of a neuron's preferred stimulus when it was shown as a match (i.e., at the end of the trial) to the response to the same stimulus when it was shown as a nonmatch on a different trial. In both cases, we measured the response of the neuron to the same stimulus. The difference between the match and nonmatch conditions is that when the stimulus is shown as a match, the animal carries a memory of that stimulus in mind. In contrast, when that same stimulus is shown as a nonmatch, no explicit memory for that stimulus is being held in mind. Our finding was that neurons in the entorhinal cortex signaled the occurrence of a matching stimulus by either decreasing or increasing their stimulus-selective response. These patterns of responses have been termed "match suppression" and "match enhancement," respectively. Because the suppressed or enhanced signals occurred well before the animal's behavioral response (120 milliseconds [msec] as latency for the match–nonmatch signal, vs. 350 msec for the behavioral response), it is plausible that these signals could be used by the animal to perform the task. Moreover, because match suppression and match enhancement were observed during both the object and spatial recognition memory tasks, this pattern of mnemonic signal appears to be common across many forms of recognition memory. Consistent with this idea, similar recognition memory signals have also been observed in the rat entorhinal cortex during the performance of an olfactory recognition memory task (Young et al., 1997). These recognition signals are common not only across tasks, but also across brain areas. Robust match–nonmatch signals have been reported in the perirhinal cortex (Miller, Li, & Desimone, 1993; Young et al., 1997), as well as in the prefrontal cortex (Miller et al., 1996).

In addition to selective match–nonmatch signals, some entorhinal neurons signaled a match–nonmatch difference for all stimuli used on a given day of testing. This response has been termed an "abstracted" match–nonmatch signal in that it signals the abstract category of "matching," regardless of the particular sample stimulus that is presented (Suzuki & Eichenbaum, 2000). Similar abstracted responses have been observed in the rat hippocampus (Wood, Dudchenko, & Eichenbaum, 1999), but are much less common in the perirhinal and prefrontal cortices. Like the selective recognition signals, abstracted recognition signals may also participate in the performance of recognition memory tasks.

Summary of Neurophysiological Findings

The findings from these neurophysiological studies make several points. First, neurons in the entorhinal cortex participate in signaling many aspects of both object and spatial recognition memory. Indeed, compared to other temporal or prefrontal areas, the entorhinal cortex conveys the widest range of sensory or mnemonic signals reported. These include stimulus-selective responses, selective working memory signals during the delay intervals of the task, and both stimulus-specific and abstracted match–nonmatch signals. Second, these findings, taken together with findings in other brain areas, show that the same kinds of match–nonmatch and working memory signals described in the entorhinal cortex are readily found across different brain areas as well as across different kinds of recognition memory tasks (i.e., object, spatial, and olfactory recognition tasks). Although similar mnemonic signals are observed across various brain areas, an important point is that these types of signals are not equally prevalent in all brain areas. For example, working memory signals are particularly prominent in the prefrontal cortex, while selective match–nonmatch signals predominate in the perirhinal cortex. The entorhinal cortex signals both selective and abstracted match–nonmatch signals, whereas abstracted signals appear to predominate in the hippocampus. Taken together, these findings suggest that all of these areas participate in the performance of recognition memory tasks, but that, depending on the particular task demands (i.e., stronger working memory component or stronger long-term memory component), some areas are more important than others.

CONCLUSIONS

The goal of this chapter has been to provide a summary of the ways in which anatomical and neurophysiological studies have contributed to our understanding of the functions of the medial temporal lobe. Important progress has been made in both lines of research. Quantitative anatomical tract-tracing techniques are providing increasingly detailed descriptions of the patterns of medial temporal lobe connections. Single-unit neurophysiological studies in behaving animals have begun to reveal the complex patterns of neural activity that underlie memory not only in the medial temporal lobe, but also in the prefrontal cortex. Multisite physiological recordings will be an important tool in determining how these interconnected areas work together to accomplish memory. A long-term goal is to map the physiological activity in both the medial temporal lobe and prefrontal cortex onto the specific connectivity of these regions, creating a "functional wiring diagram" of the memory-related areas of the brain. Continued parallel work in neuroanatomy and neurophysiology will be essential to accomplish this goal.

REFERENCES

Amaral, D. G., Insausti, R., & Cowan, W. M. (1987). The entorhinal cortex of the monkey: I. Cytoarchitectonic organization. *Journal of Comparative Neurology, 264*, 326–355.

Brodmann, K. (1909). *Vergleichende Lokalisationslehre der Grosshirnrinde.* Leipzig: Barth.

Bonon, G. von, & Bailey, P. (1947). *The neocortex of macaca mulatta.* Urbana: University of Illinois Press.

Buffalo, E. A., Ramus, S. J., Clark, R. E., Teng, E., Squire, L. R., & Zola, S. M. (1999). Dissociation between the effects of damage to perirhinal cortex and area TE. *Learning and Memory, 6*(6), 572–599.

Cohen, N. J., & Squire, L. R. (1980). Preserved learning and retention of pattern analyzing skill in amnesia: Dissociation of knowing how and knowing that. *Science, 210*, 207–209.

Eichenbaum, H., Dudchenko, P., Wood, E., Shapiro, M., & Tanila, H. (1999). The hippocampus, memory, and place cells: Is it spatial memory or a memory space? *Neuron, 23*, 209–226.

Fernandez, G., Brewer, J. D., Zhao, Z., Glover, G. H., & Gabrieli, J. D. (1999). Level of sustained entorhinal activity at study correlates with subsequent cued-recall performance: A functional magnetic resonance imaging study with high acquisition rate. *Hippocampus, 9*(1), 35–44.

Funahashi, S., Bruce, C. J., & Goldman-Rakic, P. S. (1989). Mnemonic coding of visual space in the monkey's dorsolateral prefrontal cortex. *Journal of Neurophysiology, 61,* 331–349.

Gaffan, D. (1995). Dissociated effects of perirhinal cortex ablation, fornix transection and amygdalectomy: Evidence for multiple memory systems in the primate temporal lobe. *Experimental Brain Research, 99,* 411–422.

Gaffan, D., & Murray, E. A. (1992). Monkeys (*Macaca fascicularis*) with rhinal cortex ablations succeed in object discrimination learning despite 24-hr intertrial intervals and fail at matching to sample despite double sample presentations. *Behavioral Neuroscience, 106,* 30–38.

Insausti, R., Amaral, D. G., & Cowan, W. M. (1987a). The entorhinal cortex of the monkey: II. Cortical afferents. *Journal of Comparative Neurology, 264,* 356–395.

Insausti, R., Amaral, D. G., & Cowan, W. M. (1987b). The entorhinal cortex of the monkey: III. Subcortical afferents. *Journal of Comparative Neurology, 264,* 396–408.

Jones, E. G., & Powell, T. P. S. (1970). An anatomical study of converging sensory pathways within the cerebral cortex of the monkey. *Brain, 93,* 793–820.

Leonard, B. W., Amaral, D. G., Squire, L. R., & Zola-Morgan, S. (1995). Transient memory impairment in monkeys with bilateral lesions of the entorhinal cortex. *Journal of Neuroscience, 15*(8), 5637–5659.

Maguire, E. A., Burgess, N., Donnett, J. G., Frackowiak, R. S., Firth, C. D., & O'Keefe, J. (1998). Knowing where and getting there: A human navigation network. *Science, 280,* 921–924.

Meunier, M., Bachevalier, J., Mishkin, M., & Murray, E. A. (1993). Effects on visual recognition of combined and separate ablations of the entorhinal and perirhinal cortex in rhesus monkeys. *Journal of Neuroscience, 13,* 5418–5432.

Miller, E. K., Erickson, C. A., & Desimone, R. (1996). Neural mechanisms of visual working memory in prefrontal cortex of the macaque. *Journal of Neuroscience, 16*(16), 5154–5167.

Miller, E. K., Li, L., & Desimone, R. (1993). Activity of neurons in anterior inferior temporal cortex during a short-term memory task. *Journal of Neuroscience, 13,* 1460–1478.

Mishkin, M. (1978). Memory in monkeys severely impaired by combined but not by separate removal of amygdala and hippocampus. *Nature, 273,* 297–298.

Mishkin, M., Suzuki, W. A., Gadian, D. G., & Vargha-Khadem, F. (1997). Hierarchical organization of cognitive memory. *Philosophical Transactions of the Royal Society of London, Series B, 352,* 1461–1467.

Murray, E. A., & Wise, S. P. (1996). Role of the hippocampus plus subjacent cortex but not amygdala in visuomotor conditional learning in rhesus monkeys. *Behavioral Neuroscience, 110*(6), 1261–1270.

Ramus, S. J., Zola-Morgan, S., & Squire, L. R. (1994). Effects of lesions of perirhinal cortex or parahippocampal cortex on memory in monkeys. *Society for Neuroscience Abstracts, 20,* 1074.

Ranganath, C., & D'Esposito, M. (2000). Differential response properties of prefrontal and hippocampal regions during working and long-term memory tasks. *Society for Neuroscience Abstracts, 26,* 501.

Scoville, W. B., & Milner, B. (1957). Loss of recent memory after bilateral hippocampal lesions. *Journal of Neurology, Neurosurgery and Psychiatry, 20,* 11–21.

Squire, L. R., & Zola, S. M. (1998). Episodic memory, semantic memory and amnesia. *Hippocampus, 8,* 205–211.

Suzuki, W. A., & Amaral, D. G. (1994a). Perirhinal and parahippocampal cortices of the macaque monkey: Cortical afferents. *Journal of Comparative Neurology, 350,* 497–533.

Suzuki, W. A., & Amaral, D. G. (1994b). Topographic organization of the reciprocal connections between monkey entorhinal cortex and the perirhinal and parahippocampal cortices. *Journal of Neuroscience, 14,* 1856–1877.

Suzuki, W. A., & Eichenbaum, H. (2000). The neurophysiology of memory. *Annals of the New York Academy of Sciences, 911,* 175–191.

Suzuki, W. A., Miller, E. K., & Desimone, R. (1997). Object and place memory in the macaque entorhinal cortex. *Journal of Neurophysiology, 78*, 1062–1081.

Suzuki, W. A., Zola-Morgan, S., Squire, L. R., & Amaral, D. G. (1993). Lesions of the perirhinal and parahippocampal cortices in the monkey produce long-lasting memory impairment in the visual and tactual modalities. *Journal of Neuroscience, 13*, 2430–2451.

Ungerleider, L. G., & Mishkin, M. (1982). Two cortical visual systems. In J. Ingle, M. A. Goodale, & R. J. W. Mansfield (Eds.), *Analysis of visual behavior* (pp. 549–586). Cambridge, MA: MIT Press.

Van Hoesen, G. W., & Pandya, D. N. (1975a). Some connections of the entorhinal (area 28) and perirhinal (area 35) cortices of the rhesus monkey: I. Temporal lobe afferents. *Brain Research, 95*, 1–24.

Van Hoesen, G. W., & Pandya, D. N. (1975b). Some connections of the entorhinal (area 28) and perirhinal (area 35) cortices of the rhesus monkey: III. Efferent connections. *Brain Research, 95*, 48–67.

Van Hoesen, G. W., Pandya, D. N. & Butters, N. (1972). Cortical afferents to the entorhinal cortex of the rhesus monkey. *Science, 175*, 1471–1473.

Van Hoesen, G. W., Pandya, D. N., & Butters, N. (1975). Some connections of the entorhinal (area 28) and perirhinal (area 35) cortices of the rhesus monkey: II. Frontal lobe afferents. *Brain Research, 95*, 25–38.

Vargha-Khadem, F., Gadian, D. G., Watkins, K. E., Connelly, A., Van Paesschen, W., & Mishkin, M. (1997). Differential effects of early hippocampal pathology on episodic and semantic memory. *Science, 277*, 376–380.

Wiig, K. A., & Burwell, R. D. (1998). Memory impairment on a delayed non-matching-to-position task after lesions of the perirhinal cortex in the rat. *Behavioral Neuroscience, 112*(4), 827–838.

Wood, E. R., Dudchenko, P., & Eichenbaum, H. (1999). The global record of memory in hippocampal neuronal activity. *Nature, 397*, 613–616.

Young, B. J., Otto, T., Fox, G. D., & Eichenbaum, H. (1997). Memory representation within the parahippocampal region. *Journal of Neuroscience, 17*, 5183–5195.

Zola, S. M., Squire, L. R., Teng, E., Stefanacci, L., Buffalo, E. A., & Clark, R. E. (2000). Impaired recognition memory in monkeys after damage limited to the hippocampal region. *Journal of Neuroscience, 20*, 451–463.

Zola-Morgan, S., Squire, L. R., & Amaral, D. G. (1989). Lesions of the amygdala that spare adjacent cortical regions do not impair memory or exacerbate the impairment following lesions of the hippocampal formation. *Journal of Neuroscience, 9*, 1922–1936.

Zola-Morgan, S., Squire, L. R., Amaral, D. G., & Suzuki, W. A. (1989). Lesions of perirhinal and parahippocampal cortex that spare the amygdala and hippocampal formation produce severe memory impairment. *Journal of Neuroscience, 9*, 4355–4370.

24

Neuronal Representation of Visual Long-Term Memory and Its Top-Down Executive Processing

EMI TAKAHASHI and YASUSHI MIYASHITA

Distant are the grassy plains of Mano
  in Michinoku;
men say you can conjure them
in your heart, and yet—
    —Poem sent to Otomo Yakamochi
    by LADY KASA (A.D. 730?);
    translated by LEVY (1981, p. 205)

The author of the poem quoted above, Lady Kasa, was pining for Otomo Yakamochi; she could even see a scene at distant Michinoku in her mind's eye when she thought about it, but she could not see Otomo Yakamochi, who was not so distant from her. As in this age-old poem, if we wish to see one scene that is not actually present in front of us, it is not difficult for us to imagine it with our "mind's eye." How does our "mind's eye" work? A short answer might be that visual images, or more generally our knowledge and experiences, are voluntarily recalled from memory by reactivation of their neural representations in the cerebral association cortex. In this chapter, we attempt to provide a longer, more complete description of the mechanisms underlying the encoding and retrieval of visual images.

Three questions are central to understanding these processes: (1) Where are the mnemonic representations coded, and how are they organized? (2) Which neural processes create the representations? (3) What mechanisms underlie the reactivation of the representations on demand for voluntary recall? Clinical studies in humans have suggested that long-term declarative memory is stored in the neocortical association area, which is also engaged in sensory perception (Milner, Squire, & Kandel, 1998; Squire, 1987). When electrical stimulation was applied via cortical surface electrodes placed on the temporal lobe during neurosurgery under local anesthesia, epileptic patients sometimes reported recollection of past perceptual experiences, suggesting that artificial electrical input to the putative memory storehouse might reactivate the "brain's record of auditory and visual experience" (Penfield & Perot, 1963, p. 595). Recent experimental studies in nonhuman primates have moved beyond these classical clinical observations and provided a clearer understanding of the mechanisms of visual object memory (Miyashita & Hayashi, 2000). Particular emphasis is given in this chapter to our recent findings that two types of memory retrieval signals that spread in the reverse direction to the perceptual forward signal can activate the mnemonic representation in the inferior temporal (IT) neocortex. One of these is the backward signal from the medial temporal lobe; the other is the top-down signal from the prefrontal cortex (Naya, Yoshida, & Miyashita, 2001; Tomita, Ohbayashi, Nakahara, Hasegawa, & Miyashita, 1999).

FUNCTIONAL ARCHITECTURE OF VISUAL MEMORY IN THE INFERIOR TEMPORAL CORTEX: CELL ASSEMBLIES OF PAIR-CODING NEURONS

Physical properties of objects, such as their color, texture, and shape, are analyzed along a multisynaptic occipitotemporal projection system interconnecting the striate, prestriate, and IT cortex. The IT cortex is considered to be crucial for visual perception and the recognition of objects, and is also thought to serve as the storehouse of visual associative long-term memory (Mishkin, 1982; Miyashita, 1993; Squire & Zola-Morgan, 1991). IT neurons respond selectively to complex visual patterns, and this activity is closely coupled with the conscious perception of objects (Logothetis, 1999; Miyashita & Hayashi, 2000). How then is the associative memory of visual objects represented in the IT cortex? We have examined this problem with electrophysiological and molecular biological approaches.

In experiments with monkeys, we have utilized extensively the visual pair association (PA) task, a variant of the human memory task that is sensitive to medial temporal lobe amnesia in clinical neuropsychological batteries (Miyashita, 1993; Miyashita & Hayashi, 2000). In the PA task, the subject is required to memorize many arbitrarily assigned pairs of visual stimuli, and then to retrieve from long-term memory a visual stimulus specified by another visual stimulus (Gaffan & Bolton, 1983; Murray, Gaffan, & Mishkin, 1993). We examined the anterior ventral part of the IT cortex via single-unit recordings in awake monkeys performing this task, and found a class of neurons (called "pair-coding neurons") exhibiting significantly correlated visual responses to picture pairs (Higuchi & Miyashita, 1996; Miyashita, 1988; Sakai & Miyashita, 1991). This finding gave us the first direct evidence that the activity of IT neurons could represent visual long-term memory acquired through associative learning (see Miyashita & Hayashi, 2000).

The IT cortex consists of two cytoarchitechtonically distinct but mutually interconnected areas: area TE (TE) and the perirhinal cortex (PRh). TE is located at the final stage of unimodal association areas in the ventral visual pathway that processes object vision, whereas the PRh is one of the polymodal limbic cortices that are considered to be important for memory functions (Squire & Zola-Morgan, 1991). In order to clarify functional differences between TE and the PRh, we recorded neuronal responses from both areas in monkeys performing the PA task (Naya, Yoshida, Ihara, Nagao, & Miyashita, 2000). A correlation coefficient was calculated for each stimulus-selective neuron between the cue response to a picture and the cue response to the paired associate of that picture. This coefficient, the "pair-coding index" (PCI), evaluates the degree of linkage between paired associates. The mean PCI value was significantly positive in both areas; furthermore, it was significantly greater in the PRh than in TE. Recently, we further examined the spatial distribution of such stimulus-selective neurons in the PRh and TE. We found that these neurons tended to aggregate into several clusters, and that the PRh cluster had the highest mean PCI value. We regard these clusters of pair-coding neurons as the "cell assembly" that encodes PA memory.

NEURAL CIRCUIT REORGANIZATION FOR THE FORMATION OF CELL ASSEMBLIES OF PAIR-CODING NEURONS: A MOLECULAR BIOLOGICAL STUDY IN MONKEYS

Having electrophysiologically identified the cell assembly of pair-coding neurons, we next addressed the important question of how this cell assembly is created. In light of current neurobiological theories (K. C. Martin, Barad, & Kandel, 2000; S. J. Martin, Grimwood, & Morris, 2000; Thoenen, 1995), we may assume many steps of cellular and molecular changes that ultimately create pair-coding neurons. For example, the electric activity of neurons induced by visual stimulation would be transformed into intracellular cascades of transcription factors. The cascades would activate many immediate early genes and late effector genes, which contribute to synaptogenesis and synaptic elimination and eventually to the reorganization of local neuronal networks. Reorganization of local networks can be detected electrophysiologically as a change in neuronal stimulus selectivity, typically as the emergence of the pair-coding neurons.

These cellular and molecular scenarios have been investigated most extensively in invertebrates and lower mammals (K. C. Martin et al., 2000; S. J. Martin et al., 2000). Do these scenarios also apply to cognitive memory in primates? We tackled this question by screening gene inductions during the formation of PA memory in monkeys. Molecular biological studies in monkeys must overcome various obstacles that are not present in studies with mice or invertebrates. These obstacles and some possible solutions for the obstacles are discussed in our original publications, along with details of our experimental designs (Okuno, Tokuyama, Li, Hashimoto, & Miyashita, 1999; Tokuyama, Okuno, Hashimoto, Li, & Miyashita, 2000). To overcome one of the obstacles, we used "split-brain" monkeys (i.e., monkeys whose corpus callosum [CC] and anterior commissure had been transected), enabling intra-animal comparison of gene inductions. This eliminated the potential confounding factor of genetic variation between individual monkeys.

We searched for induction of messenger ribonucleic acids (mRNAs) during the formation of visual PA memory, using a quantitative reverse transcription-polymerase chain reaction method, in which a gene of interest was coamplified with an internal standard gene; we found that the mRNA expression levels of a neurotrophin, brain-derived neurotrophic factor (BDNF), and an immediate early gene, *zif268*, were significantly up-regulated in the PRh (Tokuyama et al., 2000). We confirmed BDNF and *zif268* induction by using *in situ* hybridization. Figure 24.1 shows that BDNF mRNA-positive cells accumulated in patches in the PRh, just in the location where we had electrophysiologically found a cluster of pair-coding neurons. Neurotrophins, especially BDNF, have been proposed to mediate functional and structural synaptic modifications even in a mature nervous system (Bonhoeffer, 1996; McAllister, Katz, & Lo, 1999; Thoenen, 1995). Therefore, our findings provide the first positive evidence for the hypothesis that BDNF contributes to the reorganization of neural networks, and eventually to the formation of such cell assemblies of the pair-coding neurons in monkeys.

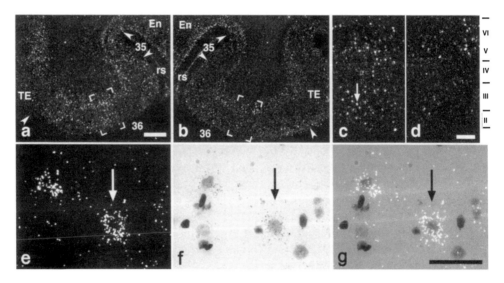

FIGURE 24.1. Gene induction in the monkey inferior temporal (IT) cortex during the formation of pair association (PA) memory, as revealed by *in situ* hybridization of brain-derived neurotrophic factor (BDNF) messenger ribonucleic acid (mRNA). (a–d) BDNF mRNA distribution in the IT gyrus of the hemisphere that learned the PA task (PA hemisphere) (a), and that in the hemisphere that learned a control visual memory task (VD hemisphere) (b). BDNF mRNA accumulated in a patch in area 36 of the PA hemisphere (framed area), but not in area 36 of the VD hemisphere. The framed areas in a and b are enlarged in c and d, respectively. BDNF mRNA-positive cells were observed in layers V–VI and in layers II–III of the PA hemisphere (c). For the arrow in c, see below (e–g). En, entorhinal cortex; 35, area 35; 36, area 36; TE, area TE; rs, rhinal sulcus. Arrowheads mark the boundaries between different cortical areas. (e–g) BDNF mRNA-positive cells in layers II–III of the PA hemisphere. Cell marked by arrow in c is enlarged and shown in darkfield (e), brightfield (f), and brightfield with epi-illumination (g). Calibration bars: 1 mm (a, b), 250 μm (c, d), 50 μm (e–g).

The figure as a whole shows that BDNF mRNA-positive cells accumulated in patches in the PRh of the PA hemisphere, just in the location where we had electrophysiologically found a cluster of pair-coding neurons. This finding provides evidence for the hypothesis that BDNF contributes to the structural reorganization of neural networks and eventually to the formation of cell assemblies of the pair-coding neurons (see text). From Tokuyama et al. (2000). Copyright 2000 by Nature America, Inc. Adapted by permission.

MEMORY RETRIEVAL PROCESSES IN THE IT CORTEX

The forward flow of visual information from TE to area 36 (A36, an immediately adjoining region in the PRh) has been considered to serve the memory-encoding process (discussed above). However, functional roles for the rich backward fiber projections from A36 to TE have not been examined. On the basis of the previous observation that IT neurons are dynamically activated by the necessity for memory recall in monkeys (Naya, Sakai, & Miyashita, 1996; Sakai & Miyashita, 1991), we have hypothesized that the backward projection participates in memory retrieval processes. We tested the hypothesis by comparing the time courses of perceptual and memory signals in TE and A36 via single-unit recording, while monkeys were performing the PA task (Naya et al., 2001). The responses of a representative A36 neuron, with stimulus-selective delay activity related to the sought target specified by a cue stimulus, are shown in Figure 24.2a. One stimulus elicited the strongest response during the cue period, and the response continued into the delay period

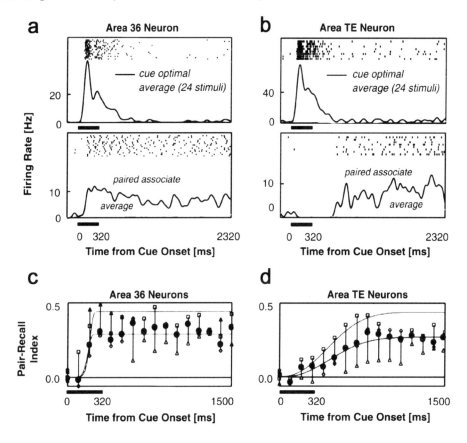

FIGURE 24.2. Neuronal activity related to memory retrieval during the PA task, as shown by a single cell in A36 (a) and in TE (b). For the raster displays (a and b), spike density functions (SDFs) were aligned at the cue onset in trials with the cue-optimal stimulus as a cue (upper panel) and in trials with its paired associate as a cue (lower panel). In the SDFs, top lines indicate responses to the cue-optimal stimulus (upper panel) or its paired associate (lower panel), and bottom lines indicate mean responses to all 24 stimuli. (c–d) Temporal dynamics of the averaged pair recall index, or PRI(t), for the population of the stimulus-selective neurons. Mean values of PRI(t) were plotted every 100 msec for A36 neurons (c) and TE neurons (d) (filled circles, total; open diamonds, monkey 1; open squares, monkey 2; open triangles, monkey 3). Top lines indicate the best-fit Weibull functions for the population-averaged PRI(t) in the two areas. Bottom lines indicate the same, but for the neurons whose PRI(t) increased above the 5% significance level. PRI(t) was defined as the partial correlation coefficient of the instantaneous firing rate at time t for each cue stimulus with the visual response to its paired-associate stimulus.

This figure shows that memory retrieval signals appeared earlier in A36, with TE neurons being later recruited to carry information about the to-be-retrieved target. It suggests that the backward projection from A36 to TE participates in memory retrieval processes. From Naya et al. (2001). Copyright 2001 by the American Association for the Advancement of Science. Adapted by permission.

(Figure 24.2a, upper panel). In the trial when the paired associate of this cue-optimal stimulus was used as a cue, the same cell started to respond during the cue period without an initial perceptual response, and maintained a tonic activity until the choice stimuli were presented (Figure 24.2a, lower panel). In TE, we also found neurons exhibiting similar target-related delay activity (Figure 24.2b). However, the time course of the delay activity of the neuron was different from the time course of the A36 neuron shown in Figure 24.2a. We examined the time course of the target-related delay activity of each neuron by considering responses to all cue stimuli. The partial correlation coefficient of the instantaneous firing rate at time t for each cue stimulus was calculated with the visual response to its paired-associate stimulus (the "pair recall index," or PRI). Stimulus-selective neurons in TE showed the slow, gradual increase of the population-averaged $PRI(t)$, which significantly differed from that in A36 (see c and d in Figure 24.2).

We also examined the perceptual signal and found that the latencies of visual response for TE neurons were significantly shorter than those for A36 neurons (TE, median 77 milliseconds [msec]; A36, median 89 msec; Kolmogorov–Smirnov test; $p < .05$). This result suggests that perceptual signals reach TE before A36, confirming their forward propagation. In contrast, as shown in Figure 24.2, memory retrieval signals appeared earlier in A36, with TE neurons being gradually recruited to carry information about the to-be-retrieved target. This means that mnemonic information spreads backward, from A36 to TE, presumably to extract PA memory from long-term storage.

TOP-DOWN MEMORY RETRIEVAL ALONG A FRONTOTEMPORAL PATHWAY

Although prefrontal lesions alone do not usually result in severe amnesia (Stuss & Benson, 1986), some neuropsychological observations indicate that the prefrontal cortex may play a role in the strategic control of memory retrieval (Incisa della Rocchetta & Milner, 1993; Moscovitch & Melo, 1997). The capacity for interhemispheric transfer through the anterior CC (Gazzaniga, 1995) also supports this view. In addition, in humans, combined lesions to the frontal and temporal lobes severely impair retrieval of old memories (Kroll, Markowitsch, Knight, & von Cramon, 1997). Behavioral experiments in macaque monkeys also suggest that interactions between the prefrontal cortex and the IT cortex are important for several visual memory tasks. Specifically, sectioning of the uncinate fascicle, a direct and reciprocal frontotemporal pathway (Ungerleider, Gaffan, & Pelak, 1989), resulted in impairments of visual associative learning and visuomotor conditional learning (Eacott & Gaffan, 1992; Gutnikov, Ma, & Gaffan, 1997).

Inspired by these observations, we have proposed the hypothesis that top-down processes originating from the prefrontal cortex can regulate the retrieval of long-term memory in the absence of bottom-up sensory input (Hasegawa, Fukushima, Ihara, & Miyashita, 1998). This hypothesis was tested in a new experimental paradigm, wherein the PA task was employed with posterior-split-brain monkeys. Monkeys underwent selective section of the splenium of the CC and the anterior commissure, which left only the anterior CC intact. We were interested in whether the prefrontal cortex could instruct the contralateral hemisphere, via the anterior CC, to retrieve long-term memory. We found that long-term memory acquired through stimulus–stimulus association did not transfer interhemispherically via the anterior CC. Nonetheless, when a visual cue was presented to one hemisphere, the anterior CC could instruct the other hemisphere to retrieve the correct stimulus specified by the cue. Two conclusions were obtained from this experiment. First, visual long-term memory is stored in the temporal cortex; second, memory retrieval is under the executive control of the prefrontal cortex, in the absence of bottom-up sensory input.

From these behavioral experiments, we had been predicting the existence of a top-down signal from the prefrontal cortex to IT cortex in memory retrieval. However, no direct neurophysiological evidence had been demonstrated before we (Tomita et al., 1999) conducted single-unit recording from the IT cortex in posterior-split-brain monkeys. The posterior-split-brain preparation enabled dissociation of the top-down signal from the bottom-up signal, as shown in Plate 24.1 (see color plates, opposite page 238). Plate 24.1a shows the bottom-up condition in the experiment. Visual stimuli (cue and choice pictures) were presented in the hemifield contralateral to the recording site in the IT cortex. The monkey had to make the correct choice specified by the cue. Fixation was required throughout a trial. It was expected that bottom-up sensory signals from the retina (black arrow) would be detected in this condition. Plate 24.1b shows the top-down condition, in which the cue stimulus was presented in the hemifield ipsilateral to the recording site. In this condition, the bottom-up sensory signal from the retina did not arrive at visual areas in the ipsilateral hemisphere (e.g., at the recording site in the ipsilateral IT cortex), and only the top-down signal (blue arrow) could activate IT neurons through feedback connections from the prefrontal cortex. Single-unit recording experiment in this configuration clearly demonstrated that in the absence of bottom-up visual inputs, single IT neurons were robustly activated by the effect of the top-down signal from the prefrontal cortex (Plate 24.1c). The top-down signal had a longer latency by about 100 msec than the bottom-up signal. The longer latency is probably attributable to multisynaptic conduction delay, reflecting the signal transformation within the prefrontal cortices. Indeed, we also demonstrated that the top-down signal was almost abolished by complete section of the anterior CC, which confirmed that the signal was transmitted not through a subcortical but through a fronto-temporal cortical pathway. The selectivity of the top-down signal suggested that the frontotemporal pathway conveyed information on semantic categorization imposed by visual stimulus–stimulus association (for details, see Tomita et al., 1999).

As described above, the top-down signal had a longer latency than the bottom-up signal. During this delay, the prefrontal cortex might prompt IT neurons to maintain cue-related information, seek out and retrieve the relevant target in the IT cortex, and also verify whether the retrieved object was the relevant one. In support of this interpretation, prefrontal neurons have been reported to share cellular specificities for visual objects stimuli with IT neurons and to show sustained responses to the object stimuli in a working memory task (Levy & Goldman-Rakic, 2000). A recent report (Rainer, Rao, & Miller, 1999) on prospective coding in prefrontal neurons similar to that found in IT neurons also supports this view. Furthermore, human PET and fMRI studies in memory retrieval tasks have shown that the prefrontal cortex is engaged in retrieval attempts, as well as in contextual monitoring or memory judgment (e.g., Buckner et al., 1998; Fletcher, Shallice, Frith, Frackowiak, & Dolan, 1998). A deeper understanding of the signal transformation within the prefrontal cortex would help to elucidate the mechanism of top-down control in memory retrieval.

CONCLUSIONS

In this chapter, we have examined neural mechanisms underlying memory retrieval and neural circuit reorganization for the formation of cell assemblies of pair-coding neurons. Our experimental data demonstrate that visual associative long-term memory is stored in the IT cortex; the IT neurons can acquire stimulus selectivity through learning, and can link representations of temporally associated stimuli. We have described these processes in detail as emergence of the pair-coding neurons in learning of the PA task. The experiments also suggest that neurotrophins, particularly BDNF, can serve as molecular mediators for the neural circuit reorganization that eventually contributes to the formation of cell assembly of the pair-coding neurons.

As discussed in this chapter, there are two signal pathways through which the mnemonic representation in the IT cortex can be activated in memory retrieval: the frontotemporal pathway and the limbic–temporal pathway. How do these two pathways cooperate during memory retrieval? Many functional neuroimaging studies have suggested that the fronto-temporal pathway is involved in retrieval effort (Lepage, Ghaffar, Nyberg, & Tulving, 2000). For example, Lepage and colleagues (2000) refer to the "retrieval mode" as a neurocognitive set, or state, in which one mentally holds in the background of focal attention a segment of one's personal past. The neural substrate of such a neurocognitive set has been identified by imaging experiments in the bilateral frontal pole (Brodmann's area [BA] 10), the bilateral frontal operculum (BA 45/47), the left dorsal prefrontal cortex (BA 8/9), and the left anterior cingulate (BA 32). However, so far, no direct anatomical and functional pathways from these areas to the temporal cortex are known. It is likely that the memory retrieval signal from these prefrontal areas is further processed in a part of the inferior prefrontal cortex, from which the direct fiber projections would reach the temporal cortex.

Another signal pathway for memory retrieval originates from the medial temporal lobe. Our neurophysiological experiments demonstrated the backward spreading of the memory retrieval signal from the PRh to the temporal neocortex (TE) with a time lag of about 300 msec. The neuronal mechanism of this long delay is not known. An attractive hypothesis suggests that the functional significance of this backward signal spreading is related to the indexing of multimodal mnemonic representations (Squire & Zola-Morgan, 1991). This pathway may play a crucial role for memory storage and retrieval for a while until memory is stored and retrieved by the hippocampus-independent system, perhaps until neocortical areas per se establish connectivity with each other. However, the nature of this indexing system is still unknown. Obtaining direct evidence for this hypothesis in animal experimentations remains a future challenge.

REFERENCES

Bonhoeffer, T. (1996). Neurotrophins and activity-dependent development of the neocortex. *Current Opinion Neurobiology, 6*, 119–126.

Buckner, R. L., Koutstaal, W., Schacter, D. L., Dale, A. M., Rotte, M., & Rosen, B. R. (1998). Functional–anatomic study of episodic retrieval: II. Selective averaging of event-related fMRI trials to test the retrieval success hypothesis. *NeuroImage, 7*, 163–175.

Eacott, M. J., & Gaffan, D. (1992). Inferotemporal–frontal disconnection: The uncinate fascicle and visual associative learning in monkeys. *European Journal of Neuroscience, 4*, 1320–1332.

Fletcher, P. C., Shallice, T., Frith, C. D., Frackowiak, R. S. J., & Dolan, R. J. (1998). The functional roles of prefrontal cortex in episodic memory: II. Retrieval. *Brain, 121*, 1249–1256.

Gaffan, D., & Bolton, J. Q. (1983). Learning of object–object associations by monkeys. *Quarterly Journal of Experimental Psychology, B35*, 149–155.

Gazzaniga, M. S. (1995). Principles of human brain organization derived from split-brain studies. *Neuron, 14*, 217–228.

Gutnikov, S. A., Ma, Y. Y. & Gaffan, D. (1997). Temporo-frontal disconnection impairs visual-visual paired association learning but not configural learning in *Macaca* monkeys. *European Journal of Neuroscience, 9*, 1524–1529.

Hasegawa, I., Fukushima, T., Ihara, T., & Miyashita, Y. (1998). Callosal window between prefrontal cortices: Cognitive interaction to retrieve long-term memory. *Science, 281,* 814–818.

Higuchi, S., & Miyashita, Y. (1996). Formation of mnemonic neuronal responses to visual paired associates in inferotemporal cortex is impaired by perirhinal and entorhinal lesions. *Proceedings of the National Academy of Sciences USA, 93,* 739–743.

Incisa della Rocchetta, A., & Milner, B. (1993). Strategic search and retrieval inhibition: The role of the frontal lobes. *Neuropsychologia, 31,* 503–524.

Kroll, N. E., Markowitsch, H. J., Knight, R. T., & von Cramon, D. Y. (1997). Retrieval of old memories: The temporofrontal hypothesis. *Brain, 120,* 1377–1399.

Lepage, M., Ghaffar, O., Nyberg, L., & Tulving, E. (2000). Prefrontal cortex and episodic memory retrieval mode. *Proceedings of the National Academy of Sciences USA, 97,* 506–511.

Levy, I. H. (Trans.). (1981). *"Man'yoshu": A translation of Japan's premier anthology of classical poetry* (Vol. 1). Princeton, NJ: Princeton University Press.

Levy, R., & Goldman-Rakic, P. S. (2000). Segregation of working memory functions within the dorsolateral prefrontal cortex. *Experimental Brain Research, 133,* 23–32.

Logothetis, N. K. (1999). Vision: A window on consciousness. *Scientific American, 281,* 69–75.

Martin, K. C., Barad, M., & Kandel, E. R. (2000). Local protein synthesis and its role in synapse-specific plasticity. *Current Opinion Neurobiology, 10,* 587–592.

Martin, S. J., Grimwood, P. D., & Morris, R. G. (2000). Synaptic plasticity and memory: An evaluation of the hypothesis. *Annual Review of Neuroscience, 23,* 649–711.

McAllister, A. K., Katz, L. C., & Lo, D. C. (1999). Neurotrophins and synaptic plasticity. *Annual Review of Neuroscience, 22,* 295–318.

Milner, B., Squire, L. R., & Kandel, E. R. (1998). Cognitive neuroscience and the study of memory. *Neuron, 20,* 445–468.

Mishkin, M. (1982). A memory system in the monkey. *Philosophical Transactions of the Royal Society of London, Series B, 298,* 83–95.

Miyashita, Y. (1988). Neuronal correlate of visual associative long-term memory in the primate temporal cortex. *Nature, 335,* 817–820.

Miyashita, Y. (1993). Inferior temporal cortex: Where visual perception meets memory. *Annual Review of Neuroscience, 16,* 245–263.

Miyashita, Y., & Hayashi, T. (2000). Neural representation of visual objects: Encoding and top-down activation. *Current Opinion in Neurobiology, 10,* 187–194.

Moscovitch, M., & Melo, B. (1997). Strategic retrieval and the frontal lobes: Evidence from confabulation and amnesia. *Neuropsychologia, 35,* 1017–1034.

Murray, E. A., Gaffan, D., & Mishkin, M. (1993). Neural substrates of visual stimulus-stimulus association in rhesus monkeys. *Journal of Neuroscience, 13,* 4549–4561.

Naya, Y., Sakai, K., & Miyashita, Y. (1996). Activity of primate inferotemporal neurons related to a sought target in pair-association task. *Proceedings of National Academy Sciences USA, 93,* 2664–2669.

Naya, Y., Yoshida, M., Ihara, T., Nagao, S., & Miyashita, Y. (2000). Spatial distribution of memory-related cells in monkey area 36 and area TE during pair-association task. *Society for Neuroscience Abstracts, 26,* 286.

Naya, Y., Yoshida, M., & Miyashita, Y. (2001). Backward spreading of memory-retrieval signal in the primate temporal cortex. *Science, 291,* 661–664. [Corrections and clarifications: *Science, 291,* 1703.]

Okuno, H., Tokuyama, W., Li, Y. X., Hashimoto, T., & Miyashita, Y. (1999). Quantitative evaluation of neurotrophin and trk mRNA expression in visual and limbic areas along the occipito-temporo-hippocampal pathway in adult macaque monkeys. *Journal of Comparative Neurology, 408,* 378–398.

Penfield, W., & Perot, P. (1963). The brain's record of auditory and visual experience. *Brain, 86,* 595–696.

Rainer, G., Rao, S. C., & Miller, E. K. (1999). Prospective coding for objects in primate prefrontal cortex. *Journal of Neuroscience, 19,* 5493–5505.

Sakai, K., & Miyashita, Y. (1991). Neural organization for the long-term memory of paired associates. *Nature, 354,* 152–155.

Squire, L. R. (1987). *Memory and brain.* New York: Oxford University Press.

Squire, L. R., & Zola-Morgan S. (1991). The medial temporal lobe memory system. *Science, 253,* 1380–1386.

Stuss, D. T., & Benson, D. F. (1986). *The frontal lobes.* New York: Raven Press.

Thoenen, H. (1995). Neurotrophins and neuronal plasticity. *Science, 270,* 593–598.

Tokuyama, W., Okuno, H., Hashimoto, T., Li, Y. X., & Miyashita, Y. (2000). BDNF upregulation during declarative memory formation in monkey inferior temporal cortex. *Nature Neuroscience, 3,* 1134–1142.

Tomita, H., Ohbayashi, M., Nakahara, K., Hasegawa, I., & Miyashita, Y. (1999). Top-down signal from prefrontal cortex in executive control of memory retrieval. *Nature, 401,* 699–703.

Ungerleider, L. G., Gaffan, D., & Pelak, V. S. (1989). Projections from inferior temporal cortex to prefrontal cortex via the uncinate fascicle in rhesus monkeys. *Experimental Brain Research, 76,* 473–484.

25

Multiple Neuronal Mechanisms for Memory in the Anterior Inferior Temporal Cortex of Monkeys

ELIZABETH A. BUFFALO
and ROBERT DESIMONE

Over the past two decades, our understanding of visual memory—how we remember and recognize visual information—has undergone a revolution similar to the dramatic changes seen in our understanding of how sensory information is processed. Sensory systems are now known to comprise a large number of separate cortical areas with complex interconnections. This complexity replaces the earlier notion of a primary sensory area with one or two cortical subsidiary areas. Likewise, recent anatomical, behavioral, and physiological studies have demonstrated that, far from being a unitary phenomenon, visual memory is accomplished in a wide variety of ways across many brain regions.

One class of memory systems supports declarative memories, which are the memories of specific facts and events. Within this category, working memory has been distinguished from long-term memory, and recognition has been distinguished from recall. Additional distinctions have been made between various material-specific processes, such as memory for faces, words, objects, spatial locations, and so on. A second class of memory systems supports nondeclarative, or implicit, memories. These include stimulus–response habits, perceptual learning, conditioning, various types of priming, and habituation. With such an abundance of kinds of memory, it is natural to ask whether they share any common physiological underpinnings.

The anterior inferior temporal (IT) cortex is an ideal place to look for the neurophysiological mechanisms that subserve various forms of visual learning and memory—both because of its position at the end of the ventral object recognition pathway in the cortex, and because of its widespread connections with other cortical and subcortical structures known to be important for memory. The visual recognition of objects depends on a ventral cortical pathway that begins in area V1, continues through areas V2, V3, and V4, and culminates in the IT cortex. The IT cortex is composed of two cytoarchitecturally and anatomically distinct regions: the perirhinal cortex, located anteriorly and ventrally; and area TE, located laterally.

In the IT cortex, cells are selective for highly complex, global object features, such as shape (Gross, 1973). This stimulus selectivity is not fixed, however, and is known to be modulated by many influences not intrinsic to the visual stimulus, such as behavioral context, relevance, experience, and attention. In this chapter, we discuss recent findings that demonstrate five ways in which neuronal activity can be modulated during the formation or expression of memory traces in the anterior IT cortex of macaque monkeys. This modulation of neural activity reflects both "top-down" and "bottom-up" influences (see Figure 25.1).

REPETITION SUPPRESSION

The most common change seen in IT neurons after experience with visual images is "repetition suppression" or "adaptive filtering" (Li, Miller, & Desimone, 1993; Miller, Gochin, &

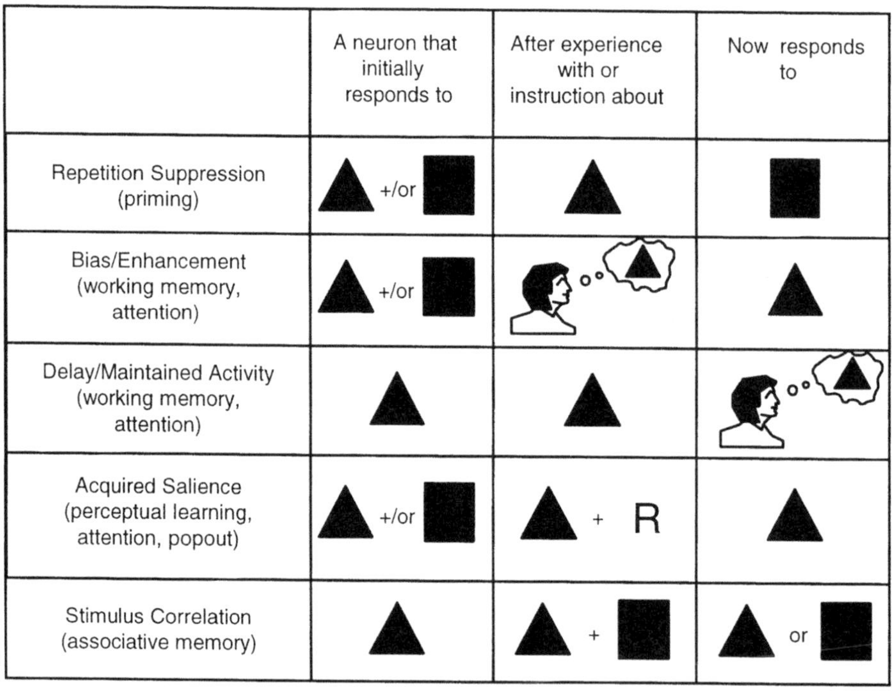

FIGURE 25.1. Schematic representation of neuronal correlates of the formation or expression of memory traces in the inferior temporal (IT) cortex. "Repetition suppression" refers to the reduction in response that occurs with repeated presentations of a stimulus. Because the neurons will continue to respond fully to novel stimuli, this will reduce the set of stimuli to which a particular neuron responds, thereby sharpening neural representations. "Bias/enhancement" refers to the increase in neuronal response to a stimulus for which the animal is actively searching or expecting. This is presumed to result from top-down feedback from neurons involved in working memory. "Delay/maintained activity" refers to the maintenance of stimulus-specific neuronal activity, when a stimulus representation is being held "online" in working memory. The icon of the person thinking of the triangle indicates that the stimulus is actively held in memory and is not actually present. "Acquired salience" is an example of a bottom-up mechanism that biases neuronal responses in favor of behaviorally relevant stimuli, when those stimuli have been repeatedly paired with reward (R). "Stimulus correlation" refers to the changes in stimulus selectivity that occur when two stimuli are paired in an associative learning task.

Gross, 1991; Miller, Li, & Desimone, 1991, 1993). Incoming sensory information is filtered by neurons according to how similar it is to information already present in either short- or long-term memory (see Figure 25.1, row 1). In monkeys, some of the IT neurons that respond selectively to particular object features, such as color or shape, give their best response to objects that contain those features but that are new, unexpected, or not recently seen. As new stimuli become familiar, synaptic weights in the cortex adjust so that the neuronal response for many cells is dampened—a case of "familiarity breeding contempt."

An example of repetition suppression can be observed in the anterior IT cortex while monkeys perform the delayed-matching-to-sample (DMS) task (Miller, Li, & Desimone, 1991). This portion of the IT cortex, the perirhinal cortex, is known to be important for visual memory (Buffalo et al., 1999; Buffalo, Ramus, Squire, & Zola, 2000; Meunier, Bachevalier, Mishkin, & Murray, 1993; Suzuki, Zola-Morgan, Squire, & Amaral, 1993; Zola-Morgan, Squire, Amaral, & Suzuki, 1989). In the standard form of the task used in our studies, a monkey was shown a sample stimulus followed, after a short delay, by a variable sequence of test stimuli. All sample and test stimuli were presented for 500 milliseconds (msec) each, separated by 700-msec delays. The monkey was rewarded for indicating whether or not any of the test stimuli matched the sample. On each trial from zero to five nonmatching stimuli intervened between the sample and the final matching test stimulus. For example, a sequence of stimuli might consist of A-B-C-D-A, with the final A being a matching test stimulus. Thus the task required recognition memory for the sample stimulus across the length of the behavioral trial.

The stimuli used in this task were complex objects, such as shapes, faces, or patterns, which elicit stimulus-selective responses from the large majority of IT cells. For about half of these stimulus-selective cells, the neural response to a visual stimulus was suppressed if it matched the test stimulus, even when several other stimuli intervened. That is, responses to test stimuli were a joint function of the sensory features of that stimulus and stored memory traces (Miller, Li, & Desimone, 1991, 1993), which is a general finding in studies of IT cells (Baylis & Rolls, 1987; Eskandar, Richmond, & Optican, 1992a, 1992b; Fahy, Riches, & Brown, 1993; Riches, Wilson, & Brown, 1991; Vogels & Orban, 1994). For example, if a cell was normally selective for stimulus A, the response to A when it was a matching test item was substantially smaller than when A appeared as a nonmatching item in the sequence (e.g., B-C-D-A-B). The degree of similarity between the sample and test stimulus that caused the suppression did not depend simply on a pixel-by-pixel comparison of the two stimuli, because the suppressive effect could be observed in many cells even when the sample and test stimuli were presented at different retinal locations, or when they differed in size (Lueschow, Miller, & Desimone, 1994).

An analysis of the time course of these effects suggests that they were generated within or before the IT cortex. The suppression of the response to matching items began extremely rapidly in the IT cortex, virtually at the onset of the visual response (within 80 msec of stimulus onset). This rapidity argues against the idea that the suppression was due to feedback to the IT cortex from other structures during the matching stimulus response. Sensitivity to repetition may be an intrinsic property of the visual cortex (Haenny & Schiller, 1988; Maunsell, Sclar, Nealey, & DePriest, 1991; Nelson, 1991).

A related suppressive effect was observed when we used stimuli in the DMS task that were initially novel to the animal (Li et al., 1993). For about a third of the cells in the IT cortex, the responses to specific sample and test stimuli declined systematically over the course of the recording session, as they became more familiar. These effects were stimulus-specific and long-lasting. That is, the reduction in response with familiarity was maintained even when several minutes and more than 100 other stimulus presentations intervened between repetitions of a given stimulus. However, the cells did not act simply as "novelty detectors," in the sense of giving their best response to any novel stimulus. Rather, both novelty and stimulus features determined the response. That is, cells gave their best response to stimuli that were both novel and had the appropriate sensory features. A study by Brown and colleagues suggests that these effects may be permanent (Fahy et al., 1993). They found that presentation of a set of stimuli on one day led to a reduced incidence of cells activated by those stimuli on a subsequent day.

Because stimulus repetition leads to response suppression for only a subpopulation of the cells in the IT cortex (about half of the stimulus-selective neurons), another way of looking at the phenomenon is that repetition leads to a smaller and *more efficient* representation of the stimulus in IT neural populations. That is, as a stimulus becomes more familiar, fewer neurons will be participating in the response to that stimulus. Direct evidence for the notion that repetition leads to smaller, more efficient representations has recently been obtained in the prefrontal cortex, which receives projections from the IT cortex (Freedman, Riesenhuber, Poggio, & Miller, 2001). After monkeys were trained to categorize computer-generated stimuli as either "cats" or "dogs," neuronal activity in the lateral prefrontal cortex reflected the category of the stimulus. After experience with the categories, almost one-third of the responsive neurons became category-selective, in that responses to stimuli in one category were suppressed relative to responses to stimuli in the other category. That is, category training led to more efficient representations because, after training, the stimuli generated responses from fewer neurons.

BIAS/ENHANCEMENT

We initially viewed repetition suppression as a general mechanism for recognition memory, within both long-term memory and working memory. Our view was that suppression results from an active memory mechanism that holds the memory of the sample "online," leading to suppressed responses when the sought-after test stimulus occurs in the sequence. However, the picture became more complicated when we studied anterior IT cells in a variant of our standard DMS task (Miller & Desimone, 1994). In the standard task, a given nonmatch test stimulus was presented only once within a given trial. For example, a particular stimulus sequence in a trial might be A-B-C-A, in which the B and the C stimuli appeared only once in the sequence. In the new variation of this task, one of the nonmatching test stimuli was repeated within the sequence (e.g., A-B-B-A). The question we asked was whether responses would be suppressed only when the sample was repeated (e.g., A), or whether responses would also be suppressed when the behaviorally irrelevant nonmatch stimulus was repeated (e.g., B). In other words, was active maintenance of the sample memory necessary for suppression to occur, or would suppression occur automatically with any stimulus repetition?

In this A-B-B-A version of the DMS task, just as in the standard version of the task described above, a class of IT neurons demonstrated repetition suppression to matching stimuli. However, these cells did not distinguish between task-relevant matches (e.g., the repetition of stimulus A) and task-irrelevant matches (e.g., the repetition of stimulus B). By contrast, another class of IT neurons gave enhanced responses only to the stimuli that matched the sample item (e.g., the final A in A-B-B-A). That is, some IT cells showed enhanced responses to stimuli that were being actively held in memory. These cells did not show enhancement for repeated intervening stimuli that were irrelevant to the task demands (e.g., the B in A-B-B-A). These results demonstrate that IT cells can be biased to give an enhanced response to the expected sample stimulus, and that this bias can span many seconds and at least several intervening stimuli (see Figure 25.1, row 2). Such a bias is presumably mediated by backward projections to the IT cortex, possibly from the prefrontal cortex (Miller, Erickson, & Desimone, 1996).

Recent evidence from Miyashita and colleagues supports this notion of feedback from the prefrontal cortex to the IT cortex (Hasegawa, Fukushima, Ihara, & Miyashita, 1998; see also Takahashi & Miyashita, Chapter 23, this volume). Monkeys were trained on a visual pair association task in which they learned to respond to an arbitrarily assigned choice picture when presented with a particular cue picture. When interhemispheric communication between the visual association cortices was prevented by transecting the splenium of the corpus callosum and the anterior commissure, monkeys were still able to associate a cue stimulus presented in one visual hemifield with its assigned choice stimulus presented in the other visual hemifield. Subsequent transection of the anterior corpus callosum (which connects the prefrontal cortices) caused performance on this task to fall to chance levels. Correspondingly, in the absence of bottom-up visual inputs, IT neurons were activated by the top-down signal from the prefrontal cortex (Tomita, Ohbayashi, Nakahara, Hasegawa, & Miyashita, 1999). These findings demonstrate interaction between the prefrontal cortex and the IT cortex in the retrieval of visual memories, and suggest that feedback projections from the prefrontal cortex to the IT cortex can support visual memory recall.

Parallel Memory Mechanisms for Short-Term Memory

Based on the results from the A-B-B-A version of the DMS task, the IT cortex contains at least two parallel mechanisms that might mediate performance in DMS tasks: an enhancement mechanism for active working memory, and a suppressive mechanism that is engaged automatically by stimulus repetition (Miller & Desimone, 1994). In monkeys performing the DMS task, both enhancement and suppression occur (in different cells) at the time of presentation of the test stimuli. Because this is the precise time when the animal must make a decision about how to respond to the test stimulus, the animal may utilize the suppression mechanism, the enhancement mechanism, or both mechanisms, depending on the specific requirements of the task. The standard version of the DMS task can be solved with either enhancement or suppression, whereas the A-B-B-A task cannot be solved by an animal relying only on the suppressive mechanism. The fact that our monkeys initially trained on the standard version of the task initially failed to distinguish between the stimulus that matched the sample and irrelevant repetitions of nonmatch stimuli in the A-B-B-A task suggests that the monkeys may have utilized the suppression mechanism when performing the standard task. More generally, the results imply that the kind of memory typically studied in behavioral and lesion studies in animals and humans may appear superficially to reflect a single phenomenon, but in fact may involve different mechanisms, depending on the specific requirements of the task, training history, and perhaps individual variables. Evidence for this idea was presented recently in a brain imaging study in humans performing the A-B-B-A task (Jiang, Haxby, Martin, Ungerleider, & Parasuraman, 2000). This study demonstrated enhanced activity in the frontal cortex, which was associated with the target and maintained across repetitions of the target. By contrast, reduced activity in the extrastriate visual cortex was associated with stimulus repetition, regardless of whether the stimulus was a target or a repeated nonmatch stimulus.

What role does the suppressive mechanism play in memory formation? Brain imaging studies using PET or fMRI in humans suggest that suppression plays a role in repetition priming, a type of implicit memory (Ungerleider, 1995). In repetition priming, experience with an item leads to faster and better performance when subjects are required to name or identify the item at a later time (Tulving & Schacter, 1990). For example, if a subject is asked to identify briefly presented drawings of objects, the subject will do so faster if he or she has seen the same drawings before. Moreover, these effects occur regardless of whether the subject actually remembers seeing the drawings before. Imaging studies have found that under conditions that lead to priming, repetition of either visually presented objects or words leads to reduced activation of cortical areas, compared to stimuli that were not seen before (Badgaiyan, Schacter, & Alpert, 1999; Buckner et al., 1995, 1998; Buckner, Koutstaal, Schacter, & Rosen, 2000; Koutstaal et al., 2001; Schacter & Buckner, 1998; Squire et al., 1992). It seems likely that the reduction in cortical activation is due to the repetition suppression effect and the shrinkage of the pool of activated cells. The fact that a smaller population of activated cells is associated with better task performance suggests that a smaller representation of a stimulus is a better representation, particularly if it is due to sharpened stimulus selectivity of the remaining cells. In this view, repetition suppression is a by-product of sharpening stimulus representations in the cortex.

DELAY/MAINTAINED ACTIVITY

Based on the results described above, we have proposed that in working memory and attentional tasks, IT neurons are biased to respond to stimuli for which they are actively searching or holding "online." When the relevant stimulus appears at the end of a delay, IT cells are primed to respond preferentially to it. What might be the source of this bias that persists throughout the delay?

A likely indicator of the bias is what has been termed "delay activity" in the IT cortex, as well as a number of other cortical areas (see Figure 25.1, row 3, and Figure 25.2). In DMS tasks, IT neurons that are selective for the features of a particular sample stimulus will typically respond to that stimulus when it is presented as a sample and then show an elevated level of activity, compared to its spontaneous firing rate, during the delay. Maintained delay activity has been observed in both versions of the DMS task described above. Consistent with studies in other laboratories (Fuster, 1990; Fuster & Jervey, 1981; Miyashita & Chang, 1988), many IT cells demonstrated stimulus-specific maintained activity in the delay interval following the sample. If a cell responded better to sample A than to sample B, it often had higher maintained activity in the delay following A than in the delay following B. However, this maintained activity was abolished after the first intervening item in the sequence. By contrast, prefrontal cells tested under the same conditions showed sample-specific delay activity that was maintained throughout the trial that was not disrupted by intervening stimuli (Miller et al., 1996). This finding suggests that the prefrontal cortex is a primary site of maintained activity in working memory, and that this signal is fed back to the IT cortex, biasing cells to respond to the expected relevant stimulus.

Working Memory Guiding Attention

It has long been accepted that attention operates as a kind of filter into working memory. Items that are attended are often held in working memory, whereas unattended items are discarded. Recent work on neural mechanisms of attention has suggested that the converse is true as well—namely, that the neural mechanisms for working memory provide a top-

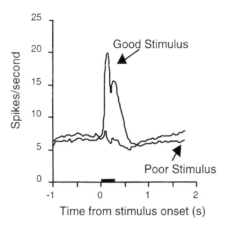

FIGURE 25.2. Delay/maintained activity. Response of a population of 88 individually recorded IT neurons at the time of the cue presentation in a visual search task. Trials with a given cue stimulus were run in blocks. Neurons showed higher delay/maintained activity both before and after the cue stimulus presentation on trials when the cue was a good stimulus for the neuron than when the cue was a poor stimulus. Adapted from Chelazzi, Duncan, Miller, and Desimone (1998).

down bias to visual areas in the ventral stream, biasing responses in favor of behaviorally relevant stimuli. Working memory therefore plays a role in determining which items in the visual field are attended.

An example of how top-down feedback to the IT cortex may bias representations comes from studies using the visual search paradigm (Chelazzi, Duncan, Miller, & Desimone, 1998; Chelazzi, Miller, Duncan, & Desimone, 1993). In those studies, while a monkey maintained fixation, a cue stimulus was presented at the fovea, followed by a delay period. After the delay, an array of two to five choice stimuli was presented extrafoveally, and the monkey was rewarded for making a saccadic eye movement to the stimulus that matched the cue stimulus (the target stimulus). The identity and location of the target stimulus varied from trial to trial (see Figure 25.3A). The array was composed of one stimulus that elicited strong responses from the cell when presented alone (good stimulus), and one or more stimuli that did not elicit strong responses when presented alone (poor stimuli).

During the delay period of this visual search task, just as in DMS tasks, IT cells showed higher maintained delay activity when a good stimulus was used as the cue than when a poor stimulus was used, consistent with the notion that feedback to the IT cortex biases activity in favor of cells coding the relevant stimulus. At the end of the delay, the initial response to the choice array was on average about the same, regardless of whether a good or poor stimulus was the target. However, within 150–200 msec of array onset and approximately 100 msec before the onset of the eye movement, the responses of most cells diverged dramatically, depending on which stimulus was the target (see Figure 25.3B). If the target was the good stimulus, the response to the array was equal to the response to the good stimulus presented alone. By contrast, if the target was a poor stimulus, the response to the array was suppressed almost to the level of response to the poor stimulus alone. In other words, cells responded to the array of stimuli as though only the target stimulus was present. In addition to providing evidence of mnemonic modulation in the IT cortex, these results support a "biased competition" model of attention (Desimone & Duncan, 1995). According to this model, when multiple stimuli appear together, they activate populations of neurons that automatically compete with one another. Attending to a stimulus biases this competition in favor of neu-

A

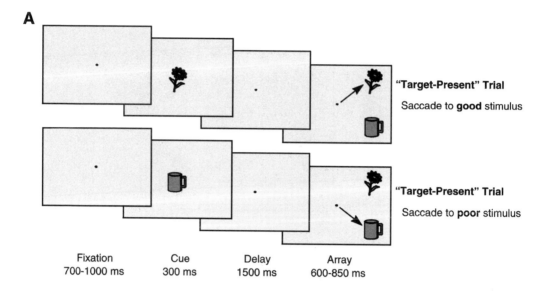

B

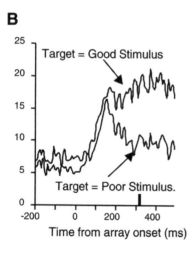

FIGURE 25.3. Bias/Enhancement. (A) Schematic representation of the visual search task. A cue stimulus was presented at the start of the trial, followed by a delay, and then by an array of stimuli. A monkey was rewarded for making a saccade to the stimulus in the array that matched the cue stimulus. On some trials, the cue target was a good stimulus for the neuron (top row); on other trials, the cue target was a poor stimulus for the neuron (bottom row). Relative locations of the good and poor stimuli in the array varied randomly from trial to trial. (B) The initial response to the choice array was about the same, regardless of which stimulus was the target stimulus. By 170 msec after stimulus onset, responses diverged dramatically, depending on whether the target stimulus was the good or poor stimulus for the neuron. This target selection effect occurred well in advance of the saccade to the target stimulus, indicated by the small vertical bar on the horizontal axis. Adapted from Chelazzi, Duncan, Miller, and Desimone (1998).

rons that respond to the attended stimulus. In the visual search task, this competition is biased in favor of the behaviorally relevant object by virtue of top-down feedback from structures involved in working memory and/or spatially directed attention, such as the prefrontal cortex (Boussaoud & Wise, 1993; Funahashi, Bruce, & Goldman-Rakic, 1989; Fuster, Bauer, & Jervey, 1982; Miller et al., 1996; Schall, Hanes, Thompson, & King, 1995). Recent data suggest that this biasing mechanism occurs even in earlier visual areas V4 and V2 (Reynolds, Chelazzi, & Desimone, 1999).

ACQUIRED SALIENCE

So far, we have described memory signals in the IT cortex that occur over relatively short intervals. However, other mechanisms have been described that are manifested over minutes, hours, or even days. Through training, an expert art historian can easily discriminate neoclassical from Romantic or Impressionist paintings. Certain artistic features that typify the various art styles immediately attract the attention of the art historian. This kind of acquired stimulus salience is demonstrated by IT neurons after long-term experience with objects (Jagadeesh, Chelazzi, Mishkin, & Desimone, 2001; see Figure 25.1, row 4). In a task of acquired salience, monkeys were repeatedly rewarded for making a saccade to a target stimulus in a two-stimulus array. This task was similar to the visual search paradigm described above, except that there was no cue stimulus at the start of the trial. The monkeys simply had to learn through trial and error which of two stimuli was the rewarded target. Once the monkeys had learned to select the rewarded stimulus reliably, the association between stimulus and reward was reversed (see A and B in Figure 25.4). As in the search task, the array consisted of one good stimulus and one poor stimulus for the neuron. When the good stimulus was the target, the response of the neuron remained high throughout the trial. By contrast, when the poor stimulus was the target, the response to the same array was suppressed strongly. This difference occurred approximately 100 msec before the eye movement to the target stimulus was made, which indicates that the information provided by these neuronal responses could have been used to guide the saccade (see C and D in Figure 25.4). Importantly, unlike the visual search task, there was no evidence for differential delay activity before the presentation of the array. In the acquired salience task, the activity of neurons was the same before the presentation of the array, regardless of which stimulus was the target. Accordingly, this finding suggests that there was no top-down feedback biasing activity in favor of the expected target. Rather, it appears that the bias in favor of the target resulted from a change in the competitive interactions between target and nontarget stimuli within (or before) the IT cortex.

Further analysis indicated that this modulation resulted from a suppression of responses to nontarget stimuli after training. From the first 10 trials of training (early phase), to the last 10 trials of training (late phase), the percentage of correct saccades increased from 55% to 89%. Correspondingly, from the early to the late phase of training, the response difference for arrays in which the good stimulus was the target versus arrays in which the poor stimulus was the target grew significantly in size. This was due to increased suppression of the neuron's response to the good stimulus when the poor stimulus was the target.

Learning also apparently changes the modular structure of the IT cortex, in that experience with a set of complex stimuli leads to an increase in the stimulus preferences of nearby cells in this cortex. For example, two nearby cells may have uncorrelated stimulus preferences prior to learning, but after as little as 1 day of experience with a set of complex stimuli, the two nearby cells may tend to respond preferentially to the same stimuli in the

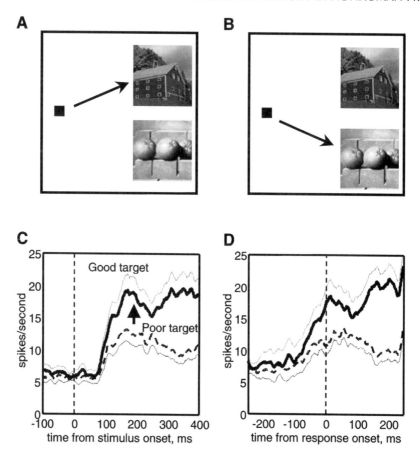

FIGURE 25.4. Acquired salience. Task learned during neurophysiological recording. A monkey maintained gaze on a fixation target (dark square); after a random delay, an array of two stimuli was presented at an unpredictable position in the peripheral visual field. The task was to learn, through trial and error, to saccade to the target stimulus in the display (A). After training with one reward contingency, the reward contingency was reversed, and the monkey relearned the task (B). Responses of a population of 55 cells to the visual array consisting of good and poor stimuli (thick lines) during correct trials locked to stimulus onset (C) and locked to saccade onset (D). Thin lines are 1 *SEM* above or below the mean. The average saccade latency is shown as the arrow at 200 msec. After training, the response to the array of stimuli was determined almost exclusively by the target stimulus. Adapted from Jagadeesh, Chelazzi, Mishkin, and Desimone (2001).

set (Erickson, Jagadeesh, & Desimone, 1999). Effects of learning on IT responses have also been shown in response to complex shapes (Kobatake, Wang, & Tanaka, 1998) and rotated views of objects (Logothetis, Pauls, & Poggio, 1995).

STIMULUS CORRELATION

Finally, mechanisms that subserve long-term stimulus correlation, for example, associative memory, have been described in the IT cortex. Associative mechanisms are engaged as a result of pairings of different sensory stimuli. In an associative learning task, monkeys

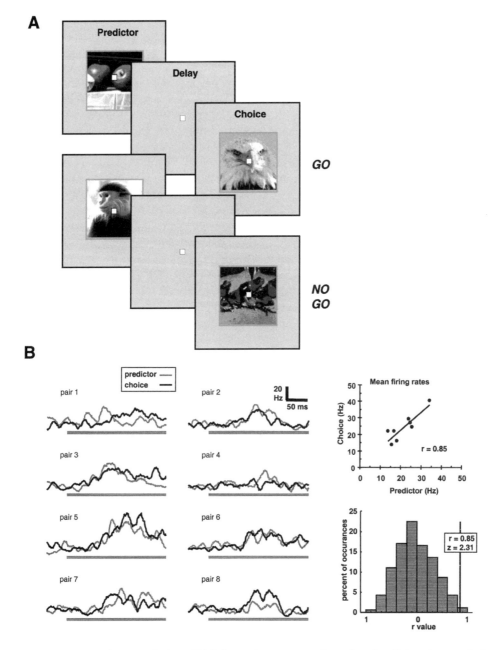

FIGURE 25.5. Stimulus correlation. (A) Schematic representation of an implicit pair association task. In this task, a predictor stimulus was presented, followed, after a delay, by a choice stimulus. The monkey was rewarded for releasing the bar on trials when the choice stimulus was a "go" stimulus and for holding a bar when the choice stimulus was a "no-go" stimulus. (B) A single neuron's responses to predictor and choice stimulus pairs. The largest responses are to both stimuli in pair 5, and the smallest responses are to both stimuli in pair 4. Each gray horizontal bar indicates the first 250 msec of stimulus presentation. Mean firing rate for each predictor stimulus was plotted against the response to the paired choice stimulus for the same cell. Response similarity was measured by the Pearson correlation coefficient for the mean. The distributions of correlation coefficients for randomly shuffled pairs were compared with the actual stimulus pairs for the same cell. Adapted from Erickson and Desimone (1999).

learn to respond to a particular choice stimulus when it is presented with an arbitrarily assigned cue stimulus. That is, they are rewarded for learning to associate the two stimuli. If two arbitrary visual stimuli occur repeatedly within a short time of each other, neurons in the IT cortex will tend to respond to both of them more commonly than would be expected by chance (Higuchi & Miyashita, 1996, Miyashita, Okuno, Tokuyama, Ihara, & Nakajima, 1996; Sakai & Miyashita, 1991; see Figure 25.1, row 5). Associative learning produces different affects in neurons in the prefrontal cortex (Rainer, Rao, & Miller, 1999).

Recently, Erickson and Desimone (1999) presented data demonstrating associative learning changes in IT neurons within a single recording session. In this study, monkeys learned to discriminate eight choice stimuli concurrently. The monkeys were rewarded for releasing a bar to half of the choice stimuli and for continuing to hold a bar for the other half of the stimuli. A predictor stimulus was presented one second before the choice stimulus was presented (see Figure 25.5A). Each choice stimulus was paired with a specific predictor stimulus for most of the trials. Occasionally, mismatched stimulus pairs were presented. Monkeys had longer response latencies on these mismatched trials, which indicated that they had learned to associate the predictors with the choice stimuli. Correspondingly, there was a significant shift in the stimulus selectivity of anterior IT neurons, such that neurons tended to respond more similarly to stimuli that were paired (see Figure 25.5B). Accordingly, unlike the other four mechanisms discussed above, changes in the IT cortex due to associative learning modulate the stimulus selectivity of individual neurons. Recent evidence from Miyashita and colleagues suggests that associative learning effects in area TE are due to feedback connections from the perirhinal portion of the IT cortex (Higuchi & Miyashita, 1996; Naya, Yoshida, & Miyashita, 2001; see also Takahashi & Miyashita, Chapter 24, this volume).

CONCLUSIONS

As we begin to understand the neural basis for visual learning and memory, it is striking how these processes are practically inseparable from the neural mechanisms of visual perception. There is no special, unitary, or extrinsic memory mechanism superimposed on the visual responses of neurons. Indeed, it is evident from the chart of memory mechanisms shown in Figure 25.1 that every mnemonic process is expressed through modulation of underlying sensory responses and activity. That is, experience-dependent modulations are simply modulations in the way the IT cortex processes or recreates visual experiences. These processes at work in the IT cortex effectively constitute acquired knowledge about the visual world.

REFERENCES

Badgaiyan, R. D., Schacter, D. L., & Alpert, N. M. (1999). Auditory priming within and across modalities: Evidence from positron emission tomography. *Journal of Cognitive Neuroscience, 11,* 337–348.

Baylis, G. C., & Rolls, E. T. (1987). Responses of neurons in the inferior temporal cortex in short term and serial recognition memory tasks. *Experimental Brain Research, 65,* 614–622.

Boussaoud, D., & Wise, S. P. (1993). Primate frontal cortex: Neuronal activity following attentional versus intentional cues. *Experimental Brain Research, 95,* 15–27.

Buckner, R. L., Goodman, J., Burock, M., Rotte M., Koutstaal, W., Schacter, D., Rosen, B., & Dale, A. M. (1998). Functional–anatomic correlates of object priming in humans revealed by rapid presentation event-related fMRI. *Neuron, 20,* 285–296.

Buckner, R. L., Koutsaal, W., Schacter, D. L., & Rosen, B. R. (2000). Functional MRI evidence for a role of frontal and inferior temporal cortex in amodal components of priming. *Brain, 123,* 620–640.

Buckner, R. L., Petersen, S. E., Ojemann, J. G., Miezin, R. M., Squire, L. R., & Raichle, M. E. (1995). Functional anatomical studies of explicit and implicit memory retrieval tasks. *Journal of Neuroscience, 15,* 12–29.

Buffalo, E. A., Ramus, S. J., Clark, R., Teng, E., Squire, L. R., & Zola, S. M. (1999). Dissociation between the effects of damage to perirhinal cortex and area TE. *Learning and Memory, 6,* 572–599.

Buffalo, E. A., Ramus, S. J., Squire, L. R., & Zola, S. M. (2000). Perception and recognition memory in monkeys following lesions of area TE and perirhinal cortex. *Learning and Memory, 7,* 375–382.

Chelazzi, L., Duncan, J., Miller, E. K., & Desimone, R. (1998). Responses of neuronal in inferior temporal cortex during memory-guided visual search. *Journal of Neurophysiology, 80,* 2918–2940.

Chelazzi, L., Miller, E. K., Duncan, J., & Desimone, R. (1993). A neural basis for visual search in inferior temporal cortex. *Nature, 363,* 345–347.

Desimone, R., & Duncan, J. (1995). Neural mechanisms of selective visual attention. *Annual Review of Neuroscience, 18,* 193–222.

Erickson, C. A., & Desimone, R. (1999). Responses of macaque perirhinal neurons during and after visual stimulus association learning. *Journal of Neuroscience, 19,* 10404–10416.

Erickson, C. A., Jagadeesh, B., & Desimone, R. (2000). Clustering of perirhinal neurons with similar properties following visual experience in monkeys. *Nature Neuroscience, 3,* 1143–1148.

Eskandar, E. N., Richmond, B. J., & Optican, L. M. (1992a). Role of inferior temporal neurons in visual memory: I. Temporal encoding of information about visual images, recalled images, and behavioral context. *Journal of Neurophysiology, 68,* 1277–1295.

Eskandar, E. N., Richmond, B. J., & Optican, L. M. (1992b). Role of inferior temporal neurons in visual memory: II. Multiplying temporal wave-forms related to vision and memory. *Journal of Neurophysiology, 68,* 1296–1306.

Fahy, F. L., Riches, I. P., & Brown, M. W. (1993). Neuronal activity related to visual recognition memory: Long-term memory and the encoding of recency and familiarity information in the primate anterior and medial inferior temporal and rhinal cortex. *Experimental Brain Research, 96,* 457–472.

Freedman, D. J., Riesenhuber, M., Poggio, T., & Miller, E. K. (2001). Categorical representation of visual stimuli in the primate prefrontal cortex. *Science, 291,* 312–316.

Funahashi, S., Bruce, C. J., & Goldman-Rakic, P. S. (1989). Mnemonic coding of visual space in the monkey's dorsolateral prefrontal cortex. *Journal of Neurophysiology, 61,* 1–19.

Fuster, J. M. (1990). Inferotemporal units in selective visual attention and short-term memory. *Journal of Neurophysiology, 64,* 681–697.

Fuster, J. M., Bauer, R. H., & Jervey, J. P. (1982). Cellular discharge in the dorsolateral prefrontal cortex of the monkey in cognitive tasks. *Experimental Neurology, 77,* 679–694.

Fuster, J. M., & Jervey, J. P. (1981). Inferotemporal neurons distinguish and retain behaviorally relevant features of visual stimuli. *Science, 212,* 952–955.

Gross, C. G. (1973). Visual functions of inferotemporal cortex. In R. Jung (Ed.), *Handbook of sensory physiology* (Vol. 7, Section 3B, pp. 451–482). Berlin: Springer-Verlag.

Hasegawa, I., Fukushima, T., Ihara, T., & Miyashita, Y. (1998). Callosal window between prefrontal cortices: Cognitive interaction to retrieve long-term memory. *Science, 281,* 814–818.

Heanny, P. E., & Schiller, P. H. (1988). State dependent activity in monkey visual cortex: I. Single cell activity in V1 and V4 on visual tasks. *Experimental Brain Research, 69,* 225–244.

Higuchi, S., & Miyashita, Y. (1996). Formation of mnemonic neuronal responses to visual paired associates in inferotemporal cortex is impaired by perirhinal and entorhinal lesions. *Proceedings of the National Academy of Sciences USA, 93,* 739–743.

Jagadeesh, B., Chelazzi, L., Mishkin, M., & Desimone, R. (2001). Learning increases stimulus salience in anterior inferior temporal cortex of the macaque. *Journal of Neurophysiology, 86,* 290–303.

Jiang, Y., Haxby, J. V., Martin, A., Ungerleider, L. G., & Parasuraman, R. (2000). Complementary neural mechanisms for tracking items in human working memory. *Science, 287*, 643–646.

Kobatake, E., Wang, G., & Tanaka, K. (1998). Effects of shape-discrimination training on the selectivity of inferotemporal cells in adult monkeys. *Journal of Neurophysiology, 80*, 324–330.

Koutstaal, W., Wagner, A. D., Rotte, M., Maril, A., Buckner, R. L., & Schacter, D. L. (2001). Perceptual specificity in visual object priming: Functional magnetic resonance imaging evidence for a laterality difference in fusiform cortex. *Neuropsychologia, 39*, 184–199.

Li, L., Miller, E. K., & Desimone, R. (1993). The representation of stimulus familiarity in anterior inferior temporal cortex. *Journal of Neurophysiology, 69*, 1918–1929.

Logothetis, J. K., Pauls, J., & Poggio, T. (1995). Shape recognition in the inferior temporal cortex of monkeys. *Current Biology, 5*, 552–563.

Lueschow, A., Miller, E. K., & Desimone, R. (1994). Inferior temporal mechanisms for invariant object recognition. *Cerebral Cortex, 4*, 523–531.

Maunsell, J. H. R., Sclar, G., Nealey, T. A., & DePriest, D. D. (1991). Extraretinal representations in area V4 in the macaque monkey. *Visual Neuroscience, 7, 561–573.*

Meunier, M., Bachevalier, J., Mishkin, M., & Murray, E. A. (1993). Effects on visual recognition of combined and separate ablations of the entorhinal and perirhinal cortex in rhesus monkeys. *Journal of Neurophysiology, 75*, 1190–1205.

Miller, E. K., & Desimone, R. (1994). Parallel neuronal mechanisms for short-term memory. *Science, 263*, 520–522.

Miller, E. K., Erickson, C. A., & Desimone, R. (1996). Neural mechanisms of visual working memory in prefrontal cortex of the macaque. *Journal of Neuroscience, 16*, 5154–5167.

Miller, E. K., Gochin, P. M., & Gross, C. G. (1991). Habituation-like decrease in the responses of neurons in inferior temporal cortex of the macaque. *Visual Neuroscience, 7*, 357–362.

Miller, E. K, Li, L., & Desimone, R. (1991). A neural mechanism for working and recognition memory in inferotemporal cortex. *Science, 254*, 1377–1379.

Miller, E. K., Li, L., & Desimone, R. (1993). Activity of neurons in anterior inferior temporal cortex during a short-term memory task. *Journal of Neuroscience, 13*, 1460–1478.

Miyashita, Y., & Chang, H. S. (1988). Neuronal correlate of pictorial short-term memory in the primate temporal cortex. *Nature, 331*, 68–70.

Miyashita, Y., Okuno, H., Tokuyama, W., Ihara, T., & Nakajima, K. (1996). Feedback signal from medial temporal lobe mediates visual associative mnemonic codes of inferotemporal neurons. *Brain Research. Cognitive Brain Research, 5*, 81–86.

Naya, Y., Yoshida, M., & Miyashita, Y. (2001). Backward spreading of the memory-retrieval signal in the primate temporal cortex. *Science, 291*, 661–664.

Nelson, S. B. (1991). Temporal interactions in the cat visual system: I. Orientation-selective suppression in the visual cortex. *Journal of Neuroscience, 11*, 344–356.

Rainer, G., Rao, C., & Miller, E. K. (1999). Prospective coding for objects in primate prefrontal cortex. *Journal of Neuroscience, 19*, 5493–5505.

Reynolds, J. H., Chelazzi, L., & Desimone, R. (1999). Competitive mechanisms subserve attention in macaque areas V2 and V4. *Journal of Neuroscience, 19*, 1736–1753.

Riches, I. P., Wilson, F. A., & Brown, M. W. (1991). The effects of visual stimulation and memory on neurons of the hippocampal formation and the neighboring parahippocampal gyrus and inferior temporal cortex of the primate. *Journal of Neuroscience, 11*, 1763–1779.

Sakai, K., & Miyashita, Y. (1991). Neural organization for the long-term memory of paired associates. *Nature, 354*, 152–155.

Schacter, D. L., & Buckner, R. L. (1998). Priming and the brain. *Neuron, 20*, 185–195.

Schall, J. D., Hanes, D. P., Thompson, K. G., & King, D. J. (1995). Saccade target selection in frontal eye field of macaque: I. Visual and premovement activation. *Journal of Neuroscience, 15*, 6905–6918.

Suzuki, W. A., Zola-Morgan, S., Squire, L. R., & Amaral, D. G. (1993). Lesions of the perirhinal and parahippocampal cortices in the monkey produce long-lasting memory impairment in the visual and tactual modalities. *Journal of Neuroscience, 13*, 2430–2451.

Squire, L. R., Ojemann, J. G., Miezin, F. M., Petersen, S. E., Videen, T. O., & Raichle, M. E. (1992). Activation of the hippocampus in normal humans: A functional anatomical study of memory. *Proceedings of the National Academy of Sciences USA, 89,* 1837–1841.

Tomita, H., Ohbayashi, M., Nakahara, K., Hasegawa, I., & Miyashita, Y. (1999). Top-down signal from prefrontal cortex in executive control of memory retrieval. *Nature, 401,* 699–703.

Tulving, E., & Schacter, D. L. (1990). Priming and human-memory systems. *Science, 247,* 301–306.

Ungerleider, L. G. (1995). Functional brain imaging studies of cortical mechanisms for memory. *Science, 270,* 769–775.

Vogels, R., & Orban, G. A. (1994). Does practice in orientation discrimination lead to changes in the response properties of macaque inferior temporal neurons? *European Journal of Neuroscience, 6,* 1680–1690.

Zola-Morgan, S., Squire, L. R., Amaral, D. G., & Suzuki, W. A. (1989). Lesions of perirhinal and parahippocampal cortex that spare the amygdala and hippocampal formation produce severe memory impairment. *Journal of Neuroscience, 9,* 4355–4370.

26

The Medial Temporal Lobe Structures and Object Recognition Memory in Nonhuman Primates

JOCELYNE BACHEVALIER, SARAH NEMANIC,
and MARIA C. ALVARADO

The development of a primate model of temporal lobe anterograde amnesia in the last two decades has been extremely influential in shaping our knowledge of the neurobiology of memory. Neuropsychological studies of amnesic patients have led to the important discovery that memory can be divided into different systems subserved by independent neural circuits. From the perspective of cognitive neuroscience, however, our understanding of memory systems requires not only direct evidence that the different memory systems do indeed exist, but also detailed characterization of the basic psychological processes and functional neural circuitries supporting each process. The findings in primates have shown that medial temporal lobe structures are responsible for certain types of memory processes (e.g., semantic, episodic, relational, spatial memory) but not others (e.g., priming, procedural, habit memory). Furthermore, within the medial temporal lobe memory system, recent studies have begun to define the specific cognitive contributions that each component of that system (e.g., the hippocampal formation per se, including the dentate gyrus, Ammon fields, and subicular complex, and the adjacent medial temporal cortex, including entorhinal, perirhinal, and parahippocampal areas) makes to memory processes (for reviews, see Murray, 2000; Suzuki, 1996; Zola-Morgan, Squire, & Ramus, 1994; see also Suzuki, Chapter 22, this volume).

This chapter explores in some detail a particular component process of the medial temporal lobe system—specifically, object recognition. The chapter begins with a brief introduction that places our experimental work in the context of other investigations of the neural substrate of object recognition memory. What follows is a review of our most recent experiments in nonhuman primates. Our strategy has been to carefully examine the specific contributions made by the hippocampal formation and the perirhinal cortex to object recognition memory, by combining manipulations of recognition memory tasks and tasks parameters with discrete damage to structures in the medial temporal lobe. Preliminary reports of our data have already appeared elsewhere (Nemanic, Alvarado, & Bachevalier, 1998, 1999, 2001).

THE MEDIAL TEMPORAL LOBE AND RECOGNITION MEMORY

"Recognition memory" is commonly defined as the ability to judge whether or not a stimulus has been encountered before (e.g., the judgment of prior occurrence; Brown, 1996). One of the first indications that the medial temporal lobe is involved in recognition memory came from patients such as H. M., who sustained resection of the medial temporal lobe as treatment for epileptic seizures (Penfield & Milner, 1958; Scoville & Milner, 1957). The hallmark postoperative deficit in these patients was an inability to recognize or recollect any information when a delay of a few minutes was interposed between study of the material and test. Severe recognition memory impairments (albeit less profound than those of H. M.) were also found in patients with anoxic ischemia resulting in neuropathology largely restricted to the hippocampal formation (Rempel-Clower, Zola, Squire, & Amaral, 1996; Zola-Morgan, Squire, & Amaral, 1986). These findings led to the proposal that the hippocampal formation is important for recognition memory and, more generally, for declarative memory.

The development of an animal model of this amnesic syndrome in nonhuman primates began with the design of a new two-choice recognition memory paradigm, the delayed-nonmatching-to-sample task (DNMS; Mishkin & Delacour, 1975), which made it possible to assess the effects of medial temporal lobe lesions on recognition memory. In this task, which employs new stimuli on each trial, an animal is trained to consistently avoid an object that has been seen a few seconds earlier in favor of a novel one that conceals a food reward. After the animal has acquired this nonmatching rule, memory capacity is taxed further by either increasing the delay between study and test, or giving the animal a list of items to remember at study. (Some studies used a different version of the same task—namely, the delayed-matching-to-sample [DMS] task, in which animals are rewarded for selecting the familiar item.) Using the DNMS task, initial work with the animal model pointed to the involvement of both the amygdaloid complex and the hippocampal formation in the amnesic syndrome, because substantial recognition impairment, at delays of 30 seconds (sec) and longer, was observed only when these two structures were removed in combination (Mishkin, 1978).

Further investigations (Zola-Morgan, Squire, & Amaral, 1989a) revealed that an electrolytic lesion of the amygdaloid complex, which spared the adjacent cortical areas, did not affect memory and did not exacerbate the recognition loss found after hippocampal formation damage alone. This finding raised the possibility that the cortical areas removed in order to access the amygdaloid complex in the original study of Mishkin (1978) might have been responsible for the severe recognition memory deficit observed. This possibility was tested directly and confirmed by the finding that damage to cortical tissue surrounding the amygdala and hippocampal formation (i.e., the perirhinal and parahippocampal cortices) was sufficient to produce a recognition loss of the same magnitude as the loss previously found when the hippocampus, amygdala, and surrounding cortical tissue were removed (Zola-Morgan, Squire, & Amaral, 1989b).

It is now appreciated that restricted damage to the perirhinal cortex, alone or in combination with damage to either the entorhinal cortex or parahippocampal area, is sufficient to produce a severe visual recognition memory impairment (Buffalo et al., 1999; Eacott, Gaffan, & Murray, 1994; Meunier, Bachevalier, Mishkin, & Murray, 1993;

Murray, 1992; Suzuki, Zola-Morgan, Squire, & Amaral, 1993; Zola-Morgan et al., 1989b; Zola-Morgan, Squire, Clower, & Rempel, 1993). Additional support for a critical role of the perirhinal cortical areas in visual recognition memory was provided by reports of recognition memory failure after cooling of this region in monkeys (George, Horel, & Cirillo, 1989; Horel, Pytko-Joiner, Voytko, & Salsbury, 1987; Horel, Voytko, & Salsbury, 1984). Furthermore, visual memory deficits after damage to ventromedial temporal cortical areas have been reported in other species, such as rodents (Bussey, Muir, & Aggleton, 1999; Mumby & Pinel, 1994; Rothblat & Kromer, 1991; Squire, 1992), and deficits have been extended to other sensory modalities, such as touch (Buffalo et al., 1999; Suzuki et al., 1993) and olfaction (Otto & Eichenbaum, 1992).

Conversely, restricted damage to the hippocampal formation that spares the adjacent cortical areas appears to have less effect on object recognition. The magnitude of recognition memory loss in these experimental studies varies from no impairment (Murray & Mishkin, 1998; Nemanic et al., 1998) to moderate impairment (Beason-Held, Rosene, Killiany, & Moss, 1999; Zola et al., 2000).

The pattern of findings from these neuropsychological studies in nonhuman primates led to the idea that the entorhinal and perirhinal cortical areas make a greater contribution to object recognition than the hippocampal formation does (Baxter & Murray, 2001; Murray, 2000). These experimental data appear to contradict data in amnesic patients showing either mild (Aggleton & Shaw, 1996) or enduring (Reed & Squire, 1997) recognition memory loss after damage to the hippocampal region. The presence of this recognition memory loss has been demonstrated even in patients with neuropathology largely limited to the CA1 field of the hippocampus (Rempel-Clower et al., 1996; Zola-Morgan et al., 1986). The only exceptions to these clinical cases are reports of good recognition memory in children with focal bilateral hippocampal damage (Gadian et al., 2000; Mishkin, Vargha-Khadem, & Gadian, 1998; Vargha-Khadem et al., 1997). Thus these divergent results indicate the need to conduct further investigations of the role of the hippocampal formation in recognition memory.

One potential limitation with the investigations in nonhuman primates reported above is that recognition memory was consistently assessed via the DNMS and DMS paradigms. Perhaps these tasks may be solved using strategies other than familiarity–novelty judgment. If so, in the absence of a fully functional hippocampus, recruitment of such strategies could support performance on the DNMS task to some extent, masking a more severe deficit in recognition memory. This idea gained support from a reinvestigation of the effects of hippocampal damage in recognition memory in humans (Reed & Squire, 1997), indicating that some recognition tasks (e.g., yes–no recognition tests) might be more sensitive than others (e.g., forced-choice recognition tests) to uncover a recognition memory impairment following hippocampal damage. Recently, we have asked whether the same idea could apply to monkeys with damage to the hippocampal region. Accordingly, we have assessed the effects of hippocampal lesions on different tasks of recognition memory. The first study (Bachevalier, Beauregard, & Alvarado, 1999) evaluated the effects of neonatal lesions of the hippocampal region (the hippocampal formation plus a portion of the parahippocampal areas TH/TF) on the DNMS task, using delays varying from 10 sec to 10 minutes. We found that the early hippocampal damage did not affect recognition memory even at delays as long as 10 minutes.

In a second study (Pascalis & Bachevalier, 1999), the same operated animals and their controls were tested in a new recognition task, the visual paired-comparison (VPC or preferential looking) task. This task is comparable to the DNMS task in that there is a familiarization phase to one object, followed by a choice phase during which the familiar object is presented together with a new one. However, in the VPC task, animals only look at the stimuli, and neither rewards nor responses toward the objects are involved. The relevant measure in this task is the amount of time spent looking at each stimulus during the choice phase. Longer duration of looking to one stimulus (generally the novel one) indicates recognition memory. Novelty preference (VPC) scores at delays from 10 to 600 sec were compared to DNMS scores at similar delays. In contrast to their good performance at all delays of the DNMS task, monkeys with neonatal hippocampal lesions displayed a strong preference for novelty at the short delays of 10 sec, but not at delays of 30 sec and longer. Given the similarities between the two recognition tasks, the findings were intriguing and raised the possibility that the DNMS task may not be as sensitive as the VPC task to recognition memory impairment (see also McKee & Squire, 1993; Zola et al., 2000). At the same time, because in our studies the neonatal hippocampal lesions were not restricted to the hippocampal formation but also included part of the parahippocampal cortical areas, the recognition memory impairment found in the VPC task might have resulted from damage to the parahippocampal cortical areas or combined damage to both regions. Accordingly, we have carried out additional studies to evaluate the effects of selective lesions of both the hippocampal formation and the perirhinal cortex on the DNMS and VPC tasks. The remainder of the chapter is a preliminary account of these data.

EXPERIMENTAL DESIGN

Young adult rhesus monkeys (*Macaca mulatta*) received either neurotoxic lesions of the hippocampal formation (group H, *n* = 4), aspiration lesions of perirhinal cortical areas 35 and 36 (group PRh, *n* = 5), or no lesions (group N, *n* = 3). All monkeys were tested on the two visual recognition tasks: first the VPC task, and then the DNMS task.

The removal of the hippocampal formation was made with 6 to 11 injections of ibotenic acid, stereotaxically guided by magnetic resonance imaging (MRI). A representative example of the hippocampal lesion is given in Figure 26.1. Aspiration lesions of the perirhinal cortex were performed according to procedures described by Meunier and colleagues (1993) and have been shown to result in a loss of recognition memory equivalent to that found after excitotoxic lesions of these cortical areas (Malkova, Bachevalier, Mishkin, & Saunders, 2001). The extent of intended damage is illustrated on coronal sections in the left panel of Figure 26.2, and the actual damage in one representative case is plotted at the same levels in the right panel of Figure 26.2.

OBJECT RECOGNITION MEMORY

Preferential Looking Task

As indicated above and illustrated in Figure 26.3, the VPC task takes advantage of the natural tendency of primates to look preferentially at novel stimuli in their environment (for more details, see Pascalis & Bachevalier, 1999).

As shown in Figure 26.4A, the unoperated control animals showed a significant preference (>60%) for looking at the novel pictures at all delays, while the operated animals gave different patterns of results. That is, whereas animals in group PRh showed preference for novelty at the 1-sec delay but not at longer delays, animals in Group H showed preference for novelty at delays as long as 30 sec but not at the longer delays. These differences were revealed by a two-way analysis of variance (group × delay), with repeated

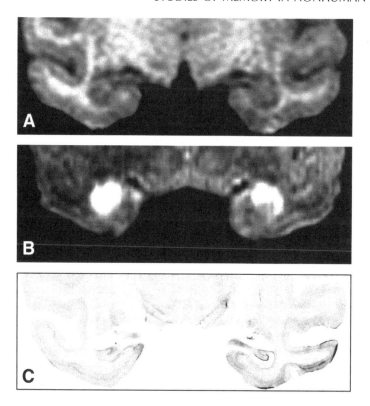

FIGURE 26.1. Coronal sections at a comparable level of the hippocampal formation. (A) Presurgical structural magnetic resonance image depicting the hippocampal formation. (B) Postsurgical Fluid Attenuated Inversion Recovery protocol (FLAIR) image depicting extent of edema/ischemia. (C) Postmortem histological section depicting the amount of cell loss.

measures for the second factor indicating a significant interaction, $F(10, 45) = 2.00$, $p < .05$. Post hoc analyses (Tukey HSD) indicated that group PRh differed significantly from group N at all delays (all p's $< .05$) except the shortest delays of 1 and 10 sec, whereas group H differed from group N only at the longest delays of 60 and 120 sec (p's $< .0001$ and .002, respectively). Interestingly, the loss of novelty preference in the operated monkeys was present despite the fact that the total time spent by the operated animals looking at the two pictures during the retention tests at each delay (mean = 4.36 and 4.25 sec for groups PRh and H, respectively) did not significantly differ from that of normal controls (mean = 4.31 sec). These results suggest that the delay-dependent loss of novelty preference in the operated groups was not related to a more general lack of interest in looking at the pictures, nor was it due to a basic inability to detect or show preference for novelty. The findings with the VPC task indicate that both the hippocampal formation and perirhinal cortex are critical for recognition memory, but that their contribution to it differs (however, see Clark, Teng, Squire, & Zola, 1997; Zola et al., 2000). Thus, while the perirhinal cortex appears to be critical for object identification and object recognition, the hippocampal formation appears to be more critical when memory of an object needs to bridge delays that exceed the normal brief capacity of the perirhinal cortex. Whether this function involves maintenance of cellular activity in the per-

Intended Lesion   **Case PRh-1**

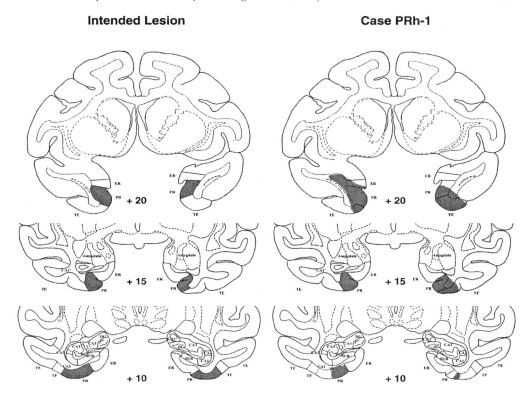

FIGURE 26.2. Coronal sections through the intended perirhinal lesions (left panel) and the perirhinal damage in one representative case (right panel). Intended and actual damage are shown in dark gray.

irhinal cortex, or permanent storage of the memory elsewhere (e.g., consolidation of information), is unclear (Nemanic, 1999).

Delayed-Nonmatching-to-Sample Task

Following the end of the VPC task, all monkeys were tested on the DNMS task. As described above, in this task each monkey had to first master the DNMS rule of displacing a novel object in favor of a familiar one it had seen 10 sec earlier. Upon acquisition of the rule, the animals were then given a performance test in which the delay between sample presentation and test was increased from 10 to 600 sec (in blocks of 100 trials each).

Only animals in group PRh were impaired on this task. Their difficulty occurred both in the acquisition of the DNMS rule and in the performance test with increasing delays (Figure 26.4B). Thus group PRh required significantly more trials (mean = 757 trials) and made more errors (mean = 240 errors) to learn the DNMS rule, as compared to groups H (average = 123 trials and 47 errors) and N (average = 125 trials and 42 errors); for trials and errors, respectively, Kruskal–Wallis $H(2) = 5.78$, $p < .05$, and $H(2) = 5.79$, $p < .05$. In addition, an analysis of variance of the performance scores indicated a significant interaction, $F(6, 27) = 3.97$, $p < .008$. Post hoc tests revealed that while group H did not differ from group N at any delay tested, group PRh differed from both at all delays (all p's < .05).

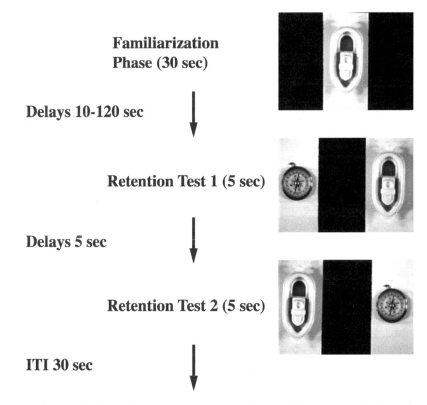

Familiarization Phase (30 sec)

Delays 10-120 sec

Retention Test 1 (5 sec)

Delays 5 sec

Retention Test 2 (5 sec)

ITI 30 sec

FIGURE 26.3. For each trial of the VPC task, the animals were first presented with a picture of an object and were required to look at the picture for a total of 30 sec. After a delay that varied from 1 to 120 sec, the picture of the familiar object was presented together with a picture of a new object for two retention tests of 5 sec each, separated by a 5-sec interval. At the end of the trial, a 30-sec period elapsed before another trial was presented in exactly the same way, using pictures of different objects for each trial. The delays were intermixed within daily testing sessions, and all animals were tested at all delays, except animals of group PRh (which were also tested at a shorter delay of 1 sec).

Discussion

Thus, on both recognition tasks, damage to the perirhinal cortex severely affected recognition memory when delays were slightly increased. These findings replicate earlier data indicating a severe loss of object recognition memory following damage to the perirhinal cortex, as measured by both the DNMS task (Buffalo et al., 1999; Eacott et al., 1994; Meunier et al., 1993; Murray, 1992) and the VPC task (Buffalo et al., 1999). By contrast, selective damage to the hippocampal formation resulted in a delay-dependent recognition deficit only in the VPC task. Thus the findings indicate that the VPC task is more sensitive to hippocampal lesions than is the DNMS task (see also Zola et al., 2000).

   The different behavioral outcomes of hippocampal lesions on the two tasks of recognition memory replicate our initial findings with neonatal nonselective hippocampal lesions (Bachevalier et al., 1999; Pascalis & Bachevalier, 1999), and suggest that the specific cognitive processes subserving each of the tasks are different (Nemanic, 1999; Pascalis & Bachevalier, 1999). For example, performance on the VPC task is based on an incidental and spontaneous tendency to direct visual attention to novel stimuli. The DNMS task, in

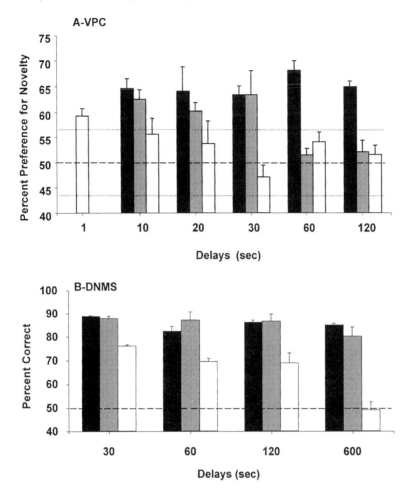

FIGURE 26.4. Performance scores on the two recognition tasks (VPC and DNMS) in monkeys with perirhinal lesions (white bars), monkeys with hippocampal lesions (gray bars), and unoperated controls (black bars).

contrast, requires cognitive abilities beyond simple recognition. That is, in the DNMS task, animals not only need to recognize whether or not the object was seen before, but also need to associate the reinforcer and the abstract quality of the object (i.e., novelty, in the case of DNMS). Given these differences between the two recognition tasks, one could speculate that in the absence of a functional hippocampus, the animals might purposely use different strategies to solve the DNMS task. These strategies may involve the active or effortful maintenance of the memory for the sample, possibly through retrospective processing or the use of a working memory buffer. If this reasoning were correct, performance on the DNMS task might be affected by hippocampal lesions if (1) much longer delays could be used, since these alternate strategies are likely to use temporary memory storage sites, and may not be able to maintain memory over protracted delays; or (2) the use of these alternate strategies during the delays was prevented. This latter possibility was tested in the following experiment.

EFFECTS OF DISTRACTORS ON DNMS PERFORMANCE

In this experiment, we tested whether the performance of monkeys with hippocampal lesions on the DNMS task would be altered by introducing a distractor during the delay period, to prevent the use of behavioral strategies to maintain the memory of the sample object. Earlier studies had already shown that retroactive interference has a deleterious effect on performance of hippocampectomized animals (Fernandez et al., 1998; Gaffan et al., 1984; Jarrard, 1975; Owen & Butler, 1981). Thus, after completion of the DNMS task, monkeys in the three groups were tested on the delay conditions of the DNMS, but now distractors were introduced at the beginning of the delay period.

Distraction type 1 was introduced at the shortest delay of 10 sec and consisted of illuminating a monkey's chamber for 3 sec. Distraction type 2 was introduced at delays of 30 to 600 sec and consisted of a motor task that required the monkey to remove a Life Saver candy from bent wires for 10 sec. For both distraction types 1 and 2, a total of 30 daily trials were given, for which one-third of the trials were distraction trials pseudo-randomly intermixed with standard DNMS trials (without distraction). Finally, distraction type 3 was introduced only at the longest delay of 600 sec and consisted of 50 trials during which the monkey was removed from the testing box, transported to its housing room, and then returned to the testing box to complete the trial.

Whereas performance of the three groups was affected by the three types of distractions, performance of the operated animals was significantly exacerbated in distraction types 1 and 3, but not distraction type 2 (Nemanic et al., 1999, in press). As shown in Table 26.1, at the short delay of 10 sec, group PRh made significantly more errors on distraction than on normal DNMS trials, relative to groups H and N (p's < .01). By contrast, at the long delay of 600 sec of distraction type 3, group H made more errors on distraction trials than on standard DNMS trials, relative to groups N and PRh (p's < .03). Thus animals with selective perirhinal lesions performed more poorly on distraction than on standard DNMS trials at the short delays, when these operated animals were still able to show some levels of recognition memory, but not at the long delays, when their performance on even the standard trials was near chance levels. These findings highlight the importance of the perirhinal cortex for recognition memory at very short delays; in addition, they illustrate that in the absence of this cortical area, other temporal structures are likely to participate in these short-term recognition processes, as revealed by the effects of distraction. By contrast, animals with selective hippocampal lesions performed normally on distraction trials at the short delays, when their recognition memory abilities were still intact, but not at the longer delays, when their recognition memory abilities were compromised (see the VPC data). This finding supports the idea that monkeys with hippocampal damage are using active, distraction-sensitive strategies to compensate for their impaired recognition memory during the long delays of the DNMS task. This latter finding suggests that recognition memory for delays up to 10 minutes could be supported by cortical areas, but that retention of information beyond this point requires the intact hippocampus, as illustrated by the effect of distraction only at long delays in animals with hippocampal lesions. The active cognitive strategies used by hippocampectomized animals to solve the DNMS task may recruit additional brain areas, such as the inferior temporal and prefrontal cortices—both of which have been shown to be important for normal performance on the standard DNMS task (Meunier et al., 1993; Meunier, Hadfield, Bachevalier, & Murray, 1996), and both of which have neurons with electrophysiological properties that could permit good performance on the DNMS task (Miller, Erickson, & Desimone, 1996; Miller, Li, & Desimone, 1991). By contrast, in recognition tasks in which increased interference acts

TABLE 26.1. Number of Errors Committed during Standard and Distraction DNMS Trials of Distraction Types 1 and 3.

Group/case	Distraction type 1		Distraction type 3	
	Standard 10 sec	Distraction 10 sec	Standard 600 sec	Distraction 600 sec
Group N				
N-1	10	6	6	22
N-2	2	0	7	8
N-3	12	8	17	10
$\bar{X}$ ($\pm$ *SEM*)	8.0 ($\pm$ 3.1)	4.7 ($\pm$ 2.4)	10.0 ($\pm$ 3.5)	13.3 ($\pm$ 4.4)
Group H				
H-1	0	2	7	26
H-2	10	12	0	22
H-3	7	12	10	30
H-4	4	2	30	24
$\bar{X}$ ($\pm$ *SEM*)	5.3 ($\pm$ 2.1)	7.0 ($\pm$ 2.9)	11.8 ($\pm$ 6.4)	25.5 ($\pm$ 1.7)
Group PRh				
PRh-1	11	24	43	42
PRh-2	29	40	43	42
PRh-3	29	32	46	40
PRh-4	10	14	36	44
PRh-5	19	34	43	44
$\bar{X}$ ($\pm$ *SEM*)	19.6 ($\pm$ 4.1)	28.8 ($\pm$ 4.5)	42.2 ($\pm$ 1.7)	42.4 ($\pm$ 0.8)

upon information just learned, the involvement of the hippocampal formation appears to be critical.

The data demonstrate that the lack of impairment on the DNMS task after selective hippocampal lesions observed in our studies may not indicate, as commonly thought, that the type of memory required for performance on the task is not impaired by the lesion; rather, it may indicate that the experimental parameters were not appropriate to detect such an impairment. These findings support many recent data from the literature suggesting that the hippocampal formation mediates systematic memory organizations based on spatial, contextual, conditional, and episodic relations, hence reducing interference and enhancing memory abilities (for a review, see Schacter & Tulving, 1994).

CONCLUSIONS

The lesion experiments reported in this chapter clearly indicate that both the perirhinal cortex and the hippocampal formation are critical for visual recognition memory processes. In the context of the data gathered over the last 10 years (as summarized above), they further confirm that these areas operate uniquely within the medial temporal lobe memory system—a notion that has recently been advanced by others (Baxter & Murray, 2001) and that has received considerable support from electrophysiological (for a review, see Brown & Xiang, 1998) and metabolic (Sybirska, Davachi, & Goldman-Rakic, 2000) studies in monkeys, as well as neuroimaging studies in humans (Lepage, Habib, & Tulving, 1998; Schacter & Wagner, 1999; Stark & Squire, 2000; Stern & Hasselmo, 1999). The major remaining challenge, however, is to clearly characterize the unique psychological and neural processes that each medial temporal lobe structure makes to memory.

ACKNOWLEDGMENTS

This work was supported in part by Grants No. MH58846 and No. MH54167 to Jocelyne Bachevalier, and by Fellowships No. MH12106 to Sarah Nemanic and No. MH10929 to Maria C. Alvarado from the National Institute of Mental Health.

REFERENCES

Aggleton, J. P., & Shaw, C. (1996). Amnesia and recognition memory: A reanalysis of psychometric data. *Neuropsychologia, 34*, 51–62.

Bachevalier, J., Beauregard, M., & Alvarado, M.C. (1999). Long-term effects of neonatal damage to the hippocampal formation and amygdaloid complex on object discrimination and object recognition in rhesus monkeys (*Macaca mulatta*). *Behavioral Neuroscience, 113*, 1127–1151.

Baxter, M. G., & Murray, E. A. (2001). Opposite relationship of hippocampal and rhinal cortex damage to delayed nonmatching-to-sample deficits in monkeys. *Hippocampus, 11*, 61–71.

Beason-Held, L. L., Rosene, D. L., Killiany, R. J., & Moss, M. B. (1999). Hippocampal formation lesions produce memory impairment in the rhesus monkey. *Hippocampus, 9*, 562–574.

Brown, M. W. (1996). Neuronal responses and recognition memory. *Seminars in the Neurosciences, 8*, 23–32.

Brown, M. W., & Xiang, J. Z. (1998). Recognition memory: Neuronal substrates of the judgement of prior occurrence. *Progress in Neurobiology, 55*, 149–189.

Buffalo, E. A., Ramus, S. J., Clark, R. E., Teng, E., Squire, L. R., & Zola, S. M. (1999). Dissociation between the effects of damage to perirhinal cortex and area TE. *Learning and Memory, 6*, 572–599.

Bussey, T. J., Muir, J. L., & Aggleton, J. P. (1999). Functionally dissociating aspects of event memory: The effects of combined perirhinal and postrhinal cortex lesions on object and place memory in the rat. *Journal of Neuroscience, 19*, 495–502.

Clark, R. E., Teng, E., Squire, L. R., & Zola, S. M. (1997). Perirhinal damage impairs memory on the visual paired-comparison task. *Society for Neuroscience Abstracts, 23*, 12.

Eacott, M. J., Gaffan, D., & Murray, E. A. (1994). Preserved recognition memory for small sets, and impaired stimulus identification for large sets, following rhinal cortex ablations in monkeys. *European Journal of Neuroscience, 6*, 1466–1478.

Fernandez, G., Weyerts, H., Schrader-Bolsche, M., Tendolkar, I., Smid, H. G., Tempelmann, C., Hinrichs, H., Scheich, H., Elger, C. E., Mangun, G. R., & Heinze, H. J. (1998). Successful verbal encoding into episodic memory engages the posterior hippocampus: A parametrically analyzed functional magnetic resonance imaging study. *Journal of Neuroscience, 18*, 1841–1847.

Gadian, D. G., Aicardi, J., Watkins, K. E., Porter, D. A., Mishkin, M., & Vargha-Khadem, F. (2000). Developmental amnesia associated with early hypoxic–ischaemic injury. *Annals of Neurology, 123*, 499–507.

Gaffan, D., Saunders, R. C., Gaffan, E. A., Harrison, S., Shields, C., & Owen, M. J. (1984). Effects of fornix transection upon associative memory in monkeys: Role of the hippocampus in learned action. *Quarterly Journal of Experimental Psychology, B36*, 173–221.

George, P. J., Horel, J. A., & Cirillo, R. A. (1989) Reversible cold lesions of the parahippocampal gyrus in monkeys result in deficits on the delayed match-to-sample and other visual tasks. *Behavioural Brain Research, 34*, 163–178.

Horel, J. A., Pytko-Joiner, D. E., Voytko, M. L., & Salsbury, K. (1987). The performance of visual tasks while segments of the inferotemporal cortex are suppressed by cold. *Brain Research, 23*, 29–42.

Horel, J. A., Voytko, M. L., & Salsbury, K. (1984). Visual learning suppressed by cooling the temporal lobe. *Behavioral Neuroscience, 98,* 310–324.

Jarrard, L. E. (1975). Role of interference in retention by rats with hippocampal lesions. *Journal of Comparative Physiology and Psychology, 89,* 400–408.

Lepage, M., Habib, R., & Tulving, E. (1998). Hippocampal PET activations of memory encoding and retrieval: The HIPER model. *Hippocampus, 8,* 313–322.

Malkova, L., Bachevalier, J., Mishkin, M., & Saunders, R. C. (2001). Neurotoxic lesions of perirhinal cortex impair visual recognition memory in rhesus monkeys. *NeuroReport, 12,* 1913–1917.

McKee, R. D., & Squire, L. R. (1993). On the development of declarative memory. *Journal of Experimental Psychology: Learning, Memory, and Cognition, 19,* 397–404.

Meunier, M., Bachevalier, J., Mishkin, M., & Murray, E. A. (1993). Effects on visual recognition of combined and separate ablations of the entorhinal and perirhinal cortex in rhesus monkeys. *Journal of Neuroscience, 13,* 5418–5432.

Meunier, M., Hadfield, W., Bachevalier, J., & Murray, E. A. (1996). Effects of rhinal cortex lesions combined with hippocampectomy on visual recognition memory in rhesus monkeys. *Journal of Neurophysiology, 75,* 1190–1205.

Miller, E. K., Erickson, C. A., & Desimone, R. (1996). Neural mechanisms of visual working memory in prefrontal cortex of the macaque. *Journal of Neuroscience, 16,* 5154–5167.

Miller, E. K., Li, L., & Desimone, R. (1991). A neural mechanism for working and recognition memory in inferior temporal cortex. *Science, 254,* 1377–1379.

Mishkin, M. (1978). Memory in monkeys severely impaired by combined but not by separate removal of amygdala and hippocampus. *Nature, 273,* 297–298.

Mishkin, M., & Delacour, J. (1975). An analysis of short-term visual memory in the monkey. *Journal of Experimental Psychology: Animal Behavior Processes, 1,* 326–334.

Mishkin, M., Vargha-Khadem, F., & Gadian, D. G. (1998). Amnesia and the organization of the hippocampal system. *Hippocampus, 8,* 212–216.

Mumby, D. G., & Pinel, J. P. J. (1994). Rhinal cortex lesions and object recognition in rats. *Behavioral Neuroscience, 108,* 11–18.

Murray, E. A. (1992). Medial temporal lobe structures contributing to recognition memory: The amygdaloid complex versus the rhinal cortex. In J. P. Aggleton (Ed.), *The amygdala: Neurobiological aspects of emotion, memory, and mental dysfunction* (pp. 453–470). New York: Wiley–Liss.

Murray, E. A. (2000). Memory for objects in nonhuman primates. In M. S. Gazzaniga (Ed.), *The new cognitive neurosciences* (pp. 753–763). Cambridge, MA: MIT Press.

Murray, E. A., & Mishkin, M. (1998). Object recognition and location memory in monkeys with excitotoxic lesions of the amygdala and hippocampus. *Journal of Neuroscience, 18,* 6568–6582.

Nemanic, S. (1999). *The effects of selective hippocampal lesions on two tasks of recognition memory in adult rhesus monkeys.* Unpublished master's thesis, University of Texas Health Science Center, Houston.

Nemanic, S., Alvarado, M. C., & Bachevalier, J. (1998). *Differential effects of selective hippocampal lesions on two visual recognition tasks in monkeys.* Paper presented at the annual meeting of the Cognitive Neuroscience Society, San Francisco.

Nemanic, S., Alvarado, M. C., & Bachevalier, J. (1999). Effects of interference on DNMS performance after selective hippocampal lesions in monkeys. *Society for Neuroscience Abstracts, 25,* 1892.

Nemanic, S., Alvarado, M. C., & Bachevalier, J. (2001). Effects of perirhinal cortical lesions on recognition memory in monkeys. *Society for Neuroscience Abstracts, 27.*

Otto, T., & Eichenbaum, H. (1992). Complementary roles of the orbital prefrontal cortex and the perirhinal–entorhinal cortices in an odor-guided delayed-nonmatching-to-sample task. *Behavioral Neuroscience, 106,* 762–775.

Owen, M., & Butler, S. (1981). Amnesia after transection of the fornix in monkeys: Long-term memory impaired, short-term memory intact. *Behavioural Brain Research, 3,* 115–123.

Pascalis, O., & Bachevalier, J. (1999). Nonselective neonatal hippocampal lesions inpair visual recognition memory when assessed by paired-comparison task but not by delayed nonmatching-to-sample task. *Hippocampus, 9,* 609–616.

Penfield, W., & Milner, B. (1958). Memory deficit produced by bilateral lesions in the hippocampal zone. *Archives of Neurology and Psychiatry, 79,* 475–497.

Reed, J. M., & Squire, L. R. (1997). Impaired recognition memory in patients with lesions limited to the hippocampal formation. *Behavioral Neuroscience, 111,* 667–675.

Rempel-Clower, N. L., Zola, S. M., Squire, L. R., & Amaral, D. G. (1996). Three cases of enduring memory impairment after bilateral damage limited to the hippocampal formation. *Journal of Neuroscience, 16,* 5233–5255.

Rothblat, L. A., & Kromer, L. F. (1991). Object recognition memory in the rat: The role of the hippocampus. *Behavioural Brain Research, 42,* 25–32.

Schacter, D. L., & Tulving, E. (Eds.). (1994). *Memory systems 1994.* Cambridge, MA: MIT Press.

Schacter, D. L., & Wagner, A. D. (1999). Medial temporal lobe activations in fMRI and PET studies of episodic encoding and retrieval. *Hippocampus, 9,* 7–24.

Scoville, W. B., & Milner, B. (1957). Loss of recent memory after bilateral hippocampal lesions. *Journal of Neurology, Neurosurgery and Psychiatry, 20,* 11–21.

Squire, L. R. (1992). Memory and the hippocampus: A synthesis from findings with rats, monkeys, and humans. *Psychological Review, 99,* 195–231.

Stark, C. E., & Squire, L. R. (2000). Functional magnetic resonance imaging (fMRI) activity in the hippocampal region during recognition memory. *Journal of Neuroscience, 20,* 7776–7781.

Stern, C. E., & Hasselmo, M. E. (1999). Bridging the gap: Integrating cellular and functional magnetic resonance imaging studies of the hippocampus. *Hippocampus, 9,* 45–53.

Suzuki, W. A. (1996). The anatomy, physiology and functions of the perirhinal cortex. *Current Opinion in Neurobiology, 6,* 179–186.

Suzuki, W. A., Zola-Morgan, S., Squire, L. R., & Amaral, D. G. (1993). Lesions of the perirhinal and parahippocampal cortices in the monkey produce long-lasting memory impairment in the visual and tactual modalities. *Journal of Neuroscience, 13,* 2430–2451.

Sybirska, E., Davachi, L., & Goldman-Rakic, P. S. (2000). Prominence of direct entorhinal–CA1 pathway activation in sensorimotor and cognitive tasks revealed by 2-DG functional mapping in nonhuman primates. *Journal of Neuroscience, 20,* 5827–5834.

Vargha-Khadem, F., Gadian, D. G., Watkins, K. E., Connelly, A., Van Paesschen, W., & Mishkin, M. (1997). Differential effects of early hippocampal pathology on episodic and semantic memory. *Science, 277,* 376–380.

Zola, S. M., Squire, L. R., Teng, E., Stefanacci, L., Buffalo, E. A., & Clark, R. E. (2000). Impaired recognition memory in monkeys after damage limited to the hippocampal region. *Journal of Neuroscience, 20,* 451–463.

Zola-Morgan, S., Squire, L. R., & Amaral, D. G. (1986). Human amnesia and the medial temporal region: enduring memory impairment following a bilateral lesion limited to field CA1 of the hippocampus. *Journal of Neuroscience, 6,* 2950–2967.

Zola-Morgan, S., Squire, L. R., & Amaral, D. G. (1989a). Lesions of the amygdala that spare the adjacent cortical regions do not impair memory or exacerbate the impairment following lesions of the hippocampal formation. *Journal of Neuroscience, 9,* 1922–1936.

Zola-Morgan, S., Squire, L. R., & Amaral, D. G. (1989b). Lesions of the hippocampal formation but not lesions of the fornix or the mammillary nuclei produce long-lasting memory impairment in monkeys. *Journal of Neuroscience, 9,* 898–913.

Zola-Morgan, S., Squire, L. R., Clower, R. P., & Rempel, N. L. (1993). Damage to the perirhinal cortex exacerbates memory impairment following lesions to the hippocampal formation. *Journal of Neuroscience, 13,* 251–265.

Zola-Morgan, S., Squire, L. R., & Ramus, S. J. (1994). Severity of memory impairment in monkeys as a function of locus and extent of damage within the medial temporal lobe memory system. *Hippocampus, 4,* 483–495.

27

Arbitrary Sensorimotor Mapping and the Life of Primates

ELISABETH A. MURRAY, PETER J. BRASTED, and STEVEN P. WISE

Chimpanzees can learn a symbolic language because they already have the necessary associative mechanisms. . . . Like all animals they must learn to make predictions about future events: the roar of the lion serves to retrieve a mental representation of the lion before the lion arrives.
—PASSINGHAM (1993, p. 240)

Compared to other types of associative memory studied in the laboratory, conditional motor learning has received relatively little attention. In formal tasks designed to assess this type of learning, one stimulus provides the context for a given action, whereas other stimuli establish contexts for different actions (Passingham, 1993). Subjects must solve the following problems: "IF input A . . . , THEN output 1 . . ." and "IF input B. . . , THEN output 2. . . ," where stimuli serve as inputs and movements as outputs. Following the terminology of propositional logic, one can term inputs "antecedents" and outputs "consequents." This kind of associative learning goes by several other names: "conditional discrimination," "conditional association," "stimulus–response association," and "habit" (a term often used synonymously with "procedural knowledge"). However, application of the last term conflicts with evidence that rapid, conditional motor learning represents a form of declarative memory in monkeys (Wise & Murray, 1999). In this chapter, we call this behavior "arbitrary sensorimotor mapping" to emphasize the general, flexible, and arbitrary nature of the linkages learned.

Arbitrary sensorimotor mapping differs importantly from other kinds of action guided by sensory inputs. In conventional sensorimotor guidance, movements are typically aimed directly at a stimulus. For example, one may grasp a grape or pluck a plum. This kind of input–output coupling involves standard sensorimotor mapping. Unlike in standard mapping, in arbitrary sensorimotor mapping no spatial algorithm relates sensory input to motor output. The mappings must be learned through experience.

Rhesus monkeys can become highly skilled at learning arbitrary sensorimotor mappings. They can learn a new mapping after one, or at most a few, presentations of a novel stimulus (Figure 27.1). In this chapter, we explore how monkeys can become so proficient at solving these problems. It takes monkeys a long time, however, to achieve this level of proficiency; because of that fact, one might argue that arbitrary sensorimotor mapping is an ability they do not use in their everyday lives. Accordingly, we also address whether laboratory experiments that examine sensorimotor mapping are relevant to the life history of monkeys. Following Passingham (1993), we contend that arbitrary sensorimotor mapping in the laboratory reflects the ability to select an appropriate action on the basis of current context, and that decisions based on context constitute an important part of a primate's life. Unlike the guidance of action by standard sensorimotor mapping, arbitrary mapping requires decisions as to which of two or more actions to take, given a particular context. Accordingly, after reviewing the laboratory data, we pose two questions. First, do nonhuman primates demonstrate comparable learning capacities in their natural habitat? Second, might their surprising abilities in the laboratory result from the transfer of natural ecological strategies to formal testing?

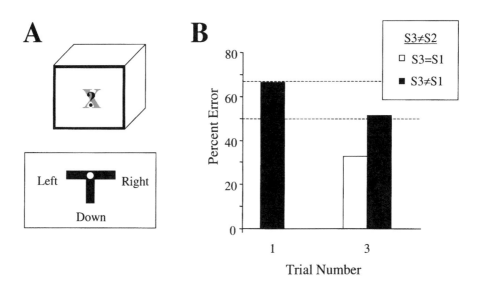

FIGURE 27.1. (A) *Top:* Schematic of a typical visual stimulus used in the arbitrary sensorimotor mapping task, presented on a video monitor. *Bottom:* View from above the joystick. After presentation of a visual stimulus, the monkey could move the joystick (white circle at "T" junction) in one of three directions. One direction was correct for that particular stimulus; the others were incorrect. (B) Percentage of error on the first and third trials of a 50-trial block. The height of the bar for trial 1 shows the average score over all such trials for four rhesus monkeys (40 trials/monkey). The percentage of errors on trial 1 is at chance level (upper dashed line). Trial 3 shows the data only for trials in which the stimulus differed from that on trial 2 (S3 ≠ S2). If the stimulus on Trial 3 was novel (filled bars)—that is, if it differed from that on both trial 1 (S3 ≠ S1) and trial 2—the monkeys chose incorrectly ~50% of the time (lower dashed line), as predicted if the monkeys were applying the change–shift strategy. If the stimulus on trial 3 was the same as that on trial 1 (S3 = S1, open bar), and thus had been seen once previously, the monkeys scored significantly better than if it was novel ($t = 3.00$, $df = 6$, $p < .03$). Thus the monkeys showed significant one-trial learning, notwithstanding the intervening trial 2. Data from Murray and Wise (1996).

IN THE LABORATORY

Arbitrary sensorimotor mapping can be distinguished from other kinds of associative learning commonly studied in the laboratory. Stimulus–reward associations, as well as sensory discriminations, can be learned by approaching stimuli according to their affective valence (i.e., their history of reinforcement, reward value, etc.). Classical conditioning (also known as Pavlovian conditioning), though having an associative nature like arbitrary sensorimotor mapping, must be based upon unconditioned reflexes. By contrast, arbitrary sensorimotor mapping relies on neither affective valence nor reflexes. It allows the association of any discriminable stimulus with any action that is in a subject's behavioral repertoire. As the monkey learns, no stimulus, movement, or target of movement gains a greater association with reward than does any other. Among the common forms of associative memory studied in the laboratory, arbitrary sensorimotor mapping most closely resembles paired-associate learning, in which both antecedents and consequents are sensory (e.g., object-to-object associations). Although arbitrary sensorimotor mapping has motor consequents rather than sensory ones, its similarity to paired-associate learning lies in the arbitrary nature of the mapping between two representations.

Most information about the neural basis of arbitrary sensorimotor mapping comes from studies of macaque monkeys and humans. Here we provide a brief overview of the topic, but the interested reader may examine other publications for further details and citations of specific findings (Murray, Bussey, & Wise, 2000; Wise & Murray, 1999). In a typical laboratory test of arbitrary sensorimotor mapping, monkeys view a two-dimensional visual stimulus on a video screen and learn to associate a movement with that stimulus. Responses may involve moving a joystick in a specific direction, touching a particular location on a touch screen, making specific responses with the hand (e.g., tapping or holding a given stimulus), or making a saccadic eye movement. A neural network involving the hippocampal system (the hippocampus, underlying parahippocampal cortex, and fornix), the basal ganglia, the basal ganglia's synaptic targets in the thalamus, the ventral and orbital prefrontal cortex, and the premotor cortex underlies the rapid acquisition of arbitrary sensorimotor mappings. Interactions of the inferior temporal cortex with the prefrontal cortex also play a role, at least for certain visuomotor mappings (Gaffan & Harrison, 1988). The latter contribution might be expected, given that these regions have direct, reciprocal connections and that the inferior temporal cortex plays a central role in shape and object vision. Lesions in any component of this set of interconnected structures affects the acquisition of arbitrary sensorimotor mappings, and these deficits do not result from difficulties in the ability either to discriminate the stimuli or to perform the responses. Thus the deficit selectively involves mapping the stimulus to the action (or the target of action). This is not to say that each of these brain regions contributes to arbitrary sensorimotor mapping in the same way; rather, it seems likely that different brain regions make different contributions. For example, the hippocampal system underlies the rapid acquisition of mappings, but is not necessary for retrieval of mappings from long-term memory or for use of certain cognitive strategies that promote learning. We explain these conclusions in more detail below.

Clinical studies have also strongly implicated both the ventrolateral prefrontal cortex and the hippocampal system in learning arbitrary sensorimotor mappings. Damage to either of these structures produces deficits on tasks assessing acquisition of such mappings. As with the monkey studies, the results demonstrate that the deficit lies specifically in mapping the stimulus to the action, as opposed to a failure in some other information-processing domain. However, as is often the case in clinical studies, the anatomical localization of lesion extent remains imprecise. For example, within the frontal cortex, the critical regions may involve the premotor cortex, the prefrontal cortex, or some combination of these regions. The contributions of neuroimaging studies to this question have been summarized elsewhere, but agree generally with the neuropsychological findings summarized here.

Figure 27.2 presents some key findings about the neural basis of arbitrary sensorimotor mapping. In studies carried out in our laboratories, we assessed both the acquisition and retention of arbitrary sensorimotor mappings in rhesus monkeys, with the aim of delineating the brain structures essential for this kind of learning. Monkeys viewed complex visual stimuli that appeared, one at a time, in the center of a video monitor. While a stimulus remained on the screen, the monkeys made a response using a joystick, which could move in only three directions (Figure 27.1A). Each stimulus mapped onto one and only one direction of joystick movement. Monkeys learned, through trial and error, to acquire novel sensorimotor mappings. In the final version of the task, the monkeys were trained on a set of three arbitrary sensorimotor mapping problems, randomly selected from trial to trial, and acquisition occurred within a single block of 50 trials. The monkeys learned all three mapping problems concurrently. They also learned to perform according to highly familiar mappings, presented in the same manner (i.e., three familiar problems were presented concurrently for a total of 50 trials). Following errors, we presented the monkeys with a limited number of correction trials, consisting of additional presentations of the stimulus that had been presented on the original trial. Under these conditions, rhesus monkeys learned very quickly, reaching a plateau of about 95% correct responses in fewer than 10 attempts at each new mapping. Figure 27.1B presents evidence for one-trial learning. Indeed, monkeys showed an equally impressive ability to learn reversals, which involved dispensing with a recently learned mapping and learning a new one for the same stimulus. After removal of the hippocampus and underlying parahippocampal cortex (H+), the monkeys' ability to learn novel mappings declined dramatically compared to their preoperative performance (Figure 27.2A, left). By contrast, they showed intact retention of the preoperatively learned, familiar mappings (Figure 27.2A, right).

These studies also showed that after gaining substantial experience with solving novel mapping problems, monkeys used at least three strategies to enhance their performance. First, on trials in which the stimulus changed from that on the previous trial, the monkeys avoided the correct response they had just made on the previous trial in favor of one of the remaining response choices. We called this strategy "change–shift". Second, after errors the monkeys used a "lose–shift" strategy on correction trials; that is, they avoided the incorrect response they had just made (Figure 27.2C). The lose–shift strategy differed from the change–shift strategy in that the former followed an error, whereas the latter followed a correctly performed trial. Finally, the monkeys used yet a third strategy, which we have termed "repeat–stay," although "win–stay" would also apply. When the stimulus remained the same from one trial to the next, the monkeys repeated the response that had led to a successful outcome on the previous trial. Experienced monkeys used all three strategies as they learned new mappings. These strategies not only improved performance scores generally, but also increased the frequency of correctly performed exemplars for each mapping, thereby presumably promoting rapid learning. Removal of H+ did not affect the use of those strategies (Figure 27.2C), even though the monkeys had a markedly reduced ability to learn novel mappings.

Removal of the ventral and orbital prefrontal cortex yielded a different pattern of results. Like monkeys with H+ removals (Figure 27.2A), monkeys with removal of the ventral

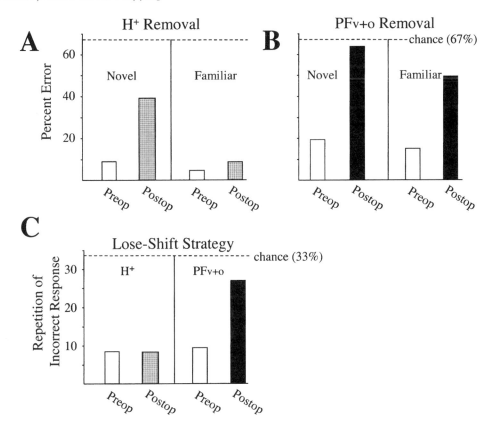

FIGURE 27.2. (A) The effect of bilateral aspiration removals of the hippocampus plus subjacent cortex (H⁺) on the acquisition of arbitrary sensorimotor mappings. Bars show asymptotic performance (i.e., mean percentage of error for the final 25 trials of a 50-trial block). A set of 120 novel arbitrary sensorimotor mappings comprised the data set for each of four monkeys, preoperatively (preop, open bars) and postoperatively (postop, shaded bars). Note that H⁺ monkeys were severely impaired in the acquisition of *novel* sensorimotor mappings (left). Data are also given for a set of 24 *familiar* mappings. Note that the monkeys showed intact retention of mappings that had been learned long before the lesion (right). (B) Comparable data for two rhesus monkeys with bilateral aspiration removals of the ventral and orbital prefrontal cortex (PFv+o). Data are in the same format as in A, except that one monkey had only 60 problems in the data set (preop, open bars; postop, black bars). These monkeys showed severe deficits in both the learning of novel mappings and the retention of familiar ones. (C) Effects of H⁺ and PFv+o lesions on a strategy. Same monkeys as in A and B. On correction trials, intact monkeys (preop) tended to shift from the initially incorrect response to one of the remaining two possibilities, thus employing a "lose–shift" strategy. Monkeys with H⁺ lesions showed the same ability postoperatively. Monkeys with PFv+o lesions lost that ability, but did not perseverate. They chose the same, incorrect response more often after the lesion than before it, but no more often than expected for a random choice among the three possible responses. Data from Murray and Wise (1996) and Murray, Bussey, and Wise (2000).

and orbital prefrontal cortex could not learn novel sensorimotor mappings as rapidly as they had before surgery (Figure 27.2B). Indeed, within a block of 50 trials, they did not improve from chance levels of performance. However, in contrast to monkeys with H⁺ damage, they also failed to retain or retrieve preoperatively learned, familiar mappings (Figure 27.2B) and had virtually no ability to employ any of the cognitive strategies outlined above (e.g., Figure 27.2C). Thus the severe deficit in arbitrary sensorimotor mapping after damage to the prefrontal cortex may have resulted either from a selective inability to employ these three strategies, or from this deficit together with an inability to learn the specific mappings (Murray et al., 2000).

The task we used provides a tool not only for studying the acquisition and retention of arbitrary mappings, but also for studying the acquisition and implementation of strategies. In this regard, we note that a three-choice task has a considerable advantage over a two-choice task. In a task with only two stimuli and two responses, after an animal performs the first trial, it may rely entirely on the repeat–stay and change–shift strategies to perform accurately, without necessarily learning the individual mappings. Thus, in the context of a lesion study, lack of impairment on such a task may result from implementation of the aforementioned strategies without any learning of the specific mappings. Outstanding questions include the generality of the neural network outlined here for other types of arbitrary mappings (such as paired-associate learning), the precise nature and contribution of the strategies, and the selective contributions of each part of the network. Finally, it should be noted that lesions in certain other structures have little or no effect on arbitrary sensorimotor mapping. For example, bilateral removals of the amygdala, most of the posterior parietal cortex, or several medial premotor areas (e.g., the supplementary motor area) fail to disrupt arbitrary sensorimotor mapping.

BEYOND THE LABORATORY

What about the natural environment of monkeys? Does arbitrary sensorimotor mapping play a role in their everyday lives? We assume for the sake of discussion that the cognitive abilities of rhesus monkeys reflect those of Old World monkeys generally. We are aware, however, that rhesus monkeys represent a noteworthy instance of ecological generalism (i.e., the ability to exploit a wide range of modified and natural environments). This fact may limit the applicability of data from rhesus monkeys to species with distinct habitat preferences and ecological specializations. Unfortunately, a comparative understanding of arbitrary mapping abilities among the primates remains a topic for future study.

In the past, the impressive laboratory abilities of nonhuman primates have not been easy to recognize in natural environments (Jolly, 1966), and field behavior has not often been considered in the light of laboratory abilities such as arbitrary mapping. Several factors may have limited a consideration of arbitrary mapping in particular, among them an aversion to reliance on learning theory and an emphasis on tool use. Tool use is at best an unsatisfactory example of arbitrary sensorimotor mapping, because the use of tools often involves a form of standard sensorimotor mapping in which the end-point effector changes from part of the animal's body to an object controlled by the animal.

Viewed in this light, it is worthwhile considering examples of field behavior that appear to incorporate aspects of arbitrary sensorimotor mapping, particularly those that appear to be learned in a natural ecological context. For instance, some vervet monkeys make different-sounding alarm calls in response to at least three different classes of predators: a "barking" call in response to leopards and other carnivores; a "cough" call for eagles and other raptors; and a "chutter" call for predatory snakes (Cheney & Seyfarth, 1990; Struhsaker, 1967). This behavior conforms to the formal definition of arbitrary sensorimotor mapping: One sensory context leads to one type of vocalization, whereas other contexts bring about different calls. The calls are arbitrary in yet another way: They do not sound like, and do not readily suggest, the referent. The responses to these calls also appear to reflect arbitrary sensorimotor mapping. Struhsaker (1967) noted that the three alarm calls mentioned above elicited three different responses: Leopard calls led nearby vervets to climb trees; eagle alarms prompted them to look skyward and then hide in bushes; and snake calls led the monkeys to stand up and look around. These behaviors, too, conform to the definition of arbitrary sensorimotor mapping: Acoustic stimuli provide the context for action.

Further studies have sought to define the influence that each call has over the response of conspecifics. When field researchers recorded the same alarm calls and later played them back in the absence of predators, each of the alarm calls elicited the typical, associated escape response (Cheney & Seyfarth, 1990). This finding suggests that vervets treat each call as a behavioral context in its own right, rather than as a threat to which they orient. In addition, each call type does more than elicit different levels of arousal, because it appears that only a call's acoustic structure, rather than its duration or amplitude, can predict the correct escape response.

Important aspects of these arbitrary mappings appear to be learned, as evidenced by young vervets that initiate unusual responses to a call or transmit inappropriate calls. For example, young vervets may give an eagle call in response to a falling leaf (Cheney & Seyfarth, 1990). Additional evidence for the view that learning is involved comes from preliminary observations by M. D. Hauser (personal communication January 15, 2001) and his colleagues of variation in vervet alarm calls. The observations summarized above come from Amboseli, Kenya, where vervets produce acoustically distinctive alarm calls in response to different classes of predators. In contrast to those vervets, Hauser and colleagues have observed that in Uganda, vervets of the same subspecies produce the same set of calls, but use them in a different way. They produce one call when a predator is near and another when it is far, but without specificity regarding the class of predator. Further evidence for learning comes from the observation that infant vervets living near swamps react much earlier in life to alarm calls used by starlings (a species that prefers swamp habitats) than do vervets that live relatively far from swamps (Hauser, 1998). Together with additional examples (Janik & Slater, 2000), these observations support the idea that experience-dependent vocalizations and responses to those vocalizations may reflect the same arbitrary sensorimotor mapping capability that can be observed in the laboratory. It seems likely that vervets learn to map distinct classes of visual inputs onto calls, as well as to map specific acoustic inputs onto different actions. Together, these sensorimotor mappings serve to decrease predation and promote defense of the kin group.

We do not mean to imply that all aspects of these behaviors are learned. For example, although the production of vocalizations by nonhuman primates can be conditioned via primary reward (Sutton & Jürgens, 1988) as well as social reinforcement (Randolph & Brooks, 1967), there is no evidence that the call structure itself can be modified (Hauser, 1996). Instead, it appears to be the context for their production that is learned. Young vervets at first produce eagle alarm calls to many things in the air, but later, through experience, learn to restrict such behavior to the context of eagle sightings (Cheney & Seyfarth, 1990).

Another possible example of arbitrary sensorimotor mapping in the field comes from studies of food-associated calling in rhesus monkeys (Hauser & Marler, 1993a, 1993b). Rhesus monkeys give five distinct calls in the context of food. They give some call types (warbles, chirps, and harmonic arches) only when in possession of a highly valued food resource, such as a coconut; they make other calls (coos and grunts) in the context of less valued food, such as cereal pellets, or in nonfood contexts. Hauser and Marler addressed the possibility that such differential calling might largely reflect motivational state, but after careful analysis they concluded that an arbitrary referential relation is also important. Their conclusion is supported by observations and experiments indicating that such factors as satiety, gender, and group membership affect call rate but not call type—as if motivation is encoded by call rate, but food quality by call type. Like the alarm call system in vervets, conspecifics react to these acoustic signals in a way that reflects the food-associated call type, with coos and grunts least likely to elicit approaches. In addition, monkeys show less aggression toward vocal food discoverers than toward silent discoverers. Hauser and Marler (1993a, p. 204) noted that one possible benefit could be "an increased access to food and an increase in the probability of successful resource defense through coalition support or kin-group defense."

Deceptive behaviors may also involve an element of arbitrary mapping. For example, a given social setting may establish the context for making or withholding some action—an idea that is inherent in at least one definition of deception. "Social tactical deception" has been defined as "(i) acts from the normal repertoire of an individual, (ii) used at low frequency and in *contexts* different from those in which it uses the high frequency (honest) version of the act, (iii) such that another familiar individual, (iv) is likely to misinterpret what the acts signify, (v) to the advantage of the actor" (Byrne & Whiten, 1988, p. 206; emphasis added). Although the low frequency of these behaviors has sometimes led to a reliance on anecdotal evidence, a wide variety of instances have been reported. For instance, after a fight between two chimpanzees, one animal limped for 1 week, but did so only in a certain context—namely, when the second animal could see him (de Waal, 1986). Cheney and Seyfarth (1990) chronicle instances of vervets' giving seemingly false leopard alarm calls during intergroup encounters. Field observers have also reported examples of animals' appearing to withhold an action selectively when in the presence of other animals, although it is sometimes problematic to distinguish the inhibition of action from a failure to notice the context for making it. de Waal (1986) notes an incident, however, in which a chimpanzee did not retrieve or react to a concealed piece of fruit until the other chimpanzees present had fallen asleep, some 3 hours later. Therefore, the animal presumably had detected the fruit, but withheld its approach response until the behavioral context changed. In an example involving copulation calls, male rhesus monkeys vocalized less frequently at the beginning of the mating season—a period of high competition for females—than later, when competition declined (Hauser, 1993). Males that called, however, had a chance for multiple matings, albeit at the risk of attack from competitors. Thus rhesus males have the capacity to suppress copulation calls in some contexts, as well as to produce them in others. It has been proposed that deception, as defined above, is driven by an animal's representation of the mental states of others rather than by associative learning, although this remains a contentious issue (Heyes, 1998; Whiten & Byrne, 1997). Arbitrary sensorimotor mappings and their reversals may underlie some aspects of deceptive behavior on either view, perhaps including the use of abstract representations (such as mental states) as a context for action.

The idea that a primate's knowledge of its social and physical environment underlies learning in the laboratory is not novel (see, e.g., Jolly, 1966; Tomasello & Call, 1997). As Tomasello and Call (1997, p. 185) suggest, "experiments in which primates relate objects to one another might be tapping skills that evolved so that primates could relate group mates to one another." They also point out (p. 185), as many have before them, that "research from the learning theory tradition has often studied skills in highly artificial circumstances that are only displayed after many hundreds, or even thousands, of experimental trials." As we have examined it, arbitrary sensorimotor mapping indeed takes many hundreds, or even thousands, of trials for monkeys to demonstrate their most impressive capabilities. Nevertheless, impressive they are. The field behaviors surveyed above suggest that arbitrary sensorimotor mapping capacities play an important role in guiding behavior according to a dynamic social context.

CONCLUDING COMMENTS

We think that arbitrary sensorimotor mapping may have some relevance to the origin of language. The quest for preadaptations for speech and language in the monkey brain has produced some progress (Ghazanfar & Hauser, 1999), but we believe that there has been undue focus on the auditory and medial frontal cortex. Because the human auditory cortex processes acoustic information for both linguistic and other purposes, and the human medial frontal cortex may be specialized for a role in generating nonverbal vocalizations (such as crying and laughing), the specific role of these areas in language is debatable. The lateral prefrontal areas of monkeys, by contrast, have many properties in common with accepted speech and language cortices. These prefrontal areas lie in a similar "geographic" relationship to the remainder of the frontal lobe: Both Broca's area in humans and the prefrontal component of the arbitrary sensorimotor mapping network in monkeys lie more or less directly in front of the orofacial representation of the motor cortex. This location is important, because it seems unlikely that evolutionary processes would dispense with one arbitrary sensorimotor mapping mechanism only to evolve another one in roughly the same place. Instead, we suggest that evolution marshaled an existing arbitrary mapping ability in the service of language (Deacon, 1998; Passingham, 1993).

But why would language evolution coopt an existing arbitrary mapping mechanism? To begin with, arbitrariness is a noted characteristic of both primate communication in general and language in particular (Hockett, 1960). A process akin to arbitrary sensorimotor mapping underlies the association of word meaning to the vocal and articulatory gestures of speech. Added to that, a different type of arbitrary mapping underlies the elicitation of word meaning by sights and sounds. The mapping of graphemes and phonemes to meaning has the same arbitrary nature as do the kinds of sensorimotor mappings discussed here. However, word comprehension more closely resembles paired-associate learning than it does arbitrary sensorimotor mapping; both the antecedent and the consequent involve nonmotor representations. It seems likely that both kinds of arbitrary mappings play a fundamental role in language—representation-to-motor mapping in speech production, and sensory-to-representation mapping in word comprehension.

Arbitrary sensorimotor mapping depends on the hippocampal system, ventrolateral prefrontal cortex, premotor cortex, and basal ganglia. Given sufficient experience, monkeys learn arbitrary mappings and their reversals with impressive speed and accuracy. We have argued that they can do so because they learn to apply knowledge and strategies useful in their natural environment to the laboratory, and that the joint function of the frontal cortex and hippocampal system underlies this capacity. Other animals can learn arbitrary sensorimotor mappings, too, but we primates seem to do it especially well—be it through daily discourse, signs and signals, or vervet vocalizations.

ACKNOWLEDGMENT

We thank Dr. Marc D. Hauser for his comments on an earlier version of this chapter.

REFERENCES

Byrne, R. W., & Whiten, A. (Eds.). (1988). *Machiavellian intelligence: Social expertise and the evolution of intellect in monkeys, apes, and humans.* Oxford: Oxford University Press.

Cheney, D. L., & Seyfarth, R. M. (1990). *How monkeys see the world: Inside the mind of another species*. Chicago: University of Chicago Press.

Deacon, T. W. (1998). *The symbolic species: The co-evolution of language and the brain*. New York: Norton.

de Waal, F. B. M. (1986). Deception in the natural communication of chimpanzees. In R. W. Mitchell & N. S. Thompson (Eds.), *Deception: Perspectives on human and non-human deceit* (pp. 221–244). Albany: State University of New York Press.

Gaffan, D., & Harrison, S. (1988). Inferotemporal–frontal disconnection and fornix transection in visuomotor conditional learning by monkeys. *Behavioural Brain Research*, 31, 149–163.

Ghazanfar, A. A., & Hauser, M. D. (1999). The neuroethology of primate vocal communication: Substrates for the evolution of speech. *Trends in Cognitive Sciences*, 3, 377–384.

Hauser, M. D. (1988). How infant vervet monkeys learn to recognize starling alarm calls: The role of experience. *Behaviour*, 105, 187–201.

Hauser, M. D. (1993). Rhesus monkey (*Macaca mulatta*) copulation calls: Honest signals for female choice? *Proceedings of the Royal Society of London*, 254, 93–96.

Hauser, M. D. (1996). *The evolution of communication*. Cambridge, MA: MIT Press.

Hauser, M. D., & Marler, P. (1993a). Food-associated calls in rhesus macaques (*Macaca mulatta*): I. Socioecological factors. *Behavioral Ecology*, 4, 194–205.

Hauser, M. D., & Marler, P. (1993b). Food-associated calls in rhesus macaques (*Macaca mulatta*): II. Costs and benefits of call production and suppression. *Behavioral Ecology*, 4, 206–212.

Heyes, C. M. (1998). Theory of mind in nonhuman primates. *Behavioral and Brain Sciences*, 21, 101–148.

Hockett, C. F. (1960). Principles of animal communication. In W. F. Lanyon & W. N. Tavolga (Eds.), *Animal sounds and communication* (pp. 392–430). Washington, DC: American Institute of Biological Sciences.

Janik, V. M., & Slater, P. J. B. (2000). The different roles of social learning in vocal communication. *Animal Behaviour*, 60, 1–11.

Jolly, A. (1966). Lemur social behavior and primate intelligence. *Science*, 153, 501–506.

Murray, E. A., Bussey, T. J., & Wise, S. P. (2000). Role of prefrontal cortex in a network for arbitrary visuomotor mapping. *Experimental Brain Research*, 133, 114–129.

Murray, E. A., & Wise, S. P. (1996). Role of the hippocampus plus subjacent cortex but not amygdala in visuomotor conditional learning in rhesus monkeys. *Behavioral Neuroscience*, 110, 1261–1270.

Passingham, R. E. (1993). *The frontal lobes and voluntary action*. Oxford: Oxford University Press.

Randolph, M. C., & Brooks, B. A. (1967). Conditioning of a vocal response in a chimpanzee through social reinforcement. *Folia Primatologia*, 5, 70–79.

Struhsaker, T. T. (1967). Auditory communication among vervet monkeys (*Cercopithecus aethiops*). In S. A. Altmann (Ed.), *Social communication among primates* (pp. 281–324). Chicago: University of Chicago Press.

Sutton, D., & Jürgens, U. (1988). Neural control of vocalization. *Comparative Primate Biology*, 4, 625–647.

Tomasello, M., & Call, J. (1997). *Primate cognition*. New York: Oxford University Press.

Whiten, A., & Byrne, R. W. (Eds.). (1997). *Machiavellian intelligence II. Extensions and evaluations*. Cambridge, England: Cambridge University Press.

Wise, S. P., & Murray, E. A. (1999). Role of the hippocampal system in conditional motor learning: Mapping antecedents to action. *Hippocampus*, 9, 101–117.

PART III

STUDIES OF MEMORY IN RODENTS AND BIRDS

Studies of small animals, especially rats and mice, take less time and are less expensive than studies in monkeys and are especially valuable when large numbers of animals are needed to explore multiple experimental conditions. Beginning in the early 1990s, the ability to genetically modify mice made it possible to relate specific genes both to synaptic plasticity and to intact animal behavior, including memory. These techniques allow one to delete specific genes in specific brain regions and also to turn genes on and off. Chapter 37 illustrates some of the first fruits of what these new techniques promise for the study of memory. Chapters 28 and 29 describe work on the role of the hippocampus in memory functions of rats. This work draws on lesions, neurophysiology, and behavior to consider declarative memory and spatial cognition. Chapter 30 describes efforts to isolate the contribution of the fornix to memory, and Chapter 31 describes initial attempts to identify separate contributions of the cell fields of the hippocampus. Chapter 32 describes how the physiology of neocortex can be shaped by sensory experience and by the cognitive state of the animal, thereby providing a neural substrate for the gradual acquisition of improved perceptual and motor skills. One neural system that has been identified as important for this process is the diffuse cholinergic projection to cortex that originates in the basal forebrain. Chapter 33 summarizes work on the links between memory, attention, and cholinergic neurons, both the neurons of nucleus basalis and those of the medial septum and the vertical limb of the diagonal band. These studies have benefited by the recent development of a toxin that permits the selective destruction of cholinergic neurons. Chapters 34 and 35 describe work showing how memory can be modulated by events that occur after learning occurs. This modulation is orchestrated by the amygdala, and can operate on hippocampus-dependent (declarative) memory as well as on neostriatum-dependent (habit) memory. Measures of neurotransmitter in hippocampus and neostriatum can predict, prior to training, which neural system will guide behavior. Chapter 36 reviews anatomical, neurophysiological, and lesion work in rats, showing how orbitofrontal cortex contributes to memory and cognition. These studies indicate a role for orbitofrontal cortex in encoding the value of a stimulus so that it can later be treated appropriately. Chapter 38 describes work on the capacity of some bird species, such as scrub jays, to cache food for later recovery by memory. Studies of this ability have provided some of the best evidence in a nonhuman animal for episodic-like memory ability, that is, memory of a unique event that includes information about what, when, and where.

28

Declarative Memory

Cognitive Mechanisms and Neural Codes

HOWARD EICHENBAUM

It is widely accepted that the hippocampus and related brain areas mediate declarative (or explicit) memory in humans (Schacter & Tulving, 1994). However, little is known about the fundamental psychological and representational mechanisms that underlie declarative memory. The aim of research in my laboratory is to identify the role of the hippocampus and related structures in declarative memory, both in terms of the underlying cognitive mechanisms (i.e., its psychological framework) and in terms of basic neuronal coding schemes (i.e., the information contained in the firing patterns of hippocampal neuronal networks).

DECLARATIVE MEMORY

One of the major breakthroughs in clarifying the nature of hippocampal involvement in memory was the demonstration of its critical role in declarative memory (Cohen & Squire, 1980; see also Eichenbaum & Cohen, 2001). Efforts to reveal the basic cognitive and neural mechanisms of declarative memory depend in part on the development of animal models in which the background history of experience can be controlled, and in which detailed biological manipulations and recordings can be accomplished. At the same time, the success of animal models depends critically on the ability to identify the basic properties of declarative memory that must be incorporated into behavioral testing. Toward this aim, we have focused on two common characterizations of declarative memory: its decomposition into episodic and semantic memory, and its accessibility to conscious recollection and support of "flexible" memory expression.

With regard to episodic and semantic memory, it is important to recognize that we acquire our conscious memories via everyday personal experiences. Thus one can view episodic memory as a "gateway" to memory through which we initially encode everyday events as they occur. There is broad agreement that the hippocampus plays a critical role in episodic memory (Vargha-Khadem et al., 1997). But processing by the hippocampal region is not limited to this component of declarative memory (Squire & Zola, 1998). Our semantic memories are largely composed of a synthesis of episodic memories, a process by which the common information that is contained within many episodic memories is organized within the framework of our knowledge about the world. Thus a possible central role of the hippocampus and associated brain areas may be both to encode episodic memories and to link them by identifying common features, thus constructing a network of memories from which semantic properties emerge.

In addition, our capacity for conscious recollection and flexible memory expression can be viewed as a natural product of the establishment of a linked episodic memory network and its semantic organization. Thus, having created a network of memories, one can envision a capacity to "surf" this network, bringing related memories to consciousness and identifying associations between memories and consequential relations among memories that are only indirectly and distantly linked. The capacity to compare and contrast memories obtained at different times in different venues has been highlighted as a central feature of declarative memory, as described by Cohen (1984). A natural consequence of such a capacity is to make inferences and generalizations from memory, also highlighted in Cohen's characterization, and so to provide for flexible expression of memories across many situations and circumstances. In humans, the process of surfing a memory network may constitute "conscious recollection." In animals, we cannot directly assess a capacity for conscious recollection. But we can create operational tests for the capacity to remember distinct experiences and to link them in support of flexible, inferential memory expression.

COGNITIVE MECHANISMS

We have been developing behavioral testing protocols that assess the capacity of rats for creating distinct representations for multiple experiences that share common elements, and for flexible, inferential expression of an organized representation of these memories. One protocol that offers a particularly good paradigm in which to examine these capacities is the "transitive inference test." The capacity for transitive inference was originally studied by Piaget (1928) in his efforts to characterize the cognitive development of young children. He initially presented subjects with a set of premises that shared overlapping elements, and then tested for the capacity to organize the premises into a larger framework that supports logical inferences among indirectly related items. For example, consider the following two premises: "Sally is more fair than Sue," and "Sue is more fair than Jane." Then one could ask, "Is Sally more fair than Jane?" The capacity to correctly confirm this logical inference depends on the extent to which the premises are remembered and linked within the larger framework "Sally > Sue > Jane," where ">" indicates "is fairer than." Furthermore, one must be able to identify the indirectly related items Sally and Jane, as well as to infer their logical relations. From the perspective of establishing a test of declarative memory, one can view the premises as a set of distinct episodic memories that can be organized within a simple one-dimensional semantic network to support flexible expression in the form of a capacity for inference between the indirectly related items. Piaget observed that this capacity emerges at about age 7 in children. Since that time, several experiments have shown that chimpanzees, monkeys, and rats can also learn this type of one-dimensional serial organization and demonstrate transitive inferences among indirectly related items (for a review, see Dusek & Eichenbaum, 1997).

Following on these successes, we (Dusek & Eichenbaum, 1997) developed a transitive inference task for rats, exploiting rodents' superb learning and memory capacities in the olfactory modality as well as their natural foraging strategies (Figure 28.1). The stimuli consisted of distinctive odorous spices added to clean playground sand through which rats dug to obtain buried cereal rewards. Animals were first presented with a series of blocks of trials involving four pairwise odor discrimination problems. Each problem was composed of two adjacent items in an arbitrarily assigned hierarchical ordering of odors. Thus subjects were initially rewarded for selecting the appropriate item in overlapping premise pairs: A > B, B > C, C > D, and D > E, where A–E are different odors and ">" indicates "is selected over." In subsequent intermediate stages of training, the number of trials in training blocks was gradually reduced, until each pair was presented only once in each sequence. Finally, all the premise pairs were presented intermixed in random order in the same session. Then, in the transitive inference testing sessions, all the premise problems were presented in random order, along with occasional probe trials that included the pair BD as the critical test of transitive inference.

Two types of control probes were also presented in this format. One probe involved the pair AE. Like the transitive probe, this pairing was novel, but it could be solved without reference to the orderly relations among the items because, during training, item A was always rewarded and item E was never rewarded. Thus an animal could be expected to choose A over E without reference to knowledge about the items intervening between them in the series. In addition, because rats would otherwise have rapidly extinguished responding to nonrewarded probe trials, the expected choice was always rewarded on each of the probe tests (B on the BD trials, and A on the AE trials). To test whether consistencies in probe performance could have been due to learning the new pairings, new odor pairs were also intermingled among premise pair trials, similar to the testing protocol used for the other types of probes.

Intact rats acquired each of the premise pairs rapidly and performed well during probe testing (Figure 28.1). In particular, normal rats made the appropriate transitive judgment between stimuli B and D about as accurately as their overall performance on the premise pairs. This finding indicates that rats have a robust capacity for transitive inference, and therefore are capable of developing and flexibly expressing a relational organization of the odor items.

The effects of two different disconnections of the hippocampus were tested. In some rats, the hippocampus was disconnected from related subcortical structures via a fornix transection. In other rats, the hippocampus was disconnected from related cortical structures by removal of the perirhinal and entorhinal cortices. Both groups of animals with hippocampal disconnections acquired the premise pairs at the normal rate and continued to perform accurately on concurrent presentations of all the premise pairs. Indeed, all groups showed a characteristic U-shaped curve in which performance was better on the end-anchored pairs—that is, pairs that included one of the consistently rewarded or nonrewarded items (A or E)—than on the inner premise pairs that did not include A or E. These observations indicate that the rats with hippocampal disconnections had somehow acquired appropriate responses to each repetitively stimulus pairing, and that their performance was sensitive to consistent reinforcement contingencies.

The most important finding was that, by contrast to their intact performance on the premise pairs, rats with either type of hippocampal disconnection showed no capacity for transitive inference (Figure 28.1). On the BD probe, they performed much worse than normal rats, and their performance was not better than would be expected by chance. In the AE control probes, intact rats and rats with either type of hippocampal disconnection accurately selected A over E, which could be guided by biases about these individual stimuli. This finding indicates that the deficit in rats with hippocampal disconnections was not due

A. Testing method

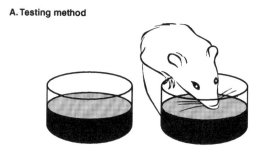

B. Protocol

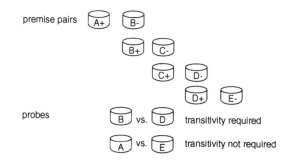

C. Results

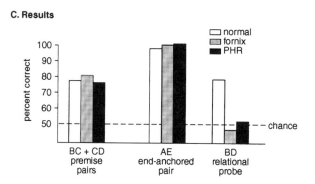

FIGURE 28.1. The transitive inference task. (A) Illustration of the rat sampling stimulus cups filled with odorized sand. (B) Illustration of the premise pairs that were presented during training, and the two key probe test pairs. The BD probe required transitivity because both items had the same reward history, whereas the AE probe could be solved without transitivity because A was always rewarded, and E was never rewarded during training. (C) Performance of normal (control) rats and rats with disconnection of the hippocampus either by transection of the fornix or ablation of the parahippocampal region (PHR). Mean response accuracy is shown for premise pairs BC and CD (from which the crtitical inference had to be made), for the AE probe, and for the critical BD probe. All animals performed well on the premise pairs and nearly perfectly on the AE pair. Normal rats performed as well on the BD probe as on the premise pairs (BC and CD), but rats with either type of hippocampal damage were severely impaired, and performed at no better than chance levels. From Eichenbaum (2001). Reprinted with permission from Eichenbaum, H. (2001). *The cognitive neuroscience of memory: An introduction.* Copyright 2001 by Oxford University Press.

merely to the novelty of the stimulus combination in a probe trial. In addition, none of the groups learned the new pairs when they were presented occasionally intermixed among presentations of premise pairs, indicating it was unlikely that performance on the BD probe was due to learning the correct choice across repetitions of that probe.

Finally, an additional and highly conservative measure was used to confirm the ability of rats to make the transitive inference. We compared the number of rats in each group that correctly chose B over D on the very first transitive probe trial, before any rewards were provided for choices on the probe. We found that 88% of normal animals made the correct transitive choice, whereas only 50% of rats with hippocampal disconnection made this choice. When all of these findings are combined, it is clear that some form of stimulus–stimulus representations can be acquired independently of the hippocampus itself. However, these representations are "hyperspecific"; that is, they can be expressed only within the confined context of a reproduction of the learning event (Schacter, 1985). Only a hippocampally mediated representation can support the flexible expression of associations among items within a larger relational organization.

NEURAL CODING

How does the hippocampus encode information such that it can support the capacity for remembering distinct experiences and linking them within a larger memory organization? A wealth of evidence indicates that hippocampal neurons respond to conjunctions of features, such as those defining spatial locations (O'Keefe, 1976), stimulus configurations (Fried, MacDonald, & Wilson 1997), and task-relevant behaviors (Berger, Alger, & Thompson, 1976). Combining these findings, we have suggested that the hippocampus encodes episodic memories as sequences of events and the places where they occur (Eichenbaum, Dudchenko, Wood, Shapiro, & Tanila, 1999). Importantly, these representations are proposed to contain two types of codings. Some involve episode-specific combinations of information, including the particular stimuli, behaviors, and places that define events unique to a particular experience. Other codings involve features of experiences that are shared across distinct episodes and therefore can serve to link them. Together the coding of distinct experiences as sequences of events and places, plus the codings of common features that connect related episodes, constitute the framework for a memory network that can support inferential memory expression.

There is substantial evidence that hippocampal neurons exhibit firing properties that include the representation of entire experiences, and include both codings that are specific to distinct experiences and codings that reflect common features among distinct episodes (see Eichenbaum et al., 1999). Virtually all experiments that have recorded the activity of hippocampal neurons in behaving animals report that the hippocampal network is continuously active, with individual cells firing for punctate periods in association with each sequential event during the flow of behavior. In addition, in virtually all situations where the behavioral sequences can be identified, the activity of individual hippocampal neurons is found to reflect both the ongoing behavior of the animal and the place where it occurs. For example, it is commonly observed that when rats perform the radial maze task, most hippocampal cells fire as an animal is moving through a particular place—either outward as the animal traverses a maze arm to obtain a reward, or inbound as the rat returns to the center of the maze (McNaughton, Barnes, & O'Keefe, 1983; Muller, Bostock, Taube, & Kubie, 1994). This combination of firing properties is not dependent on the physical structure of the maze, but occurs even in situations other than the radial maze. For example, it occurs in open fields, where the structure of the environment puts no physical constraint on the animal's movements (Markus et al., 1995; Wiener, Paul, & Eichenbaum, 1989).

In addition, there is an emerging body of evidence that hippocampal cells fire differentially in association with different kinds of experience within the same environment, such that largely different representations are constructed within the hippocampus whenever an animal appears to perceive two experiences within the environment as distinctive (Bostock, Muller, & Kubie, 1991; Gothard, Skaggs, Moore, & McNaughton, 1996; Markus et al., 1995; Skaggs & McNaughton, 1998). Importantly, in each of these situations, whereas many cells encode the events and places that are distinct to a particular type of experience, some cells encode features of the situation that are common between the experiences (Markus et al., 1995; Skaggs & McNaughton, 1998; Tanila, Shapiro, & Eichenbaum, 1997).

We (Wood, Dudchenko, & Eichenbaum, 1999) explored these properties in detail, using a protocol where rats performed the same task at several different locations in an environment. Rats were trained on a recognition memory task in which cups with scented sand were the relevant cues. On each trial a cup was placed in any of nine locations. Regardless of its location, the cup contained a reward if the odor was different from that of the previous cup (a nonmatch). Because the locations of the discriminative stimuli were varied systematically, cellular activity related to the stimuli and behavior could be dissociated from activity related to the animal's location. We found that individual hippocampal cells were active during each event during task performance, consistent with the idea that the hippocampus is involved in the representation of entire trial episodes. Some cells fired in association with highly specific combinations of stimuli, behavior, and location, consistent with the idea that the hippocampus encodes events that are unique to particular types of trial experiences. Other cells encoded a variety of the features that were common among types of trials. For example, some cells fired at a particular phase in the approach to any stimulus cup. Still others fired as a rat sampled a particular odor, regardless of its location. Others yet distinguished the match and nonmatch relationship between successive stimuli, independently of the odor or its location. And some cells fired only when the rat performed the task at a particular place, independent of the odor or its match–nonmatch status. In contrast to other characterizations of hippocampal cells as firing exclusively or primarily associated with the animal's instantaneous location (see, e.g., O'Keefe, 1999), in this situation where the same events occurred at several locations, the majority of cells with identifiable firing patterns showed specificity for nonspatial events equivalently across all locations. Furthermore, these nonspatial codings were as robust as spatial specificities observed in other cells. The combination of these observations indicates that all salient regularities of experience are captured in hippocampal neural activity; it confirms that hippocampal networks encode both complex actions and places that are unique to distinct experiences, and features that are common among them.

In addition, we (Wood, Dudchenko, Robitsek, & Eichenbaum, 2000) have found strong evidence that hippocampal networks represent distinct experiences even when spatial and behavioral features of performance are tightly controlled. In this study, rats performed a spatial alternation task in a T-maze. Each trial began with the rat at the base of the stem of the T, and commenced when the rat traversed the stem and then selected either the left- or the right-choice arm (Figure 28.2). Rewards were available at the end of each arm according to an alternation sequence. Thus a rat was required to distinguish between its left-turn and right-turn experiences, and to use its memory for the most recent experience to guide the current choice. Individual hippocampal cells fired as the rats passed through each of a sequence of locations while they traversed the maze within each trial. The key observation in this experiment was that the firing patterns of all the cells depended on

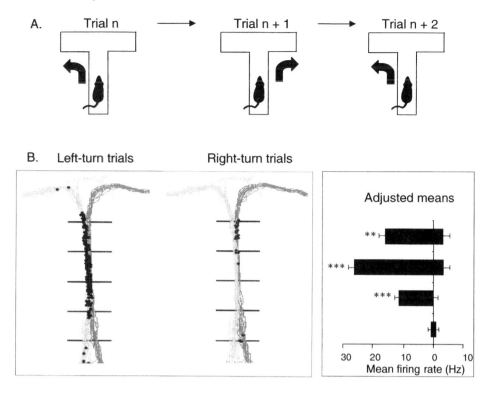

FIGURE 28.2. (A) The T-maze alternation task. In order to obtain a reward on each trial, the rat must traverse the central stem of the maze and then select the goal arm that was not visited on the previous trial. (B) Examples of a hippocampal cell that was active when a rat traversed the central stem of the T-maze. This cell fired almost exclusively as the rat performed a left-turn trial and hardly fired when the rat traversed the same location on the stem during right-turn trials. The left and middle panels show the paths taken by the animals on both trial types (light gray, left-turn trial; dark-gray, right-turn trial). The location of the rat when individual spikes occurred is indicated by dots separately for left-turn trials (left panel), and right-turn trials (middle panel). The right panel shows the mean firing rate of the cell, adjusted for variations in firing associated with the animal's speed, direction, and horizontal location, for each of four sectors of the stem. Asterisks indicate significant differences in firing rate on indicated sectors of the stem; $**p < .01$, $***p < .001$. Reprinted with permission from Eichenbaum, H. (2001). *The cognitive neuroscience of memory: An introduction.* Copyright 2001 by Oxford University Press.

whether the rat was in the midst of a left- or right-turn episode. That is, the cells fired differentially on left-turn or right-turn trials, even when a rat traveled through the same segments of the stem of the T and its overt behavior was identical on both types of trials. Indeed, detailed analyses indicated that minor variations in the animal's speed, direction of movement, or position within the relevant areas on the stem did not account for the different firing patterns on left-turn and right-turn trials for most of these cells. Although most cells showed a very strong differential activity (at least 8:1) on one trial type, some cells fired substantially when a rat was at the same point in the stem on either trial type, indicating a representation of the common spatial information between the two trial types. Thus the hippocampus encoded both the left-turn and right-turn experiences via distinct representations, and also encoded information that could link them though the common features (locations) of both experiences.

THE "MEMORY SPACE" MODEL OF DECLARATIVE MEMORY

In the experiments just described, and many more, the hippocampus has been found to play a critical role when distinct experiences must be encoded in relation to one another and linked within an organization that supports flexible, inferential memory expression. This conceptualization offers a framework for the seamless integration of capacities for episodic memory, semantic memory, and flexible memory expression as key properties of declarative memory observed in humans.

In addition, this model extends to animals as well, specifically within the domain of tests of transitive inference (Bunsey & Eichenbaum, 1996). Likewise, the findings on spatial learning can be construed as equally applicable to the model. For example, in the standard version of the Morris water maze, animals are trained on four distinct types of trials, each defined by a different starting point and swim path. These experiences contain substantial overlapping information because the swim paths from the four starting points intersect, making the same spatial information and information about movements in space common among the episodes. The representation that guides swimming from each starting point must be reconciled within a larger framework that allows an animal to find the escape platform from all of the starting points (Eichenbaum, Stewart, & Morris, 1990), and to use this framework to learn new escape locations (Steele & Morris, 1999; Whishaw & Tomie, 1997). Spatial learning of this type may be supported by a set of distinct representations of the separate swim paths, linked by codings of common information at the intersection points. In this conceptualization of spatial learning, the "space" of the maze is represented; however, the dimensions of representation are not formed in Cartesian coordinates, but rather from a set of path sequences and the intersections among them. This kind of spatial representation provides a realistic dimensional framework for a "cognitive map," and does so within a model equally applicable to spatial and nonspatial declarative memory.

The present conceptualization also offers an accounting of both the fundamental cognitive mechanisms mediated by the hippocampus and the coding scheme that underlies the proposed framework of linked episodic representations. The critical role of the hippocampus in episodic memory is envisioned as emerging from a combination of the broad range of inputs the hippocampus receives (Burwell, Witter, & Amaral, 1995; Suzuki & Amaral, 1994) and the unusually strong capacity of hippocampal neurons for plasticity that can mediate rapid encoding of conjunctions of simultaneously active inputs (Bliss & Collinridge, 1993). Thus individual hippocampal neurons are in a unique position to represent combinations of stimuli, actions, and the places where they occur as the elemental events constituting an episodic memory. In addition, because the hippocampal network is highly interconnected (Amaral & Witter, 1989), cells that fire in overlapping time periods are likely to increase their functional connectivity through the same plasticity mechanisms (McHugh, Blum, Tsien, Tonegawa, & Wilson, 1996), providing a basis for the representation of event sequences that compose the organized structure of episodic memories (see Wallenstein, Eichenbaum, Hasselmo, 1998).

Furthermore, to the extent that hippocampal cells can be reactivated by common features among different episodes, the same rapid plasticity mechanisms can shape the responses of some cells to serve as elements of multiple episodic representations, and so to link them into an integrated network. To the extent that representations of more and more experiences that contain common features are incorporated, all of the events within the network ultimately become fully interconnected. In this state the network may both provide access to the episodic memories from which it was constructed, and contain a large number of interconnections among highly repeated features common to many episodes. Such a highly interconnected network becomes virtually free of (albeit still connected to) the individual episodes of origin, and can compose the organization of a body of knowledge or semantic memory. In addition, these networks offer the capacity to link memories that are only indirectly and distantly related. This ability to "surf" the networks of episodic and semantic memory space may underlie a capacity to bring these indirectly related memories "to mind," and in this way may contribute to the experience of conscious recollection.

REFERENCES

Amaral, D. G., & Witter, M. P. (1989). The three-dimensional organization of the hippocampal formation: A review of anatomical data. *Neuroscience, 31,* 571–591

Berger, T. W., Alger, B. E., & Thompson, R. F. (1976). Neuronal substrates of classical conditioning in the hippocampus. *Science, 192,* 483–485.

Bliss, T. V. P., & Collinridge, G. L. (1993). A synaptic model of memory: Long-term potentiation in the hippocampus. *Nature, 361,* 31–39.

Bostock, E., Muller, R. U., & Kubie, J. L. (1991). Experience-dependent modifications of hippocampal place cell firing. *Hippocampus, 1,* 193–206.

Bunsey, M., & Eichenbaum, H. (1996). Conservation of hippocampal memory function in rats and humans. *Nature, 379,* 255–257.

Burwell, R. D., Witter, M. P., & Amaral, D. G. (1995). Perirhinal and postrhinal cortices in the rat: A review of the neuroanatomical literature and comparison with findings from the monkey brain. *Hippocampus, 5,* 390–408.

Cohen, N. J. (1984). Preserved learning capacity in amnesia: Evidence for multiple memory systems. In L. R. Squire & N. Butters (Eds)., *The Neuropsychology of memory* (pp. 83–103). New York: Guilford Press.

Cohen, N. J., & Squire, L. R. (1980). Preserved learning and retention of a pattern-analyzing skill in amnesia: Dissociation of knowing how and knowing that. *Science, 210,* 207–210.

Dusek, J. A., & Eichenbaum, H. (1997). The hippocampus and memory for orderly stimulus relations. *Proceedings of the National Academy of Sciences USA, 94,* 7109–7114.

Eichenbaum, H. (2001). *The cognitive neuroscience of memory: An introduction.* New York: Oxford University Press.

Eichenbaum, H., & Cohen, N. J. (2001). *From conditioning to conscious recollection: Memory systems of the brain.* New York: Oxford University Press.

Eichenbaum, H., Dudchenko, P., Wood, E., Shapiro, M., & Tanila, H. (1999). The hippocampus, memory, and place cells: Is it spatial memory or memory space? *Neuron, 23,* 1–20.

Eichenbaum, H., Stewart, C., & Morris, R .G. M. (1990). Hippocampal representation in spatial learning. *Journal of Neuroscience 10,* 331–339

Fried, I., MacDonald, K. A., & Wilson, C. L. (1997). Single neuron activity in human hippocampus and amygdala during recognition of faces and objects. *Neuron, 18,* 753–765.

Gothard, K. M., Skaggs, W. E., Moore, K. M., & McNaughton, B. L. (1996). Binding of hippocampal CA1 neural activity to multiple reference frames in a landmark-based navigation task. *Journal of Neuroscience, 16,* 823–835.

Markus, E. J., Qin, Y.-L., Leonard, B., Skaggs, W. E., McNaughton, B. L., & Barnes, C. A. (1995). Interactions between location and task affect the spatial and directional firing of hippocampal neurons. *Journal of Neuroscience, 15,* 7079–7094.

McHugh, T. J., Blum, K. I., Tsien, J. Z., Tonegawa, S., & Wilson, M. A. (1996). Impaired hippocampal representation of space in CA1-specific NMDAR1 knockout mice. *Cell, 87,* 1339–1349.

McNaughton, B. L., Barnes, C. A., & O'Keefe, J. (1983). The contributions of position, direction, and velocity to single unit activity in the hippocampus of freely-moving rats. *Experimental Brain Research, 52,* 41–49.

Muller, R. U., Bostock, E., Taube, J. S., & Kubie, J. L. (1994). On the directional firing properties of hippocampal place cells. *Journal of Neuroscience, 14*, 7235–7251.

O'Keefe, J. A. (1976). Place units in the hippocampus of the freely moving rat. *Experimental Neurology, 51*, 78–109

O'Keefe, J. A. (1999). Do hippocampal pyramidal cells signal non-spatial as well as spatial information? *Hippocampus, 9*, 352–364.

Piaget, J. (1928). *Judgment and reasoning in the child*. London: Kegan, Paul, Trench, and Trubner.

Schacter, D. L. (1985). Multiple forms of memory in humans and animals. In N. M. Weinberger, J. L. McGaugh, & G. Lynch, (Eds.), *Memory systems of the brain* (pp. 351–380). New York: Guilford Press.

Schacter, D. L., & Tulving, E. (Eds.). (1994). *Memory systems 1994*. Cambridge, MA: MIT Press.

Skaggs, W. E., & McNaughton, B. L. (1998). Spatial firing properties of hippocampal CA1 populations in an environment containing two visually identical regions. *Journal of Neuroscience, 18*, 8455–8466.

Squire, L. R., & Zola, S. M. (1998). Episodic memory, semantic memory and amnesia. *Hippocampus, 8*(3), 205–211.

Steele, R. J., & Morris, R. G. M. (1999). Delay dependent impairment in matching-to-place task with chronic and intrahippocampal infusion of the NMDA-antagonist D-AP5. *Hippocampus, 9*, 118–136.

Suzuki, W. A., & Amaral, D. G. (1994). Perirhinal and parahippocamal cortices of the macaque monkey: Cortical afferents. *Journal of Comparative Neurology, 350*, 497–533.

Tanila, H., Shapiro, M. L., & Eichenbaum, H. E. (1997). Discordance of spatial representation in ensembles of hippocampal place cells. *Hippocampus, 7*, 613–623.

Vargha-Khadem, F., Gadian, D. G., Watkins, K. E., Connelly, A., Van Paesschen, W., & Mishkin, M. (1997). Differential effects of early hippocampal pathology on episodic and semantic memory. *Science, 277*, 376–380.

Wallenstein, G. V., Eichenbaum, H., & Hasselmo, M. E. (1998). The hippocampus as an associator of discontiguous events. *Trends in Neurosciences, 21*, 315–365.

Whishaw, I. Q., & Tomie, J. (1997). Perseveration on place reversals in spatial swimming pool tasks: Further evidence for place learning in hippocampal rats. *Hippocampus, 7*(3), 361–370.

Wiener, S. I., Paul, C. A., & Eichenbaum, H. (1989). Spatial and behavioral correlates of hippocampal neuronal activity. *Journal of Neuroscience, 9*, 2737–2763.

Wood, E. R., Dudchenko, P. A., & Eichenbaum, H. (1999). The global record of memory in hippocampal neuronal activity. *Nature, 397*, 613–616.

Wood, E. R., Dudchenko, P. A., Robitsek, J. R., & Eichenbaum, H. (2000). Hippocampal neurons encode information about different types of memory episodes occurring in the same location. *Neuron, 27*, 623–633.

29

Representation of Spatial Information by Dynamic Neuronal Circuits in the Hippocampus

EDVARD I. MOSER, STIG A. HOLLUP,
and MAY-BRITT MOSER

Converging evidence suggests that the hippocampus is essential for a range of memory functions (Squire, 1992). One type of memory that depends on the hippocampus in many species is the ability to remember locations defined by landmark arrangements. There is a strong activation of the hippocampus when animals or humans recall routes that move through spatially complex environments (Bontempi, Laurent-Demir, Destrade, & Jaffard, 1999; Maguire, Frackowiak, & Frith, 1997; Maguire et al., 1998). The strongest activation is seen when the retrieved memories are recent (Bontempi et al., 1999). Lesions of the hippocampus disrupt the acquisition of spatial memory in rats (Jarrard, 1978; Morris, Garrud, Rawlins, & O'Keefe, 1982; Morris, Schenk, Tweedie, & Jarrard, 1990) as well as humans (Cave & Squire, 1991; Teng & Squire, 1999), suggesting that the integrity of the hippocampus may be necessary for encoding of new spatial memories.

What neuronal computations are responsible for the activation of the hippocampus during the processing of spatial memory? It is well established that principal cells in the hippocampus exhibit location-specific firing (O'Keefe & Dostrovsky, 1971; O'Keefe & Nadel, 1978; Wilson & McNaughton, 1993), but we know little about how this type of activity leads to spatial memory. A complete understanding of the operations by which memory is encoded, stored, and retrieved may require a multilevel approach that addresses mechanisms at the molecular, cellular, circuit, and systems levels. The present chapter reviews experiments in which we have examined the plasticity of hippocampal circuits in behaving animals by a parallel cellular and systems approach.

HIPPOCAMPAL MEMORY CIRCUITS
ARE DYNAMIC AND DISTRIBUTED

What types of neurons participate in specific hippocampal representations, and where are they located? Is memory processed by preconfigured ensembles, or are the ensembles dynamic? And are the representations localized or distributed within the hippocampus?

One clue to questions such as these is the largely parallel orientation of the excitatory pathways of the hippocampus, which repeats itself all the way from the septal pole to the temporal pole of the hippocampus (Andersen, Bliss, & Skrede, 1971; Tamamaki, Abe, & Nojyo, 1987; Tamamaki & Nojyo, 1990). These serial connections may contain the necessary circuitry for encoding, storage, and retrieval of memory, in which case a single event may be represented completely within a narrow band through the hippocampus. Different bands may represent different events and may function as semi-independent modules (Hampson, Simeral, & Deadwyler, 1999). On the other hand, these parallel pathways contain many axons that diverge from the typical direction, and there are longitudinally oriented fibers that interconnect different levels of the CA3 field and dentate hilus (Amaral & Witter, 1989; Ishizuka, Weber, & Amaral, 1990; Li, Somogyi, Ylinen, & Buzsáki, 1994). These divergent and collateral systems provide a powerful substrate for associating inputs that enter at distributed sites along the septotemporal axis of the hippocampus (Hasselmo, Schnell, & Barkai, 1995; Marr, 1971; McNaughton & Morris, 1987; Treves & Rolls, 1994). Thus the anatomical organization of the hippocampus does not indicate whether hippocampal memory representations are localized or distributed, or whether their composition is static or dynamic.

If representations are distributed, large amounts of tissue may be required for several crucial hippocampus-dependent memory functions, and small lesions may be sufficient for disrupting these operations. If the representations are localized, impairments should in most cases be seen only after substantial damage. We examined the extent of hippocampal tissue required for solving a reference memory task in the Morris water maze. Rats received hippocampal lesions of varying size and were then trained. Under these conditions, rats were able to learn in spite of damage to large fractions of the hippocampus (Moser, Moser, & Andersen, 1993; Moser, Moser, Forrest, Andersen, & Morris, 1995). If the remaining tissue was in the dorsal part of the structure, successful learning was observed when as much as 75% of the hippocampus was removed. Animals with remnants in the intermediate one-third of the hippocampus learned as well as those with a remnant in the septal one-third (Moser, Tollefsrud, Moser, & Andersen, 1997). These findings suggest that a small circuit is sufficient for acquisition of a spatial reference memory task. The same task can be acquired and retained with two nonoverlapping neuronal ensembles within the dorsal hippocampus, suggesting that spatial learning may be localized, but does not depend on a geographically constant group of neurons.

However, the fact that animals can learn with a localized network of hippocampal neurons after a partial hippocampal lesion does not imply that representations are localized in the intact brain. It is possible that spatial memory is established by whatever hippocampal circuits are available, and that representations are distributed across a large extent of the hippocampus when relevant neurons are available throughout the structure. We tested this hypothesis by first training rats to asymptotic performance levels in a Morris water maze task and then making hippocampal lesions of varying size at varying locations (Moser & Moser, 1998). Retention was tested 1 week later. If the representation were localized, performance would in most cases be compromised only after extensive damage. If it were distributed, impairments might generally be seen after small lesions as long as the entire ensemble had to be reactivated for successful retrieval. The findings support the latter alternative (see A and C in Figure 29.1). Retention was disrupted by damage to 20% or less of the total hippocampal tissue, provided that these small lesions were in the dorsal two-thirds of the hippocampus. Anterior and caudal damage to the dorsal hippocampus had similar effects. New learning was not affected in animals with lesions of this magnitude (see Figure 29.1B). When learning occurred after the lesion, the animals were able to remember the new information for at least 1 week (see Figure 29.2).

Thus, if the brain is intact during encoding, individual spatial environments are likely to be represented by highly distributed circuits. However, smaller regions can perform retention functions when the avilable circuitry during encoding is small. These results suggest that hippocampal place representations are set up dynamically. Once an ensemble is formed, its integrity is necessary for subsequent retrieval, suggesting that specific spatial information is stored across the entire ensemble. Studies of place cells have shown that these cells are organized in a nontopographical manner, with each location represented at multiple septotemporal levels of the hippocampus (Jung, Wiener, & McNaughton, 1994; O'Keefe & Nadel, 1978). The lesion data suggest that place cells at widely different levels of the structure may contribute to the same spatial representation.

SYNAPTIC PLASTICITY IN DISTRIBUTED CIRCUITS

The studies described above suggest that the formation of specific neuronal representations is a highly plastic process, but that new functional circuits remain relatively stable once they are established. What cellular mechanisms could underlie the formation of such functional circuits?

Converging evidence suggests that information is stored by activity-dependent changes in the strength of selected synapses in distributed networks of the hippocampus (Martin, Grimwood, & Morris, 2000; McNaughton & Morris, 1987). The main experimental model for activity-dependent plasticity in mammals is long-term potentiation (LTP). LTP is a long-lasting enhancement of synaptic transmission that can be induced by afferent high-frequency stimulation in all major excitatory synaptic populations of the hippocampal formation (Bliss & Lømo, 1973; Malenka & Nicoll, 1999). This type of stimulation occurs naturally during learning episodes (Larson & Lynch, 1986; Ranck, 1973) and sleep (Buzsáki, Horvath, Urioste, Hetke, & Wise, 1992), and it has been proposed that changes in synaptic strength resulting from such bursts may be necessary for formation and stabilization of memory traces (Buzsáki, 1989; Martin et al., 2000; McNaughton & Morris, 1987).

Although hippocampal LTP is possibly required for some aspects of spatial learning, it is not known how synaptic changes contribute to memory storage. It has been proposed that memories are stored as spatial patterns of potentiated and unpotentiated synapses within a distributed network, and that successful retrieval requires that the pattern of connection strengths induced by a particular learning experience be retained and reactivated (Marr, 1971; McNaughton & Morris, 1987). If so, events that interfere with the distinctness of these patterns might result in impaired retention (Figure 29.3A). We tested this idea by first training animals in the water maze, then inducing widespread LTP in the hippocampus and subsequently measuring retention (Brun, Ytterbø, Morris, Moser, & Moser, 2001). Performance was at chance levels after LTP induction, but was not affected by low-frequency control stimulation (Figure 29.3B). Saturation of the capacity for LTP was not

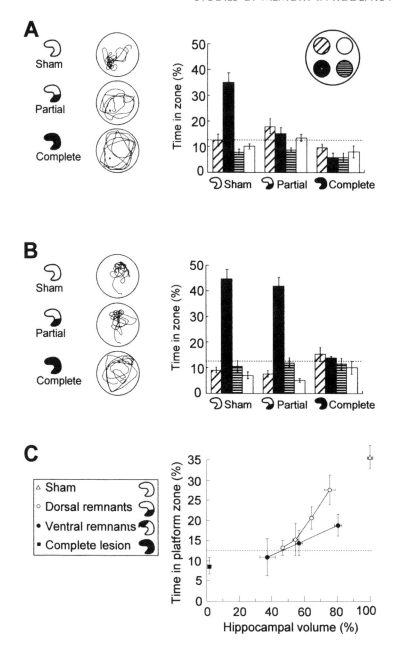

FIGURE 29.1. Impaired retention of spatial memory in a water maze after small hippocampal lesions. Rats received either complete or partial hippocampal lesions, or sham surgery. Training was conducted in two water maze environments. The lesions were made after the animals were trained to asymptotic performance in one of the environments. (A) Retention 7 days after pretraining and surgery. *Left column:* Typical swim paths. *Right column:* Time spent in a circular zone around the platform position (black) and in corresponding zones of the three other quadrants (means ± *SEM*). (B) Retention following subsequent training in a new environment (same rats). Symbols as in A. (C) Retention of the first task (A) as a function of hippocampal volume in animals with dorsal remnants (10% bins) or ventral remnants (20% bins). Stippled lines indicate chance level. From Moser and Moser (1998). Copyright 1998 by the Society for Neuroscience. Adapted by permission.

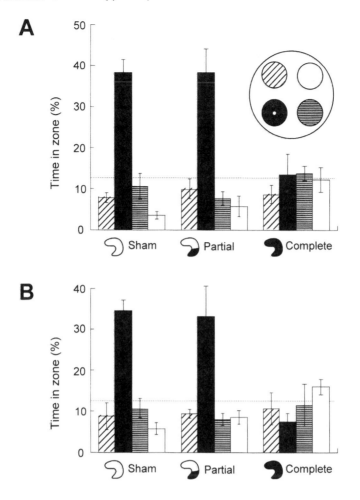

FIGURE 29.2. Retention in animals that received all training after a hippocampal lesion. Time spent in the platform zone was measured at the end of training (A) and 7 days after the last training trial (B). The lesions were of the same type as in Figure 29.1. Symbols as in Figure 29.1. From Moser and Moser (1998). Copyright 1998 by the Society for Neuroscience. Adapted by permission.

necessary for the deficit to be expressed. When LTP was blocked by an N-methly-D-aspartate receptor antagonist, memory was not attenuated (Brun et al., 2001). These data suggest that the pattern of connection strengths may be relevant for retention of spatial memory, and they are consistent with the proposal that memory is stored as distributed patterns of synaptic weights.

As in the lesion studies, the retention deficit was memory-selective. Provided that the animals had received pretraining in a different water maze, LTP did not impair new learning (Brun et al., 2001; Otnæss, Brun, Moser, & Moser, 1999). This finding suggests that there may be multiple circuits and mechanisms for spatial memory, and that knocking out one of them may not always be sufficient to result in a deficit. When plasticity is blocked in one set of hippocampal synapses, new information may be encoded by another ensemble or another mechanism. Once a memory is stored, however, maintenance of the same synaptic weight pattern is critical for retention.

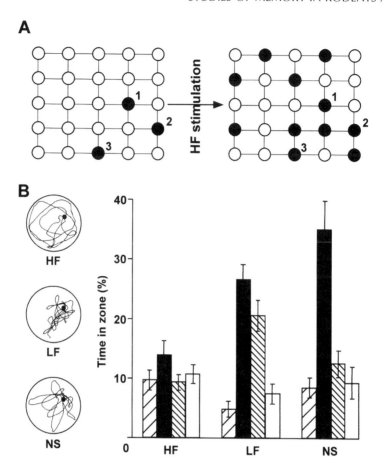

FIGURE 29.3. (A) Widespread LTP induction may disrupt the spatial pattern of potentiated and unpotentiated synapses (black and white circles, respectively) in a hippocampal neural network. *Left:* Hypothesized network after learning, showing potentiation of a few synapses (1–3). *Right:* Same network after subsequent induction of LTP. Synapses that were potentiated during learning (1–3) may not be distinguishable from those that were potentiated by electrical stimulation. (B) Effect of LTP on retention of spatial memory in a water maze (means ± *SEM*). The retention test was conducted 2 hours after stimulation was terminated. Rats that received LTP (high-frequency stimulation, HF) had apparently random search patterns. Rats that received low-frequency control stimulation (LF) performed significantly better. Symbols as in Figure 29.1. From Brun, Ytterbø, Morris, Moser, and Moser (2001). Copyright 2001 by the Society for Neuroscience. Adapted by permission.

PLASTICITY OF SPATIAL REPRESENTATIONS IN HIPPOCAMPAL PYRAMIDAL NEURONS

The data from the lesion and field potential studies suggest that hippocampal representations are highly dynamic, and thus they imply that individual neurons may exhibit significant plasticity in their firing properties. Not all cells may exhibit such plasticity, however, and different functions are likely to be performed by different cells. In order to understand how the individual neurons of a hippocampal circuit contribute to its collective functions, it would be useful to record signals from individual cells of the network as rats perform well-defined memory operations. Parallel recording from multiple separable hippocampal units has the power needed for determining whether there is a relation between firing properties of individual neurons and what the animal learns, whether different neurons perform different functions, and finally whether the observed changes in firing properties are instrumental in memory storage mediated by the hippocampus.

Most hippocampal pyramidal cells exhibit strong location-specific activity (O'Keefe & Dostrovsky, 1971). When animals explore simple environments (e.g., open fields or elevated tracks), the "place fields" of anatomically proximate hippocampal neurons collectively cover the entire environment, with an apparently equal representation of all parts of the recording arena (Wilson & McNaughton, 1993; Redish et al., 2001). However, if hippocampal neurons express information that is crucial for solving spatial memory tasks, such a homogeneous distribution would not necessarily be expected when the memory demands are increased. Trajectories from start to goal usually contain places that are more significant for successful retrieval than others—such as start locations, turning points, and goal locations—and one might ask whether neurons that contribute to retrieval of successful routes fire at such locations in particular. To approach this question, we examined whether the goal location was represented differently from the off-target areas, and whether any such differences were influenced by what was learned by the animal.

Because most spatial learning tasks are goal-directed, studies of hippocampal cells in such tasks must deal with the fact that a well-trained rat rarely visits regions that are not on the trajectory toward the goal. To study relations between pyramidal activity and memory, we developed an annular version of the Morris water maze in which all areas of the pool would be sampled by a rat, even after prolonged training. Two circular transparent walls were centered in the pool, and an escape platform was hidden at one of four possible positions within the corridor. The platform could be raised or submerged by remote control. The rats were always required to swim at least one full lap before the platform was made available. When the platform position was constant, normal animals slowed down each time they passed the target area, indicating that they knew where the platform used to be positioned. Rats with hippocampal lesions, in contrast, failed to exhibit any change in swim velocity. The lesioned rats did slow down and escape in a cued version of the task, in which a visible platform was placed on the other side of an opening in one of the corridor walls (Hollup, Kjelstrup, Hoff, Moser, & Moser, 2001). These studies suggest that the hippocampus is necessary for recognition of the goal location.

We prepared a group of animals for single-unit recording and pretrained them with either a constant or a variable platform location in the annular water maze. Signals from hippocampal pyramidal cells were recorded during several blocks of swimming, including a set of probe trials in which the platform remained unavailable for 60 seconds (Hollup, Molden, Donnett, Moser, & Moser, 2001). Most pyramidal cells had distinct, focused, and stable place fields (Figure 29.4), similar to those observed in linear environments on dry land (Gothard, Skaggs, & McNaughton, 1996; McNaughton, Barnes, & O'Keefe, 1983; O'Keefe & Recce, 1993). However, in rats that were trained with a constant platform location, a large number of neurons exhibited increased activity as the animal passed the goal area on the probe trials (Figure 29.5). Cells were more likely to have firing fields near the platform than in equally large areas elsewhere in the corridor (Figure 29.6). This effect was independent of swim direction and was expressed with all four platform positions (in different rats). The place fields did not cluster when the rats were trained with a randomly varied platform position, suggesting that the effect depended on what was learned by the animal. The data are consistent with previous claims that firing fields accumulate near salient objects or places of particular importance (Breese, Hampson, & Deadwyler, 1989; Eichen-

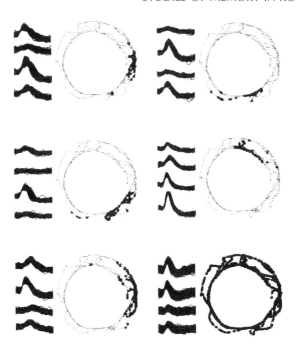

FIGURE 29.4. Place correlates of hippocampal pyramidal cells in a probe trial in an annular water maze. All cells are from the same tetrode. Individual spikes (black squares) of five pyramidal cells (first five panels) and one theta cell (bottom right panel) are superimposed on the swim path. Superimposed waveforms as recorded on each wire of the tetrode are displayed to the left of each place field. During training, the platform had always been in the southeast part of the corridor. The rat swam counterclockwise during 89.3% of the trial. From Hollup, Molden, Donnett, Moser, and Moser (2001). Copyright 2001 by the Society for Neuroscience. Adapted by permission.

baum, Kuperstein, Fagan, & Nagode, 1987; Gothard, Skaggs, Moore, & McNaughton, 1996; Hetherington & Shapiro, 1997; Wood, Dudchenko, & Eichenbaum, 1999). In the water task, however, the salient object (the platform) was not present during the recording, and so its influence on neuronal firing must have depended on associations between the remembered platform and external landmarks.

Further study showed that firing fields did not accumulate at the goal because of changes in state or ongoing behavior. Hippocampal theta activity was maintained as the rat swam over the platform. There was no difference in the power of the theta oscillations inside and outside the platform region, and there was no indication of large-amplitude irregular activity, which might have caused otherwise silent cells to fire (Buzsáki et al., 1992; Thompson & Best, 1989). Additional analyses established that there was no enhancement of firing rates as a consequence of the change in linear and angular speed in the target area. Slow swimming was not accompanied by enhanced firing when it occurred outside the platform segment (Figure 29.7). This observation confirms previous work showing that running speed does not affect background firing in place cells outside their place fields (Czurkó, Hirase, Csicsvari, & Buzsáki, 1999).

What information was actually coded by rats with firing fields in the platform area? Did they represent location only, or was the activity related to the goal characteristics of the place? On the one hand, it is possible that ordinary place fields concentrated around the platform because a rat was more attentive at this position when the spatial map was

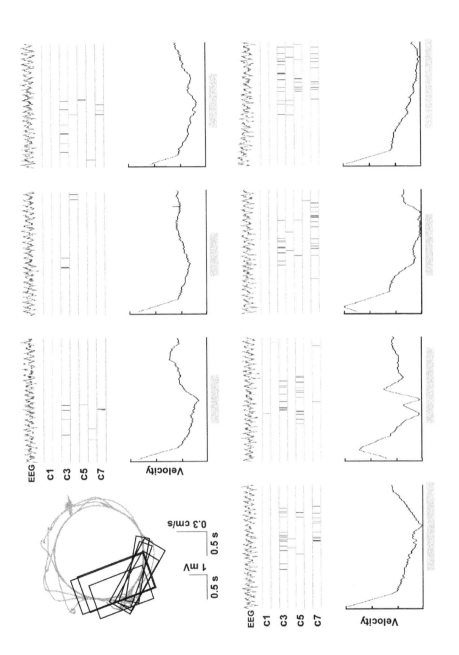

FIGURE 29.5. Enhanced activity of hippocampal neurons at the expected platform location (southwest area of the corridor). All data were recorded in the absence of the platform. *Upper left panel:* Swim path (grey). The direction was clockwise. Rectangles (black) indicate path fragments displayed to the right and below. *Remaining panels:* A total of seven fragments of 3 seconds each showing hippocampal theta activity, spike occurrence, and swim speed as a rat passed over the unavailable platform (one diagram for each crossing; seven pyramidal cells, c1–c7, in each diagram). Swimming over the platform (± 10 cm) is indicated by a grey bar below each diagram. As the rat passed over the target, there was a significant increase in the activity of several, but not all, recorded units. Swim velocity decreased, but the theta oscillations were maintained. Data from Hollup et al. (2001).

369

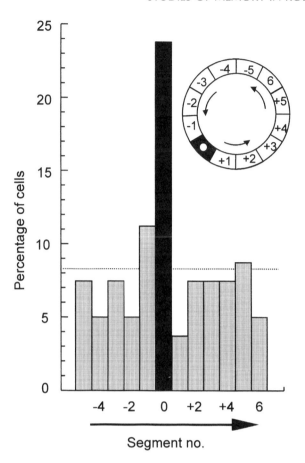

FIGURE 29.6. Distribution of firing fields during probe trials in which the platform was absent. The corridor was divided into 12 equally large segments, with the platform in the center of one of them (inset). The number of cells with firing fields in the platform segment was significantly larger than the number in any other segment (total of 80 pyramidal cells). The location of a firing field was defined as the segment with the maximum average firing rate for that cell. To avoid artifacts imposed by increased bidirectional sampling in the platform area, only data sampled in the animal's preferred swim direction (clockwise or counterclockwise) were analyzed. The chance level is indicated by a stippled line. Arrows indicate swim direction. From Hollup, Molden, Donnett, Moser, and Moser (2001). Copyright 2001 by the Society for Neuroscience. Adapted by permission.

established. On the other hand, firing in these cells may have been related to the rat's retrieval of memory about the hidden platform. These interpretations can be dissociated by a reversal test in which the goal is moved. The "attention" hypothesis predicts that activity at the old platform position should outlast the reversal and remain elevated at the original location. The "memory" hypothesis predicts that some of the firing at the platform location will follow the platform to its new position.

We have recorded neuronal activity after reversal in a limited and preliminary sample. Most place fields, including a significant fraction of those with peaks at the original platform location, remained relatively stable following the reversal. However, we identified a small number of cells that exhibited a partial shift of activity from the original platform position to the new location. Figure 29.8 shows such a cell. On the three probe tests be-

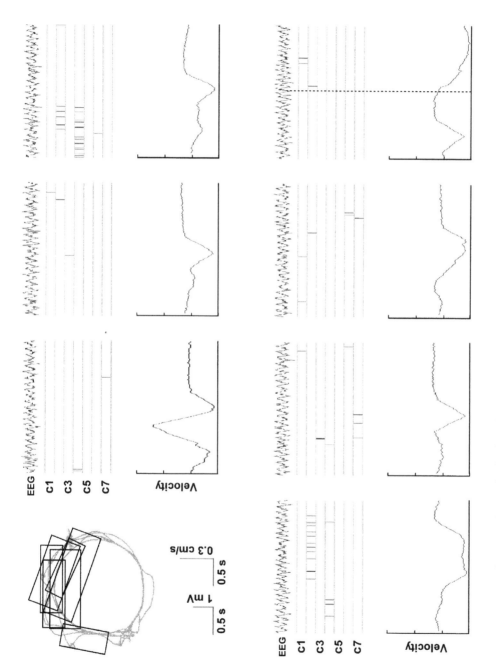

FIGURE 29.7. Unit activity during each epoch of reduced speed outside the platform area. Same trial and same symbols as in Figure 29.5. The stippled vertical line in the final diagram indicates when the rat entered the platform at a new location. The figure shows that outside the platform segment, reduced linear speed (accompanied by increased angular speed) did not lead to increased spike activity. Data from Hollup et al. (2001).

371

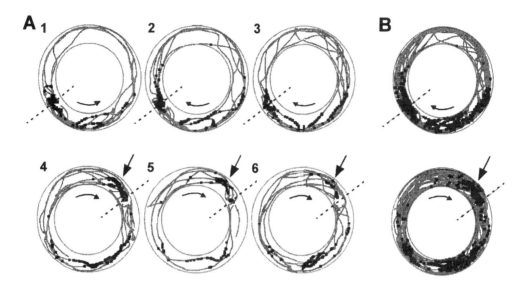

FIGURE 29.8. Firing fields of a single CA1 pyramidal cell before and after reversal of the platform position. The unit fired at the platform location before the platform was moved. (A) Firing field of the unit on probe trials before (1–3) and after (4–6) the platform was moved from southwest to northeast (symbols as in Figure 29.4). Firing rates decreased at the original target position and increased at the new position (thick arrows). (B) Superimposed firing fields from all probe tests and intervening training trials (sampled only during swimming) before (top) and after (bottom) reversal.

fore reversal, the cell fired selectively at the platform location in the southwest segment. After reversal, the cell maintained some activity at this location, but also started to fire at the new goal location in the northeast segment, where no spikes had been recorded before. This change was expressed already on the first probe test four trials after the platform had been moved. On this trial, the rat also reduced its swim velocity as it passed the target area, indicating that it had learned the new position. The spikes at the new location were likely to originate from the same cell as those recorded at the original location; however, given the limitations of current unit analysis techniques (Harris, Henze, Csicsvari, Hirase, & Buzsáki, 2000), we cannot strictly prove this point (Figure 29.9).

It remains to be established whether only cells with fields at the goal location exhibited changes in firing location. Reversal of the platform position may have caused a general remapping, with new firing correlates in many or most cells, and not only those that fired in the platform area before reversal (Bostock, Muller, & Kubie, 1991; Muller & Kubie, 1987). It is hard to make conclusive statements about the specificity of the effect without recording simultaneously from a large number of cells. To demonstrate goal-related activity specifically and unequivocally, it may be necessary to record from many tetrodes in parallel.

CONCLUSION

The studies described above were all motivated by the same question: How is memory stored in circuits of hippocampal neurons? We have shown that local circuits are capable of representing spatial information if only small areas or small numbers of synapses are available during encoding. However, when the entire hippocampal network is available at the

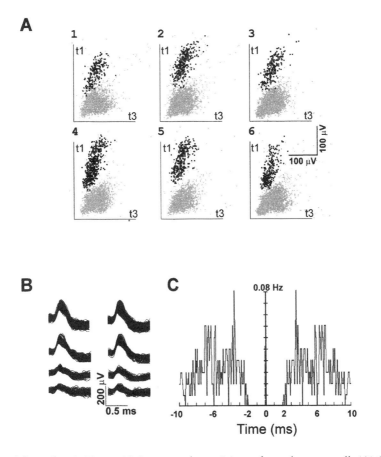

FIGURE 29.9. The spikes in Figure 29.8 appeared to originate from the same cell. (A) Scatter diagrams showing that the same unit (black) was recorded before (1–3) and after (4–6) reversal. Each panel shows peak-to-peak spike amplitudes for one pair of electrodes (t1 vs. t3) within the recording tetrode. The relatively large variation in spike amplitudes was due to strong complex spiking. Crosscorrelation analyses showed that within the range of 2–10 milliseconds, the spikes with small amplitudes tended to succeed those with larger amplitudes. (B) Superimposed waveforms from the isolated unit on each tetrode wire (left) and after (right) the platform was moved. (C) Autocorrelation analysis of the cluster in A. The absence of spikes during the refractory period (2 milliseconds) would be expected if the spikes originated from the same cell.

encoding moment, subsequent retention appears to require a widely distributed circuit within the dorsal hippocampus. The data further suggest that the maintenance of specific patterns of potentiated and unpotentiated synapses is likely to be essential for successful retention of spatial memory. Finally, learning appears to influence the distribution of firing fields in an annular water maze, suggesting that pyramidal cell activity matches the behavioral significance of places in the memory task. When an animal expected to find the platform at a constant location, a large number of place cells fired at this place. Because the platform was not present during the recording, any control that it exerted on hippocampal firing rates must have been mediated via the rat's long-term memory. The hippocampus-dependent nature of the task suggests that such memory-related activity may have had a critical function during the recognition and recall processes that took place as the animal swam over the goal location.

Little is known about the subcellular mechanisms responsible for plastic changes in firing correlates of hippocampal neurons. Long-term maintenance of place fields appears to be impaired by the same treatments that disrupt LTP in the CA1 (Kentros et al., 1998; McHugh, Blum, Tsien, Tonegawa, & Wilson, 1996); however, it is not understood how synaptic potentiation influences the signaling properties of hippocampal neurons, or how synaptic changes are encoded and retrieved by circuits of hippocampal neurons. One way to approach these issues might be to start with a direct demonstration of enhanced transmission between coupled pairs of neurons during learning. To achieve this goal, it would be essential to combine methods for parallel recording from multiple distinguishable neurons with methods for assessment of synaptic strength, and it would probably be necessary to implement the new techniques in a hippocampus-dependent memory task such as the annular water maze.

REFERENCES

Amaral, D. G., & Witter, M. P. (1989). The three-dimensional organization of the hippocampal formation: A review of anatomical data. *Neuroscience, 31,* 571–591.

Andersen, P., Bliss, T. V. P., & Skrede, K. K. (1971). Lamellar organization of hippocampal excitatory pathways. *Experimental Brain Research, 13,* 222–238.

Bliss, T. V. P., & Lømo, T. (1973). Long-lasting potentiation of synaptic transmission in the dentate area of the anaesthetized rabbit following stimulation of the perforant path. *Journal of Physiology (London), 232,* 331–356.

Bontempi, B., Laurent-Demir, C., Destrade, C., & Jaffard, R. (1999). Time-dependent reorganization of brain circuitry underlying long-term memory storage. *Nature, 400,* 671–675.

Bostock, E., Muller, R. U., & Kubie, J. L. (1991). Experience-dependent modifications of hippocampal place cell firing. *Hippocampus, 1,* 193–205.

Breese, C. R., Hampson, R. E., & Deadwyler, S. A. (1989). Hippocampal place cells: Stereotypy and plasticity. *Journal of Neuroscience, 9,* 1097–1111.

Brun, V. H., Ytterbø, K., Morris, R. G. M., Moser, M.-B., & Moser, E. I. (2001). Retrograde amnesia for spatial memory induced by NMDA receptor-mediated long-term potentiation. *Journal of Neuroscience, 21,* 356–362.

Buzsáki, G. (1989). Two-stage model of memory trace formation: A role for "noisy" brain states. *Neuroscience, 31,* 551–570.

Buzsáki, G., Horvath, Z., Urioste, R., Hetke, J., & Wise, K. (1992). High-frequency network oscillation in the hippocampus. *Science, 256,* 1025–1027.

Cave, C. B., & Squire, L. R. (1991). Equivalent impairment of spatial and nonspatial memory following damage to the human hippocampus. *Hippocampus, 1,* 329–340.

Czurkó, A., Hirase, H., Csicsvari, J., & Buzsáki, G. (1999). Sustained activation of hippocampal pyramidal cells by 'space clamping' in a running wheel. *European Journal of Neuroscience, 11,* 344–352.

Eichenbaum, H., Kuperstein, M., Fagan, A., & Nagode, J. (1987). Cue-sampling and goal-approach correlates of hippocampal unit activity in rats performing an odour-discrimination task. *Journal of Neuroscience, 7,* 716–732.

Gothard, K. M., Skaggs, W. E., & McNaughton, B. L. (1996). Dynamics of mismatch correction in the hippocampal ensemble code for space: Interaction between path integration and environmental cues. *Journal of Neuroscience, 16,* 8027–8040.

Gothard, K. M., Skaggs, W. E., Moore, K. M., & McNaughton, B. L. (1996). Binding of hippocampal CA1 neural activity to multiple reference frames in a landmark-based navigation task. *Journal of Neuroscience, 16,* 823–835.

Hampson, R. E., Simeral, J. D., & Deadwyler, S. A. (1999). Distribution of spatial and nonspatial information in dorsal hippocampus. *Nature, 402,* 610–614.

Harris, K. D., Henze, D. A., Csicsvari, J., Hirase, H., & Buzsáki, G. (2000). Accuracy of tetrode spike separation as determined by simultaneous intracellular and extracellular measurements. *Journal of Neurophysiology, 84*, 401–414.

Hasselmo, M. E., Schnell, E., & Barkai, E. (1995). Dynamics of learning and recall at excitatory recurrent synapses and cholinergic modulation in rat hippocampal region CA3. *Journal of Neuroscience, 15*, 5249–5282.

Hetherington, P. A., & Shapiro, M. L. (1997). Hippocampal place fields are altered by the removal of single visual cues in a distance-dependent manner. *Behavioral Neuroscience, 111*, 20–34.

Hollup, S., Kjelstrup, K. G., Hoff, J., Moser, M.-B., & Moser, E. I. (2001). Impaired recognition of the goal location during spatial navigation in rats with hippocampal lesions. *Journal of Neuroscience, 21*, 4505–4513.

Hollup, S., Molden, S., Donnett, J. G., Moser, M.-B., & Moser, E. I. (2001). Accumulation of hippocampal place fields at the goal location in an annular watermaze task. *Journal of Neuroscience, 21*, 1635–1644.

Ishizuka, N., Weber, J., & Amaral, D. G. (1990). Organization of intrahippocampal projections originating from CA3 pyramidal cells in the rat. *Journal of Comparative Neurology, 295*, 580–623.

Jarrard, L. E. (1978). Selective hippocampal lesions: Differential effects on performance by rats of a spatial task with preoperative versus postoperative training. *Journal of Comparative Physiology and Psychology, 92*, 1119–1127.

Jung, M. W., Wiener, S. I., & McNaughton, B. L. (1994). Comparison of spatial firing characteristics of units in dorsal and ventral hippocampus of the rat. *Journal of Neuroscience, 14*, 7347–7356.

Kentros, C., Hargreaves, E., Hawkins, R. D., Kandel, E. R., Shapiro, M., & Muller, R. U. (1998). Abolition of long-term stability of new hippocampal place cell maps by NMDA receptor blockade. *Science, 280*, 2121–2126.

Larson, J., & Lynch, G. (1986). Induction of synaptic potentiation in hippocampus by patterned stimulation involves two events. *Science, 232*, 985–988.

Li, A., Somogyi, P., Ylinen, A., & Buzsáki, G. (1994). The hippocampal CA3 network: An *in vivo* intracellular labeling study. *Journal of Comparative Neurology, 339*, 181–208.

Maguire, E. A., Burgess, N., Donnett, J. G., Frackowiak, R. S., Frith, C. D., & O'Keefe, J. (1998). Knowing where and getting there: A human navigation network. *Science, 280*, 921–924.

Maguire, E. A., Frackowiak, R. S. J., & Frith, C. D. (1997). Recalling routes around London: activation of the right hippocampus in taxi drivers. *Journal of Neuroscience, 17*, 7103–7110.

Malenka, R. C., & Nicoll, R. A. (1999). Long-term potentiation—a decade of progress? *Science, 285*, 1870–1874.

Marr, D. (1971). Simple memory: A theory of archicortex. *Philosophical Transactions of the Royal Society of London, Series B, 262*, 23–81.

Martin, S. J., Grimwood, P. D., & Morris, R. G. M. (2000). Synaptic plasticity and memory: An evaluation of the hypothesis. *Annual Review of Neuroscience, 23*, 649–711.

McHugh, T. J., Blum, K. I., Tsien, J. Z., Tonegawa, S., & Wilson, M. A. (1996). Impaired hippocampal representation of space in CA1-specific NMDAR1 knockout mice. *Cell, 87*, 1339–1349.

McNaughton, B. L., Barnes, C. A., & O'Keefe, J. (1983). The contributions of position, direction, and velocity to single unit activity in the hippocampus of freely-moving rats. *Experimental Brain Research, 52*, 41–49.

McNaughton, B. L., & Morris, R. G. M. (1987). Hippocampal synaptic enhancement and information storage within a distributed memory system. *Trends in Neurosciences, 10*, 408–415.

Morris, R. G. M., Garrud, P., Rawlins, J. N. P., & O'Keefe, J. (1982). Place navigation impaired in rats with hippocampal lesions. *Nature, 297*, 681–683.

Morris, R. G. M., Schenk, F., Tweedie, F., & Jarrard, L. E. (1990). Ibotenate lesions of hippocampus and/or subiculum: Dissociating components of allocentric spatial learning. *European Journal of Neuroscience, 2*, 1016–1028.

Moser, E. I., Moser, M.-B., & Andersen, P. (1993). Spatial learning impairment parallels the magnitude of dorsal hippocampal lesions, but is hardly present following ventral lesions. *Journal of Neuroscience, 13,* 3916–3925.

Moser, M.-B., & Moser, E. I. (1998). Distributed encoding and retrieval of spatial memory in the hippocampus. *Journal of Neuroscience, 18,* 7535–7542.

Moser, M.-B., Moser, E. I., Forrest, E., Andersen, P., & Morris, R. G. M. (1995). Spatial learning with a minislab in the dorsal hippocampus. *Proceedings of the National Academy of Sciences USA, 92,* 9697–9701.

Moser, M.-B., Tollefsrud, A., Moser, E. I., & Andersen, P. (1997). Multiple substrates for spatial learning in the rat hippocampus. *Society for Neuroscience Abstracts, 23,* 621.2.

Muller, R. U., & Kubie, J. L. (1987). The effects of changes in the environment on the spatial firing of hippocampal complex-spike cells. *Journal of Neuroscience, 7,* 1951–1968.

O'Keefe, J., & Dostrovsky, J. (1971). The hippocampus as a spatial map: Preliminary evidence from unit activity in the freely moving rat. *Brain Research, 34,* 171–175.

O'Keefe, J., & Nadel, L. (1978). *The hippocampus as a cognitive map.* Oxford: Clarendon Press.

O'Keefe, J., & Recce, M. L. (1993). Phase relationship between hippocampal place units and the EEG theta rhythm. *Hippocampus, 3,* 317–330.

Otnæss, M. K., Brun, V. H., Moser, M.-B., & Moser, E. I. (1999). Pretraining prevents spatial learning impairment following saturation of hippocampal long-term potentiation. *Journal of Neuroscience, 19,* RC49.

Ranck, J. B., Jr. (1973). Studies on single neurons in dorsal hippocampal formation and septum in unrestrained rats: Part 1. Behavoral correlates and firing repertoires. *Experimental Neurology, 41,* 461–531.

Redish, A. D., Battaglia, F. P., Chawla, M. K., Ekstrom, A. D., Gerrard, J. L., Lipa, P., Rosenzweig, E. S., Worley, P. F., Guzowski, J. F., McNaughton, B. L., & Barnes, C. A. (2001). Independence of firing correlates of anatomically proximate hippocampal pyramidal cells. *Journal of Neuroscience, 21,* RC134.

Squire, L. R. (1992). Memory and the hippocampus: A synthesis from findings with rats, monkeys, and humans. *Psychological Review, 99,* 195–231.

Tamamaki, N., Abe, K., & Nojyo, Y. (1987). Columnar organization in the subiculum formed by axon branches originating from single CA1 pyramidal neurons in the rat hippocampus. *Brain Research, 412,* 156–160.

Tamamaki, N., & Nojyo, Y. (1990). Disposition of the slab-like modules formed by axon branches originating from single CA1 pyramidal neurons in the rat hippocampus. *Journal of Comparative Neurology, 291,* 509–519.

Teng, E., & Squire, L. R. (1999). Memory for places learned long ago is intact after hippocampal damage. *Nature, 400,* 675–677.

Thompson, L. T., & Best, P. J. (1989). Place cells and silent cells in the hippocampus of freely-behaving rats. *Journal of Neuroscience, 9,* 2382–2390.

Treves, A., & Rolls, E. T. (1994). Computational analysis of the role of the hippocampus in memory. *Hippocampus, 4,* 374–392.

Wilson, M. A., & McNaughton, B. L. (1993). Dynamics of the hippocampal ensemble code for space. *Science, 261,* 1055–1058.

Wood, E. R., Dudchenko, P. A., & Eichenbaum, H. (1999). The global record of memory in hippocampal neuronal activity. *Nature, 397,* 613–616.

30

Integrating Systems for Event Memory

Testing the Contribution of the Fornix

JOHN P. AGGLETON and MALCOLM W. BROWN

THE PROBLEM

In order to understand the anatomy of amnesia, it is necessary to understand the contribution of the fornix. This tract directly connects the medial temporal lobe and the medial diencephalon, two regions that can cause anterograde amnesia when damaged. As a consequence, the fornix has been seen as a principal route linking substrates for episodic memory in the temporal lobe and diencephalon (Aggleton & Brown, 1999; Delay & Brion, 1969; Gaffan, 1992). Remarkably little is known, however, about the importance of the human fornix, in spite of its strategic location. This is principally because circumscribed pathology in this tract is exceptionally rare. This scarcity has led to a reliance on relatively few studies, where the key findings are inconsistent and where other pathologies may obscure interpretation. Whereas some individuals have seemingly normal memory following fornix damage (Cairns & Mosberg, 1951; Garcia-Bengochea & Friedman, 1987; Woolsey & Nelson, 1975), others show variable patterns of memory loss (Calabrese, Markowitsch, Harders, Scholz, & Gehlen, 1995; Cameron & Archibold, 1981; D'Esposito, Verfaellie, Alexander, & Katz, 1995; Gaffan, Gaffan, & Hodges, 1991; Geffen, Walsh, Simpson, & Jeeves, 1980; Heilman & Sypert, 1977; Hodges & Carpenter, 1991; McMackin, Cockburn, Anslow, & Gaffan, 1995; Park, Hahn, Kim, Na, & Huh, 2000; Sweet, Talland, & Ervin, 1959; Tucker, Roeltgen, Tully, Hartmann, & Boxell, 1988; Yasuno et al., 1999). In these latter cases it is often difficult to exclude the effects of ventricular enlargement, direct diencephalic damage, or indirect temporal lobe damage. Even if it is shown that fornix damage is sufficient to induce amnesia, it is unclear whether this reflects the loss of temporal lobe afferents, temporal lobe efferents, or both.

Further difficulties arise because there is still uncertainty about the specific structures within the medial temporal lobe and the medial diencephalon responsible for anterograde amnesia. This makes it harder to identify those connections of the fornix that might have a contribution to memory. A related difficulty stems from the absence of detailed anatomical information about the various pathways linking these two regions in the human brain.

377

Although it is evident that tracts such as the fornix, as well as the cingulum bundle, the inferior thalamic peduncle, and the temporopulvinar bundle of Arnold (Klingler & Gloor, 1960), all connect medial temporal and medial diencephalic structures, the precise nature of their innervations cannot be identified in the human brain (Crick & Jones, 1993). A further complication is that there may be parallel fornical and nonfornical routes that directly link the same sites (see below), as well as indirect routes between the temporal lobe and diencephalon that do not require this tract.

The present uncertainty over the role of the fornix is reflected by the fact that there are two very different models of the relationship between temporal lobe amnesia and diencephalic amnesia. In one model (the "temporal lobe memory system"), functional relationships within the temporal lobe are stressed (Eichenbaum, 2000; Squire & Knowlton, 1995). Although the fornix may convey afferents to this system, they are not crucial for its function. In the other model (the "hippocampal–diencephalic system"), additional importance is placed on information flow from the hippocampus, via the fornix, to the medial diencephalon (Aggleton & Brown, 1999; Delay & Brion, 1969; Gaffan & Gaffan, 1991). Thus in the former model (the temporal lobe memory system), any impact of fornix damage upon memory is due to hippocampal dysregulation. Furthermore, as the tract does not link the hippocampus to structures of specific importance for memory, the consequences of fornix damage are likely to be mild. In contrast, the second model (the hippocampal–diencephalic system) places the fornix in a pivotal position between key temporal and diencephalic sites, and thus fornix damage should have more disruptive effects upon memory.

In this chapter, we consider the role of the fornix in event memory. Much of the evidence comes from animal studies that are able to use techniques not applicable to humans. In this way, it has been possible to address some of the problems outlined above. At the same time, limitations are posed by the difficulty of assessing episodic-like memory in animals (Aggleton & Pearce, 2001). The resultant findings are then considered in the light of recent clinical findings.

ANATOMICAL STUDIES

Studies using axonal degeneration and axonal transport techniques have confirmed that in the monkey, the fornix provides dense inputs from the hippocampus to the medial diencephalon (Aggleton, Desimone, & Mishkin, 1986; Krayniak, Siegel, Meibach, Fruchtman, & Scrimenti, 1979; Poletti & Cresswell, 1977; Valenstein & Nauta, 1959). (Note that the term "hippocampus" is used here to refer to fields CA1–CA4, dentate gyrus, and the subiculum.) Diencephalic sites receiving hippocampal projections in the monkey include the anterior thalamic nuclei, rostral midline thalamic nuclei (including the nucleus reuniens), the lateral dorsal thalamic nucleus, the medial pulvinar nucleus, the medial and lateral mammillary nuclei, and a number of other hypothalamic nuclei. Studies using a combination of retrograde and anterograde tracers have shown that the subiculum is the principal source of these hippocampal projections (Aggleton, Desimone, & Mishkin, 1986; Krayniak et al., 1979; Swanson & Cowan, 1975). Furthermore, research combining fornix tract section with the placement of anterograde tracers in the hippocampus has demonstrated in the monkey that the fornix is the sole route for direct projections from the subiculum to the anterior thalamic nuclei, the nucleus reuniens, and other thalamic midline nuclei (Aggleton, Desimone, & Mishkin, 1986). The same exclusive use of the fornix was also found for the hippocampal inputs to the mammillary nuclei and other hypothalamic nuclei (Aggleton & Saunders, personal communication, 1997). In contrast, the inputs from the subiculum to the lateral dorsal nucleus use two routes, one via the fornix, the other via the temporopulvinar bundle (Aggleton, Desimone, & Mishkin, 1986). The inputs to the medial pulvinar solely use this latter route.

These studies have been extended recently to examine diencephalic inputs from other medial temporal sites. Projections to the thalamus were mapped in normal monkeys and in monkeys in which either the fornix or the inferior thalamic peduncle was cut prior to the injection of retrograde tracers in discrete thalamic sites (Aggleton & Saunders, 1997; Saunders, Mishkin, & Aggleton, 2001; Saunders & Rosene, 2001). These studies showed that the anterior thalamic nuclei also receive light inputs via the fornix from the presubiculum, parasubiculum, and entorhinal cortex. They also receive a very light input from the perirhinal cortex, a small component of which may use the fornix (Saunders et al., 2001). Whereas the majority of inputs to the lateral dorsal nucleus from the presubiculum and parasubiculum also use the fornix, the entorhinal projections to the lateral dorsal nucleus principally use the temporopulvinar bundle. None of the medial temporal lobe projections to the medial dorsal thalamic nucleus (from the entorhinal and perirhinal cortices) use the fornix. Instead, they rely on the inferior thalamic peduncle. These findings—along with those from a related study on the inputs from the hippocampus and parahippocampal cortices to the nucleus accumbens (Friedman, Aggleton, Saunders, & Vinsant, 1993)—reveal that for some medial temporal lobe efferents, such as those to the anterior thalamic nuclei and mammillary nuclei, the fornix is virtually the sole route. For other pathways (e.g., those to the lateral dorsal nucleus and nucleus accumbens), there are distinct, parallel routes.

A mixture of medial temporal–medial diencephalon routes is also found in the rat brain. For example, fibers from the subiculum and presubiculum to the anterior thalamic nuclei use both fornical and nonfornical routes, while those from the postsubiculum and entorhinal cortex appear to rely on nonfornical routes (Meibach & Siegel, 1977; Shibata, 1996; Van Groen & Wyss, 1990a, 1990b). Likewise, the medial temporal inputs to the lateral dorsal thalamic nucleus may solely use nonfornical routes (Shibata, 1996; Van Groen & Wyss, 1990a, 1990b). In contrast, the hippocampal inputs to the mammillary nuclei solely use the fornix (Swanson & Cowan, 1977; Van Groen & Wyss, 1990a). An overall difference between the rat and the macaque brain does, however, appear to be the greater contribution of nonfornical routes in the rat for the pathways from the subicular cortices to the thalamus.

The presence of parallel routes, which include the fornix, is also found for some of the inputs to the medial temporal lobe in both the rat and macaque brain. Perhaps most importantly, the cholinergic innervation to the hippocampal/parahippocampal regions from the basal forebrain consists of both fornical and nonfornical pathways (Amaral & Witter, 1995). An important consequence of these parallel afferent and efferent routes is that lesions of the fornix may cause only a partial disconnection of some sites. Thus, if a function that normally involves the fornix can be supported by these alternative routes, the normal contributions of the fornix may be masked even though the tract is cut.

LESION STUDIES IN ANIMALS

Comparing the effects of fornix lesions and hippocampal lesions is important, as the outcome will cast a light on their joint role in memory functions. From a consideration of the anatomy, it is evident that for some functions that involve direct hippocampal projections to the diencephalon, the effects of fornix lesions should be very similar to those of hippocampectomy. For other functions that can engage parallel routes (Aggleton, Desimone, &

Mishkin, 1986; Meibach & Siegel, 1977) or indirect pathways (e.g., via the entorhinal cortex or retrosplenial cortex), the effects should be less similar. Moreover, fornix lesions should have no direct effect on hippocampal connections with the medial pulvinar, nor should they directly affect hippocampal interactions that solely rely on inputs *from* the diencephalon (e.g., those from the thalamus via the cingulum bundle). Finally, connections between the hippocampus and the rest of the temporal lobe do not use this tract, and so they also should not be disrupted directly by fornix lesions.

In addition, some extrahippocampal regions—for example, in the monkey, the entorhinal cortex and medial perirhinal cortex (area 35)—project via the fornix. Although these projections are sparse (Saunders & Rosene, 2001), this does mean that fornix lesions could have a *more* disruptive effect than hippocampal lesions do (see, e.g., Whishaw & Jarrard, 1995). This circumstance should occur, however, only when hippocampal lesions are made by methods that spare fibers of passage, and so it is important to distinguish between conventional lesions and cytotoxic lesions of the hippocampus (cf. Goulet, Dore, & Murray, 1998).

A consideration of the behavioral effects of fornix lesions in rats accords with the predictions made from the anatomy. Thus in many instances the effects of fornix transection and hippocampectomy are qualitatively similar (Barnes, 1988). In some cases the surgeries have effects of comparable severity (e.g., Aggleton, Keith, Rawlins, Hunt, & Sahgal, 1992; Whishaw & Jarrard, 1995), but in other instances fornix lesions appear to be less disruptive (e.g., on reference memory tasks in the Morris water maze). Thus, although both hippocampal and fornix lesions impair the ability to learn the location of a submerged platform, the acquisition deficit following extensive, conventional hippocampal lesions appears much more severe than that following fornix lesions (Eichenbaum, Stewart, & Morris, 1990; Morris, Garrud, Rawlins, & O'Keefe, 1982; Warburton & Aggleton, 1999; Whishaw, Cassel, & Jarrard, 1995). Furthermore, in probe trials, rats with fimbria–fornix lesions are sometimes able to demonstrate a significant preference for the training location (Eichenbaum et al., 1990; Warburton & Aggleton, 1999; Whishaw et al., 1995), while hippocampectomized rats typically show no preference (Morris et al., 1982; Moser, Moser, Forrest, Andersen, & Morris, 1995). At first sight, this difference in performance on probe trials appears to be qualitative, but this is not necessarily so. Although cytotoxic lesions of the hippocampus proper (CA1–CA4) result in abnormal patterns of behavior in the water maze, such rats can acquire an appropriate place preference after additional training (Morris, Schenk, Tweedie, & Jarrard, 1990; Whishaw & Jarrard, 1996). Furthermore, direct comparisons between the effects of fornix lesions and cytotoxic lesions of approximately 90% of CA1–CA4 produced strikingly similar levels of deficits on place learning in a water pool (Cassel et al., 1998; Whishaw & Jarrard, 1995). Taken together, these findings indicate that fornix lesions can closely mimic lesions of CA1–CA4 on tests of spatial learning and memory. The greater disruption associated with conventional lesions (see, e.g., Morris et al., 1982) does, however, indicate that regions outside CA1–CA4 can support place learning in the absence of fornical connections.

Less frequent are those cases where fornix lesions appear to have no effect on tasks that are sensitive to hippocampectomy. These examples are instructive, as they suggest that task performance depends on the nonfornical connections of the hippocampus (e.g., on hippocampal–temporal interactions), and they may thus have a direct relevance for the two models outlined in the first section. Two examples of such tasks are configural learning and recognition memory. One study reported that hippocampal lesions (by kainic acid/colchicine), but not fornix lesions, disrupted the acquisition of negative patterning, a configural learning task (McDonald et al., 1997). A potential complication in interpreting this dissociation is that the hippocampectomized rats showed generalized overresponding, leading to possible ceiling effects. There is also the need to demonstrate formally that the normal rats were using a configural solution to solve the task (Bussey et al., 2001). A further issue is that other studies have failed to show that hippocampal lesions impair negative patterning (Davidson, McKernan, & Jarrard, 1993), thereby raising a doubt about the generality of the findings of McDonald and colleagues (1997).

In monkeys, it has been reported that recognition memory, as measured by delayed-nonmatching-to-sample (DNMS) tasks, is disrupted by hippocampal lesions (Alvarez, Zola-Morgan, & Squire, 1995; Beason-Held, Rosene, Killiany, & Moss, 1999; Zola et al., 2000), whereas fornix lesions have different effects (Bachevalier, Saunders, & Mishkin, 1985; Zola-Morgan, Squire, & Amaral, 1989). In one study, in which training occurred after surgery, the animals with fornix lesions showed an initial impairment in learning the task; following this, however, their levels of performance did not fall below those of the control animals (Zola-Morgan et al., 1989). Indeed, by the end of training, the animals with fornix lesions were significantly outperforming the control monkeys (Zola-Morgan et al., 1989). In a second DNMS study, in which training occurred prior to surgery (Bachevalier, Saunders, & Mishkin, 1985), the recognition performance of monkeys with fornix lesions did not differ significantly from that of the controls, although they did show a tendency to perform more poorly.

Further evidence for a distinction between the effects of hippocampal damage and fornix damage on tests of object recognition has come from studies of rats. In studies using either DNMS tasks or spontaneous preference tests, there is agreement that fornix lesions have no apparent effect (Clark, Zola, & Squire, 2000; Ennaceur, Neave, & Aggleton, 1996, 1997; Shaw & Aggleton, 1993). In contrast, hippocampal lesions in rats can impair tests of object recognition (Clark et al., 2000, 2001; Clark, West, Zola, & Squire, 2001; Mumby, Wood, & Pinel, 1992). These differential effects on recognition, found for both monkeys and rats, may have important implications, as tests of recognition have been regarded as key elements in a battery of behavioral tests to examine event (declarative) memory. The normal recognition performance following fornix lesions has therefore been interpreted as evidence that hippocampal connections via the fornix are not important for this form of memory (Squire & Zola-Morgan, 1991).

The significance of this difference depends on the reliability of the respective findings, and the effects of hippocampal lesions on recognition remain controversial. One study with monkeys found that extensive cytotoxic hippocampal lesions could leave DNMS performance unaffected, even at long retention delays (Murray & Mishkin, 1998). Furthermore, a meta-analysis using data from three related studies suggested a significant negative relationship between the extent of hippocampal lesion size and any DNMS performance deficit, that is, the larger the hippocampal lesion, the better the performance (Baxter & Murray, 2001b). While the validity of this meta-analysis has been challenged (Zola & Squire, 2001), within each study the correlation between lesion size and error score is negative (Baxter & Murray, 2001a). This provides a caution to the notion that the extent of hippocampal tissue damage can be directly related to a loss of recognition. This can be contrasted with the perirhinal cortex, as a separate meta-analysis found a positive correlation between the extent of cortical damage and the severity of the DNMS deficit (Baxter & Murray, 2001b). This accords with a variety of evidence highlighting the greater importance of the perirhinal cortex for recognition (Brown & Aggleton, 2001; Meunier, Bachevalier, Mishkin, & Murray, 1993; Meunier, Hadfield, Bachevalier, & Murray, 1996; Murray, 1992).

A similar situation applies to studies of object recognition by rats. As pointed out above, a number of studies have found impairments following hippocampal lesions. In contrast, other studies have reported normal object recognition memory performance after hippo-campal lesions (Aggleton, Hunt, & Rawlins, 1986; Cassaday & Rawlins, 1997; Duva et al., 1997; Mumby et al., 1996). These different patterns of results cannot be directly related to such factors as lesion size, extent of retention interval, or pre- versus postsurgical train-ing (e.g., Aggleton, Hunt, & Rawlins, 1986). As yet, it is unclear why these different re-sults are found, but one concern is the extent to which tests of object recognition are free from spatial demands (Cassaday & Rawlins, 1997; Shaw & Aggleton, 1993).

To complicate the situation further, there is evidence that fornix lesions can disrupt object recognition, but only when combined with another lesion (monkey—Bachevalier, Parkinsons, & Mishkin, 1985; rats—Ennaceur & Aggleton, 1997; Wiig & Bilkey, 1995). Thus, in monkeys neither fornix nor amygdala surgery impaired DNMS performance, but the combination produced a clear deficit (Bachevalier, Parkinsons, & Mishkin, 1985). It is important to note that this study used aspiration lesions of the amygdala, which not only affected that structure, but also disconnected additional outputs from the perirhinal cor-tex, the entorhinal cortex, and area TE (Goulet et al., 1998). One possible explanation for the results of Bachevalier, Parkinsons, and Mishkin (1985) is that there are projections from the perirhinal and entorhinal cortices that have dual routes—one via the fornix, and the other past the amygdala—to regions that can support DNMS performance (e.g., the rostral thalamus and/or prefrontal cortex). As a consequence, a combined lesion is neces-sary to produce a deficit (see also Gaffan, Parker, & Easton, 2001). Another possibility is that the partial loss of cholinergic inputs to the medial temporal lobe via the fornix un-masks a mild deficit that is difficult to detect with small group sizes. In conclusion, although some studies point to a clear dissociation between the effects of hippocampal lesions and fornix lesions on recognition tests (e.g., Clark et al., 2000), these instances are countered by those sets of studies that have failed to find differential effects. At the same time, the results of combined lesion studies indicate that the fornix carries fibers that can contribute to recognition, even though this contribution is often not necessary.

DISCONNECTION STUDIES

A quite different way of examining the possible role of the fornix in memory is to compare the effects of lesions to structures that are linked by this tract. If the consequences are similar, then it is likely that the connections via the fornix contribute to performance. A consider-ation of spatial learning in the rat reveals that this approach provides additional evidence for the importance of the fornix. Thus, just as lesions to the hippocampus (and fornix) disrupt spatial nonmatching in the T-maze and radial-arm maze, and impair place learn-ing in the Morris water maze (Barnes, 1988), so can lesions to sites linked to the hippoc-ampus via the fornix, such as the mammillary nuclei and the anterior thalamic nuclei (Aggleton & Brown, 1999; Aggleton, Neave, Nagle, & Hunt, 1995; Byatt & Dalrymple-Alford, 1996; Neave, Nagle, & Aggleton, 1997; Sutherland & Rodriguez, 1989). Further-more, lesions of the fornix, mammillary nuclei, and anterior thalamic nuclei in rats all affect scene discrimination learning in a similar way (Gaffan, Bannerman, Warburton, & Aggleton, 2001). An implication is that these regions function in an integrated manner. Consistent with this interpretation, studies of the macaque monkey have shown that lesions of the fornix, mammillary bodies, and anterior thalamic nuclei can all disrupt a concur-rent discrimination learning task in which the combination of visual objects and their lo-cation on a screen guides performance (Gaffan, 1994; Parker & Gaffan, 1997a, 1997b). It has been proposed that this task depends on attributes of episodic memory, and that the pattern of deficits provides clear evidence for the integrative action of the hippocampus, mammillary nuclei, and anterior thalamic nuclei, via the fornix, in this form of memory (Parker & Gaffan, 1997a). Additional support for this idea comes from the finding that making a fornix lesion after a lesion of the mammillary nuclei lesion has no additional effect (Parker & Gaffan, 1997a).

Although lesion studies that compare the effects of damage to sites linked by the fornix can provide indirect evidence of a functional interaction via this tract, it is necessary to use disconnection procedures to explore this issue more directly. This technique was applied to the study of spatial memory in the rat (Warburton, Baird, Morgan, Muir, & Aggleton, 2000). Unilateral lesions of the fornix were combined with unilateral lesions of the anterior thalamic nuclei in either the contralateral or ipsilateral hemisphere. In some cases the hippocampal commissure was also cut, in order to reduce the crossover of information between the two hemispheres. Although the two different fornix–thalamus surgeries produced equivalent amounts of total damage, only the crossed lesion (e.g., left fornix and right anterior thalamus) should have caused bilateral dysfunction in the anterior thalamic nuclei (if the fornix provides critical inputs to these nuclei). Behavioral tests using the T-maze (Figure 30.1), the radial-arm maze, and the Morris water maze all demonstrated that the crossed lesion did produce a greater deficit than the uncrossed lesion, but only when combined with a lesion of the hippocampal commissures (Warburton et al., 2000). These results strongly implicate connections from the hippocampus to the anterior thalamic nuclei in spatial learning, and they also show that in the rat the interhemispheric connections via the hippocampal commissure provide an effective route for information from one hemisphere to reach the diencephalon in the other hemisphere (see also Olton, Walker, & Woolf, 1982).

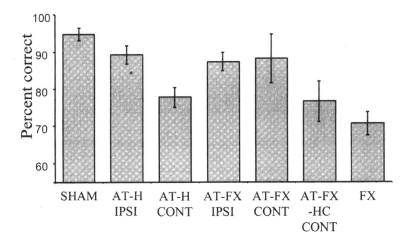

FIGURE 30.1. T-maze alternation performance of rats with various disconnection lesions. The histogram shows that impairments are caused by crossed unilateral lesions between the anterior thalamic nuclei and the hippocampus (AT+H CONT), and between the anterior thalamic nuclei and the fornix plus hippocampal commissures AT-FX-HC). Although bilateral fornix lesions (FX) also impaired performance, the remaining combinations of lesions had little or no apparent effect (AT-FX CONT, contralateral lesions of anterior thalamic nuclei and fornix, hippocampal commissures spared; AT-FX IPSI, ipsilateral lesions of anterior thalamic nuclei and fornix; AT-H IPSI, ipsilateral lesions of the anterior thalamic nuclei and hippocampus). The figure shows the mean percentage correct score and standard error over 15 sessions. Data from Warburton, Baird, Morgan, Muir, and Aggleton (2000, 2001).

To confirm this apparent hippocampal–thalamic interaction, we have used the same logic to compare the effects of crossed or ipsilateral lesions of the anterior thalamic nuclei and the hippocampus itself (Warburton, Baird, Morgan, Muir, & Aggleton, 2001). Consistent deficits were found only when the two unilateral lesions were placed in opposite hemispheres (Figure 30.1). Furthermore, the crossed lesion deficit in the Morris water maze was appreciably greater than that in the first study, which combined fornix–anterior thalamic lesions (Warburton et al., 2000, 2001). This finding suggests that there may be an additional functional contribution from the subicular, presubicular, postsubicular, and entorhinal cortices to the anterior thalamic nuclei that does not travel in the fornix. Nevertheless, these results agree with those from studies that damage the target regions themselves (Aggleton & Brown, 1999), and so they reinforce the notion that the route from the hippocampus to the anterior thalamic nuclei (and mammillary nuclei) via the fornix does support spatial processing in the rat. At the same time, these results do not preclude the possibility that projections from the anterior thalamic nuclei to the hippocampal region (via the cingulum bundle) also have an important role (Goodridge & Taube, 1997).

COMBINING IMMEDIATE EARLY GENE IMAGING WITH FORNIX LESIONS

A different way to assess the impact of fornix lesions has come with the advent of functional imaging techniques. In a recent study, we examined the effects of unilateral fornix lesions in the rat on the activity of an immediate early gene, c-*fos* (Vann, Brown, Erichsen, & Aggleton, 2000b). The expression of this gene is regarded as a general marker of neural activation (Dragunow & Faull, 1989; Herrera & Robertson, 1996; Sagar, Sharp, & Curran, 1988), although it may also have a particular role in plastic processes associated with learning (Herdegen & Leah, 1998; Tischmeyer & Grimm, 1999). In studies using this technique, the activity of multiple sites in the same brain can readily be compared at a high level of anatomical resolution, even to the level of single neurons.

Rats were first trained on a spatial working memory task in a radial-arm maze. This task was selected as it is sensitive to lesions in the hippocampus and related diencephalic sites, and training on this task also leads to increased c-*fos* activation in both the hippocampus and anterior thalamic nuclei in normal rats (Vann, Brown, & Aggleton, 2000; Vann, Brown, Erichsen, & Aggleton, 2000a; Figure 30.2, upper). In rats with unilateral fornix lesions, it was possible to examine animals that were able to perform the spatial working memory task accurately, and to compare c-*fos* expression across hemispheres in the same animals. With immunohistochemical techniques, the gene product Fos was visualized in a total of 39 brain sites (Vann et al., 2000b; Figure 30.2, lower). On the side of the fornix lesion, Fos levels were markedly reduced across the hippocampus, the entorhinal cortex, and the subicular complex (except the dorsal subiculum) when compared to the intact side. Other sites exhibiting reduced Fos included the retrosplenial cortex, the postrhinal cortex, the three anterior thalamic nuclei, the supramammillary nucleus, and the lateral septum. The prelimbic cortex was the only site to demonstrate increased Fos activity on the same side as the fornix lesion. It should be added that the mammillary nuclei could not be stained for Fos, and so no interhemispheric comparisons could be made (Vann et al., 2000b). Finally, control studies showed that fornix lesions did not affect levels of Fos when rats were resting and not in a maze.

These results demonstrate that the effects of fornix lesions extend beyond the hippocampal formation to an array of limbic sites (Vann et al., 2000b). Although not all regions

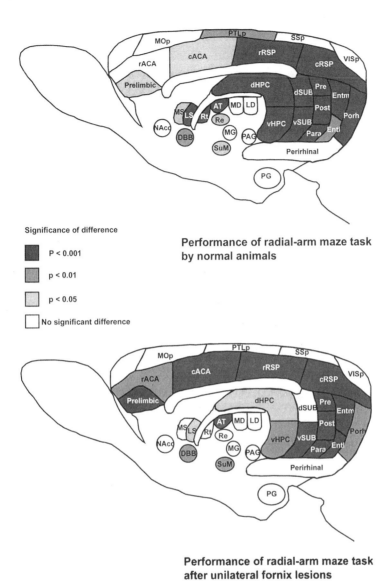

Performance of radial-arm maze task by normal animals

Significance of difference

- ■ P < 0.001
- ▨ p < 0.01
- ▢ p < 0.05
- ☐ No significant difference

Performance of radial-arm maze task after unilateral fornix lesions

FIGURE 30.2. Schematic depiction of sites showing increased Fos levels following performance of a spatial working memory task by normal rats (upper), and those sites showing abnormal Fos levels in the hemisphere with a fornix transection (lower). In both studies, the animals were run in an eight-arm radial maze, and Fos levels were measured 90 minutes after task completion. With the sole exception of the prelimbic cortex, the changes in the fornix lesion study always consisted of a decrease in Fos counts. AT, anterior thalamic nuclei; cACA, caudal anterior cingulate cortex; cRSP, caudal retrosplenial cortex; DBB, diagonal band of Broca; dHPC, dorsal hippocampus; dSUB, dorsal subiculum; Entl, lateral entorhinal cortex; Entm, medial entorhinal cortex; LD, lateral dorsal thalamic nucleus; LS, lateral septum; MD, medial dorsal thalamic nucleus; MG, medial geniculate; MOp, primary motor cortex; MS, medial septum; NAcc, nucleus accumbens; PAG, periaqueductal grey; Para, parasubiculum; PG, pontine grey; Porh, postrhinal cortex; Post, postsubiculum; Pre, presubiculum; PTLp parietal cortex; rACA, rostral anterior cingulate cortex; rRSP, rostral retrosplenial cortex; Re, nucleus reuniens; Rt, rostral reticular thalamic nucleus; SSp, primary somatosensory cortex; SuM, supramammillary nucleus; vHPC, ventral hippocampus; VISp, primary visual cortex; vSUB, ventral subiculum. Data from Vann, Brown, and Aggleton (2000) and Vann, Brown, Erichsen, and Aggleton (2000a, 2000b).

innervated by the fornix showed changes (e.g., the nucleus accumbens), a number of sites not directly innervated by the fornix were affected (e.g., the retrosplenial cortex, the postrhinal cortex). These latter changes presumably reflect primary decreases in neuronal activation in sites such as the hippocampus or the anterior thalamic nuclei, which in turn affect these additional regions. These results highlight the widespread consequences of fornix lesions and demonstrate that they do not merely produce hippocampal dysfunction. Furthermore, many of the sites that showed hypoactivity following fornix lesions were the same sites that showed increased Fos in normal rats performing the same task (Figure 30.2); that is, fornix lesions affect the very same sites that are normally recruited during task performance. It is also the case that damage to many of these same sites affects spatial memory tasks. This correspondence highlights the widespread consequences of fornix lesions. Just as the learning and performance of spatial memory tasks depend on multiple regions' functioning in a coordinated manner, so fornix lesions result in altered activity throughout the same network of regions, and cannot be regarded as merely disrupting one structure.

INTEGRATION OF ANIMAL DATA WITH HUMAN CLINICAL DATA

The potential value of studying patients with fornix damage has long been recognized, but pathology limited only to the fornix is exceptionally rare. As a consequence, there has been a reliance on single-case studies. In some cases memory appears normal (Cairns & Mosberg, 1951; Woolsey & Nelson, 1975), but in others there are variable patterns of memory loss (Calabrese et al., 1995; Cameron & Archibold, 1981; D'Esposito et al., 1995, Gaffan et al., 1991; Geffen et al., 1980; Heilman & Sypert, 1977; Hodges & Carpenter, 1991; Park et al., 2000; Sweet et al., 1959; Tucker et al., 1988; Yasuno et al., 1999). In spite of the large number of single-case studies, there appear to be no cases in which a patient has received a comprehensive cognitive assessment as well as postmortem confirmation of selective fornix damage. For this reason, there is special interest in the few group studies of fornix damage. The hope is that this approach will make it possible to identify systematically factors that might produce variations in performance. The first such study (Garcia-Bengochea & Friedman, 1987) cited 142 cases with bilateral fornix damage compiled from nine reports on fornix surgery for epilepsy. It was observed that none of these 142 patients showed a persistent memory loss. This conclusion was, however, rebutted by Gaffan and Gaffan (1991), who pointed out a series of flaws in the clinical review. These include the correction that only 38 patients (out of 142) received intended bilateral surgery, and that confirmation of the extent of these surgeries was lacking. In addition, there appeared to be no formal testing of memory, and given the epileptic status of these patients, a presurgical–postsurgical comparison would be required before an unambiguous conclusion could be reached (Gaffan & Gaffan, 1991). Since then, the largest group study has comprised six cases with varying degrees of fornix damage associated with surgery to remove a colloid cyst of the third ventricle (McMackin et al., 1995). This study found a consistent link between the extent of fornix damage, as determined by MRI, and the extent of memory impairment (McMackin et al., 1995). These investigators also reported that left fornix damage was sufficient to impair verbal memory (see also Cameron & Archibald, 1981; Tucker et al., 1988).

In view of the importance of determining the contribution of this tract to memory, we initiated a further group study consisting of 10 patients with colloid cysts (Aggleton et al., 1999). Three of these patients had bilateral fornix damage as shown by MRI, while the fornix appeared intact in the remaining seven. Although the groups with and without fornix damage did not differ on a range of factors (age, gender, surgical approach, extent of ventricular enlargement, IQ), there were marked memory differences between the two groups (Figure 30.3). Thus the three patients with bilateral fornix damage performed abnormally poorly on subtests of the Wechsler Memory Scale—Revised (WMS-R; Wechsler, 1987). These included the General Memory and Delayed Recall Indices (Figure 30.3), where their scores were comparable to those of other groups of amnesic patients (Butters et al., 1988). This was in contrast to the subjects with both fornices intact, who all achieved higher scores (Aggleton et al., 1999). The three patients with bilateral fornix damage were also severely impaired on the recall component of the Doors and People Test (Baddeley, Emslie, & Nimmo-Smith, 1994). However, there was evidence that their deficits in recognition memory, as measured by the Doors and People Test and the Warrington Recognition Memory Test (Warrington, 1984), were appreciably milder. There was, for example, a significant group × type of memory test interaction between tests of word recall and word recognition on the Doors and People Test, reflecting the much more severe deficits on the recall test (Aggleton et al., 1999). Evidence for a similar difference between recall and recognition was found in a previous group study of fornix damage following colloid cyst surgery (McMackin et al., 1995). Although it is true that tests of recognition tend to be less demanding than tests of recall, the evidence for a mild effect on recognition memory provides an intriguing link with the often preserved recognition memory found in animals with fornix lesions (see "Lesion Studies in Animals," above).

This possible correspondence between clinical and animal data was examined further by testing the 10 patients with colloid cysts (Aggleton et al., 1999) on tasks that had been developed to assess the effects of selective fornix damage in monkeys (Gaffan, 1994). For

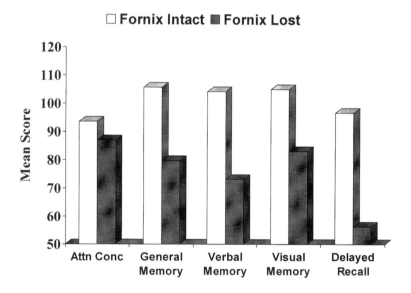

FIGURE 30.3. Mean scores on the subscales of the Wechsler Memory Scale—Revised (WMS-R) showing how fornix damage is associated with memory loss. The graph shows the mean scores for two groups of subjects who both had surgical removals of a colloid cyst. For seven subjects (white bars) the fornix was intact, for the remaining three (gray bars) it was damaged bilaterally. Data from Aggleton et al. (1999).

example, the 10 patients were tested on the same "object-in-place" task that is sensitive to lesions of the fornix, mammillary nuclei, and anterior thalamic nuclei in monkeys (Gaffan, 1994; Parker & Gaffan, 1997a, 1997b). Only the three patients with fornix damage were impaired on the object-in-place task, which is a form of concurrent discrimination (Aggleton et al., 1999). In contrast, the same three patients with fornix damage showed normal performance on the recognition of single objects in a delayed-matching-to-sample (DMS) task. Although the retention delays were only up to 20 seconds, the task was sufficiently difficult to avoid ceiling effects. Furthermore, patients with anterograde amnesia associated with more distributed pathology show clear impairments on similar DMS tasks after even shorter delays (Aggleton, Nicol, Huston, & Fairbairn, 1988; Holdstock, Shaw, & Aggleton, 1995). These findings suggest that the amnesia associated with fornix damage is more restricted than the amnesias associated with more extensive temporal lobe damage, even though the General Memory and Delayed Recall WMS-R scores can be comparable (see also Brown & Aggleton, 2001; D. Gaffan et al., 2001). At the same time, the effects of fornix lesions reveal a clear similarity to those reported for amnesic patients with partial hippocampal damage (Mayes, van Eijk, Gooding, Isaac, & Holdstock, 1999; Mayes et al., in press; Vargha-Khadem et al., 1997) or with selective mammillary nuclei damage (Dusoir, Kapur, Byrnes, McKinstry, & Hoare, 1990). The common feature in all of these studies is that the amnesic patients showed a clear loss of episodic memory combined with a relative sparing of recognition memory. For example, case Y. R. studied by Mayes and colleagues (in press) is consistently impaired on tests of recall, yet performs forced-choice item recognition tasks at normal levels, even when task difficulty rules out ceiling effects.

These results strongly indicate that fornix damage is sufficient to impair the recall of episodic information, the hallmark of anterograde amnesia. Furthermore, recent clinical studies have provided convincing evidence that damage to other components of the Papez circuit—namely, the anterior thalamic nuclei (Aggleton & Brown, 1999; Harding, Halliday, Caine, & Kril, 2000) and the mammillothalamic tract (Van der Werf, Witter, Uylings, & Jolles, 2000)—is also sufficient to induce amnesia. An issue remains concerning the severity of the memory loss associated with fornix damage and how that might affect the profile of memory impairments, such as whether it might interact with test difficulty (Manns & Squire, 1999; Reed & Squire, 1997). Nevertheless, the recent clinical findings concerning the anterior thalamic nuclei and the mammillothalamic tract (Harding et al., 2000; Van der Werf et al., 2000) serve to link temporal and diencephalic sites critical for episodic memory via the fornix. At the same time, this clinical evidence for a functional linkage between the hippocampus and the anterior thalamic nuclei has clear parallels with the outcome of lesion studies in animals into the contribution of the hippocampus, the anterior thalamic nuclei, and the fornix to spatial memory and to object-in-place memory. These animal studies include disconnection procedures, which provide more direct evidence that the hippocampus and the anterior thalamic nuclei function together in rats. There is thus a striking convergence of evidence from human and animal studies that supports the hippocampal–diencephalic model, so providing a framework for future integrated studies across species concerning the role of the fornix in event memory.

ACKNOWLEDGMENTS

We wish to acknowledge the assistance of Lorraine Awcock, Seralynne Vann, and Clea Warburton, as well as the support of the Wellcome Trust and the U.K. Medical Research Council.

REFERENCES

Aggleton, J. P., & Brown, M. (1999). Episodic memory, amnesia, and the hippocampal–anterior thalamic axis. *Behavioral and Brain Sciences, 22,* 425–489.

Aggleton, J. P., Desimone, R., & Mishkin, M. (1986). The origin, course, and termination of the hippocampothalamic projections in the macaque. *Journal of Comparative Neurology, 243,* 409–421.

Aggleton, J. P., Hunt, P. R., & Rawlins, J. N. P. (1986). The effects of hippocampal lesions upon spatial and non-spatial tests of working memory. *Behavioural Brain Research, 19,* 133–146.

Aggleton, J. P., Keith, A. B., Rawlins, J. N. P., Hunt, P. R., & Sahgal, A. (1992). Removal of the hippocampus and transection of the fornix produce comparable deficits on delayed nonmatching to position by rats. *Behavioural Brain Research, 52,* 61–71.

Aggleton, J. P., McMackin, D., Carpenter, K., Hornak, J., Kapur, N., Halpin, S., Wiles, C. M., Kamel, H., Brennan, P., Carton, S., & Gaffan, D. (1999). Differential cognitive effects of colloid cysts in the third ventricle that spare or compromise the fornix. *Brain, 123,* 800–815.

Aggleton, J. P., Neave, N. J., Nagle, S., & Hunt, P. R. (1995). A comparison of the effects of anterior thalamic, mamillary body and fornix lesions on reinforced spatial alternation. *Behavioural Brain Research, 68,* 91–101.

Aggleton, J. P., Nicol, R. M., Huston, A. E., & Fairbairn, A. F. (1988). The performance of amnesic subjects on tests of experimental amnesia in animals: Delayed matching-to-sample. *Neuropsychologia, 26,* 265–272.

Aggleton, J. P., & Pearce, J. M. (2001). Neural systems underlying episodic memory: insights from animal research. *Philosophical Transactions of the Royal Society of London, Series B, 356,* 1467–1482.

Aggleton, J. P., & Saunders, R. C. (1997). The relationship between temporal lobe and diencephalic structures implicated in anterograde amnesia. *Memory, 5,* 49–71.

Alvarez, P., Zola-Morgan, S., & Squire, L. R. (1995). Damage limited to the hippocampal region produces long lasting memory impairments in monkeys. *Journal of Neuroscience, 15,* 3796–3807.

Amaral, D. G., & Witter, M. P. (1995). Hippocampal formation. In G. Paxinos (Ed.), *The rat nervous system* (2nd ed., pp. 443–493). San Diego, CA: Academic Press.

Bachevalier, J., Parkinsons, J. K., & Mishkin, M. (1985). Visual recognition in monkeys: Effects of separate vs. combined transection of fornix and amygdalofugal pathways. *Experimental Brain Research, 57,* 554–561.

Bachevalier, J., Saunders, R. C., & Mishkin, M. (1985). Visual recognition in monkeys: Effects of transection of fornix. *Experimental Brain Research, 57,* 547–553.

Baddeley, A., Emslie, H., & Nimmo-Smith, I. (1994). *Doors and People: A test of visual and verbal recall and recognition.* Bury St. Edmunds, England: Thames Valley Test Company.

Barnes, C. A. (1988). Spatial learning and memory processes: The search for their neurobiological mechanisms in the rat. *Trends in Neurosciences, 11,* 163–169

Baxter, M. G., & Murray, E. A. (2001a). Effects of hippocampal lesions on delayed nonmatching-to-sample in monkeys: A reply to Zola and Squire. *Hippocampus, 11,* 201–203.

Baxter, M. G., & Murray, E. A. (2001b). Opposite relationship of hippocampal and rhinal damage to delayed nonmatching-to-sample deficits in monkeys. *Hippocampus, 11,* 61–71.

Beason-Held, L. L., Rosene, D. L., Killiany, R. J., & Moss, M. B. (1999). Hippocampal formation lesions produce memory impairment in the rhesus monkey. *Hippocampus, 9,* 562–574.

Brown, M. W., & Aggleton, J. P. (2001). Recognition memory: What are the roles of the perirhinal cortex and hippocampus? *Nature Reviews Neuroscience, 2,* 51–61.

Bussey, T. J., Dias, R., Redhead, E. S., Pearce, J. M., Muir, J. L,. & Aggleton, J. P. (2001). Intact negative patterning in rats with fornix or combined perirhinal and postrhinal cortex lesions. *Experimental Brain Research, 134,* 506–519.

Butters, N., Salmon, D. P., Monro, C. C., Cairns, P., Troster, A. I., & Jacobs, D. (1988). Differentiation of amnesia and demented patients with the Wechsler Memory Scale—revised. *Clinical Neuropsychology, 2,* 133–148.

Byatt, G., & Dalrymple-Alford, J. C. (1996). Both anteromedial and anteroventral thalamic lesions impair radial-maze learning in rats. *Behavioral Neuroscience, 110,* 1335–1148.

Cairns, H., & Mosberg, W. H. (1951). Colloid cyst of the third ventricle. *Surgery, Gynecology, Obstetrics, 92,* 546–570.

Calabrese, P., Markowitsch, H. J., Harders, A. G., Scholz, M., & Gehlen, W. (1995). Fornix damage and memory: A case report. *Cortex, 31,* 555–564.

Cameron, A. S., & Archibald, Y. M. (1981). Verbal memory deficit after left fornix removal: A case report. *International Journal of Neuroscience, 12,* 201.

Cassaday, H. J., & Rawlins, J. N. P. (1997). The hippocampus, objects, and their contexts. *Behavioral Neuroscience, 111,* 1228–1244.

Cassel, J.-C., Cassel, S., Galani, R., Kelche, C., Will, B., & Jarrard, L. (1998). Fimbria–fornix vs. selective hippocampal lesions in rats: Effects on locomotor activity and spatial learning and memory. *Neurobiology of Learning and Memory, 69,* 22–45.

Clark, R. E., West, A. N., Zola, S. M., & Squire, L. R. (2001). Rats with lesions of the hippocampus are impaired on the delayed nonmatching-to-sample task. *Hippocampus, 11,* 176–186.

Clark, R. E., Zola, S. M., & Squire, L. R. (2000). Impaired recognition memory in rats after damage to the hippocampus. *Journal of Neuroscience, 20,* 8853–8860.

Crick, F., & Jones, E. (1993). The backwardness of human neuroanatomy. *Nature, 361,* 109–110.

Davidson, T. L., McKernan, M. G., & Jarrard, L. E. (1993). Hippocampal lesions do not impair negative patterning: A challenge to configural association theory. *Behavioral Neuroscience, 107,* 227–234.

Delay, J., & Brion, S. (1969). *Le syndrome de Korsakoff.* Paris: Masson.

D'Esposito, N., Verfaellie, M., Alexander M. P., & Katz, D. I. (1995). Amnesia following traumatic bilateral fornix transection. *Neurology,* 1546–1550.

Dragunow, M., & Faull, R. (1989). The use of c-*fos* as a metabolic marker in neuronal pathway tracing. *Journal of Neuroscience Methods, 29,* 261–265.

Dusoir, H., Kapur, N., Byrnes, D. P., McKinstry, S., & Hoare, R. D. (1990). The role of diencephalic pathology in human memory disorder. *Brain, 113,* 1695–1706.

Duva, C. A., Floresco, S. B., Wunderlich, G. R., Lao, T. L., Pinel, J. P. J., & Phillips, A. G. (1997). Disruption of spatial but not object-recognition memory by neurotoxic lesions of the dorsal hippocampus in rats. *Behavioral Neuroscience, 111,* 1184–1196.

Eichenbaum, H. (2000). A cortico-hippocampal system for declarative memory. *Nature Reviews Neuroscience, 1,* 41–50.

Eichenbaum, H., Stewart, C., & Morris, R. G. M. (1990). Hippocampal representation in place learning. *Journal of Neuroscience, 10,* 3531–3542.

Ennaceur, A., & Aggleton, J. P. (1997). The effects of neurotoxic lesions of the perirhinal cortex combined to fornix transection on object recognition memory in the rat. *Behavioural Brain Research, 88,* 181–193.

Ennaceur, A., Neave, N. J., & Aggleton, J. P. (1996). Neurotoxic lesions of the perirhinal cortex do not mimic the behavioural effects of fornix transection in the rat. *Behavioural Brain Research, 80,* 9–25.

Ennaceur, A., Neave, N. J., & Aggleton, J. P. (1997). Spontaneous object recognition and object location memory in rats: The effects of lesions in the cingulate cortices, the medial prefrontal cortex, the cingulum bundle and the fornix. *Experimental Brain Research, 113,* 509–519.

Friedman, D. P., Aggleton, J. P., Saunders, R. C., & Vinsant, S. (1993). The organization of temporal lobe limbic inputs to the ventral striatum in macaque monkeys. *Society for Neuroscience Abstracts, 19,* 1435.

Gaffan, D. (1992). The role of the hippocampus–fornix–mammillary system in episodic memory. In L. R. Squire & N. Butters (Eds.), *Neuropsychology of memory* (2nd ed., pp. 336–346). New York: Guilford Press.

Gaffan, D. (1994). Scene-specific memory for objects: A model of episodic memory impairment in monkeys with fornix transection. *Journal of Cognitive Neuroscience, 6,* 305–320.

Gaffan, D., & Gaffan, E. A. (1991). Amnesia in man following transection of the fornix. *Brain*, *114*, 2611–2618.

Gaffan, D., Parker, A., & Easton, A. (2001). Dense amnesia in the monkey after transection of fornix, amygdala and anterior temporal stem. *Neuropsychologia*, *39*, 51–70.

Gaffan, E. A., Bannerman, D. M., Warburton, E. C., & Aggleton, J. P. (2001). Rat's processing of visual scenes: Effects of lesions to fornix, anterior thalamus, mamillary nuclei or the retrohippocampal region. *Behavioural Brain Research*, *121*, 103–117.

Gaffan, E. A., Gaffan, D., & Hodges, J. R. (1991). Amnesia following damage to the left fornix and to other sites. *Brain*, *114*, 1297–1313.

Garcia-Bengochea, F., & Friedman, W. A. (1987). Persistent memory loss following section of the anterior fornix in humans. *Surgical Neurology*, *27*, 361–364.

Geffen, G., Walsh, A., Simpson, D., & Jeeves, M. (1980). Comparison of the effects of transcortical and transcallosal removal of intraventricular tumours. *Brain*, *103*, 773–788.

Goodridge, J. P., & Taube, J. S. (1997). Interaction between the postsubiculum and anterior thalamus in the generation of head direction cell activity. *Journal of Neuroscience*, *17*, 9315–9330.

Goulet, S., Dore, F. Y., & Murray, E. A. (1998). Aspiration lesions of the amygdala disrupt the rhinal corticothalamic projection system in rhesus monkeys. *Experimental Brain Research*, *119*, 131–140.

Harding, A., Halliday, G., Caine, D., & Kril, J. (2000). Degeneration of anterior thalamic nuclei differentiates alcoholics with amnesia. *Brain*, *123*, 141–154.

Heilman, K. M., & Sypert, G. W. (1977). Korsakoff's syndrome resulting from bilateral fornix lesions. *Neurology*, *27*, 490–493.

Herdegen, T., & Leah, J. D. (1998). Inducible and constitutive transcription factors in the mammalian nervous system: Control of gene expression by Jun, Fos and Krox, and CREB/ATF proteins. *Brain Research Reviews*, *28*, 379–490.

Herrera, D. G., & Robertson, H. A. (1996). Activation of c-*fos* in the brain. *Progress in Neurobiology*, *50*, 83–107.

Hodges, J. R., & Carpenter, K. (1991). Anterograde amnesia with fornix damage following removal of IIIrd ventricle colloid cyst. *Journal of Neurology, Neurosurgery and Psychiatry*, *54*, 633–638.

Holdstock, J. S., Shaw, C., & Aggleton, J. P. (1995). The performance of amnesic subjects on tests of delayed matching-to-sample and delayed matching-to-position. *Neuropsychologia*, *33*, 1583–1596.

Klingler, J., & Gloor, P. (1960). The connections of the amygdala and of the anterior temporal cortex in the human brain. *Journal of Comparative Neurology*, *115*, 333–369.

Krayniak, P. F., Siegel, R. C., Meibach, D., Fruchtman, D. F., & Scrimenti, M. (1979). Origin of the fornix system in the squirrel monkey. *Brain Research*, *160*, 401–411.

Manns, J. R., & Squire, L. R. (1999). Impaired recognition memory of the Doors and People Test after damage limited to the hippocampal region. *Hippocampus*, *9*, 495–499.

Mayes, A. R., Isaac, C. L., Downes, J. J., Holdstock, J. S., Hunkin, N. M., Montaldi, D., MacDonald, C., Cezayirli, E. & Roberts, J. N. (in press). Memory for single items, word pairs, and temporal order of different kinds in a patient with selective hippocampal lesions. *Cognitive Neuropsychology*.

Mayes, A. R., van Eijk, R., Gooding, P. A., Isaac, C. L., & Holdstock, J. S. (1999). What are the functional deficits produced by hippocampal and perirhinal lesions? *Behavioral and Brain Sciences*, *22*, 460–461.

McDonald, R. J., Murphy, R. A., Guarraci, F. A., Gorteler, J. R., White, N. M., & Baker, A. G. (1997). Systematic comparison of the effects of hippocampal and fornix–fimbria lesions on acquisition of three configural discriminations. *Hippocampus*, *7*, 371–388.

McMackin, D., Cockburn, J., Anslow, P., & Gaffan, D. (1995). Correlation of fornix damage with memory impairment in six cases of colloid cyst removal. *Acta Neurochirugica*, *135*, 12–18.

Meibach, R. C., & Siegel, A. (1977). Thalamic projections of the hippocampal formation: Evidence for an alternative pathway involving the internal capsule. *Brain Research*, *134*, 1–12.

Meunier, M., Bachevalier, J., Mishkin, M., & Murray, E. A. (1993). Effects on visual recognition of combined and separate ablations of the entorhinal and perirhinal cortex in rhesus monkeys. *Journal of Neuroscience, 13*, 5418–5432.

Meunier, M., Hadfield, W., Bachevalier, J., & Murray, E. A. (1996). Effects of rhinal cortex lesions combined with hippocampectomy on visual recognition memory in rhesus monkeys. *Journal of Neurophysiology, 75*, 1190–1205.

Morris, R. G. M., Garrud, P., Rawlins, J. N. P., & O'Keefe, J. (1982). Place navigation impaired in rats with hippocampal lesions. *Nature, 297*, 681–683.

Morris, R. G. M., Schenk, F., Tweedie, F., & Jarrard, L. E. (1990). Ibotenate lesions of hippocampus and/or subiculum: Dissociating components of allocentric spatial learning. *European Journal of Neuroscience, 2*, 1016–1028.

Moser, M.-B., Moser, E. I., Forrest, E., Andersen, P., & Morris, R. G. M. (1995). Spatial learning with a minislab in the dorsal hippocampus. *Proceedings of the National Academy of Sciences USA, 92*, 9697–9701.

Mumby, D. G., Wood, E. R., Duva, C. A., Kornecook, T. J., Pinel, J. P. J., & Phillips, A. G. (1996). Ischemia-induced object recognition deficits in rats are attenuated by hippocampal ablation before or soon after ischemia. *Behavioral Neuroscience, 110*, 266–281.

Mumby, D. G., Wood, E. R., & Pinel, J. P. J. (1992). Object-recognition memory is only mildly impaired in rats with lesions of the hippocampus and amygdala. *Psychobiology, 20*, 18–27.

Murray, E. A. (1992). Medial temporal lobe structures contributing to recognition memory: the amygdaloid complex versus the rhinal cortex. In J.P. Aggleton (Ed.), *The amygdala: Neurobiological aspects of emotion, memory, and mental dysfunction* (pp. 453–470) New York: Wiley–Liss.

Murray, E. A., & Mishkin, M. (1998). Object recognition and location memory in monkeys with excitotoxic lesions of the amygdala and hippocampus. *Journal of Neuroscience, 18*, 6568–6582.

Neave, N., Nagle, S., & Aggleton, J. P. (1997). Evidence for the involvement of the mamillary bodies and cingulum bundle in allocentric spatial processing by rats. *European Journal of Neuroscience, 9*, 101–115.

Olton, D. S., Walker, J. A., & Woolf, W. A. (1982). A disconnection analysis of hippocampal function. *Brain Research, 233*, 241–253.

Park, S. A., Hahn, J. H., Kim, J. I., Na, D. L., & Huh, K. (2000). Memory deficits after bilateral anterior fornix infarction. *Neurology, 54*, 1379–1382

Parker, A., & Gaffan, D. (1997a). Mamillary body lesions in monkeys impair object-in-place memory: Functional unity of the fornix–mamillary system. *Journal of Cognitive Neuroscience, 9*, 512–521.

Parker, A., & Gaffan, D. (1997b). The effect of anterior thalamic and cingulate cortex lesions on object-in-place memory in monkeys. *Neuropsychologia, 35*, 1093–1102.

Poletti, C. E., & Creswell, G. (1977). Fornix system efferent projections in the squirrel monkey: An experimental degeneration study. *Journal of Comparative Neurology, 175*, 101–127.

Reed, J. M., & Squire, L. R. (1997). Impaired recognition memory in patients with lesions limited to the hippocampal formation. *Behavioral Neuroscience, 111*, 667–675.

Sagar, S. M., Sharp, F. R., & Curran, T. (1988). Expression of c-*fos* protein in brain: Metabolic mapping at cellular level. *Science, 240*, 1328–1331.

Saunders, R. C., Mishkin, M., & Aggleton, J. P. (2001). [Projections from the entorhinal cortex, perirhinal cortex, presubiculum, and parasubiculum to the medial thalamus in macaque monkeys: Identifying different pathways using disconnection techniques]. Unpublished raw data.

Saunders, R. C., & Rosene D. L. (2001). *Non-hippocampal efferents from the entorhinal (area 28) and perirhinal (area 35) cortices in the rhesus monkey: I. Subcortical projections.* Manuscript submitted for publication.

Shaw, C., & Aggleton, J. P. (1993). The effects of fornix and medial prefrontal lesions on delayed nonmatching-to-sample by rats. *Behavioural Brain Research, 54*, 91–102.

Shibata, H. (1996). Direct projections from the entorhinal area to the anteroventral and laterodorsal thalamic nuclei in the rat. *Neuroscience Research, 26*, 83–87.

Squire, L. R., & Knowlton, B. J. (1995). Memory, hippocampus, and brain systems. In M. Gazzaniga (Ed.), *The cognitive neurosciences* (pp. 825–835). Cambridge, MA: MIT Press.

Squire, L. R., & Zola-Morgan, S. (1991). The medial temporal lobe memory system. *Science, 253,* 1380–1386.

Sutherland, R. J., & Rodriguez, A. J. (1989). The role of the fornix/fimbria and some related subcortical structures in place learning and memory. *Behavioural Brain Research, 32,* 265–277.

Swanson, L. W., & Cowan, W. M. (1975). Hippocampo-hypothalamic connections: Origin in subicular cortex, not Ammon's horn. *Science, 189, 303–304.*

Swanson, L. W., & Cowan, W. M. (1977). An autoradiographic study of the organization of the efferent connections of the hippocampal formation in the rat. *Journal of Comparative Neurology, 172,* 49–84.

Sweet, W. H., Talland, G. A., & Ervin, F. R. (1959). Loss of recent memory following section of fornix. *Transactions of the American Neurological Association, 84,* 76–82.

Tischmeyer, W., & Grimm, R. (1999). Activation of immediate early genes and memory formation. *Cellular and Molecular Life Sciences, 55,* 564–574.

Tucker, D. M., Roeltgen, D. P., Tully, R., Hartmann, J., & Boxell, C. (1988). Memory dysfunction following unilateral transection of the fornix: A hippocampal disconnection syndrome. *Cortex, 24,* 465–472.

Valenstein, E. S., & Nauta, W. J. H. (1959). A comparison of the distribution of the fornix system in the rat, guinea pig, cat, and monkey. *Journal of Comparative Neurology, 113,* 337–363.

Van der Werf, Y. D., Witter, M. P., Uylings, H. B. M., & Jolles, J. (2000). Neuropsychology of infactions in the thalamus: A review. *Neuropsychologia, 38,* 613–627.

Van Groen, T., & Wyss, J. M. (1990a). The connections of the presubiculum and parasubiculum in the rat. *Brain Research, 518,* 227–243.

Van Groen, T., & Wyss, J. M. (1990b). The postsubicular cortex in the rat: Characterization of the fourth region of the subicular cortex and its connections. *Brain Research, 529,* 165–177.

Vann, S. D., Brown, M., & Aggleton, J. P. (2000). Fos expression in the rostral thalamic nuclei and associated cortical regions in response to different spatial memory tasks. *Neuroscience, 101,* 983–991.

Vann, S. D., Brown, M.W., Erichsen, J. T., & Aggleton, J. P. (2000a). Fos imaging reveals differential patterns of hippocampal and parahippocampal subfield activity in response to different spatial memory tasks. *Journal of Neuroscience, 20,* 2711–2718.

Vann, S. D., Brown, M. W., Erichsen, J. T., & Aggleton, J. P. (2000b). Using Fos imaging in the rat to determine the anatomical extent of the disruptive effects of fornix lesions. *Journal of Neuroscience, 20,* 8144–8152.

Vargha-Khadem, F., Gadian, D. G., Watkins. K. E., Connelly, A., Van Paesschen, W., & Mishkin, M. (1997). Differential effects of early hippocampal pathology on episodic and semantic memory. *Science, 277,* 376–380.

Warburton, E. C., & Aggleton, J. P. (1999). Differential deficits in the Morris water maze following cytotoxic lesions of the anterior thalamus and fornix transection. *Behavioural Brain Research, 98,* 27–38.

Warburton, E. C., Baird, A. L., Morgan, A., Muir, J. L., & Aggleton, J. P. (2000). Disconnecting hippocampal projections to the anterior thalamus produces deficits on tests of spatial memory in rats. *European Journal of Neuroscience, 12,* 1714–1726.

Warburton, E. C., Baird, A. L., Morgan, A., Muir, J. L., & Aggleton, J. P. (2001). The importance of the anterior thalamic nuclei for hippocampal function: evidence from a disconnection study in the rat. *Journal of Neuroscience, 21,* 7323–7330.

Warrington, E. K. (1984). *Recognition Memory Test.* Windsor, England: National Foundation for Educational Research–Nelson.

Wechsler, D. (1987). *The Wechsler Memory Scale—Revised.* New York: Psychological Corporation.

Whishaw, I. Q., Cassel, J.-C., & Jarrard, L. E. (1995). Rats with fimbria–fornix lesions display a place response in a swimming pool: A dissociation between getting there and knowing where. *Journal of Neuroscience, 15,* 5779–5788.

Whishaw, I. Q., & Jarrard, L. E. (1995). Similarities vs. differences in place learning and circadian activity in rats after fimbria–fornix section or ibotenate removal of hippocampal cells. *Hippocampus, 5,* 595–604.

Whishaw, I. Q., & Jarrard, L. E. (1996). Evidence for extrahippocampal involvement in place learning and hippocampal involvement in path integration. *Hippocampus, 6,* 513–524.

Wiig, K., & Bilkey, D. K. (1995). Lesions of rat perirhinal cortex exacerbate the memory deficit observed following damage to the fimbria-fornix. *Behavioral Neuroscience, 109,* 620–630.

Woolsey, R. M., & Nelson, J. S. (1975). Asymptomatic destruction of the fornix in man. *Archives of Neurology, 32,* 566–568.

Yasuno, F., Hirata, M., Takimoto, H., Taniguchi, M., Nakagawa, Y., Ikejiri, Y., Nishikawa, T., Shinozaki, K., Tanabbe, H., Sugita, Y., & Takeda, M. (1999). Retrograde temporal order amnesia resulting from damage to the fornix. *Journal of Neurology, Neurosurgery and Psychiatry, 67,* 102–105.

Zola, S. M., & Squire, L. R. (2001). Relationship between magnitude of damage to the hippocampus and impaired recognition memory in monkeys. *Hippocampus, 11,* 92–98.

Zola, S. M., Squire, L. R., Teng, E., Stefanacci, L., Buffalo, E. A., & Clark, R. E. (2000). Impaired recognition memory in monkeys after damage limited to the hippocampal region. *Journal of Neuroscience, 20,* 451–463.

Zola-Morgan, S., Squire, L. R., & Amaral, D. G. (1989). Lesions of the hippocampal formation but not lesions of the fornix or mamillary bodies produce long-lasting memory impairments in monkeys. *Journal of Neuroscience, 9,* 898–913.

31

Subregional Analysis of Hippocampal Function in the Rat

RAYMOND P. KESNER, PAUL E. GILBERT, and INAH LEE

In recent years, there has been an increasing interest in developing computational models of the hippocampus that can provide mechanisms for understanding spatial navigation and/ or processing of mnemonic information. We focus in this chapter on the role of the hippocampus in mediating memory functions. All of the computational models emphasize subregional specificity (the dentate gyrus [DG], CA3, and CA1) and mnemonic process specificity (pattern separation as a component of encoding; short-term or working memory; pattern association; pattern completion as a component of retrieval; and consolidation and intermediate memory). Both subregional and mnemonic process specificity are based mainly on anatomical and physiological recording data, and to some extent on behavioral analyses of hippocampal function (Marr, 1971; O'Reilly & McClelland, 1994; Rolls, 1996; Shapiro & Olton, 1994; Tanila, 1999). In contrast, other models of hippocampal function have assumed that the hippocampus operates as a single anatomical unit with an emphasis on one or two mnemonic processes. A few of the computational models emphasize attribute specificity, such as the representation of spatial (Kesner & Rolls, 2001; McNaughton & Nadel, 1989) or temporal (Levy, 1996; Lisman, 1999; Wallenstein, Eichenbaum, & Hasselmo, 1998) information. However, most of the computational models suggest that all attributes, including space, time, and sensory perception, are processed within the hippocampus (O'Reilly & McClelland, 1994; Rolls, 1996; Shapiro & Olton, 1994). In this chapter, we highlight behavioral analyses of hippocampal mediation of pattern separation, pattern association, and pattern completion processes based on spatial and temporal information.

PATTERN SEPARATION

It can be demonstrated that single cells within the hippocampus are activated by most sensory (including vestibular, olfactory, visual, auditory, and somatosensory) inputs, and are activated to reflect higher-order integration of sensory stimuli (Cohen & Eichenbaum,

1993). A question of importance is whether these sensory inputs have a memory representation within the hippocampus. One possible role of the hippocampus in processing sensory information may be to provide for sensory markers to demarcate a spatial location, so that the hippocampus can more efficiently mediate spatial information. That is, one of the main functions of the hippocampus may be to encode and separate spatial events from each other. This function would ensure that new, highly processed sensory information is organized within the hippocampus, and would enhance the possibility of remembering and temporarily storing one place as separate from another place. It is assumed that this is accomplished via pattern separation of event information, so that spatial events can be separated from each other and spatial interference can be reduced. This assumption is consistent with computational models of hippocampal function and cellular recording studies suggesting that the hippocampus supports pattern separation or orthogonalization of sensory input (Marr, 1971; McNaughton & Nadel, 1989; O'Reilly & McClelland, 1994; Rolls, 1996; Shapiro & Olton, 1994; Tanila, 1999). Computational models of hippocampal function suggest that pattern separation may be a function associated specifically with the DG (O'Reilly & McClelland, 1994; Rolls, 1996; Shapiro & Olton, 1994). These models propose that pattern separation is mediated by a competitive inhibitory network at the level of the DG (Rolls & Treves, 1998), as well as facilitated by sparse connections in the mossy-fiber system that connects DG neurons to CA3 neurons. The separation of patterns is accomplished due to the low probability that any two CA3 neurons will receive mossy-fiber input synapses from a similar subset of DG cells (Rolls, 1996). Shapiro and Olton (1994) also suggest that pattern separation may be facilitated by connections between CA3 and CA1.

Spatial Pattern Separation

Few behavioral experiments have been conducted to test whether the hippocampus and its subregions support spatial pattern separation. A post hoc analysis of the data from behavioral studies indicates that a deficiency in pattern separation may account for some of the behavioral deficits observed in rats with hippocampal lesions on certain spatial memory tasks. Support for this idea comes from two studies (Eichenbaum, 1996; Eichenbaum, Stewart, & Morris, 1990). When rats with fimbria–fornix lesions were trained on a water maze from a constant starting position, they learned the task as well as controls did. However, when the starting point varied on each trial, the rats with fimbria–fornix lesions displayed deficits in acquisition. In a similar study, Hunt, Kesner, and Evans (1994) demonstrated that rats with hippocampal lesions learned to enter a designated arm on an eight-arm radial maze when the arm remained constant. However, when the reward arm varied on each trial, rats with hippocampal lesions were impaired relative to controls. Moreover, McDonald and White (1995) reported deficits in animals with fornix lesions on a radial-arm maze task when the arm locations were proximal to each other. This deficit could reflect inefficient pattern separation. Rats with hippocampal lesions were impaired on these tasks when there was increased overlap or similarity among distal cues for each to-be-remembered location. Yet they performed the tasks well when the similarity was decreased. When locations are proximal as in McDonald and White's tasks, when the correct arm is varied as in Hunt and colleagues' (1994) task, or when the starting position is varied as in the task used by Eichenbaum and colleagues (1990), the locations may share many common environmental cues. In contrast, when the locations are distal or the starting point does not vary on each trial, there is minimal overlap or commonality among the environmental cues used to distinguish between the different locations. If disruption of hippocampal function results in inefficient pattern separation, then deficits on spatial tasks may occur when there is increased overlap or similarity among distal cues (and presumably increased similarity among representations within the hippocampus).

To examine directly the role of the hippocampus in separating spatial pattern information, we (Gilbert, Kesner, & DeCoteau, 1998) developed a paradigm that measured short-term memory for spatial location information as a function of spatial similarity between two spatial locations. Specifically, rats were required to remember a spatial location dependent upon environmental cues, and to differentiate between the to-be-remembered location and a different location with different degrees of similarity or overlap among the cues. Animals were tested with a cheeseboard maze apparatus and were trained on a delayed-matching-to-sample task for spatial location. Animals were trained to displace an object that was randomly positioned to cover a baited food well in one of 15 locations. The 15 locations were arranged in a row perpendicular to a start box. Following a short delay, the animals were required to choose between two objects identical to the sample object. One object was in the same location as the sample object, and the second object was in a different location among the 15 food wells. An animal was rewarded for displacing the object that was in the same position as the sample object (correct choice), but the animal received no reward for displacing the foil object (incorrect choice). Five spatial separations, from 15 cm to 105 cm, were used in the choice task to separate the correct object from the incorrect object. The animals were trained until they achieved a criterion of 75% correct across all spatial separations, and then the animals received either cortical control lesions or hippocampal lesions. Animals with cortical control lesions matched their preoperative performance, regardless of how close together or far apart the objects were located at test. In contrast, animals with hippocampal lesions were impaired at all spatial separations except the largest (105 cm). Transfer tasks demonstrated that animals tended to use environmental cues to solve this task rather than other possible strategies. These results suggested that lesions of the hippocampus decrease efficiency in spatial pattern separation. As a result, performance is impaired on trials when the objects are close together and when the spatial similarity among working memory representations is greatest.

Our (Gilbert et al., 1998) findings indicate that the hippocampus is involved in mediating spatial pattern separation. However, it is not clear from this study whether multiple subregions of the hippocampus support the separation of patterns of incoming spatial information, or whether a specific subregion may be responsible, as suggested by computational models (O'Reilly & McClelland, 1994; Rolls, 1996; Shapiro & Olton, 1994). Alternatively, if efficient separation of patterns is dependent on a functional hippocampal ensemble, then a lesion to any region of the hippocampus should impair performance on this task. To examine the role of hippocampal subregions in spatial pattern separation, we (Gilbert, Kesner, & Lee, in press) tested rats with DG or CA1 lesions on the same task. DG lesions were generated by intracranial infusions of colchicine into dorsal DG, whereas CA1 lesions were generated by intracranial infusions of ibotenic acid into dorsal CA1. The results (Figure 31.1) demonstrate that it is possible to dissociate the functions of the DG and CA1. On the spatial separation task, rats with DG lesions were significantly impaired; however, rats with CA1 lesions matched the performance of controls. The lack of a deficit in the CA1 group on the spatial task indicates that a fully intact hippocampus is not necessary for the separation of patterns of spatial information. Given that CA1 represents the primary output from the hippocampus, how can information be transmitted to other neural regions once CA1 is destroyed? This is a very important question, since other studies have also reported a lack of a deficit in spatial memory following selective damage to CA1

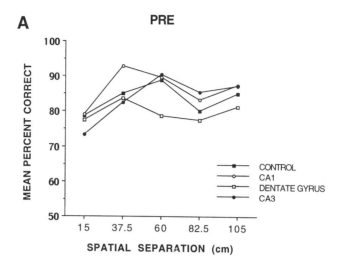

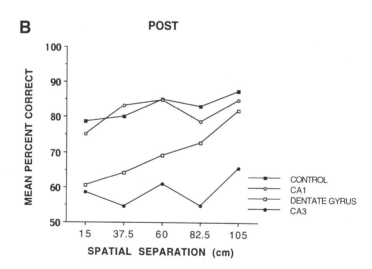

FIGURE 31.1. Spatial pattern separation. Mean percentage of correct performance as a function of spatial separation for control animals, and animals with lesions of the CA1, CA3, or DG on (A) preoperative trials and (B) postoperative trials. Data from Gilbert, Kesner, and Lee (in press).

(Davis, Colombo, & Volpe, 1988; Jarrard, 1978; Mizumori, Garcia, Raja, & Volpe, 1994). Since the CA1 lesions in the Gilbert, Kesner, and Lee (in press) study were restricted to dorsal CA1, it is possible that the sparing in ventral CA1 could support the transfer of information from CA1 out of the hippocampus. However, recent unpublished data from our laboratory have shown that rats with significant dorsal and ventral CA1 lesions perform this task as well as controls (Gilbert, Kesner, & Lee, in press). Therefore, the information does not appear to be transmitted out of the hippocampus via ventral CA1. It is suggested that the information is passed via direct CA3 extrahippocampal connections. CA3 has direct projections to the medial and lateral septal nuclei (Amaral & Witter, 1995;

Gaykema, van der Kull, Hersh, & Luiten, 1991; Risold & Swanson, 1997). The lateral septum has connections with the medial septum (Jakab & Leranth, 1995); in turn, the medial septum has projections to subiculum and eventually entorhinal cortex (Amaral & Witter, 1995; Jakab & Leranth, 1995). Thus it is possible for CA3 output to bypass the CA1 region.

In addition to behavioral data and computational models suggesting that the hippocampus may separate patterns of incoming information, there are also some physiological data. McNaughton, Barnes, Meltzer, and Sutherland (1989) examined the effects of colchicine lesions in the dorsal DG on the spatial and temporal firing characteristics of cells in the CA1 and CA3 fields. It was found that DG lesions resulted in decreased firing reliability in CA1 and CA3 neurons. If CA1 and CA3 cells are showing decreased reliability following DG lesions, then the cells may not be forming accurate representations of space. This decrease in firing reliability could reflect decreased efficiency in the DG pattern separation mechanism. A recent study by Tanila (1999) has offered cellular recording evidence for the existence of a pattern separation mechanism for generating separate representations in CA3 based on overlapping inputs. It was shown that CA3 place cells were able to maintain distinct representations of two visually identical environments and selectively reactivate either one of the representation patterns, depending on the rat's experience. The separated representations in CA3 could reflect the operation of a pattern separation mechanism at the level of the DG. In addition, CA3 may represent a temporary short-term memory buffer for patterned separated representations, based on its recurrent collateral network system (Kesner, Gilbert, & Wallenstein, 2000; Kesner & Rolls, 2001). With few exceptions, computational models of the hippocampus suggest that the CA3 region can be represented as an autoassociative network memory system that forms and temporarily stores short-term, episodic, or working memories. It is assumed that CA3 operates as an autoassociative attractor network because of recurrent excitatory connections among CA3 cells, the presence of long-term synaptic modification, and Hebbian associations, which are formed between presynaptic and postsynaptic interconnected cells. In conjunction with a set of inhibitory processes, such a network can provide a mechanism for maintaining coherent information for a short duration. In order to examine the role of the CA3 in the spatial pattern separation task, new rats with ibotenic acid lesions of the CA3 were tested in the spatial pattern separation task. The results are shown in Figure 31.1 and indicate that there was a total deficit for all spatial separations, suggesting that the CA3 region contributes to a short-term memory representation of spatial information.

Temporal Pattern Separation

Based on evidence that almost all sensory information is processed by hippocampal neurons (perhaps to provide sensory markers for time as well as space), and that the hippocampus mediates temporal information, it is likely that one of the main process functions of the hippocampus is to encode the temporal order of events. This function would ensure that newly processed sensory information is organized within the hippocampus, and would enhance the possibility of remembering and temporarily storing one event as separate from another event in time. Based on these ideas, researchers have examined the role of the hippocampus in tasks that may require the separation of temporal patterned information. Estes (1986) summarized data demonstrating that items occurring further apart in a sequence are remembered better than are temporally adjacent items. Other studies have also shown that memory performance improves as the number of items in a sequence between the test items increases (Banks, 1987; Madsen & Kesner, 1995). This phenomenon is referred to as a "temporal separation effect." It is assumed to occur because there is more interference for temporally proximal events than for temporally distant events.

Based on these findings, Chiba, Kesner, and Reynolds (1994) tested memory for the temporal order of items. In the task, each rat was given one daily trial consisting of a sample phase followed by a choice phase. During the sample phase, the animal visited each arm of an eight-arm radial maze once in a randomly predetermined order, and was given a reward at the end of each arm. The choice phase began immediately following the presentation of the final arm in the sequence. In the choice phase, two arms were opened simultaneously, and the animal was allowed to choose between the two arms. To obtain a food reward, the animal had to enter the arm that occurred earlier in the sequence that it had just followed. Temporal separations of 0, 2, 4, and 6 were randomly selected for each choice phase. These values represented the number of arms in the sample phase that intervened between the two arms that were to be used in the test phase. For example, a "0 separation" describes a condition when two arms followed each other in the sequence during the sample phase, and a "6 separation" describes a condition when visits to six different arms intervened between the two arms that were to be used in the choice phase. Once an animal reached a 75% correct criterion across all temporal separations (with the exception of the 0 separation, which rats performed at chance levels), each animal received either a hippocampal or a cortical control lesion. Following surgery, control rats matched their preoperative performance across all temporal separations. In contrast, rats with hippocampal lesions performed at chance levels across 0, 2, or 4 temporal separations, and at slightly above chance levels in the case of a 6 separation. The results suggest that the hippocampus is involved in memory for spatial location as a function of temporal separation, and that lesions of the hippocampus decrease efficiency in temporal pattern separation.

From these findings, it appears that the hippocampus is involved in mediating temporal pattern separation. However, it is not clear from this study whether multiple subregions of the hippocampus support the separation of patterns of incoming temporal information, or whether a specific subregion may be responsible for this process, as suggested by some computational models (O'Reilly & McClelland, 1994; Rolls, 1996; Shapiro & Olton, 1994). To examine the role of hippocampal subregions in temporal pattern separation, we (Gilbert, Kesner, & Lee, in press) tested rats with DG or CA1 lesions on the same task. DG lesions were generated by intracranial infusions of colchicine into dorsal DG, while CA1 lesions were generated by intracranial infusions of ibotenic acid into dorsal CA1. The results are shown in Figure 31.2 and demonstrate a dissociation in DG and CA1 functions. On the temporal separation task, rats with CA1 lesions showed impairments, whereas rats with DG lesions matched the performance of the control group. The lack of a deficit in the DG group on the temporal task indicates that a fully intact hippocampal system is not necessary for the accurate separation of patterns of temporal information. Even though this task is based on spatiotemporal information, it should be noted that the distal cues used to differentiate two adjacent arms in the eight-arm maze were an average of 104 cm apart. This distance between distal cues represents a distance that in the spatial pattern separation task described earlier did not result in a deficit in rats with DG lesions. Thus, in the temporal discrimination task, spatial pattern separation information should have been available to the rats with DG lesions. In comparison with the findings from the spatial pattern separation task, the data indicate that the DG is involved in separating spatial patterns but not temporal patterns. In contrast, CA1 is involved in separating temporal patterns but not spatial patterns. These findings appear to offer support for the computational models proposed by Rolls (1996), O'Reilly and McClelland (1994), and Shapiro

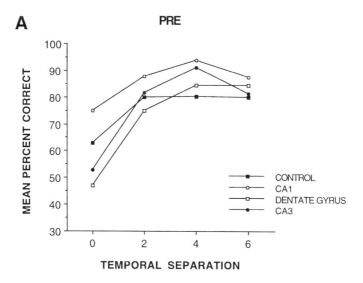

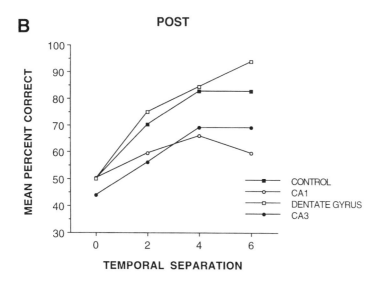

FIGURE 31.2. Temporal pattern separation. Mean percentage of correct performance as a function of temporal separation for control animals, and animals with lesions of the CA1, CA3, or DG on (A) preoperative trials and (B) postoperative trials. Data from Gilbert, Kesner, and Lee (in press).

and Olton (1994). The study represents one of the first behavioral double dissociation between subregions of the hippocampus.

Even though CA1 lesions produced a deficit in temporal pattern separation, some computational models (Levy, 1996; Lisman, 1999; Wallenstein & Hasselmo, 1997) have suggested that the CA3 region provides the means to combine separate items (spatial locations, in the experiment presented above) in a sequential fashion. These computational models have suggested that recurrent collaterals within the CA3 region can result in the activation of an asymmetrical network within CA3, which makes this area an ideal subregion of the hippocampus to code items in a temporal sequence. It was thus of interest to use the temporal order task to determine whether the CA3 region plays an important role. In this case, lesions were made using ibotenic acid injections into the CA3 region. The results are presented in Figure 31.2. The CA3 lesions impaired temporal pattern separation, just as was observed for lesions of the CA1 region. One possible explanation of this result is that the CA3 and CA1 subregions of the hippocampus work together to achieve temporal pattern separation for spatial information. CA3 may be important for associating, processing, and integrating sequential spatial information, and perhaps for maintaining a short-term representation of sequentially associated spatial information as a spatial context. Thus information may then be sent via feedforward connections to CA1, a region that directly involves chunking and temporally separating spatial information to endow this spatial context with a temporal structure of the task. Computational models and physiological data (Rolls, 1996; Skaggs, McNaughton, Wilson, & Barnes, 1996) have suggested that CA1 may play a role in compressing temporal sequences. Rolls (1996) has suggested that CA1 recodes the information represented in the CA3 network, possibly through a chunking process. We are proposing that this chunking process is facilitated by a pattern separation mechanism within CA1. Skaggs and colleagues (1996) showed electrophysiologically that the temporal structure of cell firing in CA1 becomes more compressed after initial exposure to a spatial location. In addition to asymmetrical recurrent connections within CA3, the asymmetric nature of feedforward connections from CA3 to CA1 has been known to produce a temporally specific property (e.g., negative skewness) in CA1, perhaps resulting in coding the temporal order of stimuli (Laron & Lynch, 1989; Mehta, Quirk, & Wilson, 2000). This property implicates CA1 in chunking and temporally sequencing spatial locations, reflecting the nature of the task and the environment. Thus, in the task used by Chiba and colleagues (1994), it is possible that as a rat moves down arms of the eight-arm maze, CA3 contributes by making sequential associations of spatial information and maintaining short-term memory representation of these sequential associations, and CA1 by chunking and temporally separating these spatial associations to provide a mechanism for temporal pattern separation of specific sequential units.

Although the data suggest that the hippocampus is involved in spatial and temporal pattern separation, data from our lab have demonstrated that the hippocampus is not involved in pattern separation for motor responses and reward value (Gilbert & Kesner, 2001, in press-a). Furthermore, additional data have demonstrated that the caudate nucleus and amygdala support pattern separation for motor responses and reward value, respectively (Gilbert & Kesner, 2001, in press-a). Therefore, the role of the hippocampus may be limited to spatial and temporal pattern separation.

PATTERN ASSOCIATION

It has been suggested that in addition to pattern separation, the hippocampus and its subregions support the formation of arbitrary associations, including paired-associate learning (Cohen & Eichenbaum, 1993). Rolls (1996) suggests that the hippocampus—specifically a CA3 autoassociative network—is responsible for the formation and storage of arbitrary associations. For example, information from parietal cortex regarding the location of an object may be associated with information from temporal cortex regarding the identity of an object. These two kinds of information may be projected to the CA3 region of the hippocampus to enable the organism to remember a particular object and its location.

Spatial Pattern Association

Behavioral studies have examined the effects of hippocampal lesions on the formation of arbitrary associations using paired-associate learning. Nonhuman primates and rats with hippocampal damage have been tested using paired-associate learning involving spatial stimuli. Nonhuman primates and rats with hippocampal lesions display deficits in object–place paired-associate learning (Gaffan, 1994; Gaffan & Harrison, 1989; Sziklas, Lebel, & Petrides, 1998; Sziklas & Petrides, 1996, 1999).

Our lab has designed a series of experiments to directly test the involvement of the hippocampus in spatial paired-associate learning. Rats were trained on a successive discrimination go/no-go task to examine object–place paired-associate learning. In this task, two paired associates were reinforced; these consisted of one particular object (A) in one particular location (1) and a different object (B) in a different location (2). Mispairs that were not reinforced included object A in location 2, and object B in location 1. Rats needed to learn that if an object was presented in its paired location, then the rats should displace the object to receive a reward (go); however, the rats should withhold displacing the object if it was not in its paired location (no-go). The results are shown in Figure 31.3A and indicate that rats with hippocampal lesions were, relative to controls, severely impaired in learning object–place paired associations (Gilbert & Kesner, in press-a, in press-b).

In a second task, rats were trained on a successive discrimination go/no-go task to examine odor–place paired-associate learning. In this task, the same procedure was used, except that rats needed to learn that when an odor was presented in its paired location, the rats should dig in sand mixed with the odor to receive a reward. The results are shown in Figure 31.3B and indicate that rats with hippocampal lesions were, relative to controls, severely impaired in learning odor–place paired associations (Gilbert & Kesner, in press-a, in press-b).

In a third task, rats were trained on a successive discrimination go/no-go task to examine odor–object paired-associate learning. In this task, the same procedure was used; in this task, however, the two paired associates that were reinforced consisted of one particular odor (A) and one object (1) and a different odor (B) and another object (2). Mispairs that were not reinforced included odor A and object 2, and odor B and object 1. Both the objects and the odors were presented in one fixed central location. Rats needed to learn that when the correct odor was presented simultaneously with the correct object, the rats should dig in sand mixed with the odor to receive a reward. The results are shown in Figure 31.3C and indicate that rats with hippocampal lesions acquired the odor–object task as quickly as controls (Gilbert & Kesner, in press-a, in press-b).

These data suggest that the hippocampus is clearly involved in paired-associate learning when a stimulus must be associated with a spatial location, but that the hippocampus does not appear to be important when a spatial location is not a component of the paired-associate task.

Although computational models (Rolls, 1996) suggest that the CA3 autoassociative network supports paired-associate learning, few if any behavioral studies have directly tested this hypothesis. Data from our laboratory using the above-described paradigms indicate that rats with CA3 lesions are severely impaired in object–place and object–odor paired-associate learning (see A and B in Figure 31.3). However, animals with DG or CA1 lesions learn the object–place task as well as controls do (Gilbert & Kesner, 2000). These data supports the hypothesis that CA3, but not DG or CA1, supports paired-associate learning when a stimulus must be associated with a spatial location.

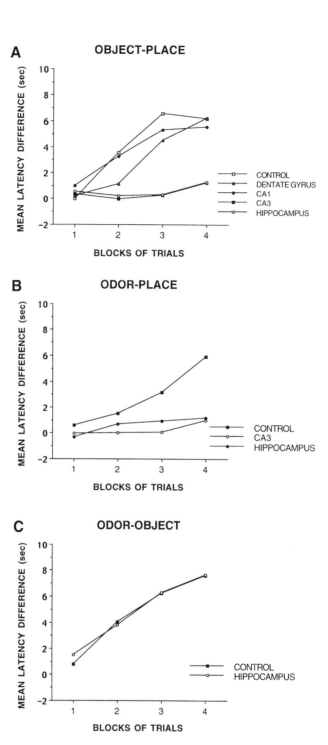

FIGURE 31.3. Spatial pattern association. Mean latency difference (latency on paired trials, subtracted from mispaired trials, with a 10-second cutoff) as a function of blocks of trials (60 trials/block) for (A) control animals and animals with hippocampus, CA1, CA3, or DG lesions on acquisition of an object–place paired-associate task; (B) control animals and animals with hippocampus or CA3 lesions on acquisition of an odor–place paired-associate task; and (C) control animals and animals with hippocampus lesions on acquisition of an odor–object paired-associate task. Data from Gilbert and Kesner (in press-a, in press-b).

Temporal Pattern Association

The hippocampus appears to contribute to some forms of temporal associative learning. For example, using an instrumental learning paradigm, Mikulka and Freeman (1975) trained rats with hippocampal lesions to select the goal box opposite their initial preference in a Y-maze following a 30-second delay. In one condition, choice of the goal box resulted in an immediate reinforcement; in the other condition, reinforcement was given after a 10-second delay. Compared to control groups, the rats with hippocampal lesions could learn the immediate but not the delayed reinforcement condition. This result suggests that the temporal processing required to associate the correct spatial location with a reward requires the hippocampus. Using a classical conditioning paradigm, Moyer, Deyo, and Disterhoft (1990) found that lesions of the hippocampus in rabbits disrupted the acquisition of eyeblink trace conditioning. In trace conditioning, a short delay intervened between the conditioned stimulus (CS) and the unconditioned stimulus (US). When, however, a US and CS overlapped in time (delay conditioning), rabbits with hippocampal damage typically performed as well as normal rabbits did. Similar learning deficits in trace fear conditioning were observed for rats with hippocampal lesions and for mice that lacked N-methyl-D-aspartate receptors in CA1 (Disterhoft, McEchron, & Tseng, 1999; Huerta, Sun, Wilson, & Tonegawa, 2000). Again, there were no deficits in a delay conditioning paradigm. Thus the hippocampus is not involved in forming all arbitrary associations, but is involved only when temporal processing is required to establish a pattern association. Further support for the importance of the CA1 region comes from the observation that CA1 pyramidal cells in rabbits given trace eyeblink conditioning exhibited a large increase in activity after both the CS and UCS early in conditioning (McEchron & Disterhoft, 1997). Thus temporal pattern associations may be mediated by the CA1 region. More research is needed to examine the role of the CA3 and DG regions in supporting temporal pattern associations. Although the data suggest that the hippocampus is involved in both spatial and temporal pattern associations, many studies have demonstrated that the hippocampus is not involved in pattern associations involving odor–odor (Bunsey & Eichenbaum, 1993; Li, Matsumoto, & Watanabe, 1999), auditory–visual (Jarrard & Davidson, 1990), visual–response (Winocur, 1991; Wise & Murray, 1999), object–object (Bingman, Strasser, Baker, & Riters, 1998; Cho & Kesner, 1995; Murray, Gaffan, & Mishkin, 1993), and odor–object (Gilbert & Kesner, 2000) associations.

PATTERN COMPLETION

It has also been suggested that the hippocampus and its subregions support pattern completion, in addition to pattern separation and pattern association. Pattern completion provides a mechanism to generate complete retrieval of well-established information based on partial or incomplete inputs. A number of computational models have proposed that autoassociative attractor networks in CA3 can perform pattern completion; that is, if a degraded version of a stimulus is presented after learning, the represented feature can be recalled from this incomplete input information (Rolls & Treves, 1998; Wallenstein et al., 1998).

Spatial Pattern Completion

It has been shown in rats that spatial cells recorded in the CA1 or hilar/CA3 subregions of the hippocampus continue to fire in the dark when visual cues are not available. This observation has been interpreted to reflect a spatial pattern completion process. It should be noted that more cells in the CA1 region than in the hilar/CA3 region displayed pattern completion (Mizumori, Ragozzino, Cooper, & Leutgeb, 1999). Similar results were reported in monkeys with spatial view cells recorded in CA1 or CA3. Again, when the view details were obscured, the spatial view cells continued to fire when the monkeys looked toward where the view had been. Again, more cells in CA1 than in CA3 displayed pattern completion (Robertson, Rolls, & Georges-Francios, 1998; Rolls, 1999).

There has been no behavioral research on the role of the hippocampus, and specifically of CA3, in pattern completion. To study pattern completion in a short-term memory paradigm, it is important that only partial or reduced information (relative to the study phase information) is presented. To examine the role of the hippocampus in mediating pattern completion, we measured short-term memory for spatial location as a function of how many components present during the study phase were removed during the test phase. Rats were tested with a cheeseboard maze apparatus on the delayed-matching-to-sample task for spatial location, as described earlier. The study phase was identical to that used in the spatial pattern separation experiment, but in this experiment, following a short delay, the animals were required to find the same location even though the object was removed. An animal was rewarded for choosing the same spatial location as the sample phase object (correct choice), but received no reward for choosing a different location (incorrect choice). In additional manipulations, the object was removed and curtains were lowered to eliminate extramaze cues (spatial condition); the object was removed and the animal was rotated seven times (vestibular condition); or the object was removed, the curtains were lowered, and the animal was rotated (spatial and vestibular condition).

Normal rats readily learned this task, and they performed well on the choice phase when the object was removed, when the curtain was lowered (spatial condition), or when the animals were rotated (vestibular condition). However, normal rats were impaired and performed at chance levels when all three manipulations (object removal plus spatial and vestibular condition) were combined. The results are shown in Figure 31.4A. After preoperative training, rats received cortical control, complete hippocampal, or CA3 lesions. The results are shown in Figure 31.4B. Control rats continued to perform the task well when any one of the cues was manipulated. In contrast, rats with complete hippocampal or CA3 lesions displayed a deficit when the object was removed or when object removal was combined with the spatial or vestibular condition. These data are consistent with proposed computational models (Hasselmo & McClelland, 1999; O'Reilly & McClelland, 1994; Rolls, 1999; Shapiro & Olton, 1994), which predict a deficit on this task following lesions of CA3. The models all suggest that an autoassociative CA3 network is responsible for the completion of patterns based on incomplete input.

Temporal Pattern Completion

In a research paradigm based on learning a hierarchy of serial or temporal ordering of pairwise discriminations (i.e., A > B, B > C, C > D, and D > E), Dusek and Eichenbaum (1997; see also Eichenbaum, Chapter 27, this volume) showed that rats with fornix lesions could accurately acquire concurrent presentations of all the pairs constituting the series. However, when a pair of items (e.g., BD) were presented that the rats had not seen, and the rats had to make a transitive inference judgment (e.g., selecting B rather than D), then rats with fornix lesions were impaired. A transitive inference judgment is thought to require memory for the temporal coding of all the items in a related sequence. It has been suggested that this process requires temporal pattern completion (Kesner et al., 2000;

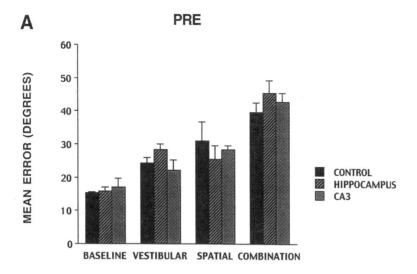

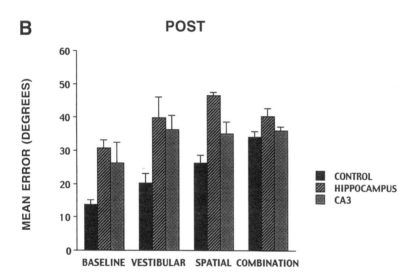

FIGURE 31.4. Spatial pattern completion. Mean error (degrees from target location) for control animals and animals with hippocampal or CA3 lesions on a spatial pattern completion task involving trials with removal of the object (baseline), removal of the object and vestibular cues (vestibular), removal of the object and spatial cues (spatial), or removal of the object, spatial cues, and vestibular cues (combination) on (A) preoperative and (B) postoperative trials.

Wallenstein et al., 1998). Subregional analyses have not yet been carried out using this paradigm, but computational models suggest that the CA1 or CA3 regions may play an important role in this process.

SUMMARY

The data discussed in this chapter are summarized in Table 31.1. It appears that, as proposed by a number of computational models, the hippocampus is involved in processing

TABLE 31.1. Behaviorally Defined Hippocampal Subregions Critical for Different Mnemonic Processes

	Mnemonic processes		
	Pattern separation	Pattern association	Pattern completion
Attributes			
Spatial	DG	CA3	CA3
Temporal	CA1	CA1	—[a]

[a]No data are yet available to clarify the role of each subregion in temporal pattern completion.

information about pattern separation, pattern association, and pattern completion. More specifically, there appears to be subregional specificity for these functions in that the DG is primarily involved in spatial pattern separation, whereas the CA3 region is involved in spatial pattern associations and spatial pattern completion. In contrast, the CA1 region is involved in temporal pattern separation and in temporal pattern associations. No data are yet available to clarify the role of each subregion in temporal pattern completion. In addition, the DG and CA3 appear to be especially important for spatial information, and CA1 for temporal information. Finally, there appears to be some process specificity in that the DG and CA1 are involved in pattern separation, whereas both CA3 and CA1 are involved in pattern association, and CA3 is involved in pattern completion. Clearly, more research is needed to develop more comprehensive computational models and more appropriate behavioral tests to further the idea of subregional (CA1, CA3, DG), process (pattern separation, pattern association, pattern completion), and attribute (spatial, temporal) specificity.

REFERENCES

Amaral, D. G., & Witter, M. P. (1995). Hippocampal formation. In G. Paxinos (Ed.), *The rat nervous system* (2nd ed., pp. 443–493). San Diego, CA: Academic Press.

Banks, W. P. (1987). Encoding and processing of symbolic information in comparitive judgements. In G. H. Bower (Ed.), *The psychology of learning and motivation: Advances in theory and research* (pp. 101–159). New York: Academic Press.

Bingman, V. P., Strasser, R., Baker, C., & Riters, L. V. (1998). Paired-associate learning is unaffected by combined hippocampal and parahippocampal lesion in homing pigeons. *Behavioral Neuroscience, 112,* 533–540.

Bunsey, M., & Eichenbaum, H. (1993). Paired associate learning in rats: Critical involvement of the parahippocampal region. *Behavioral Neuroscience, 107,* 740–747.

Chiba, A. A., Kesner, R. P., & Reynolds, A. (1994). Memory for spatial location as a function of temporal lag in rats: Role of hippocampus and medial prefrontal cortex. *Behavioral and Neural Biology, 61,* 123–131.

Cho, Y. H., & Kesner, R. P. (1995). Relational object association learning in rats with hippocampal lesions. *Behavioural Brain Research, 67,* 91–98.

Cohen, N. J., & Eichenbaum, H. B. (Eds.). (1993). *Memory, amnesia, and hippocampal function.* Cambridge, MA: MIT Press.

Davis, H. P., Colombo, P. J., & Volpe, B. T. (1988). Preoperative training effects on radial maze performance in animals with ischemia or ibotenic acid hippocampal injury. *Society for Neuroscience Abstracts, 14,* 1228.

Disterhoft, J. F., McEchron, M. D., & Tseng, W. (1999). Neurotoxic lesions of the dorsal hippocampus disrupt auditory-cued trace heart rate (fear) conditioning in rabbit. *Society for Neuroscience Abstracts, 25,* 1619.

Dusek, J. A., & Eichenbaum, H. (1997). The hippocampus and memory for orderly stimulus relations. *Proceedings of the National Academy of Sciences USA, 94,* 7109–7114.

Eichenbaum, H. (1996). Is the rodent hippocampus just for 'place'? *Current Opinion in Neurobiology, 6,* 187–195.

Eichenbaum, H., Stewart, C., & Morris, R. G. M. (1990). Hippocampal representation in place learning. *Journal of Neuroscience, 10,* 3531–3542.

Estes, W. K. (1986). Memory for temporal information. In J. A. Michon & J. L. Jackson (Eds.), *Time, mind, and behavior* (pp. 151–168). New York: Springer-Verlag.

Gaffan, D. (1994). Scene-specific memory for objects: A model of episodic memory impairment in monkeys with fornix transection. *Journal of Cognitive Neuroscience, 6,* 305–320.

Gaffan, D., & Harrison, S. (1989). Place memory and scene memory: Effects of fornix transection. *Experimental Brain Research, 74,* 202–212.

Gaykema, R. P., van der Kuil, J., Hersh, L. B., & Luiten, P. G. (1991). Pattern of direct projections from the hippocampus to the medial septum–diagonal band complex: Anterograde tracing with *Phaseolus vulgaris* leucoagglutinin combined with immunohistochemistry of choline acetyltransferase. *Neuroscience, 43,* 349–360.

Gilbert, P. E., & Kesner, R. P. (2001). [The caudate nucleus but not the hippocampus is involved in pattern separation based on response attributes.] Unpublished raw data.

Gilbert, P. E., & Kesner, R. P. (in press-a). The amygdala but not the hippocampus is involved in pattern separation based on reward value. *Neurobiology of Learning and Memory.*

Gilbert, P. E., & Kesner, R. P. (in press-b). The role of the rodent hippocampus in paired-associate learning involving associations between a stimulus and a spatial location. *Behavioral Neuroscience.*

Gilbert, P. E., & Kesner, R. P. (2000). Role of the hippocampus and hippocampal subregions in paired-associate learning. *Society for Neuroscience Abstracts, 26,* 713.

Gilbert, P. E., Kesner, R. P., & DeCoteau, W. E. (1998). The role of the hippocampus in mediating spatial pattern separation. *Journal of Neuroscience, 18,* 804–810.

Gilbert, P. E., Kesner, R. P., & Lee, I. (in press). Dissociating hippocampal subregions: A double dissociation between dentate gyrus and CA1. *Hippocampus.*

Hasselmo, M. E., & McClelland, J. L. (1999). Neural models of memory. *Current Opinion in Neurobiology, 9,* 184–188.

Huerta, P. T., Sun, L. D., Wilson, M. A., & Tonegawa, S. (2000). Formation of temporal memory requires NMDA receptors within CA1 pyramidal neurons. *Neuron, 25,* 473–480.

Hunt, M. E., Kesner, R. P., & Evans, R. B. (1994). Memory for spatial location: Functional dissociation of entorhinal cortex and hippocampus. *Psychobiology, 22,* 186–194.

Jakab, R. L., & Leranth, C. (1995). Septum. In G. Paxinos (Ed.), *The rat nervous system* (2nd ed., pp. 405–442). San Diego, CA: Academic Press.

Jarrard, L. E. (1978). Selective hippocampal lesions: Differential effects on performance by rats on a spatial task wth preoperative versus postoperative training. *Journal of Comparative and Physiological Psychology, 92,* 1119–1127.

Jarrard, L. E., & Davidson, T. L. (1990). Acquisition of concurrent conditional discriminations in rats with ibotenate lesions of hippocampus and subiculum. *Psychobiology, 18,* 68–73.

Kesner, R. P., Gilbert, P. E., & Wallenstein, G. V. (2000). Testing neural network models of memory with behavioral experiments. *Current Opinion in Neurobiology, 10,* 260–265.

Kesner, R. P., & Rolls, E. T. (2001). Role of long term synaptic modification in short term memory. *Hippocampus, 11,* 240–250.

Larson, J., & Lynch, G. (1989). Theta pattern stimulation and the induction of LTP: The sequence in which synapses are stimulated determines the degree to which they potentiate. *Brain Research, 489,* 49–58.

Levy, W. B. (1996). A sequence predicting CA3 is a flexible association that learns and uses context to solve hippocampal-like tasks. *Hippocampus, 6,* 579–590.

Li, H., Matsumoto, K., & Watanabe, H. (1999). Different effects of unilateral and bilateral hippocampus lesions in rats on the performance of radial maze and odor-paired associate tasks. *Brain Research Bulletin, 48,* 113–119.

Lisman, J. E. (1999). Relating hippocampal circuitry to function: Recall of memory sequences by reciprocal dentate–CA3 interactions. *Neuron, 22*, 233–242.

Madsen, J., & Kesner, R. P. (1995). The temporal distance effect in subjects with dementia of the Alzheimer's type. *Alzheimer's Disease and Associated Disorders, 9*, 94–100.

Marr, D. (1971). Simple memory, a theory for archicortex. *Philosophical Transactions of the Royal Society of London, Series B, 262*, 23–81.

McDonald, R. J., & White, N. M. (1995). Hippocampal and nonhippocampal contributions to place learning in rats. *Behavioral Neuroscience, 109*, 579–593.

McEchron, M. D., & Disterhoft, J. F. (1997). Sequence of single neuron changes in CA1 hippocampus of rabbits during acquisition of trace eyeblink conditioned responses. *Journal of Neurophysiology, 78*, 1030–1044.

McNaughton, B. L., Barnes, C. A., Meltzer, J., & Sutherland, R. J. (1989). Hippocampal granule cells are necessary for normal spatial learning but not for spatially-selective pyramidal cell discharge. *Experimental Brain Research, 76*, 485–496.

McNaughton, B. L., & Nadel, L. (1989). Hebb–Marr networks and the neurobiological representation of action in space. In M. A. Gluck & D. E. Rumelhart (Eds.), *Neuroscience and connectionist theory* (pp. 1–63). Hillsdale, NJ: Erlbaum.

Mehta, M. R., Quirk, M. C., & Wilson, M. A. (2000). Experience-dependent asymmetric shape of hippocampal receptive fields. *Neuron, 25*, 707–715.

Mikulka, P. J., & Freeman, F. G. (1975). The effects of reinforcement delay and hippocampal lesions on the acquisition of a choice response. *Behavioral Biology, 15*, 473–477.

Mizumori, S. J. Y., Garcia, P. A., Raja, M. A., & Volpe, B. T. (1994). Spatial- and locomotion-related neural representation in the rat hippocampus following long-term survival from ischemia. *Behavioral Neuroscience, 109*, 1081–1094.

Mizumori, S. J. Y., Ragozzino, K. E., Cooper, B. G., & Leutgeb, S. (1999). Hippocampal representational organization and spatial context. *Hippocampus, 9*, 444–451.

Moyer, J. R., Jr., Deyo, R. A., & Disterhoft, J. F. (1990). Hippocampectomy disrupts trace eyeblink conditioning in rabbits. *Behavioral Neuroscience, 104*, 243–252.

Murray, E. A., Gaffan, D., & Mishkin, M. (1993). Neural substrates of visual stimulus–stimulus association in rhesus monkeys. *Journal of Neuroscience, 13*, 4549–4561.

O'Reilly, R. C., & McClelland, J. L. (1994). Hippocampal conjunctive encoding storage, and recall: Avoiding a trade-off. *Hippocampus, 4*, 661–682.

Risold, P. Y., & Swanson, L. W. (1997). Connections of the rat lateral septal complex. *Brain Research Reviews, 24*, 115–195.

Robertson, R. G., Rolls, E. T., & Georges-Francios, P. (1998). Spatial view of cells in the primate hippocampus: Effects of removal of view details. *Journal of Neurophysiology, 79*, 1145–1156.

Rolls, E. T. (1996). A theory of hippocampal function in memory. *Hippocampus, 6*, 601–620.

Rolls, E. T. (1999). Spatial view cells and the representation of place in the primate hippocampus. *Hippocampus, 9*, 467–480.

Rolls, E. T., & Treves, A. (1998). *Neural networks and brain function.* Oxford: Oxford University Press.

Shapiro, M. L., & Olton, D. S. (1994). Hippocampal function and interference. In D. L. Schacter & E. Tulving (Eds.), *Memory systems 1994* (pp. 141–146). Cambridge, MA: MIT Press.

Skaggs, W. E., McNaughton, B. L., Wilson, M. A., & Barnes, C. A. (1996). Theta phase precession in hippocampal neuronal populations and the compression of temporal sequences. *Hippocampus, 6*, 149–172.

Sziklas, V., Lebel, S., & Petrides, M. (1998). Conditional associative learning and the hippocampal system. *Hippocampus, 8*, 131–137.

Sziklas, V., & Petrides, M. (1996). The effects of lesions to the mammillary region and the hippocampus on conditional associative learning by rats. *European Journal of Neuroscience, 8*, 106–115.

Sziklas, V., & Petrides, M. (1999). The effects of lesions to the anterior thalamic nuclei on object-place associations in rats. *European Journal of Neuroscience, 11*, 559–566.

Tanila, H. (1999). Hippocampal place cells can develop distinct representations of two visually identical environments. *Hippocampus, 9,* 235–246.

Wallenstein, G. V., Eichenbaum, H., & Hasselmo, M. E. (1998). The hippocampus as an associator of discontiguous events. *Trends in Neurosciences, 21,* 317–323.

Wallenstein, G. V., & Hasselmo, M. E. (1997). GABAergic modulation of hippocampal population activity: Sequence learning, place field development, and the phase precession effect. *Journal of Neurophysiology, 78,* 393–408.

Winocur, G. (1991). Functional dissociation of the hippocampus and prefrontal cortex in learning and memory. *Bulletin of the Psychonomic Society, 19,* 11–20.

Wise, S. P., & Murray, E. A. (1999). Role of the hippocampal system in conditional motor learning: Mapping antecedents to action. *Hippocampus, 9,* 101–117.

32

How Sensory Experience Shapes
Cortical Representations

MICHAEL P. KILGARD

Developing a comprehensive understanding of how the brain learns remains one of the greatest challenges in science. Although studies in invertebrates have established that relatively sophisticated behavior (including associative memory) can be implemented using simple synaptic plasticity rules (Glanzman, 1995), the operating principles that allow networks of millions of neurons to organize themselves and generate useful behavior remain poorly defined (Buonomano & Merzenich, 1998). Recent experiments in the mammalian sensory cortex suggest that cellular learning rules give rise to network-level rules that allow large populations of neurons to learn novel stimuli and adapt to changing situations. Greater understanding of these network-level rules will provide insight into the neural basis of learning and memory, and lead to new treatment strategies for a variety of neurological and psychiatric disorders. In this chapter, I review a series of plasticity studies that explore the principles of cortical self-organization.

SELF-ORGANIZATION IN THE CEREBRAL CORTEX

Studies of lesion-induced cortical map reorganization conducted nearly 20 years ago provided the first compelling evidence that populations of cortical neurons retain the potential for self-organization throughout adult life (for a summary of these studies, see Kaas, 1999). Further studies have revealed that cortical plasticity is not simply a specialization to facilitate recovery from injury, but rather reflects the continual optimization of cortical circuitry to meet changing behavioral demands (Merzenich, Recauzone, Jenkins, & Grajski, 1990). Behavioral experience alone is sufficient to substantially remodel the topographic maps in the primary sensory cortex. Tasks that activate a restricted region of the cortical map (e.g., a tap to a single digit or a pure tone) lead to expansion of that region of the map at the expense of neighboring areas (Jenkins, Merzenich, Ochs, Allard, & Guic-Robles, 1990; Recanzone, Merzenich, Jenkins, Grajski, & Dinse, 1992; Recanzone, Schreiner, &

Merzenich, 1993). The degree of map expansion is correlated with improvement in behavioral detection thresholds. These results suggest that cortical plasticity facilitates learning by increasing the number of cortical neurons that represent behaviorally important stimuli. This chapter evaluates and extends this hypothesis by focusing on two important questions: (1) How do neurons know *which* stimuli to learn? (2) How do they know *how* to learn them?

MECHANISMS OF EXPERIENCE-DEPENDENT CORTICAL PLASTICITY: CHOLINERGIC CONTRIBUTION

Most cellular plasticity mechanisms are controlled by neural activity. Thus it is possible that cortical map expansion is simply a consequence of the increased activity caused by the tens of thousands of stimuli delivered over the training period. This explanation was elegantly tested by exposing two groups of animals to identical acoustic and tactile stimulation, and requiring each group to respond only to information from one modality and to ignore the other (Recanzone et al., 1992, 1993). In animals that attended to the acoustic stimuli, the auditory cortex map of frequency was reorganized, while the map of the body surface in the somatosensory cortex was unchanged. In animals that attended to the tactile inputs, the opposite pattern developed. These results demonstrate that cortical plasticity is determined by the features of the sensory environment *and* the cognitive state of the animal. Clearly, neurons in sensory cortex receive detailed information about the environment via their thalamic inputs, but how do neurons evaluate which stimuli are "important"?

Cholinergic neurons in the nucleus basalis (NB) receive their inputs from the amygdala and other limbic structures, and project diffusely from the basal forebrain to the entire cerebral cortex (Mesulam, Mufson, Wainer, & Levey, 1983). Recordings in awake animals have shown that NB neurons (1) respond vigorously to both aversive and rewarding stimuli, (2) learn to respond to stimuli that predict rewards, and (3) habituate when animals become satiated (Richardson & DeLong, 1991).

Several lines of evidence suggest that these neurons activate cortical plasticity mechanisms and allow the cortex to learn behaviorally important stimuli (Hasselmo, 1995). Both cortical map plasticity and learning are disrupted in animals with NB lesions (Juliano, Ma, & Eslin, 1991; McGaughy, Everitt, Robbins, & Sarter, 2000; Webster, Hanisch, Dykes, & Biesold, 1991). Pairing a sensory stimulus with electrical activation of NB neurons causes cortical receptive fields to shift toward the paired stimulus (Bakin & Weinberger, 1996; Bjordahl, Dimyan, & Weinberger, 1998; Hars, Maho, Edeline, & Hennevin, 1993; Howard & Simons, 1994; Edeline, Hars, Maho, & Hennevin, 1994; Edeline, Maho, Hars, & Hennevin, 1994; Kilgard & Merzenich, 1998a; Tremblay, Warren, & Dykes, 1990; Webster, Rasmusson, et al., 1991). To determine more precisely how NB activity contributes to cortical map reorganization, we used electrical activation of NB neurons paired with acoustic stimulation to mimic the cholinergic and sensory inputs engaged during behavioral training.

Pairing electrical activation of the NB with a tone several hundred times per day for a month led to map reorganization that was (1) more extensive than reorganizations observed after many months of operant training, (2) specific to the tone frequency paired with NB activation, (3) progressive over the course of 4 weeks, and (4) measurable for more than 36 hours (Kilgard & Merzenich, 1998a) (Plate 32.1). These results support the idea that NB neurons instruct cortical neurons what to learn by demarcating which of the thousands of stimuli encountered in a day are behaviorally important.

LEARNING IN NATURAL SETTINGS: ADAPTIVE CORTICAL PLASTICITY—RATTLESNAKE OR HUMMINGBIRD?

Cortical map expansions allow the cortex to redistribute computational resources to focus on regions of the receptor surface that contain behaviorally relevant information. For example, the cortical representation of the ventral body surface is expanded in nursing rats (Xerri, Stern, & Merzenich, 1994). Map expansions also occur in humans following extensive training in music or Braille reading (Elbert, Pantev, Wienbruch, Rockstroh, & Taub, 1995; Sterr et al., 1998).

Despite these convincing demonstrations of cortical map reorganization, it is important to recognize that map expansion does not represent a general-purpose learning strategy. In most natural situations, relevant information is represented by the *temporal pattern* of events distributed across the cortical surface. To explore how the cortex learns to represent spatiotemporal patterns, consider for a moment an animal's first encounter with an angry rattlesnake (Figure 32.1A), and assume that either instinct or personal experience has provided this animal with an understanding that snakes can be dangerous (LeDoux, 1996).

If the animal is to avoid rattlesnakes in the future, it must (1) associate the sensory experience of the rattle with danger, and (2) improve its ability to detect the sound of the rattle. Spectral analysis reveals that the snake's rattle is a rapidly modulated, narrow-band noise centered at 6 kHz (Figure 32.1B). The simplest way to avoid rattlesnakes is to associate the repeated activation of auditory neurons tuned to 6 kHz with danger. Unfortunately, even though the snake's rattle activates a limited region of the cortical frequency map, the population of engaged neurons is by no means unique to the rattle. The same population is also activated by the threats of the much less dangerous rufous hummingbird (C and D in Figure 32.2). Confusion of these two warning sounds could lead to either needless panic or a dangerous lack of caution.

To effectively learn a new stimulus class, cortical networks must minimize the potential for confusion. It is becoming increasingly clear that multiple plasticity mechanisms contribute to modifications in cortical response properties that ensure a reliable depiction of the sensory world (Kilgard et al., 2001). In the present example, improvements could be realized via (1) receptive field plasticity to more precisely match the bandwidth of the rattle, and/or (2) temporal plasticity to shift the maximum cortical following rate closer to the 15-Hz modulation rate of the rattle. Although characteristics of the acoustic environment and similarity to previously learned sounds would determine which strategy would be most effective for coding the rattle, little is known about how the cortex determines what form of plasticity to adopt.

SENSORY EXPERIENCE DIRECTS PLASTICITY

Studies of cortical plasticity in adult monkeys have provided the clearest demonstration that the cortex can adopt dramatically different coding strategies, depending on the stimulus to be identified. Although one might initially assume that narrow receptive fields provide the most precise cortical representation, in some situations larger receptive fields appear to be more effective. Receptive fields were narrowed when New World monkeys were required to make behavioral judgments based on spectral cues (discriminating between tones of different frequency) (Recanzone et al., 1993), but were broadened when monkeys were required to make judgments about stimulus modulation rate (Recanzone et al., 1992). The simplest interpretation of these opposite results is that temporal tasks favor the development of large

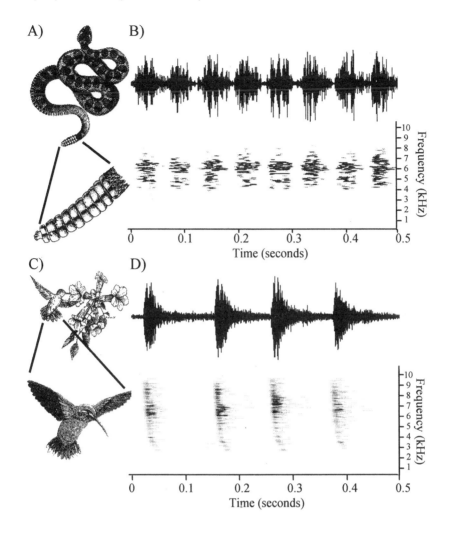

FIGURE 32.1. Acoustics of (A) Western diamondback rattlesnake and (B) rufous hummingbird threat displays. The top panel in each section displays the acoustic waveform, and the bottom panel displays the spectrogram. The two sounds have similar acoustic features, but indicate the presence of very different animals. These sounds demonstrate the potential to confuse natural sounds.

receptive fields to improve the temporal fidelity of the cortical response by allowing more neurons to be engaged, whereas spectral tasks favor the development of smaller receptive fields that provide a more fine-grained representation of the receptor surface. These results support the hypothesis that given sufficient arousal, the *form* of cortical reorganization is largely determined by the spatial and temporal characteristics of the sensory input.

Receptive Field Size

To explore in greater detail how sensory experience directs cortical plasticity, my colleagues and I evaluated receptive field size in seven groups of rats that received identical NB activation, but heard tonal stimuli with different spectral and temporal properties. Electrical activation of the NB offers several important advantages over behavioral training: (1) Motivational variability over the training interval and across animals is reduced, because animals in every group receive identical NB stimulation; (2) sensory experience can be easily controlled by varying spectral and temporal features of the acoustic environment; (3) lengthy periods of behavioral shaping are avoided; and (4) significant reorganization occurs more quickly, because habituation of NB responsiveness does not occur. Twenty-four hours after the last pairing session, cortical reorganization was quantified by recording from 50 to 100 sites in each animal.

In the first set of experiments, animals were exposed to one of two different stimulus sets. Half of the animals heard two different randomly interleaved tones several hundred times per day, paired with NB activation to simulate tone frequency discrimination training. The second group heard a rapidly modulated (15-Hz) tone with a fixed carrier frequency (pitch) to simulate training on a modulation rate task. In both groups, NB activation resulted in profound changes in receptive field size (Kilgard & Merzenich, 1998a). As in the monkey experiments, the stimuli that varied in pitch caused receptive fields to contract, while the temporally modulated stimulus caused receptive fields to expand (see a, g, and h in Figure 32.2). These results suggest that similar network-level rules exist across species to transform experience into adaptive changes in cortical response properties. These rules appear to operate as "educated guesses" about what features of a novel stimulus contain relevant information. In this case, it appears that unmodulated, spectrally diverse stimuli are assumed to contain *spectral* information, and receptive fields are narrowed to improve spectral precision. In contrast, modulated, spectrally invariant stimuli are assumed to contain *temporal* information, and receptive fields are enlarged to provide greater averaging across spectral channels.

To evaluate the hypothesis that spectral and temporal cues guide cortical plasticity, we paired sounds that were temporally modulated *and* spectrally diverse (i.e., different pitches) with identical NB activation (Kilgard et al., 2001). This "intermediate" stimulus caused significantly less receptive field expansion than the spectrally invariant stimulus, and supports the hypothesis of continuous network-level learning rules (Figure 32.2b).

This model also predicts that tone trains with very slow repetition rate and random pitch should not broaden receptive fields because the interval between tones should be so long that they should be considered unmodulated and lead to activation of the "spectral" coding strategy. To test this prediction, NB activation was paired with spectrally diverse tone trains that were modulated at two slower rates (5 and 7.5 Hz). The degree of receptive field expansion was systematically related to repetition rate (c and d in Figure 32.2). These results confirm the hypothesis that receptive field size is systematically related to temporal and spectral acoustic features that co-occur with NB activity (Figure 32.2i).

Background Stimuli

Although these results suggest that the cortex uses different receptive field strategies for certain classes of conditioned stimuli (CSs), the rattlesnake example reminds us that the optimal strategy for specific circumstances also depends upon the characteristics of background sounds in the environment. To evaluate the effect of background stimuli, NB pairing experiments were conducted with and without additional sounds that were not paired with NB activation (CSs⁻). One group of animals heard one tone frequency paired with NB activation in a silent background. The other group heard the same tone paired with the same NB

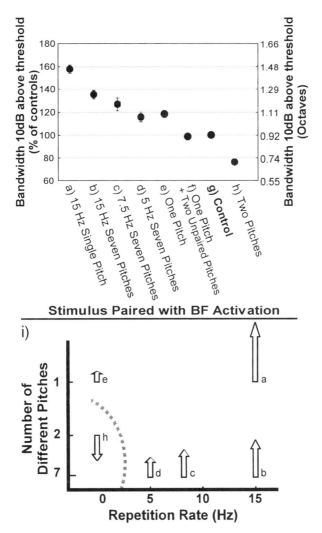

FIGURE 32.2. Receptive field size (frequency bandwidth) of A1 neurons is influenced by specific features of the auditory stimulus paired with NB activation. Mean bandwidth 10 dB above threshold with standard error (across sites) is shown. In agreement with training-induced plasticity in monkeys, receptive field size was increased by stimuli with a high degree of temporal modulation and little spectral variability (15-Hz trains of 9-kHz tones), and reduced by stimuli with more spectral diversity and no temporal modulation (i.e., two different frequencies of unmodulated tones). Pairing acoustic stimuli that shared features of each resulted in intermediate results. All experimental groups had statistically significant ($p < .05$) mean bandwidth compared to that of controls, except f. (i) The same results are replotted in schematic form to illustrate how spectral variability (y-axis) and temporal modulation (x-axis) contribute to receptive field size. The length and direction of each arrow represents the change in receptive field size shown in (a–e and h). The dotted line indicates stimuli that are predicted not to change receptive field size. From Kilgard et al. (2001). Copyright by American Physiological Society. Reprinted by permission.

stimulation; however, it also heard two other tone frequencies randomly interleaved with the paired tone, but not paired with NB activation. The presence of tonal stimuli in the background prevented the increase in receptive size that normally follows tone pairing in a quiet background (see e and f in Figure 32.2). This result suggests that pairing a single tone in a quiet background causes the cortex to adopt a strategy suitable for a simple detection task. Increasing receptive field size should decrease neural noise in a quiet background by averaging across more peripheral receptors. However, this strategy would not be adaptive in an environment filled with irrelevant tones. These results indicate that specific features of the sensory environment (including CSs+ *and* CSs−) control receptive field size and location.

Temporal Plasticity

My colleagues and I next sought to determine (1) whether temporal properties of cortical neurons can be altered by sensory experience, and (2) what stimulus features influence the development of temporal plasticity. In naïve rats, cortical neurons generally do not respond to individual stimuli presented at rates greater than 12 Hz (Kilgard & Merzenich, 1999a). We tested whether the maximum cortical following rate could be increased by pairing tones modulated at 15 Hz with NB activation. Pairing 9-kHz tone trains did not significantly alter the maximum following rate (Kilgard et al., 2001), despite dramatic receptive field plasticity (see C and D in Plate 32.1, opposite page 239). In striking contrast, the maximum following rate was increased by pairing NB stimulation with tone trains (15 Hz modulation rate) that each had a different pitch (Figure 32.3) (Kilgard & Merzenich, 1998b). This result indicates that the temporal coding strategy used by the cortex is shaped by *spectral* features of the acoustic stimulus. Specifically, it appears that the cortex adopts a map expansion strategy to better code the stimulus if tone frequency is constant, and changes its temporal characteristics only when this strategy is unavailable. To demonstrate that the changes in maximum following rate were dependent on the repetition rate of the stimuli paired with NB stimulation, we exposed two additional groups of rats to 5-Hz and 7.5-Hz trains of random carrier frequency paired with identical NB activation. These experiments confirmed that the maximum cortical following rate could be increased or decreased, depending on the sensory experience that was paired with NB activity (Figure 32.3).

Collectively, these results demonstrate that experience-dependent plasticity mechanisms can alter both receptive field structure and temporal processing in order to "fine-tune" cortical coding to match specific sensory environments. For example, cortical neurons could be made to distinguish reliably between rattlesnakes and hummingbirds by precisely adjusting the spectral and temporal filter properties of cortical neurons. It should be noted that even this "real-world" example is relatively simple, in that the sounds, like our tone trains, are periodic. Most naturally occurring stimuli are significantly more complex. Our ability to learn any of the diverse human languages indicates that the brain must be able to faithfully represent any of the spectrotemporal patterns that signify phonemes and words in each language (Kuhl, 1999).

Spectrotemporal Plasticity

In other species with rich acoustic experience, neurons have been found that are "tuned" for particular spectrotemporal transitions in their vocalizations (Esser, Condon, Suga, & Kanwal, 1997; Wang, Merzenich, Beitel, & Schreiner, 1995; Wollberg & Newman, 1972). These neurons respond strongly to the complex sequence of sounds that make up these sounds, but

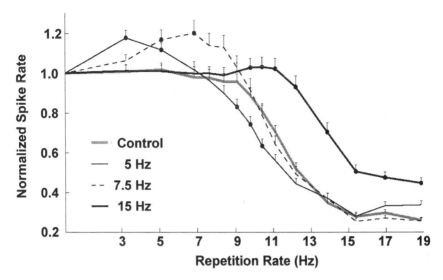

FIGURE 32.3. Sensory experience controls temporal plasticity. Lines indicate mean normalized response to tone trains of different rates. Pairing NB stimulation with 15-Hz tone trains of different carrier frequencies increased the maximum cortical following rate of A1 neurons, whereas pairing 5-Hz tone trains decreased the maximum following rate, compared to the rates of controls. The response of each site was normalized using the number of spikes evoked by the first tone in each train. Error bars indicate standard error. The rates that were significantly different from controls are marked with dots (one-way analysis of variance, Fisher's PLSD, $p < .05$). From Kilgard and Merzenich (1998b). Copyright 1998 by Nature Publishing Group. Reprinted by permission.

respond much less strongly to each of the elements in isolation. My colleagues and I have recently extended our work on simple periodic stimuli by exploring how cortical plasticity mechanisms improve the representation of transitions found in spectrotemporally complex stimuli (Kilgard & Merzenich, 1999b). We chose to investigate how the cortex learns a rapid sequence of two tones followed by a noise burst, because this sequence exhibits spectral transitions present in many natural sounds, but can be easily varied to probe the cortical representation of related sequences. As in all the previous experiments, this stimulus sequence was repeatedly paired with NB activation several hundred times per day for 4 weeks. After pairing, we found that a large proportion of cortical neurons developed response facilitation that was specific to the order of sequence elements paired with NB activation (Figure 32.4). This result extends our previous work with simple stimuli by demonstrating that neurons in the primary auditory cortex can develop responses that are specific to the spectrotemporal transitions present in complex stimuli that co-occur with NB activation.

These and earlier results provide compelling evidence that the cortex plays an active role in memory formation and continually optimizes its circuitry to improve perceptual ability. In addition, these results suggest that NB neurons instruct cortical neurons *which* stimuli are important, and that network-level rules specify *how* to learn them.

CHANGES IN AROUSAL AND BEHAVIOR CONTRIBUTE TO SELF-ORGANIZATION

One limitation of the experimental approach I have described is that the acoustic stimuli and NB activation were held constant throughout several weeks of pairing. In natural situ-

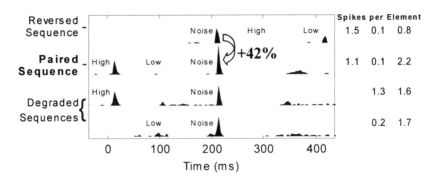

FIGURE 32.4. An example of the type of "combination-sensitive" neurons that developed in A1 after NB stimulation was paired with a high–low–noise sequence (5 kHz–12 kHz–noise burst, 100 milliseconds SOA [stimulus on set dsynchrony]). The lines under each response histogram (PSTH; peristimulustime histogram) indicate the sequence of stimuli presented. The black numbers to the right indicate the mean number of spikes evoked by each stimulus element. The noise burst exhibited a facilitated response (42% facilitation, 2.2 vs. 1.5 spikes, $p < .001$) only when it was part of the complete sequence that was paired with NB activation (see arrow). Data from Kilgard and Merzenich (1999b).

ations, learning modifies both arousal and perception, making every experience unique. To clarify the role that changes in arousal and behavior play in cortical self-organization, consider once again a hypothetical animal learning to discriminate between rattlesnake and hummingbird threats. After the first encounter with a rattlesnake, the hummingbird vocalization is likely to elicit a fear response (and NB activation) due to its physical similarity to the rattle. As a result, in the early stages of learning, both threats should be associated with NB activation. As the cortical representation of the sounds is refined, the animal should be better able to distinguish the two threats and should eventually recognize that the hummingbird vocalization does not indicate a snake is near. Gradually, the hummingbird threat should elicit less and less NB activation (Pepeu & Blandina, 1998). In addition, an improved cortical representation of the rattle should allow the animal to detect the rattle at a greater distance and to avoid dangerous close encounters. Thus in most natural circumstances cortical reorganization is self-limiting, and runaway plasticity is prevented by changes in perception and behavior (Figure 32.5).

MALADAPTIVE CORTICAL PLASTICITY—RATTLESNAKE OR GARDEN HOSE?

Although the NB experiments described above were designed to explore how sensory experience controls the form of cortical plasticity, they also provide a model of the potential consequences of unregulated plasticity. In several experiments, for example, NB-induced map expansion was so extensive that more than 90% of A1 neurons responded to the paired tone (Plate 32.1, opposite page 239) (Kilgard & Merzenich, 1998a). The potential for such profound cortical reorganization indicates that cortical plasticity must be well regulated to prevent one arousing stimulus from dominating cortical responsiveness.

Pathological brain plasticity has been implicated in a number of neurological conditions, including motor abnormalities (e.g., focal dystonia and synkinesis) and sensory dysfunction (e.g., tinnitus and chronic pain), and may be involved in many others (Byl &

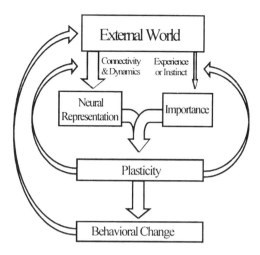

FIGURE 32.5. Working model of the interactions among perception, arousal, behavior, and plasticity.

Melnick, 1997; Friston, 1998). To clarify how plasticity mechanisms that are normally adaptive can unbalance even a healthy brain, consider the challenge of discriminating rattlesnakes from garden hoses. Whether in a primeval forest or one's own backyard, one must be able to detect snakes to avoid them. Detection is often complicated by the fact that snakes actively conceal themselves by hiding in shadows and tall grass. One way to improve the chances of detecting a hidden snake is to increase the proportion of visual cortex neurons that respond to curved or coiled objects (i.e., more "snake" neurons). There is every reason to believe that fear-induced NB activity, associated with each snake sighting, is sufficient to trigger the cortex to develop such responses.

Although more "snake-sensitive" neurons should increase the likelihood of detecting a concealed snake, they should also increase the chances of finding concealed sticks and garden hoses that resemble snakes. In the previous example, the two acoustic threats initially trigger the same fear response, but with more experience the two become separable as the sensory representation is refined. This separability is possible because, although the two sounds are similar, there are reliable physical differences between them. When sensory information is ambiguous or noisy, learning is less precise, and overgeneralization can result. As the visual system becomes more sensitive to snake-like objects, it will find more of them (especially in low-contrast environments such as tall grass, dark alleys, and brush piles). As a result, NB activation will be frequently paired with coiled garden hoses and curved sticks hidden in the grass, and the representation of snake-like objects will be further expanded. False alarms have the potential to trigger behavioral changes that may eventually contribute to the development of a full-blown phobia (Fyer, 1998). The more time one spends scanning noisy, low-contrast areas looking for snakes, the more likely one is to find something that looks like a snake and to confirm the belief that snakes abound. A lowered threshold for detecting the shape of a snake, coupled with active searching and fear, can lead to excessive plasticity and instability.

Although simplistic, this example illustrates that under certain circumstances, the same mechanisms that regulate adaptive plasticity can lead to feedback interactions that destabilize the brain. Figure 32.5 summarizes a working model of how feedback among perception, arousal, and behavior can contribute to either stability or instability. Although the experiments described in this chapter used NB activation to approximate the "importance" signal, many other systems are likely to be involved, including other projections from "higher" cortical zones and other ascending modulatory systems (Ahissar & Hochstein, 1997; Hasselmo, 1995).

CONCLUSIONS

By systematically varying the acoustic stimulus paired with electrical activation of NB neurons, my colleagues and I have documented that network-level rules operate in the cortex to transform sensory experiences into changes in cortical circuitry. Despite the unnatural method for activating NB neurons, the plasticity generated with this paradigm closely parallels natural learning (Merzenich et al., 1990). We have documented changes in map organization, receptive field size, and temporal response properties that varied systematically as spectral and temporal stimulus features were altered. The observation that cortical neurons can develop response facilitation to specific spatiotemporal patterns provides evidence that cortical self-organization sharpens the sensory representation of complex stimuli by coordinating cellular plasticity mechanisms across the cortical surface.

In addition to clarifying how networks of neurons contribute to learning and memory, a more complete understanding of the principles that guide cortical self-organization is essential to the development of treatment strategies for a variety of central nervous system disorders. Recent imaging studies suggest that cortical map plasticity is involved in tinnitus and focal dystonia (Byl, McKenzie, & Nagarajan, 2000; Muhlnickel, Elbert, Taub, & Flor, 1998), whereas degraded temporal processing is commonly observed in dyslexia (Merzenich, Wright, et al., 1996; Wright et al., 1997). Although we have seen that neurological disorders can lead to changes in perception and behavior that can maintain disordered states, there is every reason to believe that neural networks can be retrained and normal function restored (Byl & Melnick, 1997). Extensive training on a variety of temporal tasks, for example, can produce marked improvement in speech recognition and language ability in dyslexic children (Merzenich, Jenkins, et al., 1996; Tallal et al., 1996). New insight into the mechanisms of brain plasticity will undoubtedly lead to improvements in existing therapies and to the development of new approaches to treating neurological and psychiatric disorders.

ACKNOWLEDGMENTS

I am grateful to Aage Möller, Alice O'Toole, Pritesh Pandya, Navzer Engineer, Jessica Vazquez, Cherie Perroncel, Amanda Puckett, and Raluca Moucha for their comments on this chapter. I also would like to give special acknowledgment to Michael Merzenich and Christoph Schreiner. This research was supported by funds from the National Institutes of Health (NS-10414 and DC-04354), the Office of Naval Research (N00014-96-102), the National Science Foundation, and Hearing Research Inc.

REFERENCES

Ahissar, M., & Hochstein, S. (1997). Task difficulty and the specificity of perceptual learning. *Nature, 387,* 401–406.

Bakin, J. S., & Weinberger, N. M. (1996). Induction of a physiological memory in the cerebral cortex by stimulation of the nucleus basalis. *Proceedings of the National Academy of Sciences USA, 93,* 11219–11224.

Bjordahl, T. S., Dimyan, M. A., & Weinberger, N. M. (1998). Induction of long-term receptive field plasticity in the auditory cortex of the waking guinea pig by stimulation of the nucleus basalis. *Behavioral Neuroscience, 112,* 467–479.

Buonomano, D. V., & Merzenich, M. M. (1998). Cortical plasticity: From synapses to maps. *Annual Review of Neuroscience, 21,* 149–186.

Byl, N. N., McKenzie, A., & Nagarajan, S. S. (2000). Differences in somatosensory hand organization in a healthy flutist and a flutist with focal hand dystonia: A case report. *Journal of Hand Therapy, 13,* 302–309.

Byl, N. N., & Melnick, M. (1997). The neural consequences of repetition: Clinical implications of a learning hypothesis. *Journal of Hand Therapy, 10,* 160–174.

Edeline, J. M., Hars, B., Maho, C., & Hennevin, E. (1994). Transient and prolonged facilitation of tone-evoked responses induced by basal forebrain stimulations in the rat auditory cortex. *Experimental Brain Research, 97,* 373–386.

Edeline, J. M., Maho, C., Hars, B., & Hennevin, E. (1994). Non-awaking basal forebrain stimulation enhances auditory cortex responsiveness during slow-wave sleep. *Brain Research, 636,* 333–337.

Elbert, T., Pantev, C., Wienbruch, C., Rockstroh, B., & Taub, E. (1995). Increased cortical representation of the fingers of the left hand in string players. *Science, 270,* 305–307.

Esser, K. H., Condon, C. J., Suga, N., & Kanwal, J. S. (1997). Syntax processing by auditory cortical neurons in the FM-FM area of the mustached bat *Pteronotus parnellii. Proceedings of the National Academy of Sciences USA, 94,* 14019–14024.

Friston, K. J. (1998). The disconnection hypothesis. *Schizophrenia Research, 30,* 115–125.

Fyer, A. J. (1998). Current approaches to etiology and pathophysiology of specific phobia. *Biological Psychiatry, 44,* 1295–1304.

Glanzman, D. L. (1995). The cellular basis of classical conditioning in *Aplysia californica*—it's less simple than you think. *Trends in Neurosciences, 18,* 30–36.

Hars, B., Maho, C., Edeline, J. M., & Hennevin, E. (1993). Basal forebrain stimulation facilitates tone-evoked responses in the auditory cortex of awake rat. *Neuroscience, 56,* 61–74.

Hasselmo, M. E. (1995). Neuromodulation and cortical function: Modeling the physiological basis of behavior. *Behavioural Brain Research, 67,* 1–27.

Howard, M. A., III, & Simons, D. J. (1994). Physiologic effects of nucleus basalis magnocellularis stimulation on rat barrel cortex neurons. *Experimental Brain Research, 102,* 21–33.

Jenkins, W. M., Merzenich, M. M., Ochs, M. T., Allard, T., & Guic-Robles, E. (1990). Functional reorganization of primary somatosensory cortex in adult owl monkeys after behaviorally controlled tactile stimulation. *Journal of Neurophysiology, 63,* 82–104.

Juliano, S. L., Ma, W., & Eslin, D. (1991). Cholinergic depletion prevents expansion of topographic maps in somatosensory cortex. *Proceedings of the National Academy of Sciences USA, 88,* 780–784.

Kaas, J. H. (1999). The reorganization of sensory and motor maps after injury in adult mammals. In M. S. Gazzaniga (Ed.), *The new cognitive neurosciences.* Cambridge, MA: MIT Press.

Kilgard, M. P., & Merzenich, M. M. (1998a). Cortical map reorganization enabled by nucleus basalis activity. *Science, 279,* 1714–1718.

Kilgard, M. P., & Merzenich, M. M. (1998b). Plasticity of temporal information processing in the primary auditory cortex. *Nature Neuroscience, 1,* 727–731.

Kilgard, M. P., & Merzenich, M. M. (1999a). Distributed representation of spectral and temporal information in rat primary auditory cortex. *Hearing Research, 134,* 16–28.

Kilgard, M. P., & Merzenich, M. M. (1999b). Order selective plasticity in the primary auditory cortex. *Society for Neuroscience Abstracts, 25,* 391.

Kilgard, M. P., Pandya, P. K., Vazquez, J., Gehi, A., Schreiner, C. E., & Merzenich, M. M. (2001). Sensory input directs spatial and temporal plasticity in primary auditory cortex. *Journal of Neurophysiology, 86,* 326–338.

Kuhl, P. K. (1999). Language, mind, and brain: Experience alters perception. In M. S. Gazzaniga (Ed.), *The new cognitive neurosciences.* Cambridge, MA: MIT Press.

LeDoux, J. E. (1996). *The emotional brain*. New York: Simon & Schuster.

McGaughy, J., Everitt, B. J., Robbins, T. W., & Sarter, M. (2000). The role of cortical cholinergic afferent projections in cognition: Impact of new selective immunotoxins. *Behavioural Brain Research*, *115*, 251–63.

Merzenich, M. M., Jenkins, W. M., Johnston, P., Schreiner, C., Miller, S. L., & Tallal, P. (1996). Temporal processing deficits of language-learning impaired children ameliorated by training. *Science*, *271*, 77–81.

Merzenich, M. M., Recanzone, G. H., Jenkins, W. M., & Grajski, K. A. (1990). Adaptive mechanisms in cortical networks underlying cortical contributions to learning and nondeclarative memory. *Cold Spring Harbor Symposia on Quantitative Biology*, *55*, 873–887.

Merzenich, M. M., Wright, B., Jenkins, W. M., Xerri, C., Byl, N., Miller, S. L., & Tallal, P. (1996). Cortical plasticity underlying perceptual, motor, and cognitive skill development: Implications for neurorehabilitation. *Cold Spring Harbor Symposia on Quantitative Biology*, *61*, 1–8.

Mesulam, M.-M., Mufson, E. J., Wainer, B. H., & Levey, A. I. (1983). Central cholinergic pathways in the rat: An overview based on an alternative nomenclature (Ch1–Ch6). *Neuroscience*, *10*, 1185–1201.

Muhlnickel, W., Elbert, T., Taub, E., & Flor, H. (1998). Reorganization of auditory cortex in tinnitus. *Proceedings of the National Academy of Sciences USA*, *95*, 10340–10343.

Pepeu, G., & Blandina, P. (1998). The acetylcholine, GABA, glutamate triangle in the rat forebrain. *Journal of Physiology (Paris)*, *92*, 351–355.

Recanzone, G. H., Merzenich, M. M., Jenkins, W. M., Grajski, K. A., & Dinse, H. R. (1992). Topographic reorganization of the hand representation in cortical area 3b owl monkeys trained in a frequency-discrimination task. *Journal of Neurophysiology*, *67*, 1031–1056.

Recanzone, G. H., Schreiner, C. E., & Merzenich, M. M. (1993). Plasticity in the frequency representation of primary auditory cortex following discrimination training in adult owl monkeys. *Journal of Neuroscience*, *13*, 87–103.

Richardson, R. T., & DeLong, M. R. (1991). Electrophysiological studies of the functions of the nucleus basalis in primates. *Advances in Experimental Medicine and Biology*, *295*, 233–252.

Sterr, A., Muller, M. M., Elbert, T., Rockstroh, B., Pantev, C., & Taub, E. (1998). Changed perceptions in Braille readers. *Nature*, *391*, 134–135.

Tallal, P., Miller, S. L., Bedi, G., Byma, G., Wang, X., Nagarajan, S. S., Schreiner, C., Jenkins, W. M., & Merzenich, M. M. (1996). Language comprehension in language-learning impaired children improved with acoustically modified speech. *Science*, *271*, 81–84.

Tremblay, N., Warren, R. A., & Dykes, R. W. (1990). Electrophysiological studies of acetylcholine and the role of the basal forebrain in the somatosensory cortex of the cat: II. Cortical neurons excited by somatic stimuli. *Journal of Neurophysiology*, *64*, 1212–1222.

Wang, X., Merzenich, M. M., Beitel, R., & Schreiner, C. E. (1995). Representation of a species-specific vocalization in the primary auditory cortex of the common marmoset: Temporal and spectral characteristics. *Journal of Neurophysiology*, *74*, 2685–2706.

Webster, H. H., Hanisch, U. K., Dykes, R. W., & Biesold, D. (1991). Basal forebrain lesions with or without reserpine injection inhibit cortical reorganization in rat hindpaw primary somatosensory cortex following sciatic nerve section. *Somatosensory and Motor Research*, *8*, 327–346.

Webster, H. H., Rasmusson, D. D., Dykes, R. W., Schliebs, R., Schober, W., Bruckner, G., & Biesold, D. (1991). Long-term enhancement of evoked potentials in raccoon somatosensory cortex following co-activation of the nucleus basalis of Meynert complex and cutaneous receptors. *Brain Research*, *545*, 292–296.

Wollberg, Z., & Newman, J. D. (1972). Auditory cortex of squirrel monkey: Response patterns of single cells to species-specific vocalizations. *Science*, *175*, 212–214.

Wright, B. A., Lombardino, L. J., King, W. M., Puranik, C. S., Leonard, C. M., & Merzenich, M. M. (1997). Deficits in auditory temporal and spectral resolution in language-impaired children. *Nature*, *387*, 176–178.

Xerri, C., Stern, J. M., & Merzenich, M. M. (1994). Alterations of the cortical representation of the rat ventrum induced by nursing behavior. *Journal of Neuroscience*, *14*, 1710–1721.

33

The Basal Forebrain Cholinergic System and Memory

Beware of Dogma

MARK G. BAXTER and STEPHANIE L. MURG

With regard to the neuropsychology of memory, the specific function of basal forebrain cholinergic neurons has been an issue of particularly keen interest because of the marked damage to this system observed in patients with Alzheimer's disease. Efforts to understand how these neurons contribute uniquely to cognitive function have been hampered by the difficulty in producing selective lesions of this cell population. Despite recent advances in methods to produce selective neurochemical lesions, a simple description of the functional role of the cholinergic basal forebrain remains elusive. The goals of this chapter are twofold: first, to discuss some of the methodological assumptions inherent in using selective neurochemical lesions to probe the function of particular neural systems; and second, to offer potential insight into the mechanism by which these neurons may influence cognitive function, and by extension to provide a possible framework for understanding the modulation of cognition by other subcortical aminergic systems.

THEORIES OF BASAL FOREBRAIN FUNCTION: THE OLD AND THE NEW

Stated in its most simple and direct terms, the cholinergic hypothesis asserts that significant, functional disturbances in cholinergic activity occur in the brains of aged and especially demented patients, these disturbances play an important role in the memory loss and related cognitive problems associated with old age and dementia, and proper enhancement or restoration of cholinergic function may significantly reduce the severity of the cognitive loss. (Bartus, Dean, Pontecorvo, & Flicker, 1985, p. 332)

The basal forebrain cholinergic system has been thought to play a central role in cognition since the discovery over 25 years ago that cholinergic enzyme levels were sharply reduced in the brains of patients who had died of Alzheimer's disease—a condition characterized by severe cognitive deficits, including memory deficits (Bowen, Smith, White, & Davison, 1976; Perry, Perry, Blessed, & Tomlinson, 1977; Whitehouse et al., 1982). These and other findings informed the "cholinergic hypothesis of geriatric memory dysfunction," which is that loss of cholinergic input to cortical and limbic structures is the causal factor in both normal and pathological impairments in memory with aging (Bartus, Dean, Beer, & Lippa, 1982; Coyle, Price, & DeLong, 1983).

Subsequent experimental studies in laboratory animals sought to define more clearly the role that the cholinergic system plays in cognitive function. These studies supported the hypothesis that damage to the basal forebrain results in severe cognitive impairment, including impairments in learning and memory. The deficits observed were frequently attributed to loss of cholinergic neurons, even though the lesions in question damaged both cholinergic and noncholinergic basal forebrain neurons. This led to a dogma of basal forebrain function: that extensive cognitive impairment following basal forebrain lesions is due to loss of cholinergic projections from the basal forebrain to its cortical and limbic targets.

This dogma was called into question when mismatches were discovered between the extent of cholinergic damage and the extent of cognitive impairment following basal forebrain lesions. Damage to the nucleus basalis magnocellularis (NBM, where corticopetal cholinergic neurons are located) with quisqualic acid produced extensive loss of cholinergic neurons, but little impairment in learning and memory; conversely, lesions of this nucleus with ibotenic acid produced less extensive loss of cholinergic neurons, but more severe impairment in learning and memory (Markowska, Wenk, & Olton, 1990; Riekkinen, Riekkinen, & Riekkinen, 1991). In contrast, damage to the NBM consistently impaired performance in an attentional task (e.g., Muir, Everitt, & Robbins, 1994; Robbins et al., 1989). Therefore, this dogma was reformulated somewhat; it was hypothesized that cholinergic neurons in the rostral basal forebrain (the medial septum/vertical limb of the diagonal band of Broca, or MS/VDB) projecting to the hippocampus regulate learning and memory abilities, whereas those in the caudal basal forebrain projecting to the neocortex are involved in attentional processing (Dunnett, Everitt, & Robbins, 1991; Fibiger, 1991).

Consistent with this hypothesis, experiments in which neurons in the MS/VDB were destroyed by injections of neurotoxins (e.g., ibotenic acid) have found learning and memory deficits qualitatively similar to the effects of damage to target structures of the MS/VDB. For instance, ibotenic acid lesions of the MS/VDB impaired spatial learning in the Morris water maze (Hagan, Salamone, Simpson, Iversen, & Morris, 1988), similar to the effect of hippocampal damage (Morris, Garrud, Rawlins, & O'Keefe, 1982). Although these lesions were regionally discrete, the neurotoxins employed in these experiments were not selective for cholinergic neurons. Accordingly, loss of noncholinergic MS/VDB neurons could have contributed to the observed deficits.

It is apparent that a direct experimental examination of the cognitive functions of basal forebrain cholinergic neurons requires a selective neurotoxin for those cells: "Although a partial resolution can be obtained by systematic covariation of the anatomical and functional consequences of alternative toxins, the problem of lesion specificity will only be adequately resolved with the development of toxins that permit selective destruction of the cholinergic neurons alone, in the basal forebrain or elsewhere" (Dunnett, 1992, p. 359). Such a toxin was developed through the ingenious technique of targeting a ribosome-inactivating cytotoxin, saporin, to a cell surface antigen expressed by basal forebrain cholinergic neurons—the low-affinity nerve growth factor receptor (LNGFR). This was achieved by conjugating saporin to a monoclonal antibody directed against the LNGFR (Wiley, Oeltmann, & Lappi, 1991). Experiments with this toxin, 192 IgG–saporin, have suggested that these neurons do not play a central role in some aspects of learning and memory previously attributed to cholinergic MS/VDB neurons. For instance, spatial learning performance in the Morris water maze was unaffected by removal of cholinergic neurons in the MS/VDB with 192 IgG–saporin, despite a 90% loss of hippocampal choline acetyltransferase (ChAT) activity (Baxter, Bucci, Gorman, Wiley, & Gallagher, 1995). This loss of hippocampal ChAT activity was more severe than in previous studies that used less selective toxins to lesion the MS/VDB and found a spatial learning deficit (e.g., Hagan et al., 1988). A similar lack of effect of 192 IgG–saporin lesions of the MS/VDB was observed in tests of spatial working memory when histological analysis confirmed the sparing of noncholinergic neurons at the lesion site (Chappell, McMahan, Chiba, & Gallagher, 1998; McMahan, Sobel, & Baxter, 1997).

Reliable effects of selective lesions of cholinergic neurons in the NBM on attentional tasks have continued to be found (Chiba, Bucci, Holland, & Gallagher, 1995; Chiba, Bushnell, Oshiro, & Gallagher, 1999; McGaughy, Kaiser, & Sarter, 1996; Waite, Wardlow, & Power, 1999). Effects on different aspects of attentional processing have also been found following lesions of cholinergic neurons in the MS/VDB (Baxter, Gallagher, & Holland, 1999; Baxter, Holland, & Gallagher, 1997). Hence both rostral and caudal divisions of the basal forebrain appear to be involved in attentional processing. This has led to a new view of the function of basal forebrain cholinergic neurons—namely, that they are involved in attentional processing, but not in learning and memory per se:

> In brief, cortical ACh is generally hypothesized to modulate the efficacy of the cortical processing of sensory or associational information. The integrity of cortical cholinergic inputs is required for the subjects' ability to detect and select stimuli and associations for extended processing, and for the appropriate allocation of processing resources to these functions. (Sarter, Bruno, & Himmelheber, 1997, p. 107)

> . . . through the modulation of specific aspects of attention, the basal forebrain cholinergic system plays a role in optimizing behavioral performance in response to specific behavioral challenges or associative histories of stimuli. (Baxter & Chiba, 1999, p. 179)

WHAT ARE THE METHODOLOGICAL ISSUES?

The usefulness of the 192 IgG–saporin immunotoxin stems from its capacity to selectively target and efficiently destroy cholinergic neurons in the basal forebrain; therefore, in studies exploiting this unique approach, it is essential to verify both the selectivity and the completeness of the lesions on a case-by-case basis. Although it is widely accepted that rats lesioned with 192 IgG–saporin demonstrate circumscribed behavioral deficits in comparison to those lesioned with other methods (e.g., excitotoxins), unresolved questions persist regarding the functional significance of the cholinergic basal forebrain. Informed interpretation of studies that make use of any ablative strategy requires careful attention to issues of methodology, and in the case of 192 IgG–saporin, it is instructive to focus upon the features that make the toxin so appealing: the selectivity and extent of the lesions. If behavioral deficits are observed, it is critical to confirm that these effects cannot be attributed to nonselective effects of the lesions (e.g., effects on other neurochemically defined populations of cells). Conversely, if behavioral impairments are absent following the lesions, it is important to confirm that the lack of effect is not due to an incomplete lesion, or compensation by spared neural elements in the system.

Selectivity is determined by immunohistochemical assessment of the integrity of the anatomical region of interest. In addition to evaluating the depletion of cholinergic markers, it is necessary to confirm that the immunotoxic insult did not damage noncholinergic (e.g., γ-aminobutyric acid-ergic or GABAergic) cell populations. Large doses of the immunotoxin can produce nonselective damage at the lesion site, presumably by nonspecific endocytosis of the toxin protein (see Baxter, 2001, for discussion of methodological issues related to the use of 192 IgG–saporin). Variations in delivery of the toxin may also produce divergent behavioral findings. When a single large volume of 192 IgG–saporin was administered in the medial septal area, spatial working memory deficits were observed at a range of dosages (Walsh, Herzog, Gandhi, Stackman, & Wiley, 1996); however, when attempts were made to replicate this finding using multiple small septal injection sites, no functional sequelae were observed, even though cholinergic depletion was similar to that achieved by Walsh and colleagues (Chappell et al., 1998). Because 192 IgG–saporin has been reported to suppress parvalbumin expression in GABAergic septal neurons following administration of the toxin into the MS/VDB (Torres et al., 1994), it is possible that the delivery of a single large dose of the toxin to the midline (where the GABAergic neurons are located) compromised the function of these cells, leading to behavioral impairment.

Another issue, related specifically to 192 IgG–saporin, is the fact that the toxin can damage neuronal populations outside the basal forebrain. Injection of this toxin into the cerebral ventricles allows it to act upon another population of p75-expressing neurons: cerebellar Purkinje cells (Pioro & Cuello, 1988). Studies that use intracerebroventricular injections of 192 IgG–saporin commonly detect substantial impairments in spatial learning in the Morris water maze (Berger-Sweeney et al., 1994; Leanza, Nilsson, Wiley, & Björklund, 1995; Nilsson et al., 1992). Hence the interpretation of behavioral findings in such cases is subject to the same criticisms as nonspecific neurotoxic lesion methods, because the lesion extends beyond the population of interest (basal forebrain cholinergic neurons).

Along with selectivity, the extent of the lesion is of paramount importance. Verification of lesion completeness is accomplished by immunohistochemical and neurochemical assays of cholinergic markers (e.g., ChAT) in the basal forebrain region of interest. If neuronal loss is not substantial, it is difficult to draw conclusions from behavioral findings, and lack of behavioral impairment in this circumstance becomes particularly difficult to interpret. Some studies have sought to propose "thresholds" of cholinergic loss, after which functional deficits become apparent (Leanza, Nilsson, Nikkhah, Wiley, & Björklund, 1996). However, given that the cholinergic depletion in studies in which no behavioral sequelae are evident—as in those finding that rats with 192 IgG–saporin lesions of the MS/VDB are not impaired in spatial learning and memory tasks (Baxter et al., 1995, 1996; Berger-Sweeney et al., 1994; Chappell et al., 1998; Dornan et al., 1996; McMahan et al., 1997; Ricceri, Baxter, Frick, & Berger-Sweeney, 2000; Torres et al., 1994)—is greater than the depletion observed in studies that rely on nonselective neurotoxic agents and find impairment in spatial learning (e.g., Dunnett, Whishaw, Jones, & Bunch, 1987; Hagan et al., 1988; Kelsey & Landry, 1988; Kelsey & Vargas, 1993), it is reasonable to conclude that the absence of a behavioral effect is not solely due to incomplete lesions.

With regard to this issue, the relationship between amount of damage and functional impairment needs to be determined before the functional consequences of selective neurochemical lesions can be fully interpreted (for related discussion, see Olton & Markowska, 1992). For example, it is known that more than 80% loss of dopamine neurons in the substantia nigra is required before motor impairment is evident (Zigmond, Berger, Grace, & Stricker, 1989; Zigmond & Stricker, 1987). Not all systems show such functional plasticity; hippocampal lesions larger than about 20% of hippocampal volume impair spatial learning in the water maze (Moser, Moser, & Andersen, 1993). The finding of functional dissociations following selective basal forebrain cholinergic lesions casts doubt on the hypothesis that the basal forebrain cholinergic system possesses a substantial functional reserve capacity that can rapidly compensate after a lesion. In particular, the same rats that demonstrate no impairment on certain learning and memory tasks (e.g., spatial learning in the Morris water maze, or spatial working memory in the radial-arm maze; Baxter et al., 1995; McMahan et al., 1997) nevertheless demonstrate impairment in other behavioral tasks, specifically tests of attention (Baxter et al., 1997; Chiba et al., 1995). Hence the lesions are sufficiently extensive to produce functional impairment. It must be noted, however, that it remains a logical (but less parsimonious) possibility that different neurochemical effects may underlie different psychological functions of cholinergic neurons, which can differentially compensate after basal forebrain damage.

Even if differential compensation after lesions is not hypothesized, it is possible that the extent of damage to basal forebrain cholinergic neurons required to produce a functional impairment differs by behavioral function. For instance, greater than 95% damage to the basal forebrain may be required to impair learning and memory, whereas attentional impairments are manifested when damage is less severe. This would imply that cholinergic modulation may be more important for attention than for learning and memory, but not that cholinergic modulation is totally uninvolved in learning and memory. When researchers are examining this possibility, it is probably important to keep in mind that in clinical conditions such as Alzheimer's disease, cortical cholinergic depletion rarely reaches such extreme levels (e.g., Bierer et al., 1995; Etienne et al., 1986; Perry et al., 1978). Hence the effects of very extreme basal forebrain lesions may not be a relevant model of disease states in which cholinergic deficiency is evident.

A third issue (and one that is particularly difficult to resolve) is the possibility that although memory may not be impaired following selective lesions of cholinergic neurons, memory function may nonetheless be made more vulnerable to the effects of other manipulations. In one study, spatial working memory was not impaired after lesions of cholinergic neurons in the MS/VDB, but lesioned rats were more susceptible to the memory-impairing effects of intraseptal infusion of cholinergic antagonists or GABAergic agonists (Pang & Nocera, 1999). Hence, although cholinergic neurons may not be *required* for memory function, they may contribute in some way to normal mnemonic performance. This finding raises the possibility that basal forebrain cholinergic neurons may perform some functions that can be accomplished by any population of neurons within the basal forebrain, regardless of neurochemical identity, whereas other functions can be performed only by cholinergic neurons. That is, perhaps cholinergic neurons are specifically required for attentional function, but all basal forebrain neurons (whether cholinergic or noncholinergic) can subserve learning and memory functions. This would allow for the lack of effect of selective cholinergic lesions on behavioral functions that are impaired following nonspecific basal forebrain lesions and ameliorated by subsequent replacement of acetylcholine (Dickinson-Anson, Aubert, Gage, & Fisher, 1998; Winkler, Suhr, Gage, Thal, & Fisher, 1995). Results of this nature require a careful consideration of the types of questions that are answered by particular experimental approaches. Selective neurochemical lesions reveal whether a particular population of neurons is *necessary* for a particular behavioral function, but do not preclude the possibility that these neurons are ordinarily engaged in that function in normal circumstances. For instance, acetylcholine is released during performance of memory tasks (Fadda, Cocco, & Stancampiano, 2000; Ragozzino, Unick, & Gold, 1996), and increasing acetylcholine levels attenuates behavioral impairment following basal forebrain damage or inactivation (see, e.g., Degroot & Parent, 2000). These findings indicate that cholinergic neurons are active during memory tasks, and that replacement of acetylcholine is sufficient to improve memory after nonselective basal forebrain damage. But these findings do not invalidate the conclusion, drawn from studies using selective lesions of basal forebrain cholinergic neurons, that these cells are not *required* for certain forms of learning and memory.

BEWARE OF DOGMA

At face value, the "new" dogma of cholinergic basal forebrain function might be viewed as somewhat counterintuitive. Although dissociations between impairments in attention and memory have been demonstrated, it is reasonable to ask how normal memory function is sustained in the presence of disrupted attentional processing.

One possible answer to this question, proposed by Baxter and Chiba (1999), is that the effects of cholinergic lesions may be more accurately characterized as an impairment in the ability to adjust attentional processing appropriately in response to task demands than as a deficit in attention per se. Hence impaired memory function would be apparent only in situations in which attentional function is taxed in some way. Such an explanation, however, would demand a formal means of distinguishing demands on attention from demands on memory. As an example, rats with selective removal of cholinergic NBM neurons demonstrate a transient postoperative impairment in olfactory span memory, in which performance drops markedly when longer spans of stimuli must be remembered (Turchi & Sarter, 2000). These authors interpreted this deficit as reflecting an impairment in attention, due to a hypothesized dependence of working memory capacity on attentional function. However, other than the fact that the deficit follows damage to a system known to produce attentional deficits in other task paradigms, it is difficult to conclude that the memory deficit in this task stems from an impairment in attention rather than from one in memory itself. Although the hypothesis that attentional dysfunction reduces working memory capacity is entirely reasonable, this type of logic may be the first step down a slippery slope on which the interpretation of deficits observed following cholinergic lesions is constrained by the hypothesized functional role of the system. The preferred situation, of course, would be to design behavioral tasks in which influences of the lesion on different psychological processes (perception, attention, memory) could be dissociated.

Recent evidence implicates basal forebrain cholinergic neurons in cognitive functions that cannot obviously be classified as attentional. In particular, these neurons may be involved in certain types of perceptual processing, as well as in certain types of memory formation. In one recent study, the perceptual generalization between chemically related odorants was examined in rats with lesions of cholinergic neurons in the horizontal nucleus of the diagonal band of Broca (HDB), which removed cholinergic input to the olfactory bulb and piriform cortex (Linster, Garcia, Hasselmo, & Baxter, 2001). In this simple task, rats dug for a cereal reward in a cup of bedding scented with a training odorant. Probe trials compared the duration of digging in an unrewarded cup that was scented with the trained odor, a chemically related odor, or a chemically unrelated odor. The digging time on the probe trials was longest for the trained odorant and shortest for a chemically unrelated odorant. Digging times for odorants related to the trained odorant followed a generalization curve that paralleled the difference in chemical structure between the probe odorant and trained odorant (Linster & Hasselmo, 1999). Lesions of cholinergic neurons in the HDB increased generalization to chemically similar odorants, but did not affect digging times to the trained odorant or to the chemically unrelated odor (Figure 33.1; Linster et al., 2001). This effect of the cholinergic lesions is consistent with a hypothesized role of acetylcholine in sharpening receptive fields of cortical neurons (Bakin & Weinberger, 1996; Linster & Hasselmo, 1997). The behavioral effect in the generalization task was not obviously attentional in nature. Given that the attentional requirement on all the probe trials was the same, no selective effect on the chemically related odorants would be expected. Similarly, no impairment in memory was obvious, because digging times for the trained odor were equivalent between control and lesioned rats.

A second line of evidence implicates acetylcholine in memory consolidation. Rats with lesions of the MS/VDB or NBM were trained on a task involving social transmission of food preference, which requires the integrity of the hippocampal formation (Bunsey & Eichenbaum, 1995). Rats with lesions of the MS/VDB or NBM were impaired on retention of the transmitted food preferences when tested 24 hours after training (Figure 33.2A; Berger-Sweeney, Stearns, Frick, Beard, & Baxter, 2000). This impairment was highly correlated with the extent of cortical, but not hippocampal, cholinergic depletion (Figure 33.2B). This finding is consistent with converging evidence suggesting that acetylcholine may enable consolidation of long-term memories in the cortex, perhaps related to variations in acetylcholine levels during different stages of sleep (Hasselmo, 1999). Again, this impairment could not be obviously related to an impairment in attentional processing, because (at least in the MS/VDB group) immediate retention of the transmitted food preference was normal.

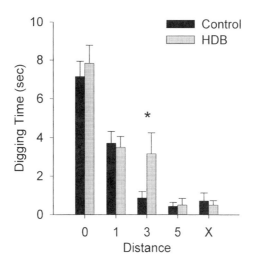

FIGURE 33.1. Effects of lesions of cholinergic neurons in the horizontal limb of the diagonal band of Broca (HDB) on odor perception. Rats were trained to dig for a reward in a cup scented with a three-carbon aliphatic aldehyde (CH_3-CH_2-CHO) and were given probe trials with the training odor, a chemically related odor (n-aliphatic aldehydes with different carbon chain lengths), or an unrelated odor (methyl salicylate). The graph shows the average digging times on probe trials (± standard errors) for all rats in both groups (black bars: sham rats, $n = 7$; gray bars: HDB-lesioned rats, $n = 6$) as a function of the difference in chain length between the conditioned odor and the test odor (0, response to trained odor; 1, 3, 5, responses to test odors differing by 1, 3, and 5 carbons from the trained odor; X, response to chemically unrelated odor). There was a significant difference between the responses of the sham-operated and HDB-lesioned rats when the tested aldehyde differed from the conditioned aldehyde by three carbons in the carbon chain. From Linster, Garcia, Hasselmo, and Baxter (2001). Copyright 2001 by the American Psychological Association. Reprinted by permission.

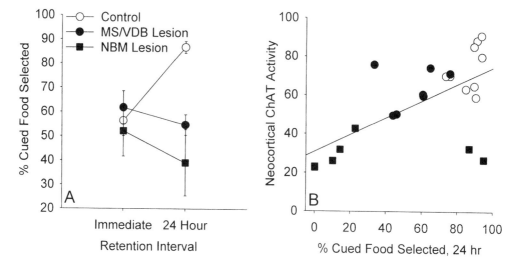

FIGURE 33.2. Effects of basal forebrain lesions (of the MS/VDB or NBM) on retention of a socially transmitted food preference. Rats were exposed to a novel flavor on the breath of a "demonstrator" rat (the "cued" flavor). Immediately after exposure to the demonstrator rat, and 24 hours later, they were allowed to eat from two cups of food—one flavored with the cued scent, the other flavored with an unfamiliar scent. (A) The percentage of cued food selected (100 × weight of cued food eaten/total weight of cued + noncued foods eaten) at two different retention intervals. There were no significant differences among the groups during the immediate trial. During the 24-hour retention trial, controls performed significantly better than both lesion groups ($p < .05$ with respect to MS/VDB and $p < .01$ with respect to NBM). (B) Correlation of performance at the 24-hour retention interval with neocortical cholinergic depletion (indexed by cortical ChAT activity). The correlation was significant ($r = .649$, $p < .01$). The correlation between 24-hour retention and hippocampal ChAT activity was not significant ($r = .099$, not shown) and was reliably smaller than the correlation between 24-hour retention and cortical ChAT activity, $t (20) = 2.021$, $p = .028$, one-tailed. From Berger-Sweeney, Stearns, Frick, Beard, and Baxter (2000). Copyright 2000 by Wiley-Liss, Inc., a subsidiary of John Wiley & Sons, Inc. Reprinted by permission.

These two examples indicate that the hypothesis that basal forebrain neurons are exclusively involved in attentional functions is incomplete. How, then, can the function of these neurons be understood? One possibility is that a unitary function of these projections at the neural level—for instance, modulating receptive field properties of cortical neurons (Bakin & Weinberger, 1996; Kilgard & Merzenich, 1998; see also Kilgard, Chapter 32, this volume), or regulating the excitability of afferent versus intrinsic projections to a dendritic field (Hasselmo & Schnell, 1994; Hasselmo, Schnell, & Barkai, 1995)—can be expressed in apparently different psychological functions at the behavioral level. Thus the effect of a basal forebrain cholinergic lesion would depend not only on the target of the cholinergic input, but on the particular behavioral situation in which cholinergic function is being tested. Therefore, it may not be possible to ascribe a unitary psychological function to these projections. This is unsatisfactory on a certain level, because in the absence of a link between particular neurobiological effects of cholinergic modulation and psychological function, it is difficult to form a priori hypotheses about when cholinergic modulation will be required for normal performance. This gap may ultimately be bridged by computational models that incorporate what is known about acetylcholine's effects at a biological level with psychological phenomena, thereby guiding behavioral experiments (see, e.g., De Rosa & Hasselmo, 2000; De Rosa, Hasselmo, & Baxter, 2001).

ACKNOWLEDGMENTS

We are grateful to Andrea Chiba and Larry Squire for their helpful comments on an earlier version of this chapter. Mark G. Baxter's research is supported by Grant No. R03-MH60089 from the National Institutes of Health, and by a Sloan Research Fellowship from the Alfred P. Sloan Foundation.

REFERENCES

Bakin, J. S., & Weinberger, N. M. (1996). Induction of a physiological memory in the cerebral cortex by stimulation of the nucleus basalis. *Proceedings of the National Academy of Sciences USA, 93*, 11219–11224.

Bartus, R. T., Dean, R. L., III, Beer, B., & Lippa, A. S. (1982). The cholinergic hypothesis of geriatric memory dysfunction. *Science, 217*, 408–417.

Bartus, R. T., Dean, R. L., III, Pontecorvo, M. J., & Flicker, C. (1985). The cholinergic hypothesis: A historical overview, current perspective, and future directions. *Annals of the New York Academy of Sciences, 444*, 332–358.

Baxter, M. G. (2001). Effects of selective immunotoxic lesions on learning and memory. In W. A. Hall (Ed.), *Methods in molecular biology: Vol. 166. Immunotoxin methods and protocols* (pp. 249–265). Totowa, NJ: Humana Press.

Baxter, M. G., Bucci, D. J., Gorman, L. K., Wiley, R. G., & Gallagher, M. (1995). Selective immunotoxic lesions of basal forebrain cholinergic cells: Effects on learning and memory in rats. *Behavioral Neuroscience, 109*, 714–722.

Baxter, M. G., Bucci, D. J., Sobel, T. J., Williams, M. J., Gorman, L. K., & Gallagher, M. (1996). Intact spatial learning following lesions of basal forebrain cholinergic neurons. *NeuroReport, 7*, 1417–1420.

Baxter, M. G., & Chiba, A. A. (1999). Cognitive functions of the basal forebrain. *Current Opinion in Neurobiology, 9*, 178–183.

Baxter, M. G., Gallagher, M., & Holland, P. C. (1999). Blocking can occur without losses in attention in rats with selective lesions of hippocampal cholinergic input. *Behavioral Neuroscience, 113*, 881–890.

Baxter, M. G., Holland, P. C., & Gallagher, M. (1997). Disruption of decrements in conditioned stimulus processing by selective removal of hippocampal cholinergic input. *Journal of Neuroscience, 17*, 5230–5236.

Berger-Sweeney, J., Heckers, S., Mesulam, M.-M., Wiley, R. G., Lappi, D. A., & Sharma, M. (1994). Differential effects on spatial navigation of immunotoxin-induced cholinergic lesions of the medial septal area and nucleus basalis magnocellularis. *Journal of Neuroscience, 14*, 4507–4519.

Berger-Sweeney, J., Stearns, N. A., Frick, K. M., Beard, B., & Baxter, M. G. (2000). Cholinergic basal forebrain is critical for social transmission of food preferences. *Hippocampus, 10*, 729–738.

Bierer, L. M., Haroutunian, V., Gabriel, S., Knott, P. J., Carlin, L. S., Purohit, D. P., Perl, D. P., Schmeidler, J., Kanof, P., & Davis, K. L. (1995). Neurochemical correlates of dementia severity in Alzheimer's disease: Relative importance of the cholinergic deficits. *Journal of Neurochemistry, 64*, 749–760.

Bowen, D. M., Smith, C. B., White, P., & Davison, A. N. (1976). Neurotransmitter-related enzymes and indices of hypoxia in senile dementia and other abiotrophies. *Brain, 99*, 459–496.

Bunsey, M., & Eichenbaum, H. (1995). Selective damage to the hippocampal region blocks long-term retention of a natural and nonspatial stimulus–stimulus association. *Hippocampus, 5*, 546–556.

Chappell, J., McMahan, R., Chiba, A., & Gallagher, M. (1998). A re-examination of the role of basal forebrain cholinergic neurons in spatial working memory. *Neuropharmacology, 37*, 481–487.

Chiba, A. A., Bucci, D. J., Holland, P. C., & Gallagher, M. (1995). Basal forebrain cholinergic lesions disrupt increments but not decrements in conditioned stimulus processing. *Journal of Neuroscience, 15*, 7315–7322.

Chiba, A. A., Bushnell, P. J., Oshiro, W. M., & Gallagher, M. (1999). Selective removal of cholinergic neurons in the basal forebrain alters cued target detection in rats. *NeuroReport, 10*, 3119–3123.

Coyle, J. T., Price, D. L., & DeLong, M. R. (1983). Alzheimer's disease: A disorder of cortical cholinergic innervation. *Science, 219*, 1184–1190.

Degroot, A., & Parent, M. B. (2000). Increasing acetylcholine levels in the hippocampus or entorhinal cortex reverses the impairing effects of septal GABA receptor activation on spontaneous alternation. *Learning and Memory, 7*, 293–302.

De Rosa, E., & Hasselmo, M. E. (2000). Muscarinic cholinergic neuromodulation reduces proactive interference between stored odor memories during associative learning in rats. *Behavioral Neuroscience, 114*, 32–41.

De Rosa, E., Hasselmo, M. E., & Baxter, M. G. (2001). Contribution of the cholinergic basal forebrain to proactive interference from stored odor memories during associative learning in rats. *Behavioral Neuroscience, 115*, 314–327.

Dickinson-Anson, H., Aubert, I., Gage, F. H., & Fisher, L. J. (1998). Hippocampal grafts of acetylcholine-producing cells are sufficient to improve behavioural performance following a unilateral fimbria–fornix lesion. *Neuroscience, 84*, 771–781.

Dornan, W. A., McCampbell, A. R., Tinkler, G. P., Hickman, L. J., Bannon, A. W., Decker, M. W., & Gunther, K. L. (1996). Comparison of site-specific injections into the basal forebrain on water maze and radial arm maze performance in the male rat after immunolesioning with 192 IgG saporin. *Behavioural Brain Research, 82*, 93–101.

Dunnett, S. B. (1992). Aging, memory, and cholinergic systems: Studies using delayed-matching and delayed-nonmatching tasks in rats. In L. R. Squire & N. Butters (Eds.), *Neuropsychology of memory* (2nd ed., pp. 357–377). New York: Guilford Press.

Dunnett, S. B., Everitt, B. J., & Robbins, T. W. (1991). The basal forebrain-cortical cholinergic system: Interpreting the functional consequences of excitotoxic lesions. *Trends in Neurosciences, 14*, 494–501.

Dunnett, S. B., Whishaw, I. Q., Jones, G. H., & Bunch, S. T. (1987). Behavioural, biochemical and histochemical effects of different neurotoxic amino acids injected into nucleus basalis magnocellularis of rats. *Neuroscience, 20*, 653–669.

Etienne, P., Robitaille, Y., Wood, P., Gauthier, S., Nair, N. P. V., & Quirion, R. (1986). Nucleus basalis neuronal loss, neuritic plaques and choline acetyltransferase activity in advanced Alzheimer's disease. *Neuroscience, 19*, 1279–1291.

Fadda, F., Cocco, S., & Stancampiano, R. (2000). Hippocampal acetylcholine release correlates with spatial learning performance in freely moving rats. *NeuroReport, 11*, 2265–2269.

Fibiger, H. C. (1991). Cholinergic mechanisms in learning, memory, and dementia: A review of recent evidence. *Trends in Neurosciences, 14*, 220–223.

Hagan, J. J., Salamone, J. D., Simpson, J., Iversen, S. D., & Morris, R. G. M. (1988). Place navigation in rats is impaired by lesions of medial septum and diagonal band but not nucleus basalis magnocellularis. *Behavioural Brain Research, 27*, 9–20.

Hasselmo, M. E. (1999). Neuromodulation: Acetylcholine and memory consolidation. *Trends in Cognitive Sciences, 3*, 351–359.

Hasselmo, M. E., & Schnell, E. (1994). Laminar selectivity of the cholinergic suppression of synaptic transmission in rat hippocampal region CA1: Computational modeling and brain slice physiology. *Journal of Neuroscience, 14*, 3898–3914.

Hasselmo, M. E., Schnell, E., & Barkai, E. (1995). Dynamics of learning and recall at excitatory recurrent synapses and cholinergic modulation in rat hippocampal region CA3. *Journal of Neuroscience, 15*, 5249–5262.

Kelsey, J. E., & Landry, B. A. (1988). Medial septal lesions disrupt spatial mapping ability in rats. *Behavioral Neuroscience, 102*, 289–293.

Kelsey, J. E., & Vargas, H. (1993). Medial septal lesions disrupt spatial, but not nonspatial, working memory in rats. *Behavioral Neuroscience, 107,* 565–574.

Kilgard, M. P., & Merzenich, M. M. (1998). Cortical map reorganization enabled by nucleus basalis activity. *Science, 279,* 1714–1718.

Leanza, G., Nilsson, O. G., Nikkhah, G., Wiley, R. G., & Björklund, A. (1996). Effects of neonatal lesions of the basal forebrain cholinergic system by 192 immunoglobulin G–saporin: Biochemical, behavioural and morphological characterization. *Neuroscience, 74,* 119–141.

Leanza, G., Nilsson, O. G., Wiley, R. G., & Björklund, A. (1995). Selective lesioning of the basal forebrain cholinergic system by intraventricular 192 IgG–saporin: Behavioural, biochemical and stereological studies in the rat. *European Journal of Neuroscience, 7,* 329–343.

Linster, C., Garcia, P. A., Hasselmo, M. E., & Baxter, M. G. (2001). Selective loss of cholinergic neurons projecting to the olfactory system increases perceptual generalization between similar, but not dissimilar, odorants. *Behavioral Neuroscience, 115,* 826–833.

Linster, C., & Hasselmo, M. (1997). Modulation of inhibition in a model of olfactory bulb reduces overlap in the neural representation of olfactory stimuli. *Behavioural Brain Research, 84,* 117–127.

Linster, C., & Hasselmo, M. E. (1999). Behavioral responses to aliphatic aldehydes can be predicted from known electrophysiological responses of mitral cells in the olfactory bulb. *Physiology and Behavior, 66,* 497–502.

Markowska, A. L., Wenk, G. L., & Olton, D. S. (1990). Nucleus basalis magnocellularis and memory: Differential effects of two neurotoxins. *Behavioral and Neural Biology, 54,* 13–26.

McGaughy, J., Kaiser, T., & Sarter, M. (1996). Behavioral vigilance following infusions of 192 IgG–saporin into the basal forebrain: Selectivity of the behavioral impairment and relation to cortical AChE-positive fiber density. *Behavioral Neuroscience, 110,* 247–265.

McMahan, R. W., Sobel, T. J., & Baxter, M. G. (1997). Selective immunolesions of hippocampal cholinergic input fail to impair spatial working memory. *Hippocampus, 7,* 130–136.

Morris, R. G. M., Garrud, P., Rawlins, J. N. P., & O'Keefe, J. (1982). Place navigation impaired in rats with hippocampal lesions. *Nature, 297,* 681–683.

Moser, E., Moser, M.-B., & Andersen, P. (1993). Spatial learning impairment parallels the magnitude of dorsal hippocampal lesions, but is hardly present following ventral lesions. *Journal of Neuroscience, 13,* 3916–3925.

Muir, J. L., Everitt, B. J., & Robbins, T. W. (1994). AMPA-induced excitotoxic lesions of the basal forebrain: A significant role for the cortical cholinergic system in attentional function. *Journal of Neuroscience, 14,* 2313–2326.

Nilsson, O. G., Leanza, G., Rosenblad, C., Lappi, D. A., Wiley, R. G., & Björklund, A. (1992). Spatial learning impairments in rats with selective immunolesion of the forebrain cholinergic system. *NeuroReport, 3,* 1005–1008.

Olton, D. S., & Markowska, A. L. (1992). The aging septo-hippocampal system: Its role in age-related memory impairments. In L. R. Squire & N. Butters (Eds.), *Neuropsychology of memory* (2nd ed., pp. 378–385). New York: Guilford Press.

Pang, K. C. H., & Nocera, R. (1999). Interactions between 192–IgG saporin and intraseptal cholinergic and GABAergic drugs: Role of cholinergic medial septal neurons in spatial working memory. *Behavioral Neuroscience, 113,* 265–275.

Perry, E. K., Perry, R. H., Blessed, G., & Tomlinson, B. E. (1977). Necropsy evidence of central cholinergic deficits in senile dementia. *Lancet, i,* 189.

Perry, E. K., Tomlinson, B. E., Blessed, G., Bergmann, K., Gibson, P. H., & Perry, R. H. (1978). Correlation of cholinergic abnormalities with senile plaques and mental test scores in senile dementia. *British Medical Journal, ii,* 1457–1459.

Pioro, E. C., & Cuello, A. C. (1988). Purkinje cells of adult rat cerebellum express nerve growth factor immunoreactivity: Light microscopic observations. *Brain Research, 455,* 182–186.

Ragozzino, M. E., Unick, K. E., & Gold, P. E. (1996). Hippocampal acetylcholine release during memory testing in rats: Augmentation by glucose. *Proceedings of the National Academy of Sciences USA, 93,* 4693–4698.

Ricceri, L., Baxter, M. G., Frick, K. M., & Berger-Sweeney, J. (2000). Preservation of reactivity to spatial novelty in adult rats after specific basal forebrain 192 IgG–saporin lesions. *Society for Neuroscience Abstracts*, 26, 1506.

Riekkinen, M., Riekkinen, P., & Riekkinen, P., Jr. (1991). Comparison of quisqualic and ibotenic acid nucleus basalis magnocellularis lesions on water-maze and passive avoidance performance. *Brain Research Bulletin*, 27, 119–123.

Robbins, T. W., Everitt, B. J., Ryan, C. N., Marston, H. M., Jones, G. H., & Page, K. J. (1989). Comparative effects of quisqualic and ibotenic acid-induced lesions of the substantia innominata and globus pallidus on the acquisition of a conditional visual discrimination: Differential effects on cholinergic mechanisms. *Neuroscience*, 28, 337–352.

Sarter, M., Bruno, J. P., & Himmelheber, A. M. (1997). Cortical acetylcholine and attention: Neuropharmacological and cognitive principles directing treatment strategies for cognitive disorders. In J. D. Brioni & M. W. Decker (Eds.), *Pharmacological treatment of Alzheimer's disease: Molecular and neurobiological foundations* (pp. 105–128). New York: Wiley.

Torres, E. M., Perry, T. A., Blokland, A., Wilkinson, L. S., Wiley, R. G., Lappi, D. A., & Dunnett, S. B. (1994). Behavioural, histochemical and biochemical consequences of selective immunolesions in discrete regions of the basal forebrain cholinergic system. *Neuroscience*, 63, 95–122.

Turchi, J., & Sarter, M. (2000). Cortical cholinergic inputs mediate processing capacity: Effects of 192 IgG–saporin-induced lesions on olfactory span performance. *European Journal of Neuroscience*, 12, 4505–4514.

Waite, J. J., Wardlow, M. L., & Power, A. E. (1999). Deficit in selective and divided attention associated with cholinergic basal forebrain immunotoxic lesion produced by 192-saporin; motoric/sensory deficit associated with Purkinje cell immunotoxic lesion produced by OX7–saporin. *Neurobiology of Learning and Memory*, 71, 325–352.

Walsh, T. J., Herzog, C. D., Gandhi, C., Stackman, R. W., & Wiley, R. G. (1996). Injection of 192 IgG–saporin into the medial septum produces cholinergic hypofunction and dose-dependent working memory deficits. *Brain Research*, 726, 69–79.

Whitehouse, P. J., Price, D. L., Struble, R. G., Clark, A. W., Coyle, J. T., & Delon, M. R. (1982). Alzheimer's disease and senile dementia: Loss of neurons in the basal forebrain. *Science*, 215, 1237–1239.

Wiley, R. G., Oeltmann, T. N., & Lappi, D. A. (1991). Immunolesioning: Selective destruction of neurons using immunotoxin to rat NGF receptor. *Brain Research*, 562, 149–153.

Winkler, J., Suhr, S. T., Gage, F. H., Thal, L. J., & Fisher, L. J. (1995). Essential role of neocortical acetylcholine in spatial memory. *Nature*, 375, 484–487.

Zigmond, M. J., Berger, T. W., Grace, A. A., & Stricker, E. M. (1989). Compensatory responses to nigrostriatal bundle injury: Studies with 6-hydroxydopamine in an animal model of parkinsonism. *Molecular and Chemical Neuropathology*, 10, 185–200.

Zigmond, M. J., & Stricker, E. M. (1987). Parkinsonism: Insights from animal models utilizing neurotoxic agents. In J. P. Coyle (Ed.), *Animal models of dementia* (pp. 1–38). New York: Liss.

34

The Amygdala Regulates Memory Consolidation

JAMES L. McGAUGH

Over a century has now passed since Müller and Pilzecker (1900) first proposed the "perseveration–consolidation hypothesis." And over half a century has passed since the publication of the first experimental studies investigating the hypothesis (Duncan, 1949). In recent decades, research using a variety of behavioral methods and many kinds of treatments affecting brain functioning has provided strong evidence supporting the consolidation hypothesis. Lasting memory is not formed instantly. Memory consolidation requires the actions of processes that occur over time (Dudai, 1996; McGaugh, 1966, 2000). The fundamental assumption underlying the research summarized briefly in this chapter is that studies investigating the effects of treatments administered after training yield important insights into the systems that regulate memory consolidation.

Findings of many studies reported over the past several decades support the following conclusions:

1. Adrenal stress hormones, as well as drugs affecting several neuromodulatory systems, enhance memory consolidation.
2. The stress hormones and drug enhancement of memory consolidation involve noradrenergic and muscarinic cholinergic activation in the amygdaloid complex.
3. The basolateral nucleus of the amygdala (BLA) is the region critically involved in mediating neuromodulatory influences on memory consolidation.
4. The BLA modulates memory consolidation by influencing memory processing in other brain regions.
5. The amygdala is involved in modulating the consolidation of many forms of memory.

MEMORY ENHANCEMENT INDUCED
BY POSTTRAINING TREATMENTS

The first experimental studies of memory consolidation used treatments such as electro-convulsive shock, and later protein synthesis inhibitors, to produce retrograde amnesia in laboratory animals (Davis & Squire, 1984; Duncan, 1949; McGaugh & Herz, 1972). As the treatments were most effective when administered shortly after learning, it seemed clear that the treatments disrupted memory consolidation. Posttraining treatments provide a highly effective technique for investigating the effects of treatments influencing memory, as brain functioning is altered only shortly *after* training. Thus effects on acquisition and retrieval that make it difficult to interpret findings when treatments are administered prior to training are obviously excluded in studies using posttraining treatments (McGaugh, 1989a).

It is also now well established that memory can be *enhanced* as well as impaired by posttraining treatments affecting brain functioning. Findings first reported several decades ago indicate that in rats and mice, posttraining systemic injections of central nervous system (CNS) stimulants enhance long-term memory for training in a variety of learning tasks (Breen & McGaugh, 1961; McGaugh, 1973; McGaugh & Herz, 1972). More recently, comparable findings have been obtained in experiments with human subjects (Soetens, D'Hooge, & Hueting, 1993). Such findings provide strong evidence that drugs can enhance memory by influencing memory consolidation (McGaugh, 1989b).

EMOTIONAL AROUSAL, ADRENAL STRESS HORMONES,
AND MEMORY CONSOLIDATION

As seen from the findings of retrograde amnesia and memory enhancement induced by posttraining treatments, the processes underlying memory consolidation are highly susceptible to modulating influences occurring after learning. This may be the case simply because it takes time for the brain to make lasting memories. Alternatively, or perhaps additionally, the slow consolidation of memory after an experience may have an adaptive role. Slow consolidation provides the opportunity for endogenously activated systems, including hormonal and brain systems, to influence the strength of the memory of an experience (Gold & McGaugh, 1975; McGaugh, 2000).

Emotionally arousing experiences are generally well remembered (Heuer & Reisberg, 1990). Extensive evidence suggests that adrenal stress hormones released by emotionally arousing experiences modulate memory consolidation. Gold and van Buskirk (1975) were the first to report that in rats, posttraining injections of the adrenal medullary hormone epinephrine enhance memory for inhibitory avoidance training. As with CNS stimulants, enhancement was produced only by injections administered shortly after training. Subsequent studies in many laboratories reported comparable findings in studies using many kinds of training tasks, including appetitively as well as aversively motivated tasks (Izquierdo & Diaz, 1983; McGaugh, 1983; McGaugh & Gold, 1989; Sternberg, Isaacs, Gold, & McGaugh, 1985). The adrenocortical stress hormone corticosterone (in the rat) also modulates memory storage (Bohus, 1994; de Kloet, 1991; Lupien & McEwen, 1997; Roozendaal, 2000; Sandi & Rose, 1994). The memory-enhancing effect of corticosterone appears to be mediated by the selective activation of glucocorticoid receptors (Oitzl & de Kloet, 1992). Thus the adrenal stress hormones epinephrine and corticosterone, which are known to have important roles at the time of a stressful event, also have a longer-lasting adaptive effect in strengthening the consolidation of memory for events that induce their release. That is, the evidence strongly suggests that they play an important role in creating strong memories of significant events (McGaugh, 1990).

INVOLVEMENT OF THE AMYGDALOID COMPLEX

Adrenal stress hormones can and no doubt do have influences throughout the brain. Corticosterone readily enters the brain. Epinephrine enters the brain poorly, if at all. This hormone appears to influence memory consolidation by activating β-adrenergic receptors on the ascending vagus (Schreurs, Seelig, & Schulman, 1986); these project to brainstem nuclei, including the nucleus of the solitary tract (Williams & McGaugh, 1993), which in turn sends noradrenergic projections to the amygdaloid complex (Ricardo & Koh, 1978). There is extensive evidence indicating that the amygdaloid complex is critically involved in mediating drug and stress hormone influences on consolidation. Early findings that posttraining electrical stimulation of the amygdala can enhance or impair memory consolidation (McGaugh & Gold, 1976) were followed by reports that posttraining intra-amygdala infusions of drugs affecting noradrenergic and opioid receptors also modulate memory consolidation (Gallagher, Kapp, Pascoe, & Rapp, 1981; Liang, Juler, & McGaugh, 1986). In addition, selective lesions of the amygdala (Cahill & McGaugh, 1991) or infusions of β-adrenoceptor antagonists into the amygdala (Liang et al., 1986) block the memory-enhancing effects of posttraining injections of epinephrine. Other findings indicated that activation of norepinephrine (NE) within the amygdala is also critical for the memory-modulating effects of GABAergic and opioid peptidergic drugs administered either systemically or directly into the amygdala. Infusions of β-adrenoceptor antagonists into the amygdala block the memory-enhancing effects of GABAergic antagonists and opiate antagonists, and also block the memory-impairing effects of GABAergic and opiate agonists (Brioni, Nagahara, & McGaugh, 1989; Introini-Collison, Nagahara, & McGaugh, 1989; McGaugh, Introini-Collison, & Nagahara, 1988).

Findings of many recent studies indicate that the BLA of the amygdala is the critical area for modulatory influences on consolidation. Memory for several kinds of training, including inhibitory avoidance and water maze spatial training, is enhanced by infusions of noradrenergic agonists administered selectively into the BLA after training (Ferry & McGaugh, 1999; Hatfield & McGaugh, 1999). In addition, glucocorticoid influences on memory consolidation require a functioning BLA. Lesions of the BLA, but not lesions of the immediately adjacent central nucleus, block the memory-modulating effects of glucocorticoids (Roozendaal & McGaugh, 1996a; Roozendaal, Portillo-Marquez, & McGaugh, 1996). Moreover, selective infusions of β-adrenergic adrenoceptor antagonists into the BLA also block glucocorticoid effects on memory consolidation (Quirarte, Roozendaal, & McGaugh, 1997) (see Figure 34.1) and infusions of a glucocorticoid agonist selectively into the BLA enhance memory consolidation (Roozendaal & McGaugh, 1997a).

These findings indicate that activation of noradrenergic receptors within the amygdala is critical for the modulation of memory consolidation by many treatments. Thus this evidence suggests that emotionally arousing learning experiences should induce the release of NE within the amygdala, and that drugs and hormones that enhance memory consolidation should enhance the release. Findings of studies using *in vivo* microdialysis and high-performance liquid chromatography to measure NE release in the amygdala strongly support these implications. Footshock comparable to that typically used in inhibitory avoidance training significantly enhances NE release (Galvez, Mesches, & McGaugh, 1996;

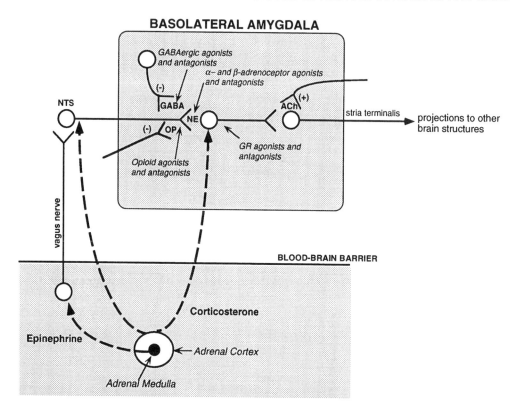

FIGURE 34.1. Schematic summary of the interactions of neuromodulatory influences regulating memory consolidation. Arousal-induced release of epinephrine from the adrenal medulla activates peripherally located β-adrenergic receptors on vagal afferents projecting to brainstem nuclei (including the nucleus of the solitary tract, NTS), which in turn send noradrenergic projections to the amygdala. Corticosterone (in the rat) readily enters the brain and can influence memory consolidation by acting at several sites. Activation of β-adrenoceptors in the (basolateral) amygdala is critical in mediating the memory-modulatory effects of both epinephrine and corticosterone. Opioid and GABAergic influences on memory are due to modulation of norepinephrine (NE) release. Noradrenergic influences require subsequent cholinergic activation within the amygdala. The amygdala influences memory by modulating consolidation occurring in other brain regions. The modulatory influences appear to be mediated largely, if not exclusively, via the stria terminalis. GR, glucocorticoid receptors; ACh, acetylcholine; OP, opioid peptides.

Quirarte, Galvez, Roozendaal, & McGaugh, 1998). Moreover, drugs and hormones that enhance memory consolidation potentiate NE release in the amygdala (Hatfield, Spanis, & McGaugh, 1999; Quirarte et al., 1998; Williams, Men, Clayton, & Gold, 1998).

Other findings suggest that noradrenergic effects require subsequent activation of muscarinic cholinergic receptors within the amygdala. Intra-amygdala infusions of muscarinic cholinergic antagonists block noradrenergic influences on memory consolidation (Dalmaz, Introini-Collison, & McGaugh, 1993; Introini-Collison, Dalmaz, & McGaugh, 1996). In addition, the BLA is a locus of muscarinic cholinergic activation critical for glucocorticoid influences on memory consolidation. Microinfusions of a cholinergic antagonist selectively into the BLA block the memory enhancement induced by systemic or intra-BLA adminstration of glucocorticoid receptor agonists (Power, Roozendaal, & McGaugh, 2000; Roozendaal, Nguyen, Power, & McGaugh, 1999).

AMYGDALA INFLUENCES ON OTHER BRAIN SYSTEMS
INVOLVED IN MEMORY CONSOLIDATION

It is clear from the findings discussed above that posttraining treatments affecting amygdala functioning influence memory consolidation. However, these findings, considered alone, do not reveal the locus of the neural processes underlying the treatment-modulated memory consolidation. Several kinds of findings suggest that the amygdala regulates memory consolidation by influencing neural processes in other brain regions (Cahill, Weinberger, Roozendaal, & McGaugh, 1999; McGaugh, 1990; McGaugh, Cahill, & Roozendaal, 1996; McGaugh, Cahill, Ferry, & Roozendaal, 2000; McGaugh, Ferry, Vazdarjanova, & Roozendaal, 2000).

Several studies using inhibitory avoidance training reported that lesions of the stria terminalis (ST), an amygdala pathway projecting to other brain regions, block the memory-modulating effects of treatments administered directly to the amygdala, including posttraining electrical stimulation of the amygdala (Liang & McGaugh, 1983a) as well as posttraining infusions of NE (Liang, McGaugh, & Yao, 1990). It is important to note that although ST lesions do not block acquisition or retention of inhibitory avoidance training, they block the memory-modulating effects of systemically administered drugs affecting adrenergic, cholinergic, and glucocorticoid receptors (Introini-Collison, Arai, & McGaugh, 1989; Introini-Collison, Miyazaki, & McGaugh, 1991; Liang & McGaugh, 1983b; Roozendaal & McGaugh, 1996b).

ST lesions also block the memory-enhancing effects induced by infusions of the cholinergic agonist oxotremorine administered into the caudate nucleus after inhibitory avoidance training (Packard, Introini-Collison, & McGaugh, 1996). The direct projections from the amygdala to the caudate (Kita & Kitai, 1990) via the ST appear to enable the memory-modulating influence of oxotremorine within the caudate nucleus. Other recent findings suggest that projections from the BLA to the nucleus accumbens via the ST are critically involved in mediating glucocorticoid effects on memory consolidation. Bilateral lesions of the nucleus accumbens, like bilateral lesions of the ST, block the enhancing effects of posttraining injections of the synthetic glucocorticoid dexamethasone on memory for inhibitory avoidance training (Setlow, Roozendaal, & McGaugh, 2000).

As is emphasized below, amygdala influences on memory are not restricted to fear-based learning or the associations of fear with cues or contexts. Several studies have found that the amygdala modulates memory consolidation in cued and spatial water maze tasks. "Double-dissociation" studies of the effects of lesions and selective drug infusions have reported that treatments affecting the caudate nucleus selectively influence cued learning, whereas treatments affecting the hippocampus selectively influence spatial learning (McDonald & White, 1993; Packard & McGaugh, 1992, 1996). For example, amphetamine infused into the caudate posttraining selectively enhances retention of cued water maze training, whereas infusions of amphetamine into the hippocampus selectively enhance retention of spatial training (Packard, Cahill, & McGaugh, 1994; Packard & Teather, 1998). Amygdala influences on memory consolidation are, however, not selective with respect to forms of learning (or types of training). Amphetamine infused into the amygdala posttraining enhances retention of both cued and spatial training. Moreover, and importantly, inactivation of the amygdala with lidocaine prior to the retention test did not block the memory enhancement induced by posttraining intra-amygdala infusions of amphetamine. Thus the amygdala is clearly not the site of the long-term memory modulated by the posttraining infusions. In contrast, when amphetamine was infused into the amygdala after training and lidocaine was infused into the caudate or hippocampus prior to the retention tests, intracaudate lidocaine infusions blocked memory enhancement in the cued task, and intrahippocampal lidocaine infusions blocked memory enhancement in the spatial task (Packard & Teather, 1998). Another recent study examining amgydala–hippocampal interactions in memory consolidation (Packard & Chen, 1999) reported that posttraining intrahippocampal infusions of glutamate enhanced rats' memory in a food-rewarded eight-arm maze. Moreover, and again importantly, posttraining intra-amygdala infusions of lidocaine blocked the enhanced memory consolidation produced by the glutamate infused into the hippocampus at the same time. Thus modulation of consolidation by a drug treatment affecting the hippocampus appears to require a functionally intact amygdala.

Comparable findings obtained in studies using inhibitory avoidance training provide further evidence that the BLA is critical for memory-modulating influences. Posttraining intrahippocampal infusions of a specific glucocorticoid agonist enhance inhibitory avoidance retention (Roozendaal & McGaugh, 1997b). Lesions of the BLA or infusions of a β-adrenoceptor antagonist or muscarinic cholinergic antagonist selectively into the BLA block the memory enhancement induced by the intrahippocampal infusions (Power et al., 2000; Roozendaal et al., 1999). These findings, considered together with those summarized above, provide strong evidence that although an intact and functioning amygdala is not critical for the retrieval of memory in the various learning tasks used, the amygdala is critical for enabling memory-modulatory influences involving other brain regions.

THE AMYGDALA'S ROLE IN MEMORY CONSOLIDATION FOR MANY KINDS OF TRAINING

As discussed above, there is considerable evidence that the amygdala modulates the consolidation of memory for many kinds of training:

Inhibitory avoidance
Y-maze discrimination training
Pavlovian contextual fear conditioning
Change in reward magnitude (CRM)
Radial maze appetitive training
Water maze spatial training
Water maze cued training

Those discussed or cited so far include inhibitory avoidance training, Y-maze discrimination training, cued and spatial water maze training, and food-rewarded eight-arm radial maze training. There is extensive evidence that the memory-modulatory influence of the amygdala is not restricted to fear-based learning. Many experiments have reported that the amygdala is involved in influencing memory for CRM (Flaherty, 1982; Salinas, Introini-Collison, Dalmaz, & McGaugh, 1997; Salinas & McGaugh, 1995, 1996; Salinas, Packard, & McGaugh, 1993; Salinas, Parent, & McGaugh, 1996). In the experiments by Salinas and colleagues, rats were first extensively trained to run to a goal box in a straight alley for a reward of 10 pellets. The reward was then reduced to 1 pellet. Significantly slower running speeds on the first few trials the next day indicated that the rats remembered the reduction in reward. Selective lesions of the BLA impaired memory for CRM (Salinas, Williams, & McGaugh, 1996). Unlike the controls, rats with BLA lesions did not run more slowly on the day after the reward was reduced to 1 pellet. Posttraining intra-amygdala infusions of lidocaine, muscimol, or the adrenoceptor antagonist propranolol also impaired CRM memory

(Salinas & McGaugh, 1995; Salinas et al., 1993, 1997), whereas infusions of the GABAergic antagonist bicuculline enhanced CRM memory (Salinas & McGaugh, 1996). These findings are comparable to those obtained in studies using inhibitory avoidance training.

Most studies of the involvement of the amygdala in learning and memory have used footshock punishment. As found with inhibitory avoidance training, posttraining intra-amygdala drug infusions modulate memory for footshock-motivated Y-maze visual discrimination training (Introini-Collison, Nagahara, & McGaugh, 1989). Posttraining amygdala infusions of drugs also modulate the retention of Pavlovian contextual fear conditioning (Liang, 1999, 2001). Furthermore, recent findings indicate that, as with inhibitory avoidance training, the BLA is selectively involved in the memory-modulatory influence of posttraining intra-amygdala drug infusions on contextual fear conditioning (Vazdarjanova & McGaugh, 1999). As noted above, posttraining intra-amygdala infusions of the muscarinic cholinergic agonist oxotremorine enhance inhibitory avoidance retention (Introini-Collison et al., 1996). In addition, posttraining intra-amygdala infusions of lidocaine impair inhibitory avoidance retention (Parent & McGaugh, 1994). In a recent experiment (Vazdarjanova & McGaugh, 1999), rats received contextual fear conditioning training, consisting of a series of footshocks delivered in one arm of a Y-maze, and were then given posttraining intra-BLA infusions of oxotremorine or lidocaine. The next day they were placed in one of the other arms of the maze, and several measures of retention were recorded: time spent "freezing," latency to enter the arm where shock was delivered and time spent in the shock arm. As indicated by all measures, the posttraining intra-BLA infusions of oxotremorine enhanced retention of contextual fear conditioning and the lidocaine infusions impaired retention. These findings provide further evidence that posttraining treatments affecting the BLA have comparable effects on memory for inhibitory avoidance training and contextual fear conditioning. It should be noted, however, that another recent study (Wilensky, Schafe, & LeDoux, 2000) confirmed previous findings (Brioni et al., 1989; Izquierdo et al., 1997; Zanatta et al., 1997) that posttraining infusions of the GABAergic agonist muscimol into the BLA impaired inhibitory avoidance retention, but reported that the infusions did not impair retention of Pavlovian contextual fear conditioning. The basis of this differential effect obtained with the two tasks remains to be clarified.

There is clear and consistent evidence that the BLA modulates memory processing involving other brain regions. However, is the BLA also a site of neural changes mediating memory, especially fear-based memory, as is hypothesized by other investigators (e.g., Davis, 2000; LeDoux, 2000)? That possibility cannot, of course, be excluded on logical grounds. However, several recent studies reporting that lesions of the amygdala (including lesions restricted to the BLA) do not prevent the acquisition or retention of fear-based learning seriously question the hypothesis that the amygdala is *the* locus of learned fear (Cahill, Vazdarjanova, & Setlow, 2000; Lehmann, Treit, & Parent, 2000; Vazdarjanova & McGaugh, 1998). Thus, although there is extensive evidence that the amygdala is involved in modulating memory consolidation, an intact amygdala does not appear to be critical for learning about and remembering dangerous events and situations.

EMOTIONAL AROUSAL, AMYGDALA ACTIVATION, AND LONG-TERM MEMORY IN HUMAN SUBJECTS

Studies of human subjects provide additional evidence consistent with the hypothesis that the amygdala is involved in modulating memory consolidation (Cahill, 2000; Cahill & McGaugh, 1998). The enhancing effect of emotional arousal on long-term memory is found in normal subjects (Cahill, Prins, Weber, & McGaugh, 1994; Heuer & Reisberg, 1990), as well as in amnesic subjects with intact amygdalae (Hamann, Cahill, McGaugh, & Squire, 1997). However, the effect is lacking in human subjects with bilateral amygdala lesions (Adolphs, Cahill, Schul, & Babinsky, 1997; Cahill, Babinsky, Markowitsch, & McGaugh, 1995). Moreover, studies using brain imaging to assess amygdala activity have reported that emotionally arousing material activates the amygdala, and that long-term memory of the material is highly correlated with the degree of amygdala activation. In an initial study using glucose PET imaging, subjects' recall of unpleasant emotionally arousing videos 3 weeks after viewing them was highly significantly correlated (+.93) with amygdala activity during viewing of the videos (Cahill et al., 1996). A subsequent study using emotionally arousing pictures and oxygen PET imaging (Hamann, Elt, Grafton, & Kilts, 1999) found that amygdala activity induced by *either* pleasant or unpleasant pictures correlated significantly with recall of the pictures one month later. A third recent study using fMRI imaging (Canli, Zhao, Brewer, Gabrieli, & Cahill, 2000) reported that subjects' memory for pictures, tested 3 weeks later, was correlated with amygdala activation during the viewing of the pictures. Finally, and most importantly, the correlation between amygdala activation and memory was greatest for the pictures that subjects rated as most emotionally intense.

CONCLUDING COMMENTS

Müller and Pilzecker's (1900) century-old memory consolidation hypothesis is abundantly supported by research findings. Lasting memories are not made instantly. They are created by the interaction of hormonal and brain systems activated by experiences. In this new century, research investigating how hormonal and brain systems act to regulate memory consolidation will no doubt provide critical insights into the neural changes underlying memory consolidation, and also identify places in the brain where memories are stored.

ACKNOWLEDGMENT

The research reported here was supported by Grant No. MH 12526 from the National Institute of Mental Health.

REFERENCES

Adolphs, R., Cahill, L., Schul, R., & Babinsky, R. (1997). Impaired declarative memory for emotional stimuli following bilateral amygdala damage in humans. *Learning and Memory*, *4*, 291–300.

Bohus, B. (1994). Humoral modulation of memory processes: Physiological significance of brain and peripheral mechanisms. In J. Delacour (Ed.), *The memory system of the brain* (Vol. 4, pp. 337–364). River Edge, NJ: World Scientific.

Breen, R. A., & McGaugh, J. L. (1961). Facilitation of maze learning with posttrial injections of picrotoxin. *Journal of Comparative and Physiological Psychology*, *54*, 498–501.

Brioni, J. D., Nagahara, A. H., & McGaugh, J. L. (1989). Involvement of the amygdala GABAergic system in the modulation of memory storage. *Brain Research*, *487*, 105–112.

Cahill, L. (2000). Modulation of long-term memory storage in humans by emotional arousal: adrenergic activation and the amygdala. In J. P. Aggleton (Ed.), *The amygdala: A functional analysis* (2nd ed., pp. 425–445). New York: Oxford University Press.

Cahill, L., Babinsky, R., Markowitsch, H., & McGaugh, J. L. (1995). The amygdala and emotional memory. *Nature*, *377*, 295–296.

Cahill, L., Haier, R., Fallon, J., Alkire, M., Tang, C., Keator, D., Wu, J., & McGaugh, J. L. (1996). Amygdala activity at encoding correlated with long-term, free recall of emotional information. *Proceedings of the National Academy of Sciences USA*, *93*, 8016–8021.

Cahill, L., & McGaugh, J. L. (1991). NMDA-induced lesions of the amygdaloid complex block the retention enhancing effect of posttraining epinephrine. *Psychobiology*, *19*, 206–210.

Cahill, L., & McGaugh, J. L. (1998). Mechanisms of emotional arousal and lasting declarative memory. *Trends in Neurosciences*, *21*, 294–299.

Cahill, L., Prins, B., Weber, M., & McGaugh, J. L. (1994). Beta-adrenergic activation and memory for emotional events. *Nature*, *371*, 702–704.

Cahill, L., Vazdarjanova, A., & Setlow, B. (2000). The basolateral amygdala complex is involved with, but is not necessary for, rapid acquisition of Pavlovian fear conditioning. *European Journal of Neuroscience*, *12*, 3044–3050.

Cahill, L., Weinberger, N. M., Roozendaal, B., & McGaugh, J. L. (1999). Is the amygdala a locus of "conditioned fear"?: Some questions and caveats. *Neuron*, *23*, 227–228.

Canli, T., Zhao, Z, Brewer, J., Gabrieli, J. D. E., & Cahill, L. (2000). Event-related activation in the human amygdala associates with later memory for individual emotional experience. *Journal of Neuroscience*, *20*, RC99.

Dalmaz, C., Introini-Collison, I. B., & McGaugh, J. L. (1993). Noradrenergic and cholinergic interactions in the amygdala and the modulation of memory storage. *Behavioural Brain Research*, *58*, 167–174.

Davis, H. P., & Squire, L. R. (1984). Protein synthesis and memory. *Psychological Bulletin*, *96*, 518–559.

Davis, M. (2000). The role of the amygdala in conditioned and unconditioned fear and anxiety. In J. P. Aggleton (Ed.), *The amygdala: A functional analysis* (2nd ed., pp. 213–287). New York: Oxford University Press.

de Kloet, E. R. (1991). Brain corticosteroid receptor balance and homeostatic control. *Frontiers in Neuroendocrinology*, *12*, 95–164.

Dudai, Y. (1996). Consolidation: Fragility on the road to the engram. *Neuron*, *17*, 367–370.

Duncan, C. P. (1949). The retroactive effect of electroshock on learning. *Journal of Comparative Physiology and Psychology*, *42*, 32–42.

Ferry, B., & McGaugh, J. L. (1999). Clenbuterol administration into the basolateral amygdala posttraining enhances retention in an inhibitory avoidance task. *Neurobiology of Learning and Memory*, *72*, 8–12.

Flaherty, C. F. (1982). Incentive contrast: A review of behavioral changes following shifts in reward. *Animal Learning and Behavior*, *10*, 409–440.

Gallagher, M., Kapp, B. S., Pascoe, J. P., & Rapp, P. R. (1981). A neuropharmacology of amygdaloid systems which contribute to learning and memory. In Y. Ben-Ari (Ed.), *The amygdaloid complex* (pp. 343–354). Amsterdam: Elsevier/North-Holland.

Galvez, R., Mesches, M., & McGaugh, J. L. (1996). Norepinephrine release in the amygdala in response to footshock stimulation. *Neurobiology of Learning and Memory*, *66*, 253–257.

Gold, P. E., & McGaugh, J. L. (1975). A single-trace, two process view of memory storage processes. In D. Deutsch & J. A. Deutsch (Eds.), *Short-term memory* (pp. 355–378). New York: Academic Press.

Gold, P. E., & van Buskirk, R. B. (1975). Facilitation of time-dependent memory processes with posttrial epinephrine injections. *Behavioral Biology*, *13*, 145–153.

Hamann, S. B., Cahill, L., McGaugh, J. L. & Squire, L. R. (1997). Intact enhancement of declarative memory for emotional material in amnesia. *Learning and Memory*, *4*, 301–309.

Hamann, S. B., Elt, T., Grafton, S., & Kilts, C. (1999). Amygdala activity related to enhanced memory for pleasant and aversive stimuli. *Nature Neuroscience*, *2*, 289–293.

Hatfield, T., & McGaugh, J. L. (1999). Norepinephrine infused into the basolateral amygdala posttraining enhances retention in a spatial water maze task. *Neurobiology of Learning and Memory*, *71*, 232–239.

Hatfield, T., Spanis, C., & McGaugh, J. L. (1999). Response of amygdalar norepinephrine to footshock and GABAergic drugs using *in vivo* microdialysis and HPLC. *Brain Research, 835,* 340–345.

Heuer, F., & Reisberg, D. (1990). Vivid memories of emotional events: The accuracy of remembered minutiae. *Memory and Cognition, 18,* 496–506.

Introini-Collison, I. B., Arai, Y., & McGaugh, J. L. (1989). Stria terminalis lesions attenuate the effects of posttraining oxotremorine and atropine on retention. *Psychobiology, 17,* 397–401.

Introini-Collison, I., Dalmaz, C., & McGaugh, J. L. (1996). Amygdala β-noradrenergic influences on memory storage involve cholinergic activation. *Neurobiology of Learning and Memory, 65,* 57–64.

Introini-Collison, I., Miyazaki, B., & McGaugh, J. L. (1991). Involvement of the amygdala in the memory-enhancing effects of clenbuterol. *Psychopharmacology, 104,* 541–544.

Introini-Collison, I. B., Nagahara, A. H., & McGaugh, J. L. (1989). Memory-enhancement with intra-amygdala posttraining naloxone is blocked by concurrent administration of propranolol. *Brain Research, 476,* 94–101.

Izquierdo, I., & Diaz, R. D. (1983). Effect of ACTH, epinephrine, β-endorphin, naloxone, and of the combination of naloxone or β-endorphin with ACTH or epinephrine on memory consolidation. *Psychoneuroendocrinology, 8,* 81–87.

Izquierdo, I., Quillfeldt, J. A., Zanatta, M. S., Quevedo, J., Schaeffer, E., Schmitz, P. K., & Medina, J. H. (1997). Sequential involvement of hippocampus and amygdala, entorhinal cortex and parietal cortex in the formation and expression of memory for inhibitory avoidance in rats. *European Journal of Neuroscience, 9,* 786–793.

Kita, H., & Kitai, S. T. (1990). Amygdaloid projections to the frontal cortex and the striatum in the rat. *Journal of Comparative Neurology, 298,* 40–49.

LeDoux, J. (2000). The amygdala and emotion: A view through fear. In J. P. Aggleton (Ed.), *The amygdala: A functional analysis* (2nd ed., pp. 289–310). New York: Oxford University Press.

Lehmann, H., Treit, D., & Parent, M. B. (2000). Amygdala lesions do not impair shock-probe avoidance retention performance. *Behavioral Neuroscience, 114,* 107–16.

Liang, K. C. (1999). Pre- or post-training injection of buspirone impaired retention in the inhibitory avoidance task: Involvement of amygdala 5-HT1A receptors. *European Journal of Neuroscience, 11,* 1491–1500.

Liang, K. C. (2001). Epinephrine modulation of memory. In P. E. Gold & W. T. Greenough (Eds.), *Memory Consolidation: Essays in honor of James L. McGaugh* (pp. 165–184). Washington, DC: American Psychological Association.

Liang, K. C., Juler, R., & McGaugh, J. L. (1986). Modulating effects of posttraining epinephrine on memory: Involvement of the amygdala noradrenergic system. *Brain Research, 368,* 125–133.

Liang, K. C., & McGaugh, J. L. (1983a). Lesions of the stria terminalis attenuate the amnestic effect of amygdaloid stimulation on avoidance responses. *Brain Research, 274,* 309–3l8.

Liang, K. C., & McGaugh, J. L. (1983b). Lesions of the stria terminalis attenuate the enhancing effect of posttraining epinephrine on retention of an inhibitory avoidance response. *Behavioural Brain Research, 9,* 49–58.

Liang, K. C., McGaugh, J. L., & Yao, H. (1990). Involvement of amygdala pathways in the influence of posttraining amygdala norepinephrine and peripheral epinephrine on memory storage. *Brain Research, 508,* 225–233.

Lupien, S. J., & McEwen, B. S. (1997). The acute effects of corticosteroids on cognition, Integration of animal and human model studies. *Brain Research Reviews, 24,* 1–27.

McDonald, R. J., & White, N. M. (1993). A triple dissociation of memory systems: Hippocampus, amygdala, and dorsal striatum. *Behavioral Neuroscience, 107,* 3–22.

McGaugh, J. L. (1966). Time-dependent processes in memory storage. *Science, 153,* 1351–1358.

McGaugh, J. L. (1973). Drug facilitation of learning and memory. *Annual Review of Pharmacology, 13,* 229–241.

McGaugh, J. L. (1983). Hormonal influences on memory. *Annual Review of Psychology, 34,* 297–323.

McGaugh, J. L. (1989a). Dissociating learning and performance: Drug and hormone enhancement of memory storage. *Brain Research Bulletin*, *23*, 339–345.

McGaugh, J. L. (1989b). Involvement of hormonal and neuromodulatory systems in the regulation of memory storage. *Annual Review of Neuroscience*, *12*, 255–287.

McGaugh, J. L. (1990). Significance and remembrance: The role of neuromodulatory systems. *Psychological Science*, *1*, 15–25.

McGaugh, J. L. (2000). Memory: A century of consolidation. *Science*, *287*, 248–251

McGaugh, J. L., Cahill, L., & Roozendaal, B. (1996). Involvement of the amygdala in memory storage: Interaction with other brain systems. *Proceedings of the National Academy of Sciences USA*, *93*, 13508–13514.

McGaugh, J. L., Cahill, L., Ferry, B., & Roozendaal, R. (2000). Brain systems and the regulation of memory consolidation. In J. J. Bolhuis (Ed.) *Brain, perception, memory: Advances in cognitive neuroscience* (pp. 233–251). Oxford: Oxford University Press.

McGaugh, J. L., Ferry, B., Vazdarjanova, A., & Roozendaal, B. (2000). Amygdala: Role in modulation of memory storage. In J. P. Aggleton (Ed.), *The amygdala: A functional analysis* (2nd ed., pp. 391–423). New York: Oxford University Press.

McGaugh, J. L., & Gold, P. E. (1976). Modulation of memory by electrical stimulation of the brain. In M. R. Rosenzweig & E. L. Bennett (Eds.), *Neural mechanisms of learning and memory* (pp. 549–560). Cambridge, MA: MIT Press.

McGaugh, J. L., & Gold, P. E. (1989). Hormonal modulation of memory. In R. B. Brush & S. Levine (Eds.), *Psychoendocrinology* (pp. 305–339). New York: Academic Press.

McGaugh, J. L., & Herz, M. J. (1972). *Memory consolidation*. San Francisco: Albion.

McGaugh, J. L., Introini-Collison, I. B., & Nagahara, A. H. (1988). Memory-enhancing effects of posttraining naloxone: Involvement of b-norarenergic influences in the amygdaloid complex. *Brain Research*, *446*, 37–49.

Müller, G. E., & Pilzecker, A. (1900). Experimentelle Beiträge zur Lehre vom Gedächtniss. *Zeitschrift für Psychologie und Physiologie der Sinners organs: Erganzungsband*, *1*, 1–288.

Oitzl, M. S., & de Kloet, E. R. (1992). Selective corticosteroid antagonist modulate specific aspects of spatial orientation learning. *Behavioral Neuroscience*, *106*, 62–71.

Packard, M. G., Cahill, L., & McGaugh, J. L. (1994). Amygdala modulation of hippocampal-dependent and caudate nucleus-dependent memory processes. *Proceedings of the National Academy of Sciences USA*, *91*, 8477–8481.

Packard, M. G., & Chen, S. A. (1999). The basolateral amygdala is a cofactor in memory enhancement produced by intrahippocampal glutamate injections. *Psychobiology*, *27*, 377–385.

Packard, M. G., Introini-Collison, I., & McGaugh, J. L. (1996). Stria terminalis lesions attenuate memory enhancement produced by intra-caudate nucleus injections of oxotremorine. *Neurobiology of Learning and Memory*, *65*, 278–282.

Packard, M. G., & McGaugh, J. L. (1992). Double dissociation of fornix and caudate nucleus lesions on acquisition of two water maze tasks: Further evidence for multiple memory systems. *Behavioral Neuroscience*, *106*, 439–446.

Packard, M. G., & McGaugh, J. L. (1996). Inactivation of hippocampus or caudate nucleus with lidocaines differentially affects expression of place and response learning. *Neurobiology of Learning and Memory*, *65*, 65–72.

Packard, M. G., & Teather, L. (1998). Amygdala modulation of multiple memory systems: Hippocampus and caudate–putamen. *Neurobiology of Learning and Memory*, *69*, 163–203.

Parent, M., & McGaugh, J. L. (1994). Posttraining infusion of lidocaine into the amygdala basolateral complex impairs retention of inhibitory avoidance training. *Brain Research*, *661*, 97–103.

Power, A. E., Roozendaal, B., & McGaugh, J. L. (2000). Glucocorticoid enhancement of memory consolidation in the rat is blocked by muscarinic receptor antagonism in the basolateral amygdala. *European Journal of Neuroscience*, *12*, 3481–3487

Quirarte, G. L., Roozendaal, B., & McGaugh, J. L. (1997). Glucocorticoid enhancement of memory storage involves noradrenergic activation in the basolateral amygdala. *Proceedings of the National Academy of Sciences USA*, *94*, 14048–14053.

Quirarte, G. L., Galvez, R., Roozendaal, B., & McGaugh, J. L. (1998). Norepinephrine release in the amygdala in response to footshock and opioid peptidergic drugs. *Brain Research*, *808*, 134–140.

Ricardo, J., & Koh, E. (1978). Anatomical evidence of direct projections from the nucleus of the solitary tract to the hypothalamus, amygdala, and other forebrain structures in the rat. *Brain Research*, *153*, 1–26.

Roozendaal, B. (2000). Glucocorticoids and the regulation of memory consolidation. *Psychoneuroendocrinology*, *25*, 213–238.

Roozendaal, B., & McGaugh, J. L. (1996a). Amygdaloid nuclei lesions differentially affect glucocorticoid-induced memory enhancement in an inhibitory avoidance task *Neurobiology of Learning and Memory*, *65*, 1–8.

Roozendaal, B., & McGaugh, J. L. (1996b). The memory-modulatory effects of glucocorticoids depend on an intact stria terminalis. *Brain Research*, *709*, 243–350.

Roozendaal, B., & McGaugh, J. L. (1997a). Glucocorticoid receptor agonist and antagonist administration into the basolateral but not central amygdala modulates memory storage. *Neurobiology of Learning and Memory*, *67*, 176–179.

Roozendaal, B., & McGaugh, J. L. (1997b). Basolateral amygdala lesions block the memory-enhancing effect of glucocorticoid administration in the dorsal hippocampus of rats. *European Journal of Neuroscience*, *9*, 76–83.

Roozendaal, B., Nguyen, B. T., Power, A., & McGaugh, J. L. (1999). Basolateral amygdala noradrenergic influence on the memory-enhancing effect of glucocorticoid receptor activation into the hippocampus. *Proceedings of the National Academy of Sciences, USA*, *96*, 11642–11647.

Roozendaal, B., Portillo-Marquez, G., & McGaugh, J. L. (1996). Basolateral amygdala lesions block glucocorticoid-induced modulation of memory for spatial learning. *Behavioral Neuroscience*, *110*, 1074–1083.

Salinas, J. A., Introini-Collison, I. B., Dalmaz, C., & McGaugh, J. L. (1997). Posttraining intra-amygdala infusions of oxotremorine and propranolol modulate storage of memory for reduction in reward magnitude. *Neurobiology of Learning and Memory*, *68*, 51–59.

Salinas, J. A., & McGaugh, J. L. (1995). Muscimol induces retrograde amnesia for changes in reward magnitude. *Neurobiology of Learning and Memory*, *63*, 277–285.

Salinas, J. A., & McGaugh, J. L. (1996). The amygdala modulates memory for changes in reward magnitude: Involvement of the amygdaloid GABAergic system. *Behavioural Brain Research*, *80*, 87–98.

Salinas, J. A., Packard, M. G., & McGaugh, J. L. (1993). Amygdala modulates memory for changes in reward magnitude: Reversible post-training inactivation with lidocaine attenuates the response to a reduction reward. *Behavioural Brain Research*, *59*, 153–159.

Salinas, J. A., Parent, M. B., & McGaugh, J. L. (1996). Ibotenic acid lesions of amygdala nuclei differentially effect the response to reductions in reward. *Brain Research*, *742*, 283–293.

Salinas, J. A., Williams, C. L., & McGaugh, J. L. (1996). Peripheral posttraining administration of 4–OH amphetamine enhances retention of a reduction in reward magnitude. *Neurobiology of Learning and Memory*, *65*, 192–195.

Sandi, C., & Rose, S. P. R. (1994). Corticosterone enhances long-term retention in one day-old chicks trained in a week passive avoidance learning paradigm. *Brain Research*, *647*, 106–112.

Schreurs, J., Seelig, T., & Schulman, H. (1986). b$_2$-adrenergic receptors on peripheral nerves. *Journal of Neurochemistry*, *46*, 294–296.

Setlow, B., Roozendaal, B., & McGaugh, J. L. (2000). Involvement of a basolateral amygdala complex—nucleus accumbens pathway in glucocorticoid-induced modulation of memory storage. *European Journal of Neuroscience*, *12*, 367–375.

Soetens, E., D'Hooge, R., & Hueting, J. E. (1993). Amphetamine enhances human-memory consolidation. *Neuroscience Letters*, *161*, 9–12.

Sternberg, D. B., Isaacs, K., Gold, P. E., & McGaugh, J. L. (1985). Epinephrine facilitation of appetitive learning: Attenuation with adrenergic receptor antagonists. *Behavioral and Neural Biology*, *44*, 447–453.

Vazdarjanova, A., & McGaugh, J. L. (1998). Basolateral amygdala is not a critical locus for memory of contextual fear conditioning. *Proceedings of the National Academy of Sciences USA, 95,* 15003–15007.

Vazdarjanova, A., & McGaugh, J. L. (1999). Basolateral amygdala is involved in modulating consolidation of memory for classical fear conditioning. *Journal of Neuroscience, 19,* 6615–6622.

Wilensky, A. E., Schafe, G. E., & LeDoux, J. E. (2000). The amygdala modulates memory consolidation of fear-motivated inhibitory avoidance learning but not classical fear conditioning. *Journal of Neuroscience, 20,* 7059–7066.

Williams, C. L., & McGaugh, J. L. (1993). Reversible lesions of the nucleus of the solitary tract attenuate the memory-modulating effects of posttraining epinephrine. *Behavioral Neuroscience, 107,* 1–8.

Williams, C. L., Men, D., Clayton, E. C., & Gold, P. E. (1998). Norepinephrine release in the amygdala following systemic injection of epinephrine or escapable footshock: Contribution of the nucleus of the solitary tract. *Behavioral Neuroscience, 112,* 1414–1422.

Zanatta, M. S., Quillfeldt, J. H., Schaeffer, E., Schmitz, P. K., Quevedo, J., Medina, J. H., & Izquierdo, I. (1997). Involvement of the hippocampus, amygdala, entorhinal cortex and posterior parietal cortex in memory consolidation. *Brazilian Journal of Medical Biology Research, 30,* 235–240.

35

Memory Modulation

Regulating Interactions between
Multiple Memory Systems

PAUL E. GOLD

The processing of information to be learned and remembered appears to occur in separate multiple memory systems that acquire different classes of information (see, e.g., Gabrieli, 1996; Nyberg & Tulving, 1996; Posner, Petersen, Fox, & Raichle, 1988; Squire, 1992; Willingham, 1999). The evidence for multiple memory systems in humans includes findings that damage to different neural systems impairs different classes of learning and memory, and that activation of different neural systems reveals participation of these systems in different classes of learning and memory.

In rodents, there is also substantial support for the view that different neural systems are responsible for processing and storing information for different types of memory. Most evidence comes from studies in which damage to one neural system interferes with one class of learning but not another, and damage to a different neural system reveals the reciprocal results. The key evidence is that damage to different brain regions impairs particular cognitive functions with sometimes extraordinary specificity. Of particular relevance are triple brain lesion × task dissociations for tasks that seem in many ways similar (e.g., motivational and sensorimotor demands), but for which specific damage to different neural systems results in apparently different and selective deficits in cognition (Kesner, Bolland, & Dakis, 1993; McDonald & White, 1993). For example, in the McDonald and White (1993) study, damage to the hippocampal formation, striatum and amygdala impaired learning on three variants of food-motivated maze learning—win–shift, win–stay, and conditioned cue preference, respectively. Thus these cleverly conceived tasks depend on the integrity of one memory system or another.

Of course, most tasks and most experiences are not as specifically linked to independent memory systems, but instead involve interplay of these systems. If separate memory systems acquire different classes of information, it becomes easy to imagine that cooperation across systems will be important in determining what new information is learned and how well it is learned. Conversely, it is also easy to imagine that if the systems compete with each other for access to information, participation of one system may interfere with learning by another system. There are several examples revealing competition between memory systems, in which damage to one system enhances the learning that is dependent on another system. Learning in the conditioned cue preference task, an amygdala-dependent task, can at times be enhanced by damage to the septohippocampal system (McDonald & White, 1995; White & McDonald, 1993). In this task, rats are first habituated to a two-arm radial maze and then are placed, on alternate days, in one of the arms; one arm is now rewarded with a large and palatable reward, and the other arm is without reward. After 8 days (four trials on each arm), a test trial is administered on which both arms are opened (unbaited), and rats can move freely between them. Trained rats show a preference for the previously baited arm. Rats with fornix lesions made prior to the habituation trials are better at learning the conditioned cue preference task than are intact rats. These findings suggest that hippocampus-dependent acquisition of place information competes with the amygdala for control of the information to be learned. More specifically, the hippocampus acquires information that is not critical to the conditioned cue preference task and may in fact be distracting or incompatible with that information. With impaired hippocampal function, the amygdala has more control over what is learned, and acquisition proceeds more quickly. Similar results have been reported in other contexts. For example, noting that ethanol often impairs learning and memory and interferes with hippocampal functions, Matthews, Ilgen, White, and Best (1999) showed that acute administration of ethanol impaired acquisition of spatial information and enhanced acquisition of nonspatial (cued) information in an eight-arm radial maze. These results are comparable to those seen in rats with fimbria–fornix lesions (Matthews & Best, 1995).

In rodents, examination of interactions between memory systems is likely to be facilitated by procedures that can evaluate activation of the different neural systems during training while they are relatively intact. Recently, we began to use measures of acetylcholine (ACh) release and extracellular glucose levels during training to monitor relative activation of different neural systems. Relating the neurochemical measures to simultaneous behavioral assessments of learning and memory has made it possible to observe both competition and cooperation between memory systems. Of particular interest, baseline ACh release levels in hippocampus and striatum predict, in advance of any training, how the brains of individual rats bias different neural systems to acquire information that will guide the rats' learned behavior. In addition, by manipulating the relative activation of different neural systems important for learning and memory, one can manipulate what information a rat will use to guide its learned performance. These experiments are described in this chapter.

GLUCOSE AND ACH MODULATION OF MEMORY PROCESSES

The examination of training-related fluctuations in extracellular glucose and ACh grew from a literature demonstrating that endogenous release of epinephrine from the adrenal medulla is an important modulator of memory processes, retroactively enhancing memory for many tasks in rodents. Because epinephrine does not enter the brain to a large extent (Axelrod, Weil-Malherbe, & Tomchick, 1959), a peripheral action of epinephrine must mediate the hormone's effects on memory. The best evidence suggests that epinephrine acts via β-adrenergic mechanisms (Cahill, Prins, Weber, & McGaugh, 1994; Gold & van Buskirk, 1978), including activation of vagal afferents to the central nervous system (Clark et al., 1998; Clark, Naritoku, Smith, Browning, & Jensen, 1999; Jensen, 2001; Williams & Clayton, 2001), or by initiating release of hepatic sources of glucose into the circulation

(Gold, 1995a). These views are not mutually exclusive, and each mechanism may contribute to epinephrine effects on memory.

The evidence supporting a role for glucose in modulation of memory formation is now extensive. In both rodents and humans, glucose administration enhances learning and memory on many tasks (Gold, 2001; Korol & Gold, 1998). In addition, direct injections of glucose into some brain areas modulate learning and memory processes. Importantly, brain extracellular glucose levels are depleted in some brain areas during training, and the depletion is blocked by glucose administration. For example, during behavioral testing on a hippocampus-dependent task, brain extracellular glucose levels decrease by as much as 40% in the hippocampus, but not in the striatum (McNay, Fries, & Gold, 2000; McNay & Gold, 1999, 2001; McNay, McCarty, & Gold, 2001). Peripheral injections of glucose, at doses that enhance learning and memory, block that depletion. Thus it appears that decreases in glucose availability to the brain regions engaged in learning and memory may limit the efficiency of memory processing, and that systemic glucose administration enhances learning and memory by maintaining brain glucose availability. Pharmacological evidence suggests that glucose may influence neural excitability by regulating potassium–adenosine triphosphate channels (Stefani & Gold, 1998, 2001; Stefani, Nicholson, & Gold, 1999).

There is also a substantial amount of evidence that glucose administration results in increases in brain ACh release in a manner that contributes to the effects of glucose on memory. The next section of this chapter describes studies of training-related fluctuations in ACh levels in different neural systems. These experiments represent an approach directed at using profiles of ACh release in different brain areas while rats are engaged in learning and memory tasks, to observe interactions between neural systems. When combined, the results provide a form of functional imaging of ACh release as a marker of relative activation of different memory systems. In this way, the experiments afford an opportunity to integrate the precise cognitive roles of multiple independent memory systems identified on the basis of brain damage with the apparently broad cognitive roles of hormonal and neurotransmitter modulators of memory formation (Gold, 1995b; Gold, McIntyre, McNay, Stefani, & Korol, 2001).

MODULATORS OF MEMORY AS SELECTORS OF LEARNING STRATEGIES

Typically, interpretation of modulation of learning and memory centers on pharmacological mechanisms by which hormones and neurotransmitters strengthen and weaken recent memories. When one is considering systemically administered treatments, this interpretation is readily supported by a large set of experiments. For example, when epinephrine or glucose is administered systemically near the time of training, similar effects are evident on learning and memory in many very different tasks (cf. Gold, 1995b). These broad effects contrast strikingly with the findings from studies of multiple memory systems, as described above.

Recent experiments have addressed the empirical difference between the relatively global effects seen in modulation of memory with the more restrictive effects seen with lesions. One set of experiments involved direct injections of drugs into different neural systems, with the goal of modulating the level of participation of different neural systems in learning and memory. For example we (Chang & Gold, 2001) tested the effects of injections of lidocaine, a local anesthetic, into the hippocampus prior to training on two similar four-arm radial maze tasks with comparable difficulty and comparable sensorimotor and motivational demands. One is a hippocampus-dependent place task, in which the goal arm is kept constant and the other three arms are randomly used as start arms. The other is a striatum-dependent response task in which, regardless of room position, the goal arm is entered by making a specific turn (i.e., right or left) when exiting a randomly selected start arm. Consistent with predictions from lesion studies (e.g., Matthews & Best, 1995), lidocaine injections into the hippocampus resulted in impaired acquisition of the place version of the maze and, conversely, enhanced acquisition of the response task. These findings suggest that increases and decreases in the hippocampal contribution to learning change the outcome of competition between hippocampal and striatal memory systems.

Drug injections have also been used to increase the participation of different neural systems during learning. Packard and Teather (1999) showed that direct injections of glutamate into the hippocampus or striatum enhanced learning and memory for the place or cue version, respectively, of a swim task, mirroring the effects of lesions of the hippocampus and striatum on these tasks. Another experiment involved training rats on a four-arm cross-shaped maze that can be solved with either place or response strategies (Packard, 1999). Intrahippocampal or intrastriatal injections of glutamate differentially enhanced learning place or response, respectively. These findings complement those observed earlier showing that lidocaine injections into the hippocampus or striatum impair the use of place or response solutions to the maze (Packard & McGaugh, 1996).

Another approach to studying the relative contributions of different neural systems to learning and memory is to examine activation of those systems during learning. We have completed a series of experiments in which ACh release, measured in *in vivo* microdialysis samples collected during behavioral testing, is used as a marker of activation of hippocampal and striatal systems. In earlier experiments, we found that release of hippocampal ACh increased when rats were tested for spatial working memory in spontaneous alternation tasks. Moreover, when injected systemically or directly into the medial septum, morphine impaired performance on a three-arm maze and also reduced ACh release in the hippocampus (Ragozzino & Gold, 1995).

Similarly, glucose, injected systemically at a dose that enhances performance on a similar (four-arm) maze, augmented the increase in ACh release in the hippocampus seen during behavioral testing without drug treatment (Ragozzino, Unick, & Gold, 1996; Figure 35.1). Note (left panel) that systemic injections of glucose enhanced alternation performance in a typical inverted-U manner. Measures of ACh release obtained in microdialysis samples from the same animals during behavioral testing revealed, first, that behavioral testing resulted in a substantial increase in ACh release in the hippocampus; and, second, that the increase was potentiated in a similar inverted-U dose–response curve by glucose injections. These findings are consistent with the view that activation of hippocampal processing, marked here by an increase in the release of ACh, is important for this hippocampus-dependent task.

More recently, we have measured ACh release to mark the level of activation of several memory systems during learning. One experiment was based on the finding that damage to the hippocampus can enhance the learning of an amygdala-dependent conditioned cue preference task. In this case, ACh release in the hippocampus was *negatively* correlated with acquisition (McIntyre, Pal, Marriott, & Gold, in press)—a finding consistent with evidence (McDonald & White, 1995; White & McDonald, 1993) that fornix lesions enhance performance on this task (Figure 35.2). These findings suggest that the extent of hippocampal activation, using ACh release as a marker, predicts the extent to which acquisition of an amygdala-dependent task will be impaired.

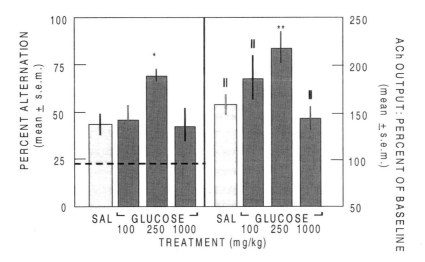

FIGURE 35.1. *Left panel:* Effects of systemic injections of glucose on spontaneous alternation performance (four-arm maze). *Right panel:* Effects of behavioral testing and of glucose injections on release of ACh in the hippocampus. Note that glucose had similar inverted-U dose–response curves for effects on alternation scores and on ACh release. From Ragozzino, Unick, and Gold (1996). Copyright 1996 by the National Academy of Sciences, USA. Reprinted by permission.

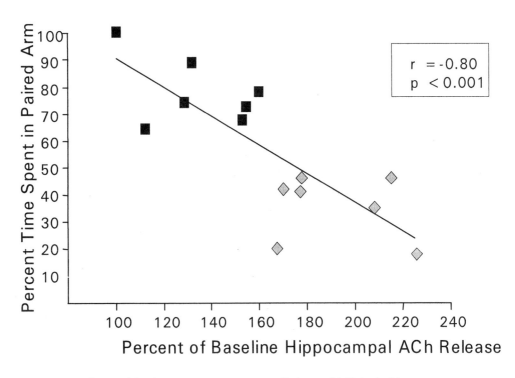

FIGURE 35.2. Competition between memory systems. Release of ACh in the hippocampus was negatively correlated with learning in an amygdala-dependent conditioned place preference task ($r = -.80$, $p = .0007$). From McIntyre, Pal, Marriott, and Gold (in press). Copyright 2001 by the Society for Neuroscience. Reprinted by permission.

In another experiment (McIntyre, Marriott, & Gold, 2001a), we examined ACh release in the amygdala during testing on a hippocampus-dependent spontaneous alternation task. In this case, the correlation between amygdala ACh release and performance of the hippocampus-dependent task did not reveal competition, but instead showed cooperation between the systems. As shown in Figure 35.3, there was a positive correlation between ACh release in the amygdala and scores on the hippocampus-dependent spontaneous alternation task.

Thus, when ACh release is interpreted as a marker of activation of neural systems, there appears to be asymmetry in the way different neural systems coordinate their processing of new information. The findings of the studies of ACh release suggest that hippocampal activation interferes with learning of information that is dependent on the amygdala (or striatum), whereas amygdala activation promotes learning of information that is dependent on the hippocampus. Thus, although the findings that lesions of the amygdala can interfere with acquisition of specific tasks supports a contribution of the amygdala to learning (cf. Davis, 1997; Fanselow & LeDoux. 1999), our findings support the view that the contribution of the amygdala is to modulate memory processing in other brain areas, including the hippocampus (e.g., Cahill, Weinberger, Roozendaal, & McGaugh, 1999; Ferry, Roozendaal, & McGaugh, 1999; Gold, Rose, & Hankins, 1978; Packard, Cahill, & McGaugh, 1994; Vazdarjanova & McGaugh, 1999).

Although tasks can be designed to be largely dependent on one or another memory system, most tasks are dependent on more than one neural system to process learning and memory. When one is examining one memory system at a time, it is relatively easy to imagine modulating the contribution of each system to its own class of learning. However, when two or more memory systems are important to learning a task, the issue becomes more complex. The possibility arises that by regulating the relative contributions of multiple systems to memory, modulators will bias cognitive processing toward or away from one learning

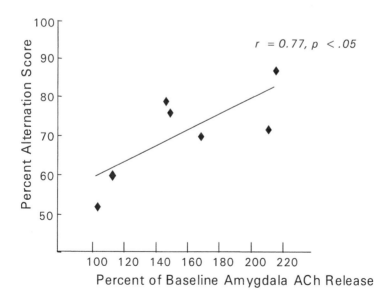

FIGURE 35.3. Cooperation between memory systems. Release of ACh in the amygdala was positively correlated with hippocampus-dependent alternation performance. From McIntyre, Marriott, and Gold (2001a).

strategy as opposed to another. Regulation of multiple memory systems in this way may modulate not only the strength of what is learned, but also the quality of what is learned.

We have begun to examine interactions between memory systems by examining ACh release while rats were trained on a task we term the "ambiguous T-maze." This task has a long history and a recent resurgence of interest (Barnes, 1988; Barnes, Nadel, & Honig, 1980; Packard, 1999; Packard & McGaugh, 1996; Restle, 1957; Tolman, Ritchie, & Kalish, 1947). In the T-maze, a rat is trained to approach a single goal arm. This response can be learned using either response (turn right, egocentric) strategies or place (go to the arm on a particular side of the room, allocentric) strategies. Which strategy a rat has used for learning can be assessed on probe trials after training. On probe trials, a rat is tested on the T-maze with the start arm rotated 180 degrees. The rat then displays what it learned by returning either to the arm reached by making the same turn in the maze or to the arm located in the same place in the room. The response versus place strategies are likely to be caudate- versus hippocampus-dependent (Cook & Kesner, 1988; Kesner et al., 1993; Mitchell & Hall, 1988; Packard, 1999; Packard & McGaugh, 1996). Acquisition of this task is also sensitive to hormonal influences: Female rats show a preference for place learning at proestrus (high estrogen) and a preference for response learning at estrus (low estrogen) (Korol, Couper, McIntyre, & Gold, 1996)—findings consistent with learning rates on mazes that can be learned best using either place or response strategies, but not both (Korol & Kolo, in press).

Using this task, we have examined in some detail training-related changes in ACh release in samples collected simultaneously from the hippocampus and striatum. In our experiments, male rats were divided about evenly in terms of showing response or place choices on the probe trials. Using *in vivo* microdialysis, we collected samples simultaneously from the hippocampus and from the striatum in individual rats before, during, and after training on the maze (McIntyre, Marriott, & Gold, 2001b). During training, ACh release increased in both the hippocampus and striatum, regardless of the strategy each rat used. However, the profiles of the increases in ACh release in the hippocampus and striatum were different, depending on what each rat learned (i.e., predicting the strategy revealed on the probe trial). When measured during training, those rats that were later found to be accomplishing place learning had significantly greater increases in ACh release in the hippocampus than did the rats that were later found to be accomplishing response learning. Those rats that showed response learning had greater increases in the striatum than did the rats that showed place learning, though this difference was not statistically significant (Figure 35.4).

However, when the ratios of changes in ACh release in the hippocampus and striatum were compared, there was a clear pattern distinguishing rats that learned via place strategies from those that learned via response strategies. An unexpected finding was obtained when ACh release was measured at baseline (i.e., *before* learning). In baseline samples collected during the hour prior to training, those rats that would later adopt a place strategy for learning had higher ratios of hippocampus–striatum ACh release than did the rats that would later use a response strategy (Figure 35.5). These results suggest that extracellular ACh levels in the hippocampus and striatum of naive rats reveal individual differences in the function of memory systems, and that these differences predict what will be learned by different animals trained on the same task.

These findings fit well with the extensive literature demonstrating involvement of cholinergic systems, particularly the septohippocampal cholinergic system, to learning and memory (e.g., Brioni, Decker, Gamboa, Izquierdo, & McGaugh, 1990; Chrobak, Stackman, & Walsh, 1989; Dougherty, Turchin, & Walsh, 1998; Givens & Olton, 1995; Markowska,

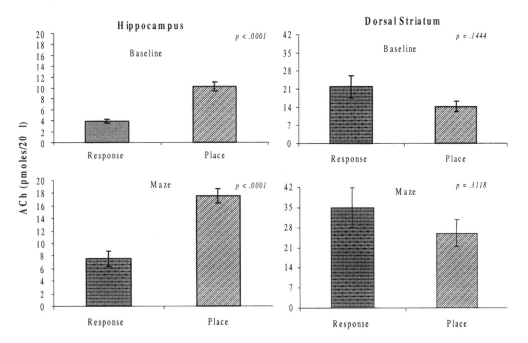

FIGURE 35.4. ACh levels in the hippocampus and dorsal striatum at baseline and during training on the ambiguous T-maze. Rats were separated into those that showed, on probe trials conducted after training to criterion, place or response strategies. In both brain areas and for all rats regardless of strategy used, ACh release increased above baseline when rats were trained on the maze. Both before and during training, those rats that used place strategies at the time of criterion performance had levels of ACh release in hippocampus higher than those of rats that used response strategies. The opposite relationship was seen in the striatum, though this was not statistically significant. From McIntyre, Marriott, and Gold (2001b).

Olton, & Givens, 1995; Mizumori, Perez, Alvarado, Barnes, & McNaughton, 1990; Olton, Wenk, & Markowska, 1991). Systemic and direct brain injections of cholinergic receptor agonists or antagonists reliably enhance or impair learning and memory, respectively (cf. Everitt & Robbins, 1997; Gold, 1995a, 1995b; Olton et al., 1991; Olton & Markowska, 1992). Such findings have provided the bases for several models of learning and memory relating cholinergic functions to learning and memory (e.g., Hasselmo & Bower, 1993; Myers et al., 1996).

CONCLUSIONS

Collecting microdialysis samples online for measurement of ACh release during training makes it possible to observe the relative activation of different neural systems during learning. Moreover, assessing ACh release in different neural systems prior to training makes it possible to identify biases within and across neural systems that influence what information is most readily learned. For example, baseline ACh release reveals the preferred learning strategy that will be selected at the time of training. Although there has been substantial attention to the study of individual differences in learning ability, these recent results suggest that one can also study the biological underpinnings of individual differences in what is learned.

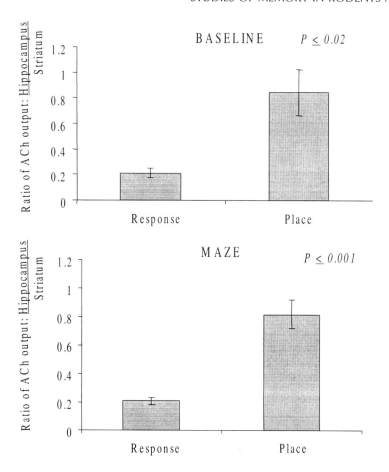

FIGURE 35.5. Ratios of ACh release in the hippocampus and striatum at baseline and during maze training. Note that those rats that showed response strategies at the time they reached criterion performance (9/10 correct) on the T-maze had ratios significantly lower, both at baseline and during training, than did rats that showed place strategies. From McIntyre, Marriott, and Gold (2001b).

The findings lead naturally to a more fundamental question: What establishes the biasing of the memory systems that will preferentially be tapped when a new experience is encountered? Although genetic influences may be important, another possibility is that individual differences in ACh release in different neural systems may reflect prior experience. In our experiments, the prior history of each rat is not controlled. Is it possible that past success at solving tasks with a particular strategy leads to a brain that is biased toward use of that same strategy? According to this view, neuromodulatory influences may themselves be plastic (metamodulation?; Katz & Edwards, 1999)—able to be modified by prior experience, and thereby changing the bias between neural systems involved in learning and memory. Such changes in the balance between memory systems might produce a condition in which acquisition of a skill based on one memory system would lead to preferential selection of that previously successful memory system when faced later with a new cognitive challenge. To the extent that successes follow successes, the end product is that the modulators of memory acting to bias cognitive processing at a systems level will steer the individual toward some strategies and away from others, producing individual differences in memory strategies and hence in abilities.

The ability to measure release of neurotransmitters at once in different memory systems of behaving rats opens new directions for studies of modulation of learning and memory. When such studies are combined with direct pharmacological manipulations of different memory systems, it is now possible to create profiles, akin to functional imaging, of the interactive participation of multiple neural systems in creating new memories.

ACKNOWLEDGMENTS

Preparation of this chapter and of much of the research from my laboratory described here was supported by grants from the National Institute on Aging (No. AG 07648), the National Institute of Neurological Disorders and Stroke (No. NS 32914), the U.S. Department of Agriculture (No. 00-35200-9839), and the Alzheimer's Disease and Related Disorders Association.

REFERENCES

Axelrod, J., Weil-Malherbe, H., & Tomchick, R. (1959). The physiological disposition of ^{3}H-epinephrine and its metabolite metanephrine. *Journal of Pharmacology and Experimental Therapeutics, 127,* 251–256.

Barnes, C. A. (1988). Aging and the physiology of spatial memory. *Neurobiology of Aging, 9,* 563–568.

Barnes, C. A., Nadel, L., & Honig, W. K. (1980). Spatial memory deficit in senescent rats. *Canadian Journal of Psychology, 34,* 29–39.

Brioni, J. D., Decker, M. W., Gamboa, L. P., Izquierdo, I., & McGaugh, J. L. (1990). Muscimol injections in the medial septum impair spatial learning. *Brain Research, 522,* 227–234.

Cahill, L., Prins, B., Weber, M., & McGaugh, J. L. (1994). Beta-adrenergic activation and memory for emotional events. *Nature, 371,* 702–704.

Cahill, L., Weinberger, N. M., Roozendaal, B., & McGaugh, J. L. (1999). Is the amygdala a locus of "conditioned fear"? Some questions and caveats. *Neuron, 23,* 227–228.

Chang, Q., & Gold, P. E. (2001). *Intra-hippocampal lidocaine injections impair acquisition of a place task but facilitate acquisition of a response task in rats.* Manuscript in preparation.

Chrobak, J. J., Stackman, R. W., & Walsh, T. J. (1989). Intraseptal administration of muscimol produces dose-dependent memory impairments in the rat. *Behavioral and Neural Biology, 52,* 357–369.

Clark, K. B., Naritoku, D. K., Smith, D. C., Browning, R. A., & Jensen, R. A. (1999). Enhanced recognition memory following vagus nerve stimulation in human subjects. *Nature Neuroscience, 2,* 94–98.

Clark, K. B., Smith, D. C., Hassert, D. L., Browning, R. A., Naritoku, D. K., & Jensen, R. A. (1998). Post-training electrical stimulation of vagal afferents with concomitant vagal efferent inactivation enhances memory storage processes in the rat. *Neurobiology of Learning and Memory, 70,* 364–373.

Cook, D., & Kesner, R. P. (1988). Caudate nucleus and memory for egocentric localization. *Behavioral and Neural Biology, 49,* 332–343.

Davis, M. (1997). Neurobiology of fear responses: The role of the amygdala. *Journal of Neuropsychiatry and Clinical Neuroscience, 9,* 382–402.

Dougherty, K. D., Turchin, P. I., & Walsh, T. J. (1998). Septocingulate and septohippocampal cholinergic pathways: Involvement in working/episodic memory. *Brain Research, 810,* 59–71.

Everitt, B. J., & Robbins, T. W. (1997). Central cholinergic system and cognition. *Annual Review of Psychology, 48,* 649–684.

Fanselow, M. S., & LeDoux, J. E. (1999). Why we think plasticity underlying Pavlovian fear conditioning occurs in the basolateral amygdala. *Neuron, 23,* 229–232.

Ferry, B., Roozendaal, B., & McGaugh, J. L. (1999). Role of norepinephrine in mediating stress hormone regulation of long-term memory storage: A critical involvement of the amygdala. *Biological Psychiatry, 46,* 1140–1152.

Gabrieli, J. D. E. (1996). Memory systems analyses of mnemonic disorders in aging and age-related disorders. *Proceedings of the National Academy of Sciences USA, 93,* 13534–13540.

Givens, B., & Olton, D. S. (1995). Bidirectional modulation of scopolamine induced working memory impairments by muscarinic activation of the medial septal area. *Neurobiology of Learning and Memory, 63,* 269–276.

Gold, P. E. (1995a). The role of glucose in regulating brain and cognition. *American Journal of Clinical Nutrition, 61,* S987–S995.

Gold, P. E. (1995b). Modulation of emotional and non-emotional memories: Same pharmacological systems, different neuroanatomical systems. In J. L. McGaugh, N. M. Weinberger, & G. S. Lynch (Eds.), *Brain and memory: Modulation and mediation of neural plasticity* (pp. 41–74). New York: Oxford University Press.

Gold, P. E. (2001). Drug enhancement of memory in aged rodents and humans. In M. E. Carroll & J. B. Overmier (Eds.), *Animal research and human health: Advancing human welfare through behavioral science* (pp. 293–304). Washington, DC: American Psychological Association.

Gold, P. E., McIntyre, C., McNay, E., Stefani, M. R., & Korol, D. L. (2001b). Neurochemical referees of dueling memory systems. In P. E. Gold & W. T. Greenough (Eds.), *Memory consolidation: Essays in honor of James L. McGaugh—A time to remember* (pp. 219–248). Washington, DC: American Psychological Association.

Gold, P. E., Rose, R. P., & Hankins, L. L. (1978). Retention impairment produced by unilateral amygdala stimulation: Reduction by posttrial amygdala stimulation. *Behavioral Biology, 22,* 515–523.

Gold, P. E., & van Buskirk, R. B. (1978). Effects of α- and β-adrenergic receptor antagonists on post-trial epinephrine modulation of memory: Relationship to post-training brain norepinephrine concentrations. *Behavioral Biology, 24,* 168–184.

Hasselmo, M. E., & Bower, J. M. (1993). Acetylcholine and memory. *Trends in Neurosciences, 16,* 218–222.

Jensen, R. (2001). Neural pathways mediating the modulation of learning and memory by arousal. In P. E. Gold & W. T. Greenough (Eds.), *Memory consolidation: Essays in honor of James L. McGaugh—A time to remember* (pp 129–140). Washington, DC: American Psychological Association.

Katz, P. S., & Edwards, D. H. (1999). Metamodulation: the control and modulation of neuromodulation. In P. S. Katz (Ed.), *Beyond neurotransmission: Neuromodulation and its importance for information processing* (pp. 349–381). New York: Oxford University Press.

Kesner, R. P., Bolland, B. L., & Dakis, M. (1993). Memory for spatial locations, motor responses, and objects: Triple dissociation among the hippocampus, caudate nucleus, and extrastriate visual cortex. *Experimental Brain Research, 93,* 462–470.

Korol, D. L., Couper, J. M., McIntyre, C. K., & Gold, P. E. (1996). Learning strategies across the estrous cycle in female rats. *Society for Neuroscience Abstracts, 22,* 1386.

Korol, D. L., & Gold, P. E. (1998). Glucose, memory and aging. *American Journal of Clinical Nutrition, 67,* 764S–771S.

Korol, D. L., & Kolo, L. L. (in press). Estrogen-induced changes in place and response learning in young adult female rats. *Behavioral Neuroscience.*

Markowska, A. L., Olton, D. S., & Givens, B. (1995). Cholinergic manipulations in the medial septal area: Age-related effects on working memory and hippocampal electrophysiology. *Journal of Neuroscience, 15,* 2063–2073.

Matthews, D. B., & Best, P. J. (1995). Fimbria/fornix lesions facilitate the learning of a nonspatial response task. *Psychonomic Bulletin and Review, 2,* 113–116.

Matthews, D. B., Ilgen, M., White, A. M., & Best, P. J. (1999). Acute ethanol administration impairs spatial performance while facilitating nonspatial performance in rats. *Neurobiology of Learning and Memory, 72,* 167–179.

McDonald, R. J., & White, N. M. (1993). A triple dissociation of memory systems: Hippocampus, amygdala and dorsal striatum. *Behavioral Neuroscience, 107,* 3–22.

McDonald, R. J., & White, N. M. (1995). Information acquired by the hippocampus interferes with acquisition of the amygdala-based conditioned-cue preference in the rat. *Hippocampus, 5,* 189–197.

McIntyre, C. K., Marriott, L. K., & Gold, P. E. (2001a). *Cooperation between memory systems: Acetylcholine release in the amygdala correlates positively with good performance on a hippocampus-dependent task.* Manuscript in preparation.

McIntyre, C. K., Marriott, L. K., & Gold, P. E. (2001b). *Individual differences in learning strategy predicted by brain acetylcholine release in rats.* Manuscript submitted for publication.

McIntyre, C. K., Pal, S. N., Marriott, L. K., & Gold, P. E. (in press). Competition between memory systems: Acetylcholine release in the hippocampus correlates negatively with good performance on an amygdala-dependent task. *Journal of Neuroscience.*

McNay, E. C., Fries, T. M., & Gold, P. E. (2000). Decreases in rat extracellular hippocampal glucose concentration associated with cognitive demand during a spatial task. *Proceedings of the National Academy of Sciences USA, 97,* 2881–2885.

McNay, E. C., & Gold, P. E. (1999). Extracellular glucose concentrations in the brain. *Journal of Neurochemistry, 73,* 2222–2223.

McNay, E. C., & Gold, P. E. (2001). Age-related differences in hippocampal extracellular fluid glucose concentration during behavioral testing and following systemic glucose administration. *Journal of Gerontology: Biological Sciences, 56A,* B66–B71.

McNay, E. C., McCarty, R. M., & Gold, P. E. (2001). Fluctuations in glucose concentration during behavioral testing: Dissociations both between brain areas and between brain and blood. *Neurobiology of Learning and Memory, 75,* 325–337.

Mitchell, J. A., & Hall, G. (1988). Learning in rats with caudate–putamen lesions: Unimpaired classical conditioning and beneficial effects of redundant stimulus cues on instrumental and spatial learning deficits. *Behavioral Neuroscience, 102,* 504–514.

Mizumori, S. J. Y., Perez, G. M., Alvarado, M. C., Barnes, C. A., & McNaughton, B. L. (1990). Reversible inactivation of the medial septum differentially affects two forms of learning in rats. *Brain Research, 528,* 12–20.

Myers, C. E., Ermita, B. R., Harris, K., Hasselmo, M., Solomon, P., & Gluck, M. A. (1996). A computational model of cholinergic disruption of septohippocampal activity in classical eyeblink conditioning. *Neurobiology of Learning and Memory, 66,* 51–66.

Nyberg, L., & Tulving, E. (1996). Classifying human long-term memory: Evidence from converging dissociations. *European Journal of Cognitive Psychology, 8,* 163–183.

Olton, D. S., & Markowska, A. L. (1992). The aging septo-hippocampal system: Its role in age-related memory impairments. In L. R. Squire & N. Butters (Eds.), *Neuropsychology of memory* (2nd ed., pp. 378–385). New York: Guilford Press.

Olton, D. S., Wenk, G. L., & Markowska, A. M. (1991). Basal forebrain, memory and attention. In R. T. Richardson (Ed.), *Activation to acquisition: Functional aspects of the basal forebrain cholinergic system* (pp. 247–262). Boston: Birkhaüser.

Packard, M. G. (1999). Glutamate infused posttraining into the hippocampus or caudate–putamen differentially strengthens place and response learning. *Proceedings of the National Academy of Sciences USA, 96,* 12881–12886.

Packard, M. G., Cahill, L., & McGaugh, J. L. (1994). Amygdala modulation of hippocampal-dependent and caudate nucleus-dependent memory processes. *Proceedings of the National Academy of Science USA, 91,* 8477–8481.

Packard, M. G., & McGaugh, J. L. (1996). Inactivation of hippocampus or caudate nucleus with lidocaine differentially affects expression of place and response learning. *Neurobiology of Learning and Memory, 65,* 65–72.

Packard, M. G., & Teather, L. A. (1999). Dissociation of multiple memory systems by posttraining intracerebral injections of glutamate. *Psychobiology, 27,* 40–50.

Posner, M. I., Petersen, S. E., Fox, P. T., & Raichle, M. E. (1988). Localization of cognitive operations in the human brain. *Science, 240,* 1627–1631.

Ragozzino, M. E., & Gold, P. E. (1995). Glucose injections into the medial septum reverse the effects of intraseptal morphine infusions on hippocampal acetylcholine output and memory. *Neuroscience, 68,* 981–988.

Ragozzino, M. E., Unick, K. E., & Gold, P. E. (1996). Hippocampal acetylcholine release during memory testing in rats: Augmentation by glucose. *Proceedings of the National Academy of Sciences, 93,* 4693–4698.

Restle, F. (1957). Discrimination of cues in mazes: A resolution of the "place-vs.-response" question. *Psychological Review, 64,* 217–228.

Squire, L. R. (1992). Memory and the hippocampus: A synthesis from findings with rats, monkeys, and humans. *Psychological Review, 99,* 195–231.

Stefani, M. R., & Gold, P. E. (1998). Intra-septal injections of glucose and glibenclamide attenuate galanin-induced spontaneous alternation performance deficits in the rat. *Brain Research, 813,* 50–56.

Stefani, M. R., & Gold, P. E. (2001). Intra-hippocampal infusions of K-ATP channel modulators influence spontaneous alternation performance: Relationships to acetylcholine release in the hippocampus. *Journal of Neuroscience, 21,* 609–614.

Stefani, M. R., Nicholson, G. M., & Gold, P. E. (1999). ATP-sensitive potassium channel blockade enhances spontaneous alternation performance in the rat: A potential mechanism for glucose-mediated memory enhancement. *Neuroscience, 93,* 557–563.

Tolman, E. C., Ritchie, B. F., & Kalish, D. (1947). Studies in spatial learning: V. Response learning vs. place learning by the non-correction method. *Journal of Experimental Psychology, 37,* 285–292.

Vazdarjanova, A., & McGaugh, J. L. (1999). Basolateral amygdala is involved in modulating consolidation of memory for classical fear conditioning. *Journal of Neuroscience, 19,* 6615–6622.

White, N. M., & McDonald, R. J. (1993). Acquisition of a spatial conditioned place preference is impaired by amygdala lesions and improved by fornix lesions. *Behavioural Brain Research, 55,* 269–281.

Williams, C. L., & Clayton, E. C. (2001). Contribution of brainstem structures in modulating memory storage processing. In P. E. Gold and W. T. Greenough (Eds.), *Memory consolidation: Essays in honor of James L. McGaugh—A time to remember* (pp. 141–164). Washington, DC: American Psychological Association.

Willingham, D. B. (1999). The neural basis of motor-skill learning. *Current Directions in Psychological Science, 8,* 178–182.

36

The Orbitofrontal Cortex

Modeling Prefrontal Function in Rats

GEOFFREY SCHOENBAUM, BARRY SETLOW, and MICHELA GALLAGHER

A common functional identity is determined by the same type of structure and connections, whatever the mammal examined. . . . Stratigraphic analogy, grossly appreciated in Nissl or Weigert preparations, constitutes a valuable data point, but it is not completely decisive or infallible.
—RAMÓN Y CAJAL (1922/1988, p. 524)

In histological preparations, a signature granular cell layer distinguishes a broad expanse of the prefrontal cortex positioned rostral to the motor cortex in both human and nonhuman primate brains. Although cytoarchitectonic criteria originally provided a basis for defining cortical areas (Brodmann, 1909), it was recognized in early writings that "functional identity" of structures between different species would ultimately depend on data (then largely unavailable) regarding specific anatomical connections and physiology rather than "stratigraphic analogy" (Ramón y Cajal, 1922/1988). Since the middle of the last century, the definition of the prefrontal cortex has been influenced by a wealth of new information on neuroanatomical connections gained from tract-tracing studies (see Preuss, 1995, for a review). As Ramón y Cajal envisioned, these new data indicate that prefrontal areas share functions in different species, even in the absence of a granular cell layer.

Early on, Rose and Woolsey (1949) proposed that projections from the mediodorsal thalamus (MD) defined the prefrontal cortex. Indeed, the cytoarchitectonic definition of the prefrontal cortex in the nonhuman primate corresponded well with the topography of innervation from the MD. Since then, it has become clear that an additional defining feature of the prefrontal cortex is its rich interconnections with other brain systems, including other "association" areas of the posterior and temporal neocortex, limbic structures such as the hippocampus and amygdala, and major efferent projections to the striatum (Ongur & Price, 2000; Preuss, 1995). This connectional anatomy has provided an important basis for further subdividing regions of the prefrontal cortex and guiding functional analysis of prefrontal systems. The prefrontal cortex in the primate, which constitutes nearly a third of the neocortex, is now widely recognized to comprise three main subdivisions: a dorsolateral region (Brodmann's cytocarchitectonic area 46 and lateral parts of areas 8, 9, 10, and 11), a medial region (areas 12, 24, and 32), and finally an orbitofrontal region (areas 13, 47, and inferior aspects of areas 10, 11, and 13) (Fuster, 2000). This chapter focuses on the orbitofrontal division of the prefrontal cortex, providing an overview of recent research that suggests strong functional homologies between the orbitofrontal cortex in the primate brain and a region in the rat brain that shares similar anatomical connectivity.

In the rat, the MD can be divided into three segments (Groenewegen, 1988; Krettek & Price, 1977a). Projections from the medial and central segments of the MD define a region that includes orbital areas and the ventral and dorsal agranular insular cortices (Groenewegen, 1988; Kolb, 1984; Krettek & Price, 1977a; Leonard, 1969). These MD regions in the rat receive direct afferents from the amygdala, the medial temporal lobe, and the ventral pallidum/ ventral tegmental area; olfactory input from the piriform cortex additionally innervates the central MD segment (Groenewegen, 1988; Krettek & Price, 1977a; Ray & Price, 1992). The primate orbitofrontal region is defined by the projections of the medially located, magno-cellular MD division (Goldman-Rakic & Porrino, 1985; Kievit & Kuypers, 1977; Russchen, Amaral, & Price, 1987). Like the medial and central segments of the rat MD, this region of the primate MD also receives afferents from limbic structures such as the amygdala and regions in the medial temporal lobe, olfactory structures such as the piriform cortex, and the ventral pallidum (Russchen et al., 1987). These data indicate that a defined region in the rat cortex is likely to receive input from the thalamus very similar to that reaching the primate orbitofrontal cortex. Based in part on this pattern of input, the projection fields of the medial and central MD in the orbital and agranular insular areas of the rat prefrontal cortex have been proposed as homologous to the primate orbitofrontal region (Groenewegen, 1988; Leonard, 1969; Ongur & Price, 2000; Preuss, 1995).

Other neuroanatomical studies in the past two decades have confirmed that in addition to receiving projections from MD regions, the orbitofrontal cortex in the rat has direct connections with a number of other structures resembling those found in the primate brain. Perhaps most notable are reciprocal connections with the basolateral complex of the amygdala, a region thought to be involved preferentially in affective or motivational aspects of learning (Davis, 2000; Everitt & Robbins, 1992; Gallagher & Holland, 1999; LeDoux, 1995; see also McGaugh, Chapter 33, this volume). In primates, these connections (Price, Russchen, & Amaral, 1987) have been invoked to explain certain similarities in behavioral abnormalities resulting from damage to either the orbitofrontal cortex or the amygdala (see, e.g., Damasio, 1994; Fuster, 1997; Gaffan & Murray, 1990; Jones & Mishkin, 1972). Reciprocal connections between the basolateral amygdala and areas within the rat orbitofrontal cortex (Kita & Kitai, 1990; Kolb, 1984; Krettek & Price, 1977b; Shi & Cassell, 1998) suggest that interactions between these structures may have a similar importance for regulation of behavioral functions in rats as well.

Additional similarities between rat and primate connectional anatomy provide another basis for functional parallels involving the orbitofrontal cortex. For example, in both species the orbitofrontal cortex provides a strong efferent projection to the ventral striatum, overlapping with innervation from limbic structures such as the amygdala and subiculum (Groenewegen, Berendse, Wolters, & Lohman, 1990; Groenewegen, Vermeulen-Van der Zee, te Kortschot, & Witter, 1987; Haber, Kunishio, Mizobuchi, & Lynd-Balta, 1995; McDonald, 1991). In fact, the specific circuitry connecting the orbitofrontal region, limbic structures, and ventral striatum represents a striking parallel across species that suggests possible similarities in functional interaction among these major components of the forebrain (Groenewegen et al., 1990; McDonald, 1991; O'Donnell, 1999).

Of course, obvious differences in corticocortical connections of the orbitofrontal region are evident in comparisons of primates and rats, in line with the expansion of cortical processing systems in the primate brain. The rat orbitofrontal cortex is nonetheless multimodal with respect to input from cortical sensory processing streams (Kolb, 1990; Ongur & Price, 2000; Reep, Corwin, & King, 1996). In addition, the orbitofrontal cortex receives direct projections from the piriform cortex as well as from olfactory-related MD regions in both species (Barbas, 1993; Carmichael, Clugnet, & Price, 1994; Cinelli, Moyano-Ferreyra, & Barragan, 1985; Price et al., 1991; Takagi, 1986; Yarita, Iino, Tanabe, Kogure, & Takagi, 1980).

The conservation of many features of anatomical connectivity across species provides a strong foundation for studies of functional similarities. Such an approach has already revealed that homologies in connectional circuits between the primate and rat orbitofrontal regions are accompanied by homologies in function and in information processing. From these data, it appears that in both rats and primates, the orbitofrontal cortex serves a role in the strategic use of motivational information that is encoded with reference to prior experience, current context, and expectations regarding predicted events. This functional description of the orbitofrontal cortex provides a basis for its central role in guiding goal-directed behavior and may be tied to broader conceptualizations of the role of the prefrontal cortex in executive function—a topic we return to at the end of this chapter.

FROM CLINICAL DESCRIPTIONS TO EXPERIMENTAL PARADIGMS FOR ORBITOFRONTAL FUNCTION

The most famous clinical case, which set the stage for much subsequent investigation, was that of Phineas Gage, a railroad foreman in the 1800s who suffered a traumatic injury thought to involve the orbitofrontal region (Damasio, 1994; Harlow, 1868). Following his injury, Gage became unable to continue productive work and exhibited a remarkable change in personality, characterized by socially impulsive behavior. Descriptions of patients with damage to the orbitofrontal cortex have continued to identify maladaptive actions as a hallmark of the clinical syndrome. In nonhuman primates and rats, damage to the orbitofrontal cortex likewise produces behavioral abnormalities in a social context. A seemingly invariable consequence of such lesions in monkeys is a loss of social rank (Butter, Mishkin, & Mirsky, 1968; Butter & Snyder, 1972). It has also been noted that rats display abnormalities in social behavior and changes in aggressiveness after orbitofrontal damage (Kolb, 1984; Kolb & Nonneman, 1974).

Socially inappropriate and impulsive behaviors after orbitofrontal damage were initially studied as instances of a more general manifestation of "disinhibition." Indeed, early experimental studies focused on deficits in response inhibition as the hallmark of damage to orbitofrontal cortex (Mishkin, 1964). For example, primates with orbitofrontal lesions are impaired in acquisition or reversal of discriminations in which cues are paired with reinforcement, and where different responses must be executed to receive rewards (Butter, 1969; Diaz, Robbins, & Roberts, 1996; Gaffan & Murray, 1990; Jones & Mishkin, 1972; Tanabe, Yarita, Iino, Ooshima, & Takagi, 1975). Typically the behavioral deficit is manifested as an inability to withhold inappropriate responses, and impairment is particularly apparent on tasks or in situations that require a modification of the normal response set or tendency (Mishkin, 1964). The important distinction made in these studies was that impairment was in the persistence of an old (or prepotent) pattern of responding, rather than in an inability to learn new patterns (Jones & Mishkin, 1972).

Deficits in discrimination performance are also observed in rats after damage to the orbitofrontal cortex. For example, rats with orbitofrontal lesions are impaired at discriminations involving olfactory cues (Eichenbaum, Clegg, & Feeley, 1983; Whishaw, Tomie, & Kolb, 1992). Impaired performance on discriminations is observed despite normal odor detection, and, like primates with orbital lesions, rats exhibit perseverative responding (Eichenbaum et al., 1983). Rats are also impaired at using odor cues to guide performance in a delayed-nonmatching task (Otto & Eichenbaum, 1992) and in object discrimination performance (DeCoteau, Kesner, & Williams, 1997). The olfactory modality used in this research with rats exploits the heavy involvement of the rat orbitofrontal cortex in olfactory processing. Encoding of olfactory information is also well documented by single-cell recording in the monkey orbitofrontal cortex (Rolls, Critchley, Mason, & Wakeman, 1996; Tanabe, Iino, & Takagi, 1975; Thorpe, Rolls, & Maddison, 1983).

Although response inhibition was an important theme early on, more recent research, noting the connections of the orbitofrontal cortex with the amygdala, has focused on alterations in motivational and affective processes as a key component of the behavioral deficits associated with orbitofrontal damage. In support of this general perspective, a syndrome similar to that seen after orbital damage, in which monkeys lose social rank, has also been observed after damage to the amygdala (Rosvold, Mirsky, & Pribram, 1954; but see Emery et al., 2001). Further support for this perspective has come from a series of recent laboratory investigations with patients and from experimental studies using monkeys and rats.

In work with patients, Bechara, Damasio, Tranel, and Damasio (1997) devised a gambling task in which observations of behavioral performance were made along with measures of autonomic arousal. In this experimental setting, as in their lives, patients with orbitofrontal damage were prone to making disadvantageous decisions. Notably, they also failed to display measures of increased autonomic arousal that were routinely observed in control subjects prior to choices that were likely to be costly, in comparison with choices that led to more reliable gains. Although these deficits appear to be specific to damage in the orbitofrontal region within the prefrontal cortex (Bechara, Damasio, Tranel, & Andersen, 1998), they are also observed in patients with amygdala damage (Bechara, Damasio, Damasio, & Lee, 1999). These findings are consistent with the idea that the orbitofrontal cortex plays a critical role in processing motivational information that is based on prior experience and that processing in this region provides a strategic guide for expectations about predicted events. Moreover, the evidence suggests that this function depends on orbitofrontal interconnections with the amygdala.

Alongside the intriguing findings from such research with patients, other recent studies have shown that interference with normal function of this circuitry in animals (monkeys and rats) can selectively impair goal-directed behavior, when such deficits are isolated from other performance- and learning-related factors. These studies have employed learning tasks that permit associations between cues to be assessed, along with the current incentive value of events or outcomes predicted by those cues. These associations between cues, responses, or contextual information and the incentive properties of outcomes provide an important basis for the expectancy that guides goal-directed behavior.

One such task (Figure 36.1) exploits the ability of rats to modify responses toward a goal based on information about the value of the predicted outcome. Initially, rats are trained to expect food delivery at a food cup following presentation of a 10-second light conditioned stimulus (CS). As a consequence of learning, rats approach the food cup in the presence of the light CS (Figure 36.1A). In a second phase of the protocol (Figure 36.1B), rats are given food, identical to that delivered in the learning task, in their home cage;

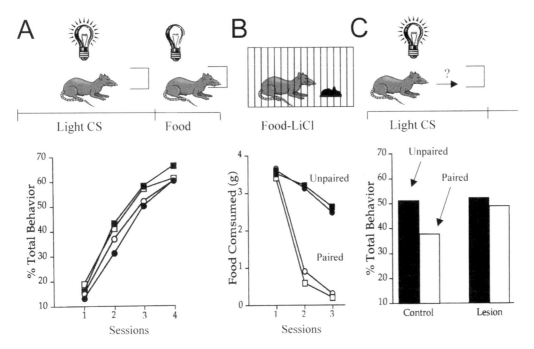

FIGURE 36.1. Effects of neurotoxic lesions of orbitofrontal cortex on performance in a devaluation task. As illustrated (A, upper panel), control rats and rats with bilateral neurotoxic lesions of orbitofrontal cortex were trained to associate a conditioned stimulus (light CS) with an unconditioned stimulus (food US). Over several sessions (1–4), both lesioned (circles) and control (squares) rats developed a conditioned response at the food cup to the light (A, lower panel). This food cup response is represented as the percentage of total behavior. There was no effect of the lesion on the development of the food cup response. The rats then received presentations of the food item in their home cages, followed by illness induced by lithium chloride (LiCl) injection (B, upper panel). Some rats in each group received paired presentations of food and illness (filled circles and squares), while others received unpaired presentations (open circles and squares). Rats that received paired presentations stopped consuming the food item (B, lower panel). Again, no effect of the lesions was observed. The following day the rats were returned to the training environment, and conditioned responses to the light cue were measured (C, upper panel). When exposed to the light CS (C, lower panel), control rats that had received paired presentations of food and illness reduced conditioned responses to the food cup relative to unpaired controls. Rats with orbitofrontal lesions did not show this decrease in conditioned responding as a result of reinforcer devaluation. From Gallagher et al. (1999). Copyright 1999 by the Society for Neuroscience. Adapted by permission.

consumption of this food is followed by induction of illness by injection of lithium chloride. Rats thus acquire a taste aversion and subsequently refrain from consumption of the food that led to illness. In the final phase of the experimental protocol, the effects of "devaluation" of the food are assessed on goal-directed behavior in the original training apparatus (Figure 36.1C). Control rats reduce their responding toward the food cup in the presence of the light CS in nonreinforced trials. In contrast, rats with orbitofrontal damage (Gallagher, McMahan, & Schoenbaum, 1999) fail to show this change in food cup responses after food devaluation (Figure 36.1C). This deficit is notable because lesioned rats, like normal rats, refrain from consuming the food that led to illness (Figure 36.1B). Thus rats with orbitofrontal damage can inhibit a prepotent response (i.e., food consumption), but they fail to use this information to guide behavior in response to cues that predict the devalued food. Like patients in the gambling task, rats with orbitofrontal damage continue to make responses that will lead to an undesirable outcome. It is also notable that in rats, as in human clinical cases, the behavioral deficit in modifying goal-directed responses after orbitofrontal damage is reproduced by damage to the amygdala (Hatfield, Han, Conley, Gallagher, & Holland, 1996). In the case of rats, this deficit is observed after highly selective neurotoxic lesions of the basolateral amygdala, the origin of direct projections to the orbitofrontal cortex.

Other research using devaluation protocols has demonstrated the involvement of amygdala–orbitofrontal circuitry in monkeys. In those studies, a change in incentive value was induced by selectively overfeeding a food item that was used as a reinforcer. After such satiation, normal monkeys were less likely to select a visually presented object that had been reinforced with the "devalued" food in earlier discrimination training. This change in responding, however, was absent in monkeys that had lesions of the amygdala (Malkova, Gaffan, & Murray, 1997) or lesions that disconnected the amygdala and orbitofrontal regions (Baxter, Parker, Lindner, Izquierdo, & Murray, 2000). As in rats, monkeys with damage to this circuitry appear to be unable to use the motivational guidance provided by an expected outcome to guide goal-directed behavior. In the next section, we consider studies of information encoding by orbitofrontal neurons, which may serve as a basis for the adaptive regulation of goal-directed behavior that appears to be organized by this region.

HOMOLOGIES IN INFORMATION PROCESSING BETWEEN THE RAT AND PRIMATE ORBITOFRONTAL CORTEX

A number of recording studies have been conducted in recent years examining the properties of orbitofrontal neurons in monkeys and rats while they perform relevant behavioral tasks. The results of these investigations suggest strong similarities in the properties of orbitofrontal neurons across species and in the features of information encoding that are likely to serve as a basis for the critical role of the orbitofrontal cortex in guiding goal-directed behavior.

Some of the earliest recording studies in the orbitofrontal cortex noted the importance of the biological significance of stimuli in determining the firing properties of neurons. For example, although neurons do respond to specific olfactory cues (Schoenbaum & Eichenbaum, 1995a; Tanabe, Iino, & Takagi, 1975; Yonemori et al., 2000), they appear to be most responsive to odors with some biological importance, such as odors of urine, feces, or other animals (Onoda, Imamura, Obota, & Iino, 1984). Food odors and visual features of food items also evoke activity in orbitofrontal neurons (Thorpe et al., 1983). Moreover, such responses are sensitive to motivational state. For example, satiation decreases the responsiveness of orbitofrontal neurons to food-related cues (Critchley & Rolls, 1996b).

In monkeys, neutral cues that signal rewarding or aversive contingencies also strongly activate orbitofrontal neurons (Critchley & Rolls, 1996a; Rosenkilde, Bauer, & Fuster, 1981; Thorpe et al., 1983; Tremblay & Schultz, 1999). Similarly, the orbitofrontal cortex in rats appears to encode the acquired significance of cues. For example, in rats trained to perform an eight-odor go/no-go discrimination task, many orbitofrontal neurons fired selectively during sampling of the odor cues (Figure 36.2). In this task, rats learned that four of the odors were reinforced (water was provided to thirsty rats), while the other four odors were not reinforced (Schoenbaum & Eichenbaum, 1995a, 1995b). As illustrated in Figure 36.2, odor-responsive activity recorded in well-trained rats typically discriminated among odor cues on the basis of their association with reinforcement rather than their sensory properties. Similar findings have been reported in primates trained to perform an

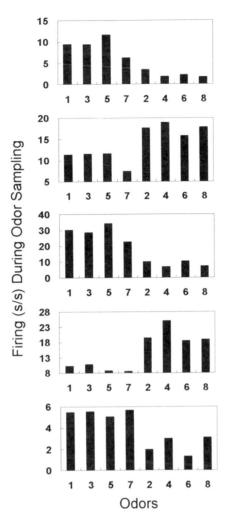

FIGURE 36.2. Encoding of associated outcome rather than sensory features of cues in the orbito-frontal cortex, revealed by neural activity during odor sampling. Neurons in the rat orbitofrontal cortex were recorded during performance of an eight-odor go/no-go odor discrimination task. On each trial, one odor was presented. After odor sampling, a response could be made at a nearby fluid well for a water reward. Four odors were positive, indicating that a response would be rewarded; four odors were negative, indicating that no reward would be given for responding. Rats were well trained on the discrimination prior to recording, responding to positive odors and rarely to negative odors. Activity in orbitofrontal cortex is shown in spikes/second during odor sampling for five different neurons. Each panel shows activity for a different neuron to each of the eight different odors presented in each session. Positive odors 1+, 3+, 5+, and 7+ are on the left of each panel, and negative odors 2-, 4-, 6-, and 8- are on the right of each panel. Note that the cells responded to all positive or all negative odors and did not distinguish between odors that were associated with the same outcome. From Schoenbaum and Eichenbaum (1995b). Copyright 1995 by the American Physiological Society. Adapted by permission.

odor discrimination task (Critchley & Rolls, 1996a). Orbitofrontal neurons also respond similarly to different complex visual cues (different pattern stimuli) that signal the same reward (Tremblay & Schultz, 1999). It is important to note that neurons in the orbitofrontal cortex are not solely attuned to the positive or rewarding significance of cues. For example, as shown in Figure 36.2, several neurons fire most strongly to odors associated with nonreinforcement; other studies (Critchley & Rolls, 1996a; Schoenbaum, Chiba, & Gallagher, 1999) have reported that orbitofrontal neurons are selectively active during sampling of cues associated with an aversive outcome (delivery of aversive saline in monkeys or quinine in rats).

The notion that neurons in the orbitofrontal cortex are specialized for encoding the motivational significance or value of the events associated with cues is consistent with evidence that the orbitofrontal cortex activity established in associative learning is dramatically affected when contingencies are modified. In an odor discrimination task for rats in which different odors predicted either sucrose or quinine, reversal of the reinforcement contingencies altered the encoding properties of neurons (Figure 36.3), thereby indicating the dependence of neural activity on the value (rewarding or aversive) of the predicted events (Schoenbaum et al., 1999). Reversal training in monkeys likewise alters the responsiveness of orbitofrontal neurons to olfactory cues (Rolls et al., 1996). In addition, it has been shown that the encoding properties of orbitofrontal neurons in monkeys are altered by more subtle variations in the incentive value of predicted outcomes. For example, orbitofrontal neurons respond more strongly to cues that predict preferred food items than to cues predicting less preferred food items (Tremblay & Schultz, 1999). This encoding can also reflect relative preferences among the items that are available at a given time. For example, a neuron that fires more robustly to the cue predicting a preferred outcome in one block of trials will decrease firing to that cue in a subsequent trial block when a more preferred reward is introduced (Tremblay & Schultz, 1999). The dependence of encoding during cue presentation on relative preference has yet to be tested in rats. However, other important features of encoding that reflect the anticipation of expected rewards during delay intervals can be observed in both species.

Orbitofrontal neurons are active in both rats and primates during short delays interposed between responses and delivery of reinforcement (Schoenbaum et al., 1998; Tremblay & Schultz, 1999, 2000a), or in some cases during delays between cue presentation and responses to instructions preceding reinforcer delivery (Hikosaka & Watanabe, 2000). This activity appears to encode expectancy of an impending outcome, independently of the response made to gain access to the outcome (Figure 36.4). Like neuronal activity during presentation of predictive cues, differential firing during delays emerges with learning (Schoenbaum, Chiba, & Gallagher, 1998; Schoenbaum et al., 1999; Tremblay & Schultz, 2000b) and is linked to the incentive value rather than to the specific identity of the impending reward (Hikosaka & Watanabe, 2000; Tremblay & Schultz, 1999, 2000a). The dependence of these correlates on the incentive value of the reward appears to distinguish anticipatory delay activity in the orbitofrontal cortex from similar activity in dorsolateral prefrontal regions (Hikosaka & Watanabe, 2000; Watanabe, 1996).

In each of these studies, it is particularly interesting, given the multimodal input to the orbitofrontal cortex, that neural encoding of incentive value appears to be independent of the physical attributes of either the signaling event or the impending outcome. For example, cues with different physical features (different odors or different complex visual stimuli) can evoke similar responses when those cues predict similar rewards (Schoenbaum & Eichenbaum, 1995a; Tremblay & Schultz, 1999). Moreover, neuronal firing in anticipation of reinforcers differs according to incentive value rather than the nature of the re-

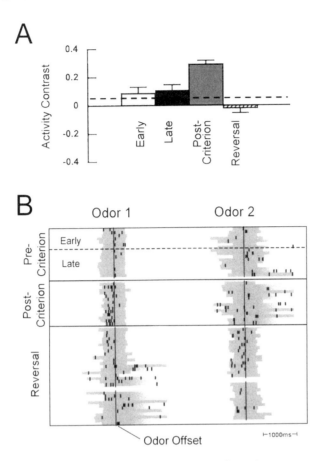

FIGURE 36.3. Representation of incentive value in the orbitofrontal cortex, revealed by neural activity during discrimination and reversal training. Neurons in the rat orbitofrontal cortex were recorded during acquisition and reversal of new two-odor discrimination problems in a go/no-go paradigm. On each trial, an odor was presented. Responses after sampling of the positive odor resulted in delivery of a sucrose solution; responses after sampling of the negative odor resulted in delivery of a quinine solution. Rats were presented with a novel odor pair in each session. Neural activity was recorded as the rats learned to withhold responses to the negative cue to avoid the quinine solution during accurate performance, and then during reversal training where the reinforcers paired with the odor cues were switched. (A) Contrast in population activity during odor sampling calculated for the 96 of 328 orbitofrontal neurons that exhibited selective firing to odor cues during accurate performance. Differential activity in these cells (illustrated in B) developed only during odor sampling in the postcriterion phase of prereversal training and disappeared after reversal. Activity contrast was calculated as the difference in firing to positive and negative odors, referenced to the polarity of this difference during postcriterion trials, and normalized by the sum of those rates in each training phase. The dotted line represents a baseline value calculated from neural activity recorded between trials. Selectivity in this population of neurons differed significantly from baseline only during the postcriterion phase. (B) An example of a neuron with differential firing during odor sampling that developed during acquisition of the discrimination and was evident only before reversal. Neural activity is shown for representative trials in raster format. Trials are shown sequentially for each odor. Activity on each trial began with odor onset, was synchronized to odor offset, and ended with a response or after 1,500 milliseconds for no-go trials (faded). This cell developed selective firing to odor 1 in the postcriterion trial block, during accurate performance on the discrimination. This selective response diminished rapidly after reversal and disappeared. From Schoenbaum et al. (1999). Copyright 1999 by the Society for Neuroscience. Adapted by permission.

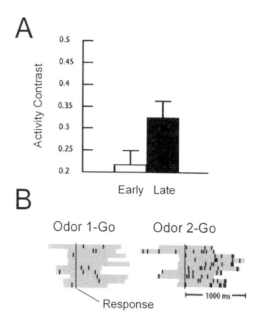

FIGURE 36.4. Representation of incentive value in the orbitofrontal cortex during delays after cue sampling and during the response at the fluid well up to the time of reinforcer delivery. Neurons were recorded in the same experiment illustrated in Figure 36.3. (A) Contrast in population activity during the delay after responding at the fluid well but before reinforcer delivery, calculated for the 74 of 328 orbitofrontal neurons that exhibited selective firing during this period (illustrated in B). Selective firing during the delay in this population of neurons developed rapidly during training and increased significantly with learning between the early and late phases of precriterion training. Activity contrast was calculated by comparing firing during the delay on positive and negative trials, as described for Figure 36.3. (B) This figure shows an example of a neuron that did not fire differentially during odor sampling but did fire differentially later in each trial—namely, during a brief delay after a response had been made but before reinforcement was delivered. This selective activity appeared to anticipate delivery of the quinine solution. Neural activity is shown for representative trials in raster format. Trials are shown sequentially for each odor. Activity on each trial began with odor offset, was synchronized to the response at the fluid well, and ended with reinforcer delivery. Only go responses made during precriterion training are shown. From Schoenbaum et al. (1999). Copyright 1999 by Macmillan. Adapted by permission.

ward (Hikosaka & Watanabe, 2000). The independence of encoding in the orbitofrontal cortex from the physical features of cues is also evident for more abstract "cues." For example, firing in the orbitofrontal cortex can encode incentive value based on apparent conjunctions between places and odors (Lipton, Alvarez, & Eichenbaum, 1999), or based on whether the odor matches one presented on the preceding trial (Ramus & Eichenbaum, 2000). Such encoding is prominent when the demands of the task require those features to guide performance. For example, in the study by Ramus and Eichenbaum (2000), rats sampled an odor on each trial and were rewarded for responding if the odor did not match the sampled odor on the immediately preceding trial. Although odor identity was important in determining whether a match was made, the identity of the odor was not, by itself, correlated with outcome. In this setting, a high proportion of neurons recorded in the orbitofrontal cortex (64%) had differential activity, depending on whether the odor sampled was a match or a nonmatch. Few cells fired selectively to odors based on their identity, and almost no neurons fired independently of whether an odor was a match. Thus orbitofrontal neurons are capable of representing more abstract conjunctions between cues if these representations are reliably associated with outcomes.

The features of information encoding by orbitofrontal neurons illustrated by these recording studies are consistent with the view that in both rats and nonhuman primates, this region serves a role in the strategic use of motivational information that is encoded in reference to prior experience, current context, and expectations about predicted events. Moreover, the close relationship of encoding to the incentive value of expected outcomes is consistent with a central role of the orbitofrontal cortex in guiding goal-directed behavior based on how incentive value and outcomes are represented. Impairments in devaluation studies in both rats and monkeys with orbitofrontal lesions, as well as the maladaptive responses made by neurological patients with orbitofrontal damage, may reflect the loss of such representations or the inability to use them effectively to guide behavior.

CONCLUSIONS

New evidence indicates that the orbitofrontal region is especially important for prospective encoding of outcome value. This role is evident in the effect of lesions, which impair behaviors that depend on the appropriate use of that information, and in the properties of orbitofrontal neurons, which represent incentive value independent of the physical attributes of predicted events. Recent research demonstrates a remarkable parallel across primates and rats in this characteristic of the orbitofrontal region, providing a basis for functional homology across species.

The incentive value of anticipated events encoded in the orbitofrontal cortex is likely to be used in conjunction with information represented in other prefrontal regions to guide behavior. For example, cells in the primate dorsolateral prefrontal cortex represent physical features of information in the environment, including object identity and spatial location (Wilson, Scalaidhe, & Goldman-Rakic, 1993). The information used to guide behavior therefore has a distributed representation, with specialization in different prefrontal regions, at least in part, reflecting differences in connectivity with other cortical and subcortical systems. Although we have emphasized the importance of orbitofrontal connections with the amygdala in this chapter (see also Gallagher et al., 1999; Schoenbaum et al., 1998, 1999), the influence of connections with other structures is also evident in the properties of orbitofrontal neurons (Lipton et al., 1999; Ramus & Eichenbaum, 2000; Schoenbaum & Eichenbaum, 1995a). As in other prefrontal regions, representations in the orbitofrontal cortex generally develop with accurate task performance (Asaad, Rainer, & Miller, 2000; Rainer, Assad, & Miller, 1998; Schoenbaum & Eichenbaum, 1995b; Schoenbaum et al., 1999), and neural activity persists during delays to anticipate outcomes (Hikosaka & Watanabe, 2000; Schoenbaum et al., 1998; Tremblay & Schultz, 1999). Within a framework that assigns a role for the prefrontal cortex in executive functions, the orbitofrontal cortex may now be viewed as an important component of the prefrontal system. Additional comparative research will help to illuminate both the similarities and distinctive features of the prefrontal cortex across mammalian species.

REFERENCES

Asaad, W. F., Rainer, G., & Miller, E. K. (2000). Task-specific neural activity in the primate prefrontal cortex. *Journal of Neurophysiology, 84,* 451–459.

Barbas, H. (1993). Organization of cortical afferent input to orbitofrontal areas in the rhesus monkey. *Neuroscience, 56,* 841–864.

Baxter, M. G., Parker, A., Lindner, C. C. C., Izquierdo, A. D., & Murray, E. A. (2000). Control of response selection by reinforcer value requires interaction of amygdala and orbitofrontal cortex. *Journal of Neuroscience, 20,* 4311–4319.

Bechara, A., Damasio, H., Damasio, A. R., & Lee, G. P. (1999). Different contributions of the human amygdala and ventromedial prefrontal cortex to decision-making. *Journal of Neuroscience, 19,* 5473–5481.

Bechara, A., Damasio, H., Tranel, D., & Andersen, S. W. (1998). Dissociation of working memory from decision making within the human prefrontal cortex. *Journal of Neuroscience, 18,* 428–437.

Bechara, A., Damasio, H., Tranel, D., & Damasio, A. R. (1997). Deciding advantageously before knowing the advantageous strategy. *Science, 275,* 1293–1294.

Brodmann, K. (1909). *Vergleichende Lokalisationslehre der Grosshirnrhinde.* Leipzig: Barth.

Butter, C. M. (1969). Perseveration and extinction in discrimination reversal tasks following selective frontal ablations in *Macaca mulatta. Physiology and Behavior, 4,* 163–171.

Butter, C. M., Mishkin, M., & Mirsky, A. F. (1968). Emotional responses toward humans in monkeys with selective frontal lesions. *Physiology and Behavior, 3,* 213–215.

Butter, C. M., & Snyder, D. R. (1972). Alterations in aversive and aggressive behaviors following orbital frontal lesions in rhesus monkeys. *Acta Neurobiologiae Experimentalis, 32,* 525–565.

Carmichael, S. T., Clugnet, M.-C., & Price, J. L. (1994). Central olfactory connections in the macaque monkey. *Journal of Comparative Neurology, 346,* 403–434.

Cinelli, A. R., Moyano-Ferreyra, H., & Barragan, E. (1985). Reciprocal functional connections of the olfactory bulbs and other olfactory related areas with the prefrontal cortex. *Brain Research Bulletin, 19,* 651–661.

Critchley, H. D., & Rolls, E. T. (1996a). Olfactory neuronal responses in the primate orbitofrontal cortex: Analysis in an olfactory discrimination task. *Journal of Neurophysiology, 75,* 1659–1672.

Critchley, H. D., & Rolls, E. T. (1996b). Hunger and satiety modify the responses of olfactory and visual neurons in the primate orbitofrontal cortex. *Journal of Neurophysiology, 75,* 1673–1686.

Damasio, A. R. (1994). *Descartes' error.* New York: Putnam.

Davis, M. (2000). The role of the amygdala in conditioned and unconditioned fear and anxiety. In J. Aggleton (Ed.), *The amygdala: A functional analysis* (2nd ed., pp. 213–288). Oxford: Oxford University Press.

DeCoteau, W. E., Kesner, R. P., & Williams, J. M. (1997). Short-term memory for food reward magnitude: The role of the prefrontal cortex. *Behavioural Brain Research, 88,* 239–249.

Diaz, R., Robbins, T. W., & Roberts, A. C. (1996). Dissociation in prefrontal cortex of affective and attentional shifts. *Nature, 380,* 69–72.

Eichenbaum, H., Clegg, R. A., & Feeley, A. (1983). Reexamination of functional subdivisions of the rodent prefrontal cortex. *Experimental Neurology, 79,* 434–451.

Emery, N. J., Capitanio, J. P., Mason, W. A., Machado, C. J., Mendoza, S. P., & Amaral, D. G. (2001). The effects of bilateral lesions of the amygdala on dyadic social interactions in rhesus monkeys (*Macaca mulatta*). *Behavioral Neuroscience, 115,* 515–544.

Everitt, B. J., & Robbins, T. W. (1992). Amygdala–ventral striatal interactions and reward-related processes. In J. Aggleton (Ed), *The amygdala: Neurological aspects of emotion, memory, and mental dysfunction* (pp. 401–429). New York: Wiley.

Fuster, J. M. (1997). *The prefrontal cortex* (3rd ed.). New York: Lippincott–Raven.

Fuster, J. M. (2000). The prefrontal cortex of the primate: A synopsis. *Psychobiology, 28,* 125–131.

Gaffan, D., & Murray, E. A. (1990). Amygdalar interaction with the mediodorsal nucleus of the thalamus and the ventromedial prefrontal cortex in stimulus–reward associative learning in the monkey. *Journal of Neuroscience, 10,* 3479–3493.

Gallagher, M., & Holland, P. (1999). Amygdala circuitry in attentional and representational processes. *Trends in Cognitive Sciences, 3,* 65–73.

Gallagher, M., McMahan, R. W., & Schoenbaum, G. (1999). Orbitofrontal cortex and representations of incentive value in associative learning. *Journal of Neuroscience, 19,* 6610–6614.

Goldman-Rakic, P. S., & Porrino, L. J. (1985). The primate mediodorsal (MD) nucleus and its projection to the frontal lobe. *Journal of Comparative Neurology, 242,* 535–560.

Groenewegen, H. J. (1988). Organization of the afferent connections of the mediodorsal thalamic nucleus in the rat, related to the mediodorsal–prefrontal topography. *Neuroscience, 24,* 379–431.

Groenewegen, H. J., Berendse, H. W., Wolters, J. G., & Lohman, A. H. M. (1990). The anatomical relationship of the prefrontal cortex with the striatopallidal system, the thalamus and the amygdala: Evidence for a parallel organization. *Progress in Brain Research, 85,* 95–118.

Groenewegen, H. J., Vermeulen-Van der Zee, E., te Kortschot, A., & Witter, M. P. (1987). Organization of the projections from the subiculum to the ventral striatum in the rat: A study using anterograde transport of *Phaseolus vulgaris* leucoagglutinin. *Neuroscience, 23,* 103–120.

Haber, S. N., Kunishio, K., Mizobuchi, M., & Lynd-Balta, E. (1995). The orbital and medial prefrontal circuit through the primate basal ganglia. *Journal of Neuroscience, 15,* 4851–4867.

Harlow, J. M. (1868). Passage of an iron bar through the head. *Publications of the Massachusetts Medical Society, 2,* 329–346.

Hatfield, T., Han, J.-S., Conley, M., Gallagher, M., & Holland, P. (1996). Neurotoxic lesions of basolateral, but not central, amygdala interfere with Pavlovian second-order conditioning and reinforcer devaluation effects. *Journal of Neuroscience, 16,* 5256–5265.

Hikosaka, K., & Watanabe, M. (2000). Delay activity of orbital and lateral prefrontal neurons of the monkey varying with different rewards. *Cerebral Cortex, 10,* 263–271.

Jones, B., & Mishkin, M. (1972). Limbic lesions and the problem of stimulus–reinforcement associations. *Experimental Neurology, 36,* 362–377.

Kievit, J., & Kuypers, H. G. J. M. (1977). Organization of the thalamo-cortical connexions to the frontal lobe in the rhesus monkey. *Experimental Brain Research, 29,* 299–322.

Kita, H., & Kitai, S. T. (1990). Amygdaloid projections to the frontal cortex and the striatum in the rat. *Journal of Comparative Neurology, 298,* 40–49.

Kolb, B. (1984). Functions of the frontal cortex of the rat: A comparative review. *Brain Research Reviews, 8,* 65–98.

Kolb, B. (1990). Organization of the neocortex of the rat. In B. Kolb & R. C. Tees (Eds.), *The cerebral cortex of the rat* (pp. 21–33). Cambridge, MA: MIT Press.

Kolb, B., & Nonneman, A. J. (1974). Frontolimbic lesions and social behavior in the rat. *Physiology and Behavior, 13,* 637–643.

Krettek, J. E., & Price, J. L. (1977a). The cortical projections of the mediodorsal nucleus and adjacent thalamic nuclei in the rat. *Journal of Comparative Neurology, 171,* 157–192.

Krettek, J. E., & Price J. L. (1977b). Projections from the amygdaloid complex to the cerebral cortex and thalamus in the rat and cat. *Journal of Comparative Neurology, 172,* 225–254.

LeDoux, J. E. (1995). Emotion: Clues from the brain. *Annual Review of Psychology, 46,* 209–235.

Leonard, C. M. (1969). The prefrontal cortex of the rat: I. Cortical projection of the mediodorsal nucleus. II. Efferent connections. *Brain Research, 12,* 321–343.

Lipton, P. A., Alvarez, P., & Eichenbaum, H. (1999). Crossmodal associative memory representations in rodent orbitofrontal cortex. *Neuron, 22,* 349–359.

Malkova, L., Gaffan, D., & Murray, E. A. (1997). Excitotoxic lesions of the amygdala fail to produce impairment in visual learning for auditory secondary reinforcement but interfere with reinforcer devaluation effects in rhesus monkeys. *Journal of Neuroscience, 17,* 6011–6020.

McDonald, A. J. (1991). Organization of the amygdaloid projections to the prefrontal cortex and associated striatum in the rat. *Neuroscience, 44,* 1–14.

Mishkin, M. (1964). Perseveration of central sets after frontal lesions in monkeys. In J. M. Warren & K. Akert (Eds.), *The frontal granular cortex and behavior* (pp. 219–241). New York: McGraw-Hill.

O'Donnell, P. (1999). Ensemble coding in the nucleus accumbens. *Psychobiology, 27,* 187–197.

Onoda, N., Imamura, K., Obota, F., & Iino, M. (1984). Responses selectivity of neocortical neurons to specific odors in the rabbit. *Journal of Neurophysiology, 52*, 638–652.

Ongur, D., & Price, J. L. (2000). The organization of networks within the orbital and medial prefrontal cortex of rats, monkeys and humans. *Cerebral Cortex, 10*, 206–219.

Otto, T., & Eichenbaum, H. (1992). Complementary roles of the orbital prefrontal cortex and the perirhinal–entorhinal cortices in an odor-guided delayed-nonmatching-to-sample task. *Behavioral Neuroscience, 106*, 762–775.

Preuss, T. M. (1995). Do rats have prefrontal cortex?: The Rose–Woolsey–Akert program reconsidered. *Journal of Cognitive Neuroscience, 7*, 1–24.

Price, J. L., Carmichael, S. T., Carnes, K. M., Clugnet, M.-C., Kuroda, M., & Ray, J. P. (1991). Olfactory input to the prefrontal cortex. In J. Davis & H. Eichenbaum (Eds.), *Olfaction: A model system for computational neuroscience* (pp. 101–120). Cambridge, MA: MIT Press.

Price, J. L., Russchen, F. T., & Amaral, D. G. (1987). The limbic region: II. The amygdaloid complex. In A. Bjorklund, T. Hokfelt, & L. W. Swanson (Eds.), *Handbook of chemical neuroanatomy: Vol. 5. Integrated systems of the CNS* (Pt. I, pp. 279–388). Amsterdam: Elsevier.

Rainer, G., Asaad, W. F., & Miller, E. K. (1998). Selective representation of relevant information by neurons in the primate prefrontal cortex. *Nature, 393*, 577–579.

Ramón y Cajal, S. (1988). Studies on the fine structure of the regional cortex of rodents: 1. Suboccipital cortex (retrosplenial cortex of Brodmann). In J. DeFelipe & E. G. Jones (Eds. & Trans.), *Cajal on the cerebral cortex: An annotated translation of the complete writings* (pp. 524–546). New York: Oxford University Press. (Original work published 1922)

Ramus, S. J., & Eichenbaum, H. (2000). Neural correlates of olfactory recognition memory in the rat orbitofrontal cortex. *Journal of Neuroscience, 20*, 8199–8208.

Ray, J. P., & Price, J. L. (1992). The organization of the thalamocortical connections of the mediodorsal thalamic nucleus in the rat, related to the ventral forebrain–prefrontal cortex topography. *Journal of Comparative Neurology, 323*, 167–197.

Reep, R. L., Corwin, J. V., & King, V. (1996). Neuronal connections of orbital cortex in rats: Topography of cortical and thalamic afferents. *Experimental Brain Research, 111*, 215–232.

Rolls, E. T., Critchley, H. D., Mason, R., & Wakeman, E. A. (1996). Orbitofrontal cortex neurons: Role in olfactory and visual association learning. *Journal of Neurophysiology, 75*, 1970–1981.

Rose, J. E., & Woolsey, C. L. (1949). Organization of the mammalian thalamus and its relationships to the cerebral cortex. *Electroencephalography and Clinical Neurophysiology, 1*, 391–403.

Rosenkilde, C. E., Bauer, R. H., & Fuster, J. M. (1981). Single cell activity in ventral prefrontal cortex in behaving monkeys. *Brain Research, 209*, 375–394.

Rosvold, H. E., Mirsky, A. F., & Pribram, K. H. (1954). Influence of amygdalectomy on social behavior in monkeys. *Journal of Comparative and Physiological Psychology, 47*, 173–178.

Russchen, F. T., Amaral, D. G., & Price, J. L. (1987). The afferent input to the magnocellular division of the mediodorsal thalamic nucleus in the monkey, *Macaca fascicularis*. *Journal of Comparative Neurology, 256*, 175–210.

Schoenbaum, G., Chiba, A. A., & Gallagher, M. (1998). Orbitofrontal cortex and basolateral amygdala encode expected outcomes during learning. *Nature Neuroscience, 1*, 155–159.

Schoenbaum, G., Chiba, A. A., & Gallagher, M. (1999). Neural encoding in orbitofrontal cortex and basolateral amygdala during olfactory discrimination learning. *Journal of Neuroscience, 19*, 1876–1884.

Schoenbaum, G., & Eichenbaum, H. (1995a). Information coding in the rodent prefrontal cortex: I. Single neuron activity in orbitofrontal cortex compared with that in piriform cortex. *Journal of Neurophysiology, 74*, 733–750.

Schoenbaum, G., & Eichenbaum, H. (1995b). Information coding in the rodent prefrontal cortex. II. Ensemble activity in orbitofrontal cortex. *Journal of Neurophysiology, 74*, 751–762.

Shi, C.-J., & Cassell, M. D. (1998). Cortical, thalamic, and amygdaloid connections of the anterior and posterior insular cortices. *Journal of Comparative Neurology, 399*, 440–468.

Takagi, S. F. (1986). Studies on the olfactory nervous system of the Old World monkey. *Progress in Neurobiology, 27*, 195–250.

Tanabe, T., Iino, M., & Takagi, S. F. (1975). Discrimination of odors in olfactory bulb, pyriform–amygdaloid areas, and orbitofrontal cortex of the monkey. *Journal of Neurophysiology, 38*, 1284–1296.

Tanabe, T., Yarita, H., Iino, M., Ooshima, Y., & Takagi, S. F. (1975). An olfactory projection area in orbitofrontal cortex of the monkey. *Journal of Neurophysiology, 38*, 1269–1283.

Thorpe, S. J., Rolls, E. T., & Maddison, S. (1983). The orbitofrontal cortex: Neuronal activity in the behaving monkey. *Experimental Brain Research, 49*, 93–115.

Tremblay, L., & Schultz, W. (1999). Relative reward preference in primate orbitofrontal cortex. *Nature, 398*, 704–708.

Tremblay, L., & Schultz, W. (2000a). Reward-related neuronal activity during go–no go task performance in primate orbitofrontal cortex. *Journal of Neurophysiology, 83*, 1864–1876.

Tremblay, L., & Schultz, W. (2000b). Modifications of reward expectation-related neuronal activity during learning in primate orbitofrontal cortex. *Journal of Neurophysiology, 83*, 1877–1885.

Watanabe, M. (1996). Reward expectancy in primate prefrontal neurons. *Nature, 382*, 629–632.

Whishaw, I. Q., Tomie, J.-A., & Kolb, B. (1992). Ventrolateral prefrontal cortex lesions in rats impair the acquisition and retention of a tactile–olfactory configural task. *Behavioral Neuroscience, 106*, 597–603.

Wilson, F. A. W., Scalaidhe, S. P. O., & Goldman-Rakic, P. S. (1993). Dissociation of object and spatial processing domains in primate prefrontal cortex. *Science, 260*, 1955–1958.

Yarita, H., Iino, M., Tanabe, T., Kogure, S., & Takagi, S. F. (1980). A transthalamic olfactory pathway to orbitofrontal cortex in the monkey. *Journal of Neurophysiology, 43*, 69–85.

Yonemori, M., Nishijo, H., Uwano, T., Tamura, R., Furita, I., Kawasaki, M., Takashima, Y., & Ono T. (2000). Orbital cortex neuronal responses during an odor-based conditioned associative task in rats. *Neuroscience, 95*, 691–703.

37

Genetics of Memory in the Mouse

MARK MAYFORD and EDWARD KORZUS

The mouse and human genomes each consist of approximately 35,000 individual genes. This limited complement of molecular components is sufficient to develop a functioning nervous system containing on the order of 10^{15} synaptic connections and capable of the myriad mental abilities with which we are all familiar. Understanding of the molecular mechanisms by which the mammalian brain develops and functions in the adult has been facilitated by several technical advances in the genetic manipulation of the mouse that have occurred over the past decade. These techniques, collectively referred to as "reverse genetics," allow one to begin with a gene of interest and to generate a mouse in which that gene has been deleted or has been altered in function through the introduction of subtle mutations. The resulting mouse can be bred, and the offspring, each carrying the same specific molecular lesion, can be studied at various levels of analysis—from the cellular to the systems to the behavioral level—to determine the consequences of the genetic alteration.

In the area of cognitive neuroscience, much effort has focused on elucidating the cellular and molecular mechanisms of learning and memory. In 1973 synaptic connections within the rabbit hippocampus were shown to undergo long-term potentiation (LTP), a form of activity-dependent synaptic plasticity, which displays a number of features that make it a plausible cellular mechanism for information storage in the brain (Bliss & Lomo, 1973). The approach in the mouse has been to pinpoint genes that are important for the generation of LTP and to produce "knockout" mice in which that gene has been deleted. These animals are then tested to identify the expected deficits in LTP and to evaluate the impact of these deficits on various learning and memory tasks. Mice carrying targeted deletions of the genes encoding Ca^{2+}/calmodulin-dependent protein kinase II (CamKII), the *fyn* tyrosine kinase, the N-methyl-D-aspartate (NMDA) receptor R1 subunit (NR1), and the cyclic adenosine monophosphate (cAMP)-responsive element-binding (CREB) factor all exhibited deficits in LTP measured in the CA1 region of the hippocampus (Bourtchuladze et al., 1994; Grant et al., 1992; Silva, Paylor, Wehner, & Tonegawa, 1992; Silva, Stevens, Tonegawa, & Wang, 1992; Tsien, Huerta, & Tonegawa, 1996). When tested for spatial memory in the water maze paradigm—the best-characterized hippocampus-dependent task in rodents—the mutant mice were impaired. However, when LTP at other synapses in the hippocampus was disrupted by genetic manipulations, including CA3 mossy-fiber LTP

(PKA-Cβ1⁻ mutant) and LTP at synapses of the perforant path onto the dentate gyrus granule cells (Thy-1⁻ mutant), spatial memory ability remained intact (Huang et al., 1995; Nosten-Bertrand et al., 1996). These initial results tended to support a role for LTP, at least in the CA1 region of the hippocampus, and demonstrated the power of the genetic approach to generate animal models for cognitive studies.

REGULATED GENETIC MODIFICATION

Although the genetic approach offers the ability to alter almost any known gene, there are several difficulties with the interpretation of complex phenotypes in a standard knockout mouse. First, because the gene is deleted in all cells that would normally express it, it is difficult to determine whether a given behavioral phenotype results from alterations observed in just one brain region (such as the hippocampus) or from the effect of the gene deletion on other brain structures. In addition, as behavioral scientists are well aware, performance of a learning and memory task does not depend on a single process; it also requires proper sensory and motor function, as well as the appropriate motivation and attention to performance of the task. Moreover, memory itself can be divided into a number of phases: the initial encoding of information; a consolidation period, where memory can be reorganized and its cellular and anatomical substrates altered; and a final phase, where the information must be accessed and used to guide behavior during retrieval. It is often difficult to determine which of these various processes is altered in a knockout mouse. For example, an animal may lack LTP in the hippocampus but fail in a spatial memory task because of a subtle alteration in perception due to lack of the gene in the sensory cortex. Finally, because the gene is absent for the entire developmental history of the animal, one cannot ascribe a given behavioral or electrophysiological phenotype to a direct requirement for the gene product in the adult animal; the phenotype may result from an indirect effect on neuronal development. These difficulties have led investigators to develop new technology to allow for both anatomical and temporal control over genetic modifications in the mouse (Mayford & Kandel, 1999). These techniques permit genes to be turned on and off at precise times and in limited subsets of neurons within the brain.

ARE NMDA RECEPTORS ESSENTIAL FOR MEMORY FORMATION?

Although the signaling mechanisms recruited for the induction of stable, long-lasting LTP are complex, Figure 37.1 shows a simple model (for a review, see Malenka & Nicoll, 1999) for the initial induction of LTP that forms the basis of the genetic experiments discussed below. According to this model, the induction of LTP in the Schaffer collateral pathway of CA1 neurons of the hippocampus requires activation of NMDA receptors. The Ca^{2+} signal produced by NMDA receptor activation is then transduced into a long-lasting increase in synaptic strength through activation of CamKII and phosphorylation, or insertion, of α-amino-3-hydroxy-5-methyl-4-isoxazole-4-propionic acid (AMPA)-type glutamate receptors. The current flux of the phosphorylated receptors is enhanced, resulting in a greater depolarization in response to future glutamate signals.

Deletion of the NMDA receptor subunit NR1 via a standard gene knockout approach eliminates NMDA currents throughout the nervous system and results in early neonatal lethality (Forrest et al. 1994; Li, Erzurumlu, Chen, Jhaveri, & Tonegawa, 1994). In order to circumvent this problem and study the role of NMDA receptors in adult learning and

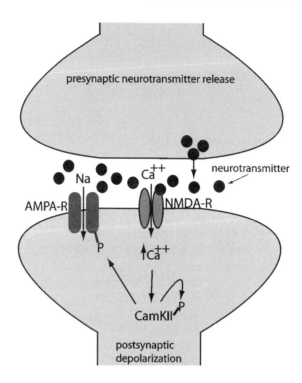

FIGURE 37.1. A model for LTP induction. Schematic representation of a current model for the initial induction of LTP. When glutamate is released concurrently with postsynaptic depolarization, NMDA receptors are activated. The increase in Ca^{2+} in the postsynaptic dendritic spine activates CamKII, which becomes constitutively active through autophosphorylation. The prolonged activation of the kinase leads to elevated phosphorylation of AMPA-type glutamate receptors, which in turn enhances the current flux through these receptors.

memory, Tsien and colleagues (Tsien, Chen, et al., 1996; Tsien, Huerta, & Tonegawa, 1996) have used a conditional gene knockout approach as outlined in Figure 37.2. Cre recombinase is an enzyme capable of deleting DNA sequences that are flanked by two small 34 bp recognition sequences called loxP sites. The conditional knockout approach uses two separate lines of mice. In the first mutant line, a portion of the gene encoding NR1 is flanked by two loxP sites placed in introns using homologous recombination in embryonic stem cells. This modification of the gene, often referred to as "floxing," typically does not produce any phenotypic effect, since the loxP sites are small and hidden in introns. The second line is a transgenic mouse that expresses Cre recombinase under the control of the CamKIIα promoter, which normally directs expression into excitatory forebrain neurons. Separately, the two genetic modifications are silent. However, when the mice are bred together such that two copies of the floxed NR1 gene and the CamKIIα–Cre transgene are now in the same mouse, the NR1 gene is deleted, but only in those cells that express Cre recombinase. Remarkably, the functional activity of Cre recombinase in these mutant animals is restricted to CA1 neurons, even though the CamKIIα promoter has a much broader spectrum of expression. Thus in mice carrying both genetic modifications (CA1–NR1 knockout mice), the NR1 gene is deleted only in the CA1 neurons of the hippocampus. It is unclear why the knockout is limited to the CA1 neurons, although it probably involves the requirement of a certain threshold level of Cre to induce recombination. Never-

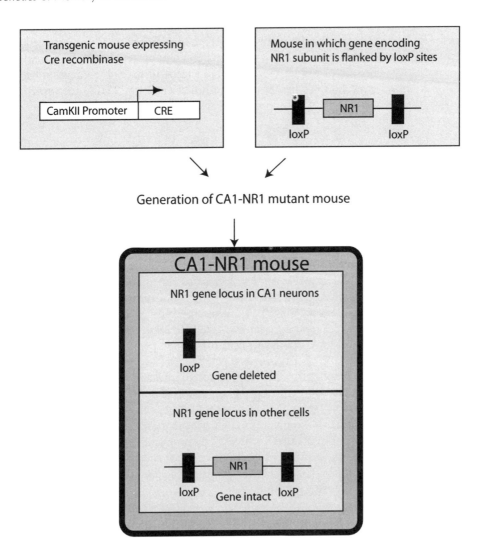

FIGURE 37.2. Conditional NMDA receptor knockout strategy. Two genetic modifications are introduced into a single mouse. The conditional knockout mouse carries a transgene in which the Cre recombinase is expressed from the CamKIIα promoter as well as two floxed NR1 loci. Expression of the Cre recombinase results in deletion of the NR1 gene in CA1 pyramidal neurons. In all other cells of this mutant mouse, the NR1 gene remains intact. Data from Tsien, Chen, et al. (1996) and Tsien, Huerta, and Tanegawa (1996).

theless, this small bit of serendipity provides a very interesting model with which to investigate the role of NMDA-dependent LTP in learning and memory.

An electrophysiological analysis of CA1–NR1 knockout mice clearly showed, as expected, a requirement for NMDA receptors in the induction of LTP (Tsien, Huerta, & Tonegawa, 1996). LTP was absent in the CA1 neurons that lacked the NR1 gene. However, normal LTP could be produced in the dentate gyrus granule cells of the hippocampus where NR1 was expressed normally. To test the impact of this highly specific impairment in synaptic plasticity on cognitive function, the mice were tested for hippocampus-dependent spatial memory in the water maze task. Although the mice performed normally in a simple cued version of the task, they were severely impaired on the spatial version of the same task. Subsequent studies of these mice revealed deficiencies in other hippocampal (but nonspatial) tasks, such as social transmission of food preference, object recognition, and contextual fear conditioning (Rampon et al., 2000). These studies confirmed a role for NMDA receptors in LTP induction at CA1 synapses and for hippocampus-dependent forms of memory.

CAMKII SIGNALING IN LTP AND MEMORY

Although NMDA receptor activation is the first step in the induction of LTP, it is the Ca^{2+} signal produced by the receptor that is thought to mediate the biochemical changes underlying LTP. How is a brief Ca^{2+} signal lasting on the order of 1 second converted into a long-lasting physiological change lasting many days? CamKII is a major Ca^{2+}-dependent protein kinase that is concentrated in dendritic spines and has the capacity to convert short-lasting Ca^{2+} signals into long-lasting biochemical changes (Braun & Schulman, 1995). Though CamKII is normally inactive in the absence of Ca^{2+} and calmodulin, upon exposure to Ca^{2+} the enzyme becomes active and is able to phosphorylate protein substrates. Among the best substrates for CamKII are other subunits of CamKII itself, and upon autophosphorylation at a key regulatory amino acid (Thr286), the kinase activity becomes Ca^{2+}-independent. Thus brief Ca^{2+} elevation can produce prolonged CamKII activation through autophosphorylation at Thr286.

To test the role of CamKII autophosphorylation in LTP and memory, Giese, Fedorov, Filipkowski, and Silva (1998) introduced a point mutation into the CamKIIα gene, converting Thr286 to Ala and thereby preventing autophosphorylation. This mutation eliminated the ability of the kinase to convert to the Ca^{2+}-independent form, but preserved its ability to become active in the presence of Ca^{2+}. The mutant mice showed a disruption of LTP in CA1 neurons across a range of stimulation frequencies and failed in the spatial memory version of the water maze. These results suggested a role for CamKII activation in LTP induction and memory formation.

Is CamKII activation sufficient to induce LTP at hippocampal synapses and does altering LTP acutely in the adult animal interfere with memory formation? In order to address this question, Mayford and colleagues (1996) used the tetracycline (TET) system to induce, in transgenic animals, expression of a mutant Ca^{2+}-independent form of the kinase. In this mutant, Thr286 is converted to Asp, thereby mimicking the effect of autophosphorylation and producing a kinase that is continuously active. The TET system allows for both anatomical and temporal control over the expression of the CamKII–Asp286 transgene, as outlined in Figure 37.3. The TET system for gene regulation involves the use of a recombinant transcription factor known as the tetracycline transactivator (tTA). tTA is a hybrid molecule consisting of the TET repressor from *E. coli* fused to a VP16 transcriptional activation domain from the virus SV40 (Gossen & Bujard, 1992). This molecule functions as a eukaryotic transcription activator that can be inhibited by TET analogues such as doxycycline (DOX). Two different lines of transgenic animal are generated to obtain TET-regulated gene expression in mice. In the first line, the CamKII promoter is used to drive expression of tTA into excitatory forebrain neurons. In the second line of mice, the gene of interest—in this case, the mutant CamKII–Asp286—is fused to a promoter that binds tTA. When both transgenes are introduced into the same animal through mating, tTA will activate expression of the CamKII–Asp286 transgene, and introduction of DOX into the animal's diet will suppress that expression.

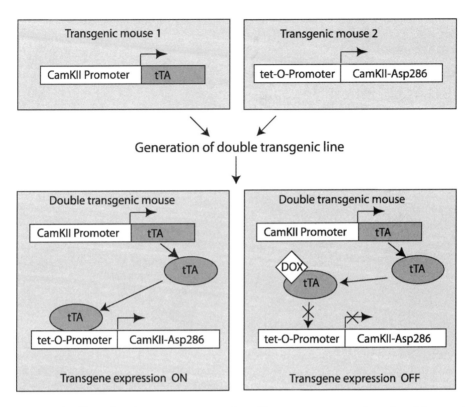

FIGURE 37.3. TET-regulated transgene expression. Two transgenes are introduced into a single mouse to obtain regulation. In the double transgenic mouse, the CamKIIα promoter drives expression of the tTA transcription factor into excitatory forebrain neurons, and tTA in turn activates expression of the mutant CamKII–Asp286 transgene via the tet-O-promoter. When these animals are fed the TET analogue doxycycline (DOX), the DOX binds to tTA, causing it to dissociate from the tet-O-promoter and thereby suppressing expression of the CamKII–Asp286 transgene. Data from Mayford et al. (1996).

The CamKII–Asp286 mice showed elevated levels of CamKII activity but no increase in basal synaptic transmission, as might be expected if LTP had been induced by the activation of the kinase alone. In addition, LTP induction by high-frequency (100-Hz) stimulation was unaltered. These results suggested that activation of CamKII is not sufficient to induce LTP (although see Pettit, Perlman, & Malinow, 1994). LTP is generally induced in hippocampal slices by short bursts of 100-Hz stimulation. However, long-lasting synaptic plasticity is also induced by lower frequencies of stimulation. Thus stimulation at 5 and 10 Hz will produce small amounts of LTP, whereas stimulation at 1 Hz produces long-term depression (LTD). Thus there is a correlation between the frequency of synaptic stimulation and the size and direction of synaptic change, with high frequencies producing LTP and low frequencies producing LTD. When the CamKII–Asp286 mice were examined in the lower-frequency range, they showed a shift in this frequency response function in the range of 5–10 Hz, such that LTP was impaired and LTD was enhanced (Figure 37.4A; Mayford et al., 1996; Mayford, Wang, Kandel, & O'Dell, 1995). When expression of the CamKII–Asp286 transgene was suppressed by feeding the animals DOX, the electrophysiological impairment was reversed.

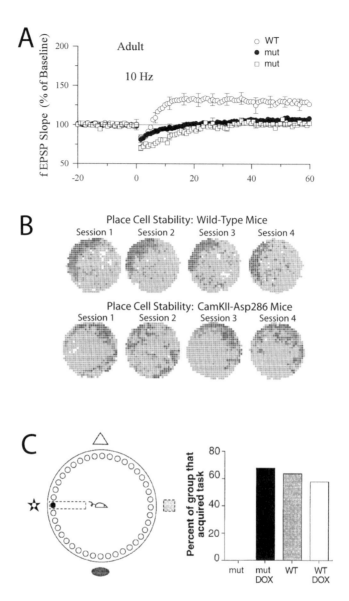

FIGURE 37.4. Multilevel analysis of a genetically modified mouse. (A) Field excitatory postsynaptic potential (EPSP) slopes were measured before and after 10-Hz stimulation of hippocampal slices at CA3–CA1 synapses. This protocol produced a long-lasting potentiation of synaptic transmission in wild-type slices (WT), but failed to potentiate slices from two different lines of CamKII–Asp286 mice (mut). (B) Action potential firing frequency from four successive recording sessions for a single place cell measured in wild-type mice (top row) and CamKII–Asp286 mice (bottom row). Firing rates are partitioned into six bins and usually color-coded in ascending order: yellow, orange, red, green, blue, and purple (presented here in a gray scale). Place fields recorded from wild-type animals were stable and remained in a similar position across the four consecutive sessions. The positional firing patterns recorded in transgenic animals were unstable. (C) Effect of CamKII–Asp286 transgene expression on spatial memory formation assessed in the Barnes circular maze. The Barnes maze (left panel) is an open disk with 40 holes in at the perimeter. Beneath one hole is a darkened escape tunnel that the mice must find by using distal cues located on the walls of the room. Expression of the CamKII–Asp286 transgene resulted in an impairment in acquisition of the task. Suppression of transgene expression by administration of DOX reversed this impairment. Panel A from Mayford et al. (1996). Copyright 1996 by the American Association for the Advancement of Science. Reprinted by permission. Panel B from Rotenberg et al. (1996). Copyright 1996 by Elsevier Science. Adapted by permission.

The impairment in hippocampal LTP in the 5- to 10-Hz frequency range is particularly interesting from a behavioral point of view. It has been quite difficult to demonstrate behaviorally induced, LTP-like phenomena in the hippocampus, possibly because information in any given behavioral task is sparsely encoded and is thus unlikely to affect a sufficient number of synapses for detection. Therefore, we do not know the patterns of natural activity that animals might use to encode behaviorally relevant information. However, in the hippocampus there is a rhythmic oscillation in the 5- to 10-Hz range known as the theta rhythm, which is present when rodents explore a novel environment (Smythe, Colom, & Bland, 1992). If LTP is used to encode spatial information in the hippocampus, the hippocampus is likely to use some pattern of activity at this frequency. Moreover, the CamKII–Asp286 mice have a reversible plasticity deficit specifically in this frequency range. The CamKII–Asp286 mutant mice exhibited a deficit in spatial memory on the Barnes circular maze (Figure 37.4C). This deficit in spatial memory was completely reversed by suppression of transgene expression. These results suggested that both the electrophysiological and behavioral effects of the transgene are due to the acute action of the gene in adult animals, rather than to an irreversible developmental defect.

MEMORY RETRIEVAL

Temporally regulated genetic modification not only provides the ability to dissociate developmental effects of a mutation from adult effects, but also allows for the dissection of the various stages of memory encoding, consolidation, and retrieval. An example of this type of use of the system is shown in Figure 37.5. Here a line of TET-regulated CamKII–Asp286 mice was studied that expresses the transgene exclusively in the striatum and lateral amygdala (Mayford et al., 1996). The lateral amygdala is a critical component of the circuitry recruited for Pavlovian fear conditioning. In this task, animals are given a series of tone–shock pairings and learn to fear both the apparatus in which training occurred (context conditioning) and the tone that predicts the shock (cued conditioning) (LeDoux, 1995). Animals in which the transgene was active during training could learn neither the cued nor the context version of this task, but when the transgene was suppressed, learning and memory were normal. Those animals that learned the task with the transgene off were next divided into two groups in which the transgene was either reactivated or maintained in the off state. When the transgene was reactivated after the initial learning, the animals showed memory impairment. This was unlikely to reflect a performance deficit, because the animals showed normal unconditioned fear responses; the impairment was more likely to reflect a disruption in memory storage or retrieval processes. These results demonstrate, in a preliminary way, the utility of regulated genetic modification in the study of behavior. Regulation offers some of the temporal advantages of the pharmacological approach, while providing for a greater specificity and breadth of possible molecular intervention.

WHAT CAN WE LEARN FROM MOUSE MUTANTS ABOUT HIPPOCAMPAL MEMORY FOR SPACE?

In the two examples discussed thus far, deficits in CA1 hippocampal LTP were associated with deficits in spatial learning. Although LTP may be one mechanism for encoding memories, it is the impact of these synaptic changes on the pattern of neuronal firing that ulti-

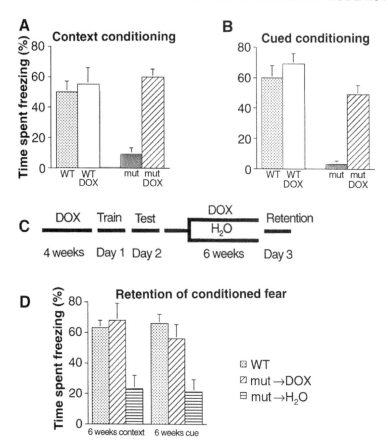

FIGURE 37.5. Regulated transgene expression for the study of memory storage and retrieval. Fear conditioning is a simple form of associative learning in which a tone (cue) or novel environment (context) is associated with an aversive stimulus. Both cued and contextual fear conditioning depend on the integrity of the amygdala, whereas lesions of the hippocampus can selectively impair the contextual version of this task. Here a group of animals expressing the CamKII–Asp286 transgene (mut) exclusively in the striatum and lateral amygdala was examined. The mice showed a severe impairment in both the contextual (A) and cued (B) versions of this task, which could be reversed when the transgene was suppressed by administration of DOX. (C) Time line representing administration of DOX and behavioral training and testing sessions for the experiment in D. (D) When transgenic animals were trained with the CamKII–Asp286 transgene suppressed, mice showed no differences in fear conditioning compared to wild-type animals. After training, the transgene was turned on for over 6 weeks (mut → H₂O), and the animals were tested again and compared to a control group in which the transgene remained off (mut → DOX). Expression of the transgene after an animal learned the task reduced freezing, thereby indicating impairment in memory storage or retrieval. From Mayford et al. (1996). Copyright 1996 by the American Association for the Advancement of Science. Reprinted by permission.

mately controls behavior. What can be learned about the impact of these mutations on this systems property of the hippocampus?

Excitatory neurons in the hippocampus encode information about space. These neurons, known as "place cells," fire action potentials selectively when an animal is in a particular location in its environment. The summed activity of many thousands of neurons is thought to form a spatial representation of that particular environment. New environments induce different patterns of cell firing, such that new place fields form within minutes and are stable for many weeks.

The discovery that CamKII–Asp286 mutant mice show a disruption in spatial learning as well as in LTP expression prompted the study of place cells in these animals (Rotenberg, Mayford, Hawkins, Kandel, & Muller, 1996). Mice were fitted with chronically implanted extracellular recording electrodes and allowed to explore a cylindrical environment for 15 minutes while the activity of individual neurons was recorded. The frequency of firing at each location in the environment is shown in Figure 37.4B. Analysis of place fields formed in the CA1 region in the CamKII–Asp286 transgenic mice revealed several abnormalities compared to the place fields of wild-type mice. Although the transgenic mice had place cells, their positional firing pattern was weaker and less compact. Perhaps more striking with regard to the observed spatial memory deficit was the instability of the place fields over time. As exemplified by the difference in firing patterns between sessions 1 and 2 in Figure 37.4B, the place fields in the mutant mice shifted over time, whereas the wild-type animals showed stable place fields over all recording sessions. It seems clear that this type of instability in spatial representation would make it difficult to form a long-term memory for location.

A similar series of experiments was performed on NR1–CA1 knockout mice (McHugh, Blum, Tsien, Tonegawa, & Wilson, 1996). In these mice, the place fields appeared to be unaltered and stable over time. However, a disruption was observed in the correlation in firing that is normally seen between cells that encode overlapping spatial locations. Such a disruption might be expected to lead to degradation in the spatial map that arises from coordinated firing of large groups of cells at each particular location in space. Thus, in two cases, mutant mice with an impairment in LTP showed deficits in the encoding of spatial information by hippocampal neurons and in spatial memory formation. It is tempting to conclude that the LTP deficits caused the place cell deficits, which in turn led to impaired spatial memory. However, as discussed below, it is not always the case that inhibition of LTP in the hippocampus results in impairments in spatial memory.

IS LTP A CELLULAR MECHANISM OF MEMORY STORAGE?

Is LTP a cellular mechanism of memory storage? This question, as phrased here, is somewhat imprecise. First, LTP is an artificially induced phenomenon measured in brain slices, and it is produced with patterns of electrical stimuli that do not normally occur in the brain. Second, there are many different types of memory that depend on different anatomical structures and possibly on different cellular mechanisms. A more appropriate way to phrase the question, so that it is addressable by the experiments discussed here, is as follows: Is there a cellular mechanism of neuronal plasticity that uses mechanisms similar to LTP and is required in the CA1 region of the hippocampus for spatial memory formation in rodents? The results discussed thus far are consistent with such an interpretation. However, these data are correlative. When interpreting results from the analysis of a mutant mouse that lacks LTP and also lacks spatial memory, one can conclude that the mutation causes both the LTP and the memory phenotypes, but one cannot conclude that one phenotype causes the other.

This correlation between LTP at CA1 synapses and spatial memory formation has been challenged by several recent experiments. As shown in Figure 37.1, the simple model of LTP induction postulates that the final step in induction is the phosphorylation of AMPA-type glutamate receptors. To test this idea, Zamanillo and colleagues (1999) generated a knockout in the major AMPA-type glutamate receptor subunit (GluR1). As expected, these mice showed a complete lack of LTP in the CA1 region of hippocampal slices. Surprisingly, the GluR1 knockout mice exhibited normal spatial memory. Recently, a second knockout mouse in which the gene for CamKIV was deleted also showed a lack of long-lasting LTP but appeared to have normal spatial memory (Ribar et al., 2000).

A series of pharmacological experiments have also called into question the role of NMDA-dependent LTP in the encoding of spatial memories (Bannerman, Good, Butcher, Ramsay, & Morris, 1995; Saucier & Cain, 1995). Although it had been known for some time that intrahippocampal infusions of NMDA receptor blockers at levels sufficient to block the induction of LTP impaired spatial memory in naive rats (Davis, Butcher, & Morris, 1992), these newer experiments found that if animals were pretrained in the water maze, their ability to encode new spatial memories was insensitive to NMDA blockade. Specifically, rats were trained in a spatial version of the water maze in one room and then moved to an unfamiliar room for training in a second water maze. Those animals that received pretraining performed the second spatial memory task normally, even though hippocampal LTP was pharmacologically blocked by inhibition of NMDA receptors. However, the hippocampus was still required for learning the second task, as bilateral hippocampal lesion resulted in a severe spatial memory deficit on the second maze (Bannerman et al., 1995). Thus the hippocampus itself is required for spatial learning in the circumstances studied here, but LTP in the hippocampus is not.

Do these results disprove the hypothesis that LTP is a cellular mechanism of memory storage? The results certainly indicate that LTP in the CA1 region of the hippocampus is not always essential for spatial memory formation. However, it is still possible that LTP is used under most conditions to store information, but that other mechanisms can substitute for LTP in some mutant animals or following certain types of pretraining (Moser & Moser, 2000). For example, in a delayed-matching-to-place paradigm in the water maze, pretraining did not protect the memory from disruption by NMDA receptor blockade (Steele & Morris, 1999). Moreover, recent experiments demonstrate that if wild-type rats are trained in a spatial memory task, and following encoding of the memory LTP is produced indiscriminately by electrical stimulation of the hippocampus, then the memory is disrupted (Brun, Ytterbø, Morris, Moser, & Moser, 2001). This finding suggests that under normal circumstances information may be encoded by LTP-like synaptic weight changes, and that if the relative synaptic weights are subsequently altered, then the memory can be erased. However, if yet-to-be-identified mechanisms can sometimes substitute for LTP in the coding of memories, the LTP hypothesis becomes difficult to test conclusively without a clearer understanding of the circumstances under which those alternative mechanisms are able to operate.

NEW DIRECTIONS IN NEUROGENETICS

We have focused in this chapter on the use of genetically modified mice to dissect the molecular mechanisms of learning and memory. The work has primarily centered on the notion that LTP is a cellular mechanism of information encoding in the brain, and that mice designed to lack LTP should exhibit some impairment in memory; clearly, this relationship fails to hold under some circumstances. However, the usefulness of genetic manipulation in the mouse is not dependent on the validity of the LTP hypothesis. Mice carrying single-gene mutations provide clues to understanding normal brain development and function, and identify candidate genes that may contribute to genetic forms of retardation and cognitive disorders in human beings. The key is to understand how a given alteration in a single gene leads to cognitive dysfunction and what kind of dysfunction is present.

Several approaches and principles can guide attempts to understand the mechanisms by which genetic alterations affect cognitive function. The use of regulated genetic modification allows one to dissociate the effects of a gene on neural development from acute effects on the adult brain. Moreover, when gene expression is altered at the various stages of memory encoding, consolidation, and recall, the effect of the gene on memory can be more precisely defined. This approach also provides useful controls for sensory, motor, and motivational effects. A second important consideration is the anatomy of the genetic alteration. Ideally, the genetic change would be introduced into a single cell type and in a single anatomically defined region of the brain. Although the performance of a complex learning and memory task involves processing in many brain areas, from sensory inputs to motor outputs, precise anatomical restriction of mutations allows one to focus on the computations performed at one location in this processing stream. This advantage is best exemplified by the analysis of the CA1–NR1 knockout mice. Here the CA3 input to CA1 yielded a coordinated pattern of place cell firing, whereas the output from the mutant CA1 revealed a disruption in the coordination of place cell firing (McHugh et al., 1996). The isolation of new promoter elements to drive more restricted patterns of gene expression should facilitate the molecular anatomical study of memory.

A clear understanding of learning and memory will require delineation of the cellular mechanisms that neurons use to encode information. This requirement is particularly difficult to satisfy. The approach of genetics is to let the molecules guide one to the cellular mechanisms. Although only a single gene is specifically altered in knockout and transgenic mice, it is clear that this gene does not act in isolation, and that there will probably be compensatory changes in the expression of other genes. The successful sequencing of the mouse and human genomes, combined with the development of DNA microarrays or "gene chips," provides a method for characterizing the compensatory changes in any gene that occurs in response to the mutation of a single gene (Lee & Lee, 2000). The use of this technology should provide a detailed understanding of the molecular alterations in neurons of transgenic and knockout mice, and should thus provide new insights into the mechanisms by which behavior is altered.

Finally, one of the drawbacks of the reverse genetic approach is that it is driven by the decision of which genes one chooses to mutate. If the underlying assumptions are wrong, then the resulting mutant mice may be uninformative. An alternative approach being taken by a number of investigators is to apply a classical forward genetic approach to complex behaviors in the mouse. In this case mice are treated with a chemical mutagen, and large numbers of offspring are tested for alterations in behaviors, including impairments in learning and memory. Once a mutant is identified, the responsible gene defect is isolated via classical genetic mapping techniques. The primary drawback of this approach is the historic difficulty in identifying which gene has been altered. The resurgence of interest in this approach has been fueled by the sequencing of the mouse genome, by the increase in the number of genetic markers, and by the development of high-throughput mapping techniques. These developments should make the forward genetic approach faster and more cost-effective than in the past, with the advantage that very few assumptions need be made about the underlying mechanisms of the behavior of interest.

REFERENCES

Bannerman, D. M., Good, M. A., Butcher, S. P., Ramsay, M., & Morris, R. G. (1995). Distinct components of spatial learning revealed by prior training and NMDA receptor blockade. *Nature*, *378*, 182–186.

Bliss, T. V., & Lomo, T. (1973). Long-lasting potentiation of synaptic transmission in the dentate area of the anaesthetized rabbit following stimulation of the perforant path. *Journal of Physiology (London)*, 232, 331–356.

Bourtchuladze, R., Frenguelli, B., Blendy, J., Cioffi, D., Schutz, G., & Silva, A. J. (1994). Deficient long-term memory in mice with a targeted mutation of the cAMP-responsive element-binding protein. *Cell*, 79, 59–68.

Braun, A. P., & Schulman, H. (1995). The multifunctional calcium/calmodulin-dependent protein kinase: From form to function. *Annual Review of Physiology*, 57, 417–445.

Brun, V. H., Ytterbø, K., Morris, R. G., Moser, M.-B., & Moser, E. I. (2001). Retrograde amnesia for spatial memory induced by NMDA receptor-mediated long-term potentiation. *Journal of Neuroscience*, 21, 356–362.

Davis, S., Butcher, S. P., & Morris, R. G. (1992). The NMDA receptor antagonist D-2-amino-5-phosphonopentanoate (D-AP5) impairs spatial learning and LTP *in vivo* at intracerebral concentrations comparable to those that block LTP *in vitro*. *Journal of Neuroscience*, 12, 21–34.

Forrest, D., Yuzaki, M., Soares, H. D., Ng, L., Luk, D. C., Sheng, M., Stewart, C. L., Morgan, J. I., Connor, J. A., & Curran, T. (1994). Targeted disruption of NMDA receptor 1 gene abolishes NMDA response and results in neonatal death. *Neuron*, 13, 325–338.

Giese, K. P., Fedorov, N. B., Filipkowski, R. K., & Silva, A. J. (1998). Autophosphorylation at Thr286 of the alpha calcium–calmodulin kinase II in LTP and learning. *Science*, 279, 870–873.

Gossen, M., & Bujard, H. (1992). Tight control of gene expression in mammalian cells by tetracycline-responsive promoters. *Proceedings of the National Academy of Sciences USA*, 89, 5547–5551.

Grant, S. G, O'Dell, T. J., Karl, K. A., Stein, P. L., Soriano, P., & Kandel, E. R. (1992). Impaired long-term potentiation, spatial learning, and hippocampal development in *fyn* mutant mice. *Science*, 258, 1903–1910.

Huang, Y. Y., Kandel, E. R., Varshavsky, L., Brandon, E. P., & Qi, M., Idzerda, R. L., McKnight, G. S., & Bourtchouladze, R. (1995). A genetic test of the effects of mutations in PKA on mossy fiber LTP and its relation to spatial and contextual learning. *Cell*, 83, 1211–1222.

LeDoux, J. E. (1995). Emotion: Clues from the brain. *Annual Review of Psychology*, 46, 209–235.

Lee, P. S., & Lee, K. H. (2000). Genomic analysis. *Current Opinion in Biotechnology*, 11, 171–175.

Li, Y., Erzurumlu, R. S., Chen, C., Jhaveri, S., & Tonegawa, S. (1994). Whisker-related neuronal patterns fail to develop in the trigeminal brainstem nuclei of NMDAR1 knockout mice. *Cell*, 76, 427–437.

Malenka, R. C., & Nicoll, R. A. (1999). Long-term potentiation—a decade of progress? *Science*, 285, 1870–1874.

Mayford, M., Bach, M. E., Huang, Y. Y., Wang, L., Hawkins, R. D., & Kandel, E. R. (1996). Control of memory formation through regulated expression of a CamKII transgene. *Science*, 274, 1678–1683.

Mayford, M., & Kandel E. R. (1999). Genetic approaches to memory storage. *Trends in Genetics*, 15, 463–470.

Mayford, M., Wang J., Kandel E. R., & O'Dell, T. J. (1995). CamKII regulates the frequency-response function of hippocampal synapses for the production of both LTD and LTP. *Cell*, 81, 891–904.

McHugh, T. J., Blum, K. I., Tsien, J. Z., Tonegawa, S., & Wilson, M. A. (1996). Impaired hippocampal representation of space in CA1-specific NMDAR1 knockout mice. *Cell*, 87, 1339–1349.

Moser, M.-B., & Moser, E. I. (2000). Pretraining and the function of hippocampal long-term potentiation. *Neuron*, 26, 559–561.

Nosten-Bertrand, M., Errington, M. L., Murphy, K. P., Tokugawa, Y., & Barboni, E., Kozlova, E., Michalovich, D., Morris, R. G., Silver, J., Stewart, C. L., Bliss, T. V., & Morris, R. J. (1996). Normal spatial learning despite regional inhibition of LTP in mice lacking Thy-1. *Nature*, 379, 826–829.

Pettit, D. L., Perlman, S., & Malinow, R. (1994). Potentiated transmission and prevention of further LTP by increased CamKII activity in postsynaptic hippocampal slice neurons. *Science, 266,* 1881–1885.

Rampon, C., Tang, Y. P., Goodhouse, J., Shimizu, E., Kyin, M., & Tsien, J. Z. (2000). Enrichment induces structural changes and recovery from nonspatial memory deficits in CA1 NMDAR1-knockout mice. *Nature Neuroscience, 3,* 238–244.

Ribar, T. J., Rodriguiz, R. M., Khiroug, L., Wetsel, W. C., Augustine, G. J., & Means, A. R. (2000). Cerebellar defects in Ca2+/calmodulin kinase IV-deficient mice. *Journal of Neuroscience, 20,* RC107.

Rotenberg, A., Mayford, M., Hawkins, R. D., Kandel, E. R., & Muller, R. U. (1996). Mice expressing activated CaMKII lack low frequency LTP and do not form stable place cells in the CA1 region of the hippocampus. *Cell, 87,* 1351–1361.

Saucier, D., & Cain, D. P. (1995). Spatial learning without NMDA receptor-dependent long-term potentiation. *Nature, 378,* 186–189.

Silva, A. J., Paylor R., Wehner, J. M., & Tonegawa, S. (1992). Impaired spatial learning in alpha-calcium–calmodulin kinase II mutant mice. *Science, 257,* 206–211.

Silva, A. J, Stevens, C. F., Tonegawa, S., & Wang, Y. (1992). Deficient hippocampal long-term potentiation in alpha-calcium–calmodulin kinase II mutant mice. *Science, 257,* 201–206.

Smythe, J. W., Colom, L. V., & Bland, B. H. (1992). The extrinsic modulation of hippocampal theta depends on the coactivation of cholinergic and GABA-ergic medial septal inputs. *Neuroscience and Biobehavioral Reviews, 16,* 289–308.

Steele, R. J., & Morris R. G. (1999). Delay-dependent impairment of a matching-to-place task with chronic and intrahippocampal infusion of the NMDA-antagonist D-AP5. *Hippocampus, 9,* 118–136.

Tsien, J. Z., Chen, D. F., Gerber, D., Tom, C., Mercer, E. H., Anderson, D. J., Mayford, M., & Kandel, E. R. (1996). Subregion- and cell type-restricted gene knockout in mouse brain. *Cell, 87,* 1317–1326.

Tsien, J. Z, Huerta, P. T., & Tonegawa, S. (1996). The essential role of hippocampal CA1 NMDA receptor-dependent synaptic plasticity in spatial memory. *Cell, 87,* 1327–1338.

Zamanillo, D., Sprengel, R., Hvalby, O., Jensen, V., Burnashev, N., Rozov, A., Kaiser, K. M., Koster, H. J., Borchardt, T., Worley, P., Lubke, J., Frotscher, M., Kelly, P. H., Sommer, B., Andersen, P., Seeburg, P. H., & Sakmann, B. (1999). Importance of AMPA receptors for hippocampal synaptic plasticity but not for spatial learning. *Science, 284,* 1805–1811.

38

Testing Episodic-Like Memory in Animals

NICOLA S. CLAYTON and DANIEL P. GRIFFITHS

The idea that there are many forms of memory or memory systems was first suggested by Maine de Biran over 200 years ago and he went to great lengths to explain these ideas (see Maine de Biran, 1929; Schacter & Tulving, 1994). Despite this, it is really during the past 30 years that the taxonomy of memory systems has proliferated (see, e.g., Weiskrantz, 1990; Squire, Knowlton, & Musen, 1993). Of all these categories, episodic memory is the only one that has been thought to be unique to humans (see, e.g., Tulving, 1983). Episodic memory involves the encoding and storage of memories concerned with unique, personal experiences and their subsequent recall (Tulving, 1983). According to Tulving's classical definition, episodic memory "receives and stores information about temporally dated episodes or events, and temporal–spatial relations among these events" (Tulving, 1972, p. 385). Thus episodic memory provides information about the "what" and "when" of events ("temporally dated experiences"), as well as "where" they happened ("temporal–spatial relations"). Episodic memory is also the most fragile type of memory: It is the last to be acquired in childhood (Perner & Ruffman, 1995; Pillemer & White, 1989), the first to be lost as we age (Herlitz & Forsell, 1996; Nilsson, Backman, Erngrund, & Nyberg, 1997), and the most susceptible to brain traumas (see, e.g., Milner, Corkin, & Teuber, 1968; Scoville & Milner, 1957) and neurodegenerative diseases such as Alzheimer's disease (see, e.g., Henderson, Paganini-Hill, Emanuel, Dunn, & Buckwalter, 1994; Kimura, 1995; Sherwin, 1988). Tests of episodic memory capabilities are therefore used as behavioral markers for the onset of these debilitating diseases of the mind.

Many researchers have suggested that episodic memory is unique to humans (Tulving & Markowitsch, 1998), in part because of the reliance on language for testing this type of recall. Recent work on memory for cache sites in food-storing jays, however, provides a working model for testing components of episodic memory in animals in the absence of language (Clayton & Dickinson, 1998). These findings provide an exciting new model for bridging the gap between human and animal studies of memory.

STUDYING EPISODIC MEMORY IN ANIMALS

Tulving and Markowitsch (1998) define episodic memory, at least in part, in terms of the conscious experience of recollection. This definition makes it impossible to demonstrate this form of memory in animals, because there are no agreed-upon behavioral markers of conscious experience. Other attempts to define episodic memory without reference to consciousness do not resolve this problem. Morris and Frey (1997) asserted that to show event memory (a synonym for episodic memory), "a task should distinguish between changes in behaviour that occur because an animal remembers some prior event and changes that merely happen because some prior event has occurred" (p. 1495). This definition also lacks an agreed-upon behavioral measure of the experience of recollection.

The dilemma can be resolved to some degree by adopting Tulving's (1972) original definition of episodic memory when referring to animals: the retrieval of information about "where" a unique event took place, "what" occurred during the episode, and "when" it happened. The merit of this definition is that the simultaneous retrieval and integration of information about these three features of a single, unique experience may be demonstrated behaviorally in animals, without the need for language. Contemporary definitions of episodic memory require a demonstration of "autonoetic" consciousness (Tulving & Markowitsch, 1998). This special kind of self-knowing awareness differs from the "noetic" consciousness that is involved with the retrieval of nonepisodic declarative information. The distinction is based on the fact that human subjects can distinguish between recalling past personal experience and remembering an impersonal declarative fact. In view of this, the two types of consciousness can be defined operationally in terms of remembering and knowing; remembering a specific event requires autonoetic consciousness, whereas knowing a fact is noetic in nature. Remembering getting soaked in the rain in Cambridge last Monday is an example of episodic memory, but knowing that it often rains in England is not. In the absence of language, this feature of episodic memory is impossible to demonstrate in animals. We therefore refer to an animal's ability to fulfill the behavioral criteria regardless of autonoetic consciousness as "episodic-like" memory (Clayton & Dickinson, 1998).

Elsewhere (Griffiths, Dickinson, & Clayton, 1999), we have reviewed possible examples of episodic memory in animals and their alternative accounts (see Table 38.1). Typically, the memory tasks that have been used either (1) require the animal to remember only a single feature of the episode, as opposed to integrating information about several features; or (2) give the animal repeated training experiences, so that the animal need not remember a single specific past experience. The animal can often solve the task by simply recognizing which object is the most familiar, as opposed to recalling the specific features of an event. For example, monkeys can be trained to choose between two complex objects on the basis of whether they are the same as (delayed-matching-to-sample [DMS] tasks) or different from (delayed-nonmatching-to-sample [DNMS] tasks) an object they were shown some time previously. Although the animal may have recalled the events episodically, the simpler explanation is that the monkey learned to choose—or avoid—the most familiar object. There is a distinct difference between the feeling that a stimulus is familiar and an episodic recollection of where and when it has been seen before (Aggleton & Brown, 1999; Mandler, 1980); thus a face can appear highly familiar without any recall of where and when one has previously met its owner. Because the monkeys are required to recognize a stimulus, but not to recollect where and when it had been seen, these matching tasks are readily solved by familiarity rather than episodic recall. If the animals solve the task by familiarity rather than episodic recall, then they should learn the task more quickly when novel objects are used. Mishkin and Delacour (1975) did find that the monkeys learned more rapidly when novel objects were used, supporting this account.

A different approach is to consider cases in nature in which an animal might benefit from the capacity to remember the "what, where, and when" of individual past episodes.

TABLE 38.1. Episodic and Declarative Memory: Defining Features

Declarative memory (episodic and semantic common features)	Episodic memory (unique features)
• Large, complex, and highly structured, with fast encoding operations. • Can receive factual information through different sensory modalities and internally generated sources. • Stored information is representational (isomorphic with what is in the world) and propositional (can be described symbolically). • Information has truth value, can be accessed and expressed flexibly, and can be used as a basis for inferences. • Processing is highly sensitive to context. • System is cognitive (as opposed to behavioral): Information can be "thought about." • Behavioral expression of retrieval products is optional rather than obligatory. • System interacts closely with other brain and behavior systems, such as language, emotion, affect, and reasoning. • Dependent on medial temporal lobe and diencephalic structures such as the thalamic nuclei.	• Concerned with conscious recollection of specific past experiences. • Is oriented, at the time of retrieval, to the past. • Is accompanied by "autonoetic" consciousness, which enables "remembering" (relating to personal experience) as opposed to "knowing." • Embedded relationship with semantic ("knowing" memory: Episodic remembering always implies semantic knowing, whereas knowing does not imply remembering. • Development occurs later than semantic abilities in children. • More vulnerable to a number of brain pathologies and aging. • Is dependent on frontal lobes in a way that declacative memory is not: Episodic retrieval is associated with changes in regional cerebral blood flow in right prefrontal cortex rarely caused by semantic recall. • Unique to humans?

Note. Data from Tulving and Markowitsch (1998) by Griffiths, Dickinson, and Clayton (1999).

These criteria are probably met by several behaviors (Clayton & Griffiths, in press). One candidate is food caching: Having hidden hundreds of seeds throughout its territory, an animal relies on memory to recover its caches, weeks, or even months later (Shettleworth, 1995). Although it is well established that food-storing species remember the location of their caches, there are good reasons to believe that they encode much richer representations of their caches, including what the contents are and whether or not these items are perishable (see, e.g., Griffiths & Clayton, 2001). In order to fulfill the behavioral criteria for episodic memory, animals must be able to encode information about a caching or recovery episode based on a single, personal experience that occurred in the past, and then accurately recall the information about what, where, and when this particular past event occurred.

EPISODIC-LIKE MEMORY IN FOOD-STORING BIRDS

In a series of experiments, we used a food-caching paradigm to examine the episodic-like memory capabilities of scrub jays. We tested their ability to keep track of the fate of their caches either in terms of remembering what was cached, where, and whether or not it had been recovered; or in terms of whether or not the cached items had perished. In order to ensure that each episode was unique, the birds cached and recovered from trial-unique trays. The experimental procedure is illustrated in Figure 38.1. The first experiment assessed how richly the events that occur during a caching episode are encoded by contrasting memory for caching with that for recovery. Both caching and recovery episodes involve memory for the location and content of the same food items, but the episodes differ in terms of

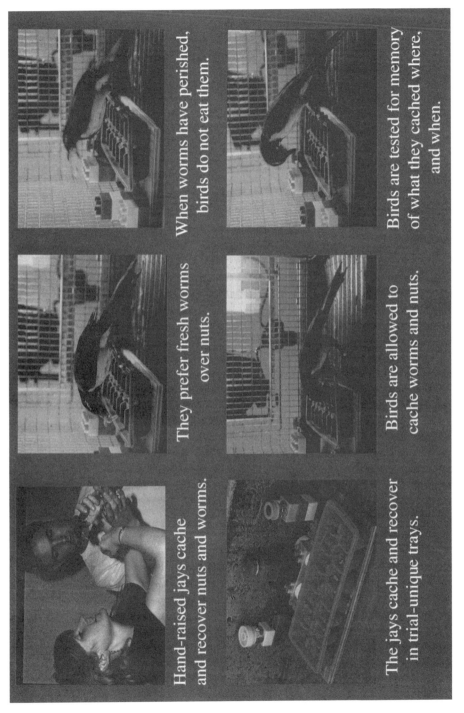

Hand-raised jays cache and recover nuts and worms.

They prefer fresh worms over nuts.

When worms have perished, birds do not eat them.

The jays cache and recover in trial-unique trays.

Birds are allowed to cache worms and nuts.

Birds are tested for memory of what they cached where, and when.

FIGURE 38.1. A photograph of one of the food-caching experiments using scrub jays (*Aphelocoma coerulescens*). Hand-raised subjects cached both worms and peanuts in plastic ice-cube trays, which consisted of a 2 × 7 array of cube molds filled with sand, each of which was a potential cache site. The trays were attached to a wooden board and were surrounded by a visuospatially distinct structure made of Legos. Different trays were used on every trial, and were placed in the birds' home cage at the time of caching and recovery.

which type of action is performed (namely, caching or recovering caches) and whether the food cache is intact at the end of the episode (after caching) or whether the cache site is now empty (after recovery).

The birds were first allowed to cache peanuts in one side of two different trays, and to cache dog biscuits in the other side of both trays. They were then allowed to recover the peanuts from one tray and to recover the dog biscuits from the other tray. In a final test, both sides of both trays were presented to the birds simultaneously. Caches were removed prior to this test trial and the trays were filled with fresh sand, so that no extraneous cues were present and the birds therefore had to rely on their memory. If they could remember what type of food they had cached in each of the sites, could recall what they had recovered from each site, and could integrate these two sources of information, then during the test trial birds ought to go to the tray that should still contain their preferred food (Clayton & Dickinson, 1999a).

The relative preference of the foods at recovery was manipulated by prefeeding the jays with one of the two food types, because prefeeding of a specific food selectively reduces the subsequent value of that food in terms of both eating and caching (Clayton & Dickinson, 1999b). They were prefed peanuts or dog biscuits in powdered form, to ensure that they could not cache during the prefeeding phase. Those that had been prefed peanuts preferentially searched in the cache sites in which they had cached dog biscuits, and selectively searched only in those sites from which the birds had not recovered dog biscuits during the previous recovery phase (i.e., the intact dog biscuit sites). Likewise, those birds that had been prefed dog biscuits preferentially searched in the intact peanut sites. This ability to encode what action occurred, and whether a cache site still contains food, enables an animal to keep track of "what" is cached and "where" across a series of caching and recovery episodes (Clayton & Dickinson, 1999a).

The behavioral criterion for episodic memory also requires the animal to recall information about "when" the caching episode occurred. We addressed this issue in a series of experiments by asking whether jays could remember "when" as well as "what" and "where." Jays in the "degrade" group were given the opportunity to learn that certain perishable food types (such as worms) degrade with time. Jays in the "replenish" group did not have the opportunity to learn that these perishable foods degrade over time, because fresh food was put in place of the degraded food prior to recovery. The birds were then allowed to choose between two types of cache sites on the basis of whether or not their contents were likely to have perished, based on the time since caching.

The jays were allowed to cache perishable worms and nonperishable peanuts either in two sides of the same tray (Clayton & Dickinson, 1998) or in two different trays (Clayton & Dickinson, 1999b). During a series of four training trials, the jays were allowed to recover their caches either 4 or 124 hours later. The birds in the degrade group rapidly learned to avoid sites where they had cached perishable worms if the retention interval was such that the worms would have degraded (124 hours); they preferred to recover the nonperishable peanuts that they had previously cached. This switch in preference to recover peanuts as opposed to worms was apparent after just two or three trials. When the worms had been cached only 4 hours earlier, so that they had not had time to degrade, then the jays in the degrade group preferentially recovered worms over their alternative, nonperishable food caches. Birds in the replenish group, which did not have the chance to learn about perishability, preferentially recovered the worms regardless of the retention interval between caching and recovery, and there was no change in behavior across trials.

As in the previous experiment, the caches were removed prior to the recovery test trials, to establish whether or not jays could remember where and when the worms and peanuts had been cached. Performance on the test trials gave the same results as during training: Birds in the replenish group always preferred to search in worm sites, whereas birds in the degrade group preferred to search worm sites if the worms had been cached only 4 hours earlier but searched in peanut sites if the worms had been cached 124 hours earlier. The results of this second experiment suggest that the birds could remember not only what they cached where, but also the relative time since a particular caching event took place (Clayton & Dickinson, 1998, 1999c).

It could be argued, however, that the birds only needed to remember "where" and "when" they cached, because birds in the degrade group could learn to search in the locations where they remembered caching worms 4 hours previously and to avoid those sites if they remembered caching them 124 hours earlier, so that searches to the peanut sites were simply default responses. To determine whether the jays could remember the contents of the caches as well as where they cached and when, a third experiment was conducted in which the same birds cached peanuts (P) and perishable mealworms (M) on P/M trials, and cached peanuts (P) and perishable crickets (C) on P/C trials (Clayton, Yu, & Dickinson, 2001). The trays were always trial-unique, and both the side of the tray in which they cached the various foods, and the order in which they cached peanuts and perishable items, were counterbalanced across trials. On each trial, the birds were allowed to cache the perishable items in one side of the tray and the nonperishable items in the opposite side of the same tray. The jays then recovered their caches from the tray after retention intervals of 4, 28, and 100 hours, but the perishable mealworms decayed at a faster rate than the crickets.

During training trials, birds in the degrade group learned that the mealworms were only fresh 4 hours after caching, whereas crickets were fresh after 4 and 28 hours, but degraded after a retention interval of 100 hours. As in the previous experiment, birds in the replenish group always encountered unperished food items. Preliminary feeding tests had established that jays prefer both perishable food items over peanuts, but that they like mealworms more than crickets. It was hypothesized that all the birds should selectively recover mealworms on P/M trials and crickets on P/C trials, when those items were fresh. The jays in the degrade group should switch their preference to peanuts when the mealworms were cached 28 or 100 hours earlier on P/M trials, and when the crickets were cached 100 hours earlier on P/C trials. The birds were given only four P/C and P/M trials at each retention interval, because the birds in the degrade group acquired this information about rates of perishability after just two or three trials of each type. The jays in the degrade group reversed their search preference when the retention interval was such that the perishable foods would have degraded, even on test trials in which no food was present at recovery. These results established that the jays relied on memory as opposed to visual, olfactory, or tactile cues that might emanate directly from the sand covering the hidden food.

Without further training, the birds were given a further test trial (i.e., no food present during recovery) after they had cached mealworms in one side of the tray and crickets in the other side of the same tray—a caching condition that they had not experienced previously. On this test trial, they were allowed to search for these caches either 4 hours later (when both foods were still fresh) or 28 hours later (when the mealworms had decayed but the crickets were still fresh). Since jays prefer fresh mealworms over crickets, it was predicted that the birds in the replenish group should always search preferentially in the sites in which they had cached the mealworms. If they could apply their knowledge about the relative perishability profiles of mealworms and crickets derived from earlier P/M and P/C trials to this novel M/C trial, the degrade group should search selectively for mealworms when these had been cached 4 hours ago, but switch to searching for crickets when the mealworms had been cached 28 hours previously. The results confirmed these expectations, demonstrating that the birds could remember not only where and when they hid their caches, but also enough information about the contents of the caches to allow them to distinguish between mealworm and cricket cache sites. Furthermore, the results suggest that the birds could flexibly use the information learned in one context and apply it to a new caching condition.

In order to search preferentially for mealworms during the 4-hour test trials and for crickets during the 28-hour test trials, at the time of recovery birds in the degrade group must have been able to recognize the trays in which they had cached mealworms and crickets earlier. Like many other tests of memory, the problem is that this task can be solved either by recollection or by familiarity. Familiarity is an automatic process based on the perceptual characteristics of the stimuli that allows an individual to distinguish previously experienced stimuli from novel ones, but does not require recollection of any of the details of the original presentation of the stimuli. Thus the jays may have based their decision of when to search for worms on the relative familiarity of the two trays, as opposed to recalling what they cached where and when. If this were the case, then birds in the degrade group could have learned to search in mealworm sites on the 4-hour trials (when the tray was relatively familiar), and learned to search in cricket sites when the tray had not been seen for 28 hours (and was therefore relatively unfamiliar).

To test whether the jays could remember what, where, and when in the absence of using tray familiarity as a cue, the same birds were given a further pair of test trials in which they cached mealworms in one side of the tray and crickets in the other side of the same tray. On the M-C trial, birds cached mealworms first; then, instead of caching crickets immediately afterward, there was a retention interval of 24 hours between the two caching events, followed by a further gap of 4 hours before the recovery test phase (in which no food was present, so we could test for memory). Thus the mealworms were 28 hours old and the crickets were only 4 hours old at the time of recovery on the M-C trial. The reverse order of caching was enforced on the C-M trial, so that the crickets were 28 hours old and the mealworms were still fresh, having been cached only 4 hours earlier. If the birds in the degrade group were relying on familiarity to solve the task, then they should preferentially search for mealworms on both M-C and C-M trials, because on both recovery test trials the tray had been seen only 4 hours earlier. By contrast, if the birds remembered how long ago each type of food had been cached, then they should only search for mealworm cache sites on C-M trials (when the mealworms had been cached 4 hours earlier) and switch to cricket caches on M-C trials (when the mealworms had been cached 28 hours earlier and should therefore have degraded). The degrade group showed this switch in preference from mealworm sites on C-M trials to cricket sites on M-C trials; as expected, the replenish group always searched in mealworm sites. We therefore conclude that the birds in the degrade group must have remembered the time at which they cached the mealworms, and in a way that cannot be explained by relative familiarity of the trays (Clayton et al., 2001).

Taken together, these results show that jays can episodically recall what was cached, where it was cached, and when this particular caching event occurred in the past. In addition to remembering information about the "what, where, and when" of a caching event, jays can also remember what they recovered and from where, differentiate between memories of caching and recovering, and update the information about the current status of their caches, based on whether or not they have already recovered that particular cache. When all this information is integrated together, it is sufficient to enable a jay to isolate what was cached and what was recovered, where, and how long ago; functionally, the animal has enough information to recall the episode of caching a specific item (Griffiths et al., 1999). These results fulfill the behavioral criteria for episodic memory (Tulving, 1983).

A MAMMALIAN MODEL

The extent to which these behavioral features of episodic-like memory in birds resemble human episodic memory remains an open question. Clearly, there is a pressing need to develop experimental tests of episodic-like memory in other species, particularly non-human mammals This task is important, because common features of memory in species whose evolution diverged millions of years ago may point to fundamental mechanisms of how the brain learns and retains information. The last shared ancestor between birds and humans lived about 250 million years ago. The fact that some birds at least are capable of episodic-like memory opens up new avenues of research concerning where and how episodic memory is formed and stored in the brain. It may therefore help us understand how space, time, and events are represented and remembered in the brain.

Many rodents store and recover food. Laboratory rats, for example, will readily cache in captivity if deprived of food (see, e.g., Hunt & Willoughby, 1939; Wolfe, 1939). Given the excitement and potential power of transgenic and knockout procedures for investigating the genetic and molecular bases of learning and memory in laboratory rodents, not to mention the wealth of knowledge about the anatomy and neurophysiology of the rodent hippocampus, an obvious next step is to develop a rat or mouse model of episodic-like memory based on the food-caching bird paradigm. The development of a rodent model system could make an important contribution to our understanding of the neural, molecular, and behavioral mechanisms of mammalian episodic memory (see Griffiths & Clayton, 2001). It may also provide exciting new approaches for exploring the treatment of human subjects suffering from memory deficits.

We have carried out two (hitherto unreported) studies on memory for caches in rats. The rats were maintained on a reversed short-day light cycle, with training taking place in the dark phase. All animals were male, and were kept on a 23-hour deprivation schedule. These conditions are optimal for inducing caching behavior (Vander Wall, 1990). To demonstrate that the rats were capable of caching food items and accurately recovering them in the lab, they were placed in an arena and allowed to explore four trial-unique caching trays, which were placed one at a time in the arena for 5 minutes each. Each tray was put in a distinct spatial location, and walls of Legos placed around each tray made them visually and topographically unique. The rats were given the opportunity to eat and cache dog biscuits in only one of the trays. The bowl of dog food kibbles was placed in the center of the arena; rather than eating directly from the bowl, rats typically carried the food to the safety of the tray, which was placed at the center of one of the walls of the arena. There they ate a few kibbles and then cached several more in the wood shavings within the tray. Each rat was then removed from the arena and placed back in its home cage. All four trays were returned simultaneously 24 hours later. To induce cache recovery behavior, the hungry rat was simply allowed back into the arena, and no food was present other than that which the animal had cached previously within the tray. The experimenter observed the rat's behavior during a 10-minute recovery period by looking through the observation window.

After three training trials, the rats were given a test trial in which no food was available during recovery. As with the jay studies, this procedure ensured that the rats had to rely on memory, instead of using any visual or olfactory cues that might signal the location of the food. In both training and test trials, the number of looks in each tray, the number of entries into each tray, and the time spent in each tray were recorded. A look was recorded when a rat faced the tray with its eye level above that of the Lego walls. An entry was only recorded as soon as the rat's front paws touched the sawdust, and an entry was deemed to be over when the rat's back paws left the tray (Figure 38.2).

The results of the probe test showed that the probability that the rats made their first look in the correct tray was significantly greater than that expected from random searching (binomial test, $p = .0129$). As shown in the top panel of Figure 38.3, the rats entered the correct tray significantly more often than the other three trays combined (two-sample, one-tailed t test, $t = 3.6$, $df = 7$, $p = .0044$). The bottom panel of Figure 38.3 also shows that the rats spent significantly more time in the correct tray than the other three trays combined (two-sample, one-tailed t test, $t = 3.4$, $df = 7$, $p = .0057$). Furthermore, the time spent per visit in the correct tray was significantly greater than the mean time spent in each of the other three trays ($t = 3.4$, $df = 7$, $p = .0057$).

Once it was shown that rats could cache and accurately recover these cached items using memory alone, a second experiment was conducted to show that rats could also remember the location and identity of two different food types. In Experiment 2, the rats were given the opportunity to explore four trays in succession, but the procedure differed from the first experiment in that the rats could eat and cache in two of the trays; they cached banana chips in one tray and Brazil nuts in a different tray. During the recovery phase of the training trials, they were allowed to explore the four trays simultaneously and to eat and recover any cached food from the two trays. After seven training trials, a test trial was conducted in the same way as Experiment 1, with one difference. Immediately prior to the recovery phase, rats were prefed either banana chips or Brazil nuts for 1 hour. Rather than relying on an intrinsic preference for one food over the other, we therefore devalued one of the two food types by allowing the animals to eat only one of the two food types, so that they became sated on that specific food but would still consume a second food type. If the rats remembered which food was cached where, then, as a result of specific satiety, they should preferentially search for the food that had not been prefed.

The results clearly showed that this pattern was observed: The probability that the rats made their first look in the correct tray was significantly greater than that expected from random searching (binomial test, $p = .0013$). As shown in Figure 38.4, the rats made more entries into the tray containing the non-prefed food caches than into the tray in which they had cached the prefed food (matched-pair t test, $t = 3.6$, $df = 8$, $p = .007$), and spent more time in the non-prefed food tray relative to the prefed tray ($t = 4.615$, $df = 8$, $p = .017$). These results show that rats can remember the location and specific contents of their food caches. The question remains as to whether they can also integrate information about how long ago the caches were made. If they can, then they satisfy the behavioral criteria for possessing episodic-like memory in the same way that jays do—by demonstrating that they can recall specific, trial-unique events about what they buried in the sand, as well as where and when they cached it.

IMPLICATIONS

There is a large gap between human and animal studies of memory, and in particular the extent to which nonhuman animals possess episodic-like memory. This is principally attributable to the absence of suitable tasks that can isolate episodic memory, without the reliance on language for testing episodic recall. We now believe, however, that the food-caching paradigm tests the ability of an animal to recall what happened, where, and when,

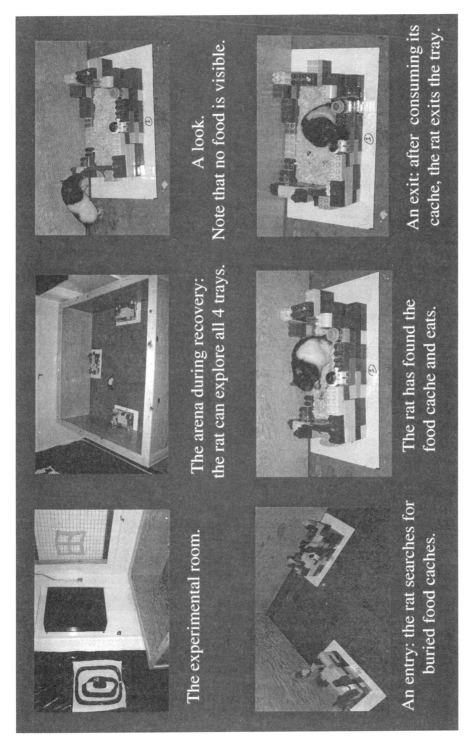

The experimental room.

The arena during recovery:
the rat can explore all 4 trays.

A look.
Note that no food is visible.

An entry: the rat searches for
buried food caches.

The rat has found the
food cache and eats.

An exit: after consuming its
cache, the rat exits the tray.

FIGURE 38.2. Cache recovery behavior in rats. The photographs show the experimental setup during the recovery phase of a trial. In this experiment, the rat is tested for its ability to remember which one of four trays contains food. The rat can freely explore all four trays. We recorded the total number of looks each rat made, the number of looks before entering each tray, and the total time spent in each tray.

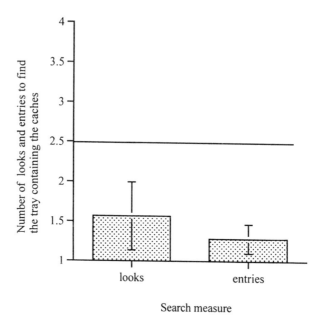

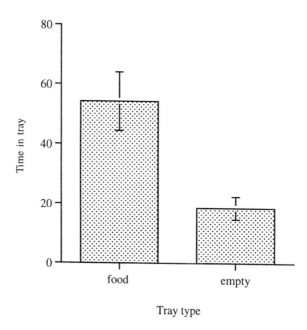

FIGURE 38.3. The results of the first food-caching memory paradigm in rats, which tested whether the animals could remember the locations of their caches. The top panel shows the mean and standard error of the number of entries to the tray in which each rat had cached and to the other trays on the test trial in which no food was present during recovery. The bottom panel shows the mean and standard error of the amount of time spent in the trays.

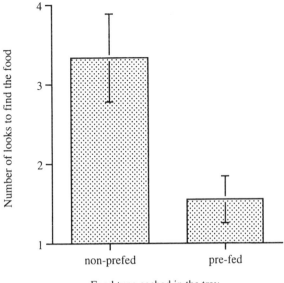

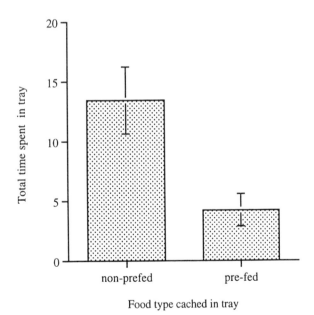

FIGURE 38.4. The results of the second food-caching memory paradigm in rats, which tested whether the animals could remember the contents and locations of their caches. The top panel shows the mean and standard error of the number of entries to the tray containing the non-prefed food. The bottom panel shows the mean and standard error of the amount of time spent in the prefed and non-prefed trays.

based on a trial-unique experience. The fact that this paradigm can be adapted for rats opens up the possibility of investigating the neural basis of episodic-like memory.

Possible Neurobiological Studies

Human amnesia studies suggest that the hippocampus plays a crucial role in the recall of episodic memory (e.g., Vargha-Khadem et al., 1997; Zola-Morgan, Squire, & Amaral, 1986). The hippocampus has also been heavily implicated in solving spatial tasks in animals (Eichenbaum, Dudchenko, Wood, Shapiro, & Tanila, 1999; Morris, Garrud, Rawlins, & O'Keefe, 1982; O'Keefe & Nadel, 1978) and in humans (Maguire et al., 2000). Although spatial memory may contribute to the "where" component of episodic memory, the question remains as to what cognitive mechanisms relate spatial and episodic memory. One possibility is that the hippocampus is critical for integrating the individual components that need to be remembered to perform a "what, where, and when" task, resulting in an understanding of the relationships between stimuli (see, e.g., Eichenbaum et al., 1999). In this regard, it is important to note that rodents with selective hippocampal lesions are deficient in learning some nonepisodic tasks, including spatial tasks (such as learning the location of the hidden platform in a water maze—see, e.g., Morris et al., 1982) and nonspatial tasks (which involve learning and inferring the relationships between odors—see, e.g., Bunsey & Eichenbaum, 1996; Dusek & Eichenbaum, 1997).

The food-caching memory paradigm provides an interesting model with which to test these dissociations. It contains a strong spatial component—that is, "where" the food is hidden. It is therefore reasonable to assume that the hippocampus is involved in processing the spatial element of the episodic-like memory task. If we were to lesion the hippocampus and test the animals on the task as it stands, they may fail to solve the task due to an incapability to process episodic-like information. A simpler explanation, however, would be that they merely cannot remember where they cached the food in the absence of the hippocampus. This potential confound may not apply to the food-caching memory paradigm in rodents, however, because in all of the experiments with rats described in this chapter, the rats were aided in the memory task of relocating the food by the presence of a variety of cues that differed in both location and features—both on the walls of the experimental room in which the rats were tested, and on caching trays whose Lego walls had unique topographies and color patterns. In terms of the experiments performed, the presence of these different types of cues does not detract from the conclusion that the rats used some form of memory to relocate the cached food.

Given the fragility of episodic memory, an understanding of how the hippocampus is involved in the various stages of memory processing may provide new avenues for the treatment of human patients suffering from age-induced memory loss and neurodegenerative diseases of the mind. The advantage of using the food-caching memory model is that we can test involvement of the hippocampus and other interconnected brain regions in the integration of information about "what, where, and when," as well as the individual components of this memory.

Tests of Episodic Memory That Do Not Rely on Language

One advantage of the food-caching memory paradigm is that it does not rely on language for testing episodic recall. In principle, this paradigm could also be adapted to test human memory. Given that episodic memory is probably the last form of memory to be acquired in humans, it has been difficult to determine the extent to which this form of memory is developmentally dependent upon language skills. We believe that this model could be used to investigate the development of episodic memory in children, and therefore provide an alternative or addition to the deferred imitation task that has been used so successfully to test the ability of young children to remember specific past events (Bauer, 1996). In the deferred imitation task, a child observes an adult perform a sequence of actions using a variety of props. After a delay, the child is given the opportunity to imitate what he or she has seen the demonstrator do, using the same props. Bauer and her colleagues have shown that children as young as 13 months of age can remember these specific events and accurately imitate the sequence of prop-related actions performed by the demonstrator, even over time periods of several months (for a review, see Bauer, 1996).

Developing the jay episodic-like memory task may have the potential to provide some exciting new developments in this area, because it may allow experimenters to test when the various components of episodic memory develop in young children (e.g., whether memories for "when" develop later than memories for "what" and "where"). Such tests can also be used to test not only whether young children are able to remember the order in which a specific sequence of actions occurred, but also how that information might be flexibly deployed to solve new problems. Some tests of this nature, which are based on the experiments with scrub jays, are already underway (J. Russell, personal communication, November 2000). The children see an experimenter place an attractive toy in one of two empty boxes and then place a second identical toy in the other box. The experimenter then removes one of the toys, so that only one box still contains a toy; 30 minutes later, the child is allowed to choose one of the two boxes. Children above 21 months of age consistently choose the box containing the toy (i.e., significantly above-chance-level performance), whereas those 18 months of age perform at chance levels, and those below 18 months of age are below chance-level performance. Russell suggests that the ability to remember events develops at about 18 months of age, and that the below-chance-level performance of the younger children is due to the fact that they have learned that the box that the experimenter uses twice is more strongly associated with toys, even though after the second visit the box no longer contains a toy. The "what, where, and when" paradigm used for jays could also be adapted for tests of human memory. To determine when children are able to recall the "when" as well as the "what" and "where" of an event, subjects of different ages could be allowed to hide various treats and recover them after different time intervals. Imagine the scenario in which a child hides a slice of chocolate cake under one box, and a sealed packet of graham crackers under another box. When given the choice of selecting just one of the hidden items, a child with episodic-like memory capabilities should recover the slice of chocolate cake after a short interval, but should choose the biscuits over a longer time interval, when the cake has become stale. This type of task would allow one to test the rate at which memory for events develops, without the confound of language development.

The food-caching task could also be used to test the memory capabilities of adult and young patients with speech difficulties (e.g., aphasia). The development of an effective test of episodic memory in language-impaired patients would allow us to distinguish between neurological deficits that cause language impairments and those resulting in a disruption of episodic memory. The challenge for the future is to develop other tasks that may capture some of the critical features of episodic memory that do not rely on language, thereby providing the opportunity to investigate the neural bases of episodic-like memory, and the similarities and differences between this form of memory and that possessed by healthy human adults. This in turn may provide invaluable insights into how and why episodic memory has evolved in humans, and why it is so fragile.

ACKNOWLEDGMENTS

This research was supported by grants from the National Institutes of Health (No. NS35465 and No. NOT-99-022), the Whitehall Foundation, the American Federation for Aging Research, the University of California–Davis faculty research fund, and the Grindley Fund to N. S. Clayton. D. P. Griffiths was supported by the Whitehall Foundation and the Grindley Fund. We thank all the undergraduate student interns in Clayton's lab who assisted in running the rat and jay experiments. We also thank Jennifer Greig for technical assistance, and Tony Dickinson, Nathan Emery, Nick Mackintosh, Jim Russell, and Dan Schacter for helpful comments on this chapter.

REFERENCES

Aggleton, J. P., & Brown, M. W. (1999). Episodic memory, amnesia and the hippocampal–anterior thalamic axis. *Behavioral and Brain Sciences, 22*, 425–444.

Bauer, P. J. (1996). What do infants recall of their lives?: Memory for specific events by one- to two-year-olds. *American Psychologist, 51*, 29–41.

Bunsey, M., & Eichenbaum, H. (1996). Conservation of hippocampal memory functions in rats and humans. *Nature, 379*, 255–257.

Clayton, N. S., & Dickinson, A. (1998). Episodic-like memory during cache recovery by scrub jays. *Nature, 395*, 272–274.

Clayton, N. S., & Dickinson, A. (1999a). Memory for the content of caches by scrub jays. *Journal of Experimental Psychology: Animal Behavior Processes, 25*(1), 82–91.

Clayton, N. S., & Dickinson, A. (1999b). Motivational control of food storing in the scrub jay *Aphelocoma coerulescens*. *Animal Behaviour, 57*, 435–444.

Clayton, N. S., & Dickinson, A. (1999c). Scrub jays (*Aphelocoma coerulescens*) remember when as well as where and what food items they cached. *Journal of Comparative Psychology, 113*, 403–416.

Clayton, N. S., Yu, K., & Dickinson, A. (2001). Scrub jays (*Aphelocoma coerulescens*) can form integrated memory for multiple features of caching episodes. *Journal of Experimental Psychology: Animal Behavior Processes, 27*, 17–29.

Dusek, J. A., & Eichenbaum, H. (1997). The hippocampus and memory for orderly stimulus relations. *Proceedings of the National Academy of Sciences USA, 94*, 7109–7114.

Eichenbaum, H., Dudchenko, P., Wood, E., Shapiro, M., & Tanila, H. (1999). The hippocampus, memory, and place cells: Is it spatial memory or a memory space? *Neuron, 23*, 209–226.

Griffiths, D. P., & Clayton, N. S. (2001). Testing episodic memory in animals: A new approach. *Physiology and Behavior, 73*, 1–8.

Griffiths, D. P., Dickinson, A., & Clayton, N. S. (1999). Declarative and episodic memory: What can animals remember about their past? *Trends in Cognitive Sciences, 3*(2), 74–80.

Henderson, V. W., Paganini-Hill, A., Emanuel, C. K., Dunn, M. E., & Buckwalter, J. G. (1994). Estrogen replacement therapy in older women: Comparisons between Alzheimer's disease cases and nondemented control subjects. *Archives of Neurology, 51*, 896–899.

Herlitz, A., & Forsell, Y. (1996). Episodic memory deficit in elderly adults with suspected delusional disorder. *Acta Psychiatrica Scandanavica, 93*, 355–361.

Hunt, J. M., & Willoughby, R. R. (1939). The effect of frustration on hoarding in rats. *Psychosomatic Medicine, 1*, 309–310.

Kimura, D. (1995). Estrogen replacement therapy may protect against intellectual decline in postmenopausal women. *Hormones and Behavior, 29*, 312–321.

Maguire, E. A., Gadian, D. G., Johnsrude, I. S., Good, C. D., Ashburner, J., Frackowiak, R. S., & Firth, C. D. (2000). Navigation-related structural changes in the hippocampus of taxi drivers. *Proceedings of the National Academy of Sciences USA, 98,* 4398–4403.

Maine de Biran. (1929). *The influence of habit on the faculty of thinking* (M. D. Boehm, Trans.). Baltimore: Williams & Williams.

Mandler, G. (1980). Recognizing: The judgement of previous experience. *Psychological Review, 87,* 252–271.

Milner, B., Corkin, S., & Teuber, H. L. (1968). Further analysis of the hippocampal amnesic syndrome: Fourteen year follow up study of H. M. *Neuropsychologia, 6,* 215–234.

Mishkin, M., & Delacour, J. (1975). An analysis of short-term visual memory in the monkey. *Journal of Experimental Psychology: Animal Behavior Processes, 1,* 326–334.

Morris, R. G. M., Garrud, P., Rawlins, J. N. P., & O'Keefe, J. (1982). Place navigation impaired in rats with hippocampal lesions. *Nature, 297,* 681–683.

Morris, R. G. M., & Frey, U. (1997). Hippocampal synaptic plasticity: Role in spatial learning or the automatic recording of attended experience? *Phiosophical Transactions of the Royal Society of London, Series B, 352,* 1489–1503

Nilsson, L.-G., Backman, L., Erngrund, K., & Nyberg, L. (1997). The Betula prospective cohort study: Memory, health and aging. *Aging and Cognition, 1,* 1–36

O'Keefe, J., & Nadel, L. (1978). *The hippocampus as a cognitive map.* Oxford: Clarendon Press.

Perner, J., & Ruffman, T. (1995). Episodic memory and autonoetic consciousness: Developmental evidence and a theory of childhood amnesia. *Journal of Experimental Child Psychology, 59,* 516–548.

Pillemer, D. B., & White, S. H. (1989). Childhood events recalled by children and adults. *Advances in Child Development and Behaviour, 21,* 297–340.

Schacter, D. L., & Tulving, E. (1994). What are the memory systems of 1994? In D. L. Schacter & E. Tulving (Eds.), *Memory systems 1994* (pp. 1–38). Cambridge, MA: MIT Press.

Scoville, W. B., & Milner, B. (1957). Loss of recent memory after bilateral hippocampal lesions. *Journal of Neurology, Neurosurgery and Psychiatry, 20,* 11–21.

Sherwin, B. B. (1988). Estrogen and/or androgen replacement therapy and cognitive functioning in surgically menopausal women. *Psychoneuroendocrinology, 13,* 345–357.

Shettleworth, S. J. (1995). Memory in food-storing birds: From the field to the Skinner box. In E. Alleva, A. Fasolo, H.-P. Lipp, & L. Nadel (Eds.), *Behavioral brain research in naturalistic and semi-naturalistic settings: Proceedings of NATO Advanced Study Institute Series, Maratea, Italy* (pp. 158–179). The Hague, The Netherlands: Kluwer Academic.

Squire, L. R., Knowlton, B., & Musen, G. (1993). The structure and organization of memory. *Annual Review of Psychology, 44,* 453–496.

Tulving, E. (1972). Episodic and semantic memory. In E. Tulving & W. Donaldson (Eds.), *Organization of memory* (pp. 381–403). New York: Academic Press.

Tulving, E. (1983). *Elements of episodic memory.* Oxford: Clarendon Press.

Tulving, E., & Markowitsch, H. J. (1998). Episodic and declarative memory: Role of the hippocampus. *Hippocampus, 8*(3), 198–204.

Vander Wall, S. B. (1990). *Food hoarding in animals.* Chicago: University of Chicago Press.

Vargha-Khadem, F., Gadian, D. G., Watkins, K. E., Connelly, A., Van Paesschen, W., & Mishkin, M. (1997). Differential effects of early hippocampal pathology on episodic and semantic memory. *Science, 277,* 376–380.

Weiskrantz, L. (1990). Problems of learning and memory: One or multiple memory systems? *Philosophical Transactions of the Royal Society of London, Series B, 329,* 99–108.

Wolfe, J. B. (1939). An exploratory study of food-storing in rats. *Journal of Comparative and Physiological Psychology, 28,* 97–108.

Zola-Morgan, S., Squire, L. R., & Amaral, D. G. (1986). Human amnesia and the medial temporal lobe region: Enduring memory impairment following a bilateral lesion limited to field CA1 of the hippocampus. *Journal of Neuroscience, 6,* 2950–2967.

INDEX